Radiotherapy in Clinical Practice

To 'Shelagh'

Radiotherapy in Clinical Practice

Edited by

H. F. Hope-Stone, FRCR
Consultant Radiotherapist and Oncologist, Department of Radiotherapy and Oncology, The London Hospital

Butterworths
London Boston Durban Singapore Sydney Toronto Wellington

First published, 1986

British Library Cataloguing in Publication Data

Radiotherapy in clinical practice.

1. Radiotherapy
I. Hope-Stone, H. F.
615.8'42 RM847

ISBN 0-407-00320-7

Library of Congress Cataloging in Publication Data

Radiotherapy in clinical practice.

Includes bibliographies and index.
1. Cancer — Radiotherapy. I. Hope-Stone, H. F.
[DNLM: 1. Neoplasms — radiotherapy. QZ 269 R1295]
RC271.R3R338 1985 616.99'40642 85-21315
ISBN 0-407-00320-7

Photoset by Illustrated Arts Limited, Sutton, Surrey
Printed and bound in Great Britain at the University Press, Cambridge

Preface

Radiotherapy — the word used to describe one method of treating mainly malignant disease — has now become linked with oncology, and indeed many individuals and even departments have changed their titles to reflect this association. Nevertheless, the art or science of radiotherapy is still a very specialized one, although no one would wish to practise it in total isolation from the wider context of oncology. Radiotherapists still see an amazingly broad spectrum of disease, and in this age of super-specialization might therefore be described as the last remaining 'general clinicians' in the hospital environment.

This book describes in some detail how radiotherapeutic techniques have evolved over the past 50 years to treat both malignant disease and occasionally benign conditions, particularly in the UK. The problems of treating patients with these diseases are also discussed in very general terms in the wider oncological context, but without going into the details of surgical and chemotherapeutic approaches. The intention has been to provide both the experienced practitioner and the trainee with a source book of information. By using it to plan and treat their patients they will no longer need to look up detailed references in often esoteric journals. As the treatment of cancer needs a broad approach, however, a physicist, a radiographer and an oncologist have been asked to describe how they contribute to the management of patients. It is therefore hoped that the book will help to crystallize thought on the management of mainly malignant disease by this very specialized form of therapy.

I would like to thank my two secretaries, Miss S.E.A. Gibby, and Miss A. Barrington-Jones, for all their help in the preparation and revision of the manuscripts, and also to thank my colleague, Dr B. S. Mantell, for his useful advice both initially and subsequently on the form and content of the book.

H.F. Hope-Stone

Contributors

S. J. Arnott, FRCS, FRCR
Consultant Radiotherapist, St Bartholomew's Hospital, London; formerly Senior Lecturer in Radiotherapy, University of Edinburgh, Edinburgh

D. Ash, MRCP, FRCR
Consultant in Radiotherapy and Oncology, Cookridge Hospital, Leeds

D. G. Bratherton, MA, MBBChir, FRCR
Consultant Radiotherapist, Addenbrookes Hospital, Cambridge

Pauline Curtis, HDCR(T)
Meyerstein Institute of Radiotherapy and Oncology, The Middlesex Hospital, London

J. M. Henk, MA, MBBChir, FRCR
Consultant in Radiotherapy and Oncology, Department of Radiotherapy and Oncology, The Royal Marsden Hospital, London

H. F. Hope-Stone, FRCR
Consultant Radiotherapist and Oncologist, Department of Radiotherapy and Oncology, The London Hospital

A. M. Jelliffe, MD, FRCP, FRCR
Director, British National Lymphoma Investigation, The Middlesex Hospital, London

S. C. Klevenhagen, BSc, MSc, PhD, CPhys, FInstP
Chief Physicist, Department of Medical Physics, The London Hospital; Honorary Lecturer, University of London

G. Mair, FRCR
Consultant Radiotherapist and Oncologist, Department of Radiotherapy and Oncology, The London Hospital

B. S. Mantell, MRCP, FRCR
Consultant Radiotherapist and Oncologist, The London Hospital and The London Chest Hospital; Honorary Senior Lecturer, Cardiothoracic Institute, University of London

R. T. D. Oliver, MD, FRCP
Reader in Medical Oncology, Department of Medical Oncology, The London Hospital; Honorary Consultant to St Bartholomew's and St Peter's Hospitals, London

P. N. Plowman, MA, MD, MRCP, FRCR
Consultant in Radiotherapy and Oncology to St Bartholomew's Hospital and The Hospital for Sick Children, London

T. J. Priestman, MD, FRCP, FRCR
Consultant in Radiotherapy and Clinical Oncology, Dudley Road and Queen Elizabeth Hospitals, Birmingham

M. L. Sutton, MA, BM, BCh, MRCP, DMRT, FRCR
Consultant Radiotherapist, Christie Hospital and Holt Radium Institute, Withington, Manchester

J. S. Tobias, MD, MRCP, FRCR
Consultant in Radiotherapy and Oncology, Department of Radiotherapy and Oncology, University College Hospital, London

Contents

1 Some clinical aspects of radiobiology
M. L. Sutton 1

2 The role of radiosensitizers
J. M. Henk 19

3 Urological malignancies
H. F. Hope-Stone 27

4 Breast cancer
J. S. Tobias 69

5 Cancer of the head and neck
J. M. Henk 93

6 Soft tissue and bone sarcomas
S. J. Arnott 124

7 Intrathoracic tumours
B. S. Mantell 145

8 Hodgkin's disease and non-Hodgkin's lymphomas
A. M. Jelliffe 177

9 Gynaecological radiotherapy
M. L. Sutton 203

10 Tumours in children
P. N. Plowman 238

11 Haematological malignancy in the adult
G. Mair 258

12 Skin malignancy
D. G. Bratherton 280

13 Tumours of the endocrine system
P. N. Plowman 300

14 Gastrointestinal carcinomas
T. J. Priestman 316

15 Malignant disease of the central nervous system
H. F. Hope-Stone 337

16 Interstitial therapy
D. Ash 369

17 The management of benign conditions
B. S. Mantell 384

18 The management of patients: a radiographer's viewpoint
Pauline Curtis 400

19 The role of the physicist in radiotherapy
S. C. Klevenhagen 411

20 Medical and radiotherapeutic oncology: the interaction
R. T. D. Oliver 432

Index

1

Some clinical aspects of radiobiology

M. L. Sutton

Introduction

'It was precisely this notion of infinite series which in the sixth century BC led the Greek philosopher Zeno to conclude that since an arrow shot towards a target first had to cover half the distance, and then half the remainder, and then half the remainder after that, and so on *ad infinitum,* the result was that although an arrow is always approaching its target, it never quite gets there, and Saint Sebastian died of fright.

(Slightly modified from *Jumpers*, Tom Stoppard)

Of all the clinical disciplines, radiotherapy probably has the most secure scientific foundations. There is now a huge literature on the submolecular, subcellular, and tissue events which mediate the immediate and delayed effects of irradiation; indeed, looked at differently, radiation has proved an extremely controllable, flexible, and measurable tool in elucidating the mechanisms of tissue reponses to injury in general, and in demonstrating many phenomena of the cell cycle and cell kinetics of tissues. All radiotherapists require a knowledge of radiobiology, directly comparable with the physician's need to be familiar with pharmacological concepts. Many practising radiotherapists hold ambivalent views about the true value of radiobiological research, and are uneasy about applying laboratory-derived principles when designing novel therapeutic strategies. There is ample justification for this mistrust — to date the achievements of radiobiology have been almost exclusively interpretative, and predictive successes of radiobiology are difficult to identify. Radiotherapists in training commonly encounter radiobiology simultaneously with the introduction or re-introduction of the physics of radiation, and this encourages the study of biological effects of radiation to proceed from the submolecular towards the tissue level. It is taught that the single-dose cell survival curve becomes exponential after a certain dose is exceeded, which obscures rather than illuminates the everyday reality of radiation-induced tumour cure. Tumours are eradicated by irradiation; they do not, nor did Saint Sebastian, die of fright. There used to be a fashion for postulating unspecified 'host' mechanisms, often vaguely immunological, which were supposedly responsible for eradicating the last remaining cells in tumours. The fact that cell-survival curves were not demonstrated to be other than exponential throughout their entire range was simply due to constraints imposed on laboratory experiments by the test systems originally available.

There are many comprehensive and recent accounts of 'classical' radiobiology, and it is not the present author's intention that this chapter should be a superficial restatement of now very familiar material, widely accessible elsewhere. Instead, a limited number of topics of contemporary clinical radiotherapeutic interest or relevance are discussed from a broadly radiobiological stance.

They are:

(1) Novel fractionation schemes
(2) The dose-rate effect
(3) Dose-modifying chemical adjuvants.

Desirability of two dose level trials

All these situations illustrate well the need to design trials which are guaranteed to permit comparison of different methods of treatment in terms of the equivalence of the morbidity that they cause. The true value of such radiobiologically-inspired developments as for example, hyperbaric oxygen and fast neutrons, has been obscured because so often the apparent superiority of the novel treatment has been accompanied by increased morbidity: when this is the case, it can justifiably be argued that by increasing the radiation dose in the conventional arm of a trial to a level which would raise its morbidity to the level seen in the novel arm of the trial, similar advantages in local tumour control would be observed. Some ingenious but ultimately unconvincing solutions have been offered to circumvent the difficulties experienced in evaluating inadequately designed trials. For example, the results of the Medical Research Council's trial of fast-neutron therapy have been expressed as the ratio of treatment complications to the uncomplicated local tumour controls in the neutron and low l.e.t. arms of the trial, with conclusions favourable to fast-neutron treatment (Catterall and Bewley, 1979); unfortunately these conclusions have not been confirmed by other reports (Duncan *et al.*, 1984, 1985).

In a small prospective randomized trial of fast neutrons in stage II and III carcinoma of the bladder, carried out at the Christie Hospital, Manchester (Pointon, Read and Greene, 1985), neutrons were not demonstrably superior to photons in bringing about local control. An important feature of this trial was that the novel (i.e. fast neutron) treatment was given at two doses, and the current trial of remote afterloading at accelerated dose rate is similarly designed (*see* Chapter 9). The purpose of having two dose levels in the novel arm of any trial is to demonstrate a portion of the two dose-response curves for local control and complication: interpolation or limited extrapolation between the four data points (*Figure 1.1*) permits identification of that dose which

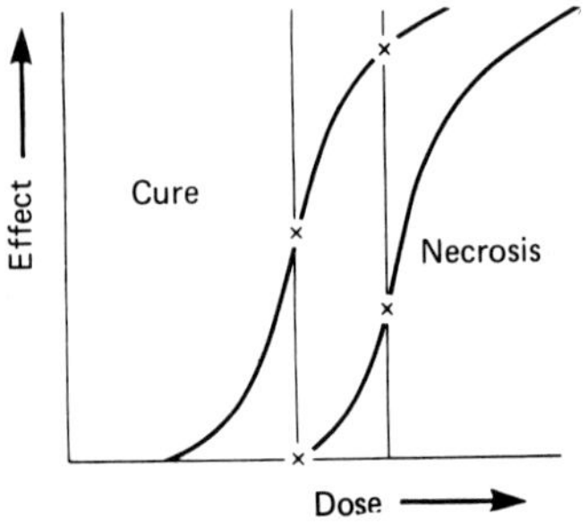

Figure 1.1 Treatments carried out at two appropriately different doses generate relevant portions of the cure and complication dose-effect curves

would be associated with identical incidence of morbidity in both sides of the trial. *Figure 1.2* illustrates a situation in which the novel treatment is superior to the conventional one, whereas *Figure 1.3* illustrates the converse. Much of the now very extensive literature on the concurrent administration of cytotoxic drugs and irradiation is worthless, as equivalent morbidity was only occasionally achieved (either by good luck or judgement), instead of being virtually guaranteed by appropriate trial design. It seems not unlikely that truly effective radiosensitizers of hypoxic cells may shortly become available, and it is essential that the lessons learnt (or perhaps not learnt) from previous experience with hyperbaric oxygen are applied. In this situation, it is likely that a reduction in total dose will be necessary for patients receiving sensitizers, to prevent the anticipated enhancement of normal tissue effects (*see below*). Estimates of the magnitude of this dose reduction are only approximate, and accordingly two-dose level studies are the only scientific means of ensuring that the clinically relevant values are established.

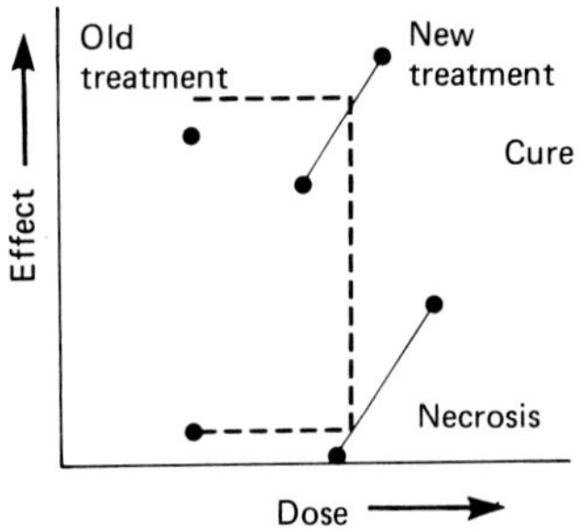

Figure 1.2 The new treatment is truly superior to the old treatment, i.e. more cure for the equivalent damage ('necrosis')

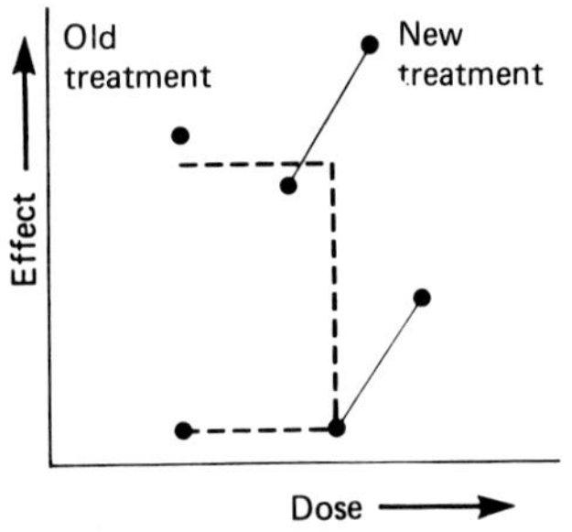

Figure 1.3 The new treatment is inferior to the old, i.e. less cure for the equivalent damage

Single-dose dose-effect curves are steep (*Figure 1.4*), irrespective of the end-point chosen — for example, tumour cure or late necrosis. With increasing fractionation, as the fraction size decreases, the curve retains its sigmoid shape but becomes progressively less steep (*Figure 1.5*). Successful empirically-derived clinical treatment regimens differ widely. Manchester commonly exploits 3-week radical treatments of 15 fractions of a size approaching 370 cGy (Easson and Pointon, 1985): perhaps more widely adopted are regimens of 30 fractions of 200 cGy administered over 5 or 6 weeks. The steepness of the whole-tissue dose response curves (for both normal and malignant tissues) is less for the protracted regimens than for shorter ones. Expressed differently, in short regimens, the dose is more critical in determining the response than in longer ones. This may be of

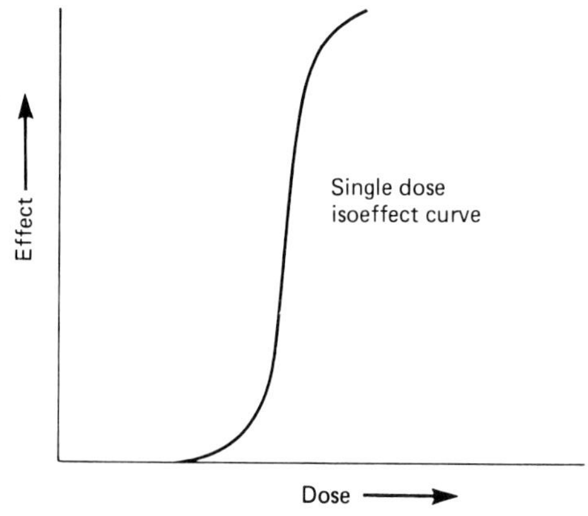

Figure 1.4 Single dose dose-effect curves are sigmoid and steep, with a rapidly rising near-linear middle portion

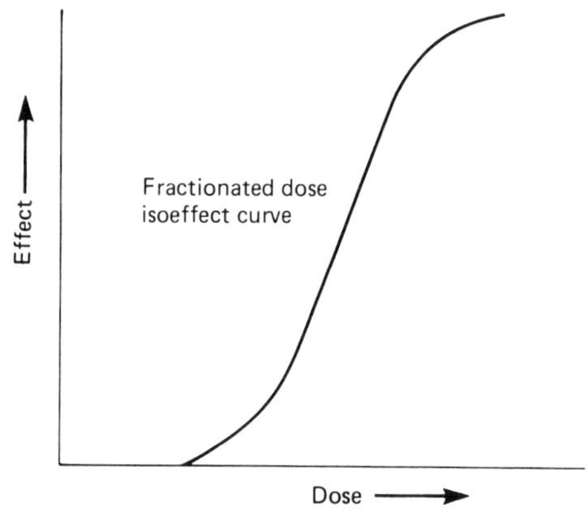

Figure 1.5 With fractionation, the sigmoid shape and the near-linear middle portion remain, but the slope is less steep throughout the range

considerable significance in determining what ought to be the disparity between the doses in two-dose level studies. Relatively less steep, protracted regimens may be capable of supporting dose differences of the order of 15%, and may indeed require such differences to demonstrate an adequate range of tissue effects; a 15% dose range in trials resulting in steeper and more critical dose-response curves would clearly be unacceptable, for at the higher dose, late morbidity would be excessive, whereas at the lower dose seriously inadequate tumour control would be equally likely.

In some clinical, and in many experimental situations, dose-effect differences are reliably detectable when doses differ by as little as 3–4%; treatment regimens resulting in steep dose-response curves of high criticality cannot be ethically compatible with dose differences much greater than 7–8%. Until the concept of two-dose level studies in 'innovative' treatment arms gains wider acceptance, it will not be possible to suggest appropriate dose ranges for the commonly-employed regimens in current use. In the two Manchester trials referred to above, the dose range has been ± 3.5% of the dose in the novel arms of the trials which would be anticipated to generate levels of morbidity close to those generated by the reference (usually the conventional) arms of the trials. Undeniably, the success of two-dose level studies depends to some extent on percipience or luck associated with the choice of the anticipated optimum (equi-morbid) dose for the novel treatment.

When novel treatments involve alterations in the total dose, as when known or potentially dose-modifying agents are combined with radiotherapy, the record of laboratory-derived radiobiological predictions is unfortunately far from unblemished, but the development of whole-tissue experimental systems increasingly less remote from clinical practice is leading to increasing confidence in accepting the recommendations of those radiobiologists working with such systems. Parenthetically, it may be noted that the dose reduction suggested from murine experiments designed to be pertinent to dose-rate changes imposed by the adoption of a remote afterloading system (*see below*), was much larger than most clinicians were initially disposed to accept, but 4 years' experience appears to indicate that the radiobiologically-inspired recommendations were closer to reality than the experientially derived predictions of a large body of clinical radiotherapists.

Response of normal tissue

In collaboration with an experimental radiobiologist whose experiments have always been directed towards clinically relevant targets, the present author once attempted to write a chapter about radiobiology which as a matter of principle declined to show a single-dose response curve (Sutton and Hendry, 1984). In that chapter it was the intention to avoid introductory pages containing over familiar diagrams which we felt would quickly overwhelm the tolerance of the reader. Clinically inappropriate notions derived from such curves have turned many practising radiotherapists away from radiobiology. However, single-dose response curves are relevant to fractionated X-ray treatments, most of which have been empirically derived. Reference to the early segment of the single-dose response curve (*Figure 1.6*) indicates that the fraction size of most treatments is not on the linear and therefore predictable part of the curve; numerically small increments of dose have disproportionately large effects in terms of cell killing. One of the main responsibilities of clinical radiobiology ought to be to devise means whereby treatments of different fraction size, over all time, and total dose can be equated. Whereas in the single-dose cell survival curve there is a precise end point, in the clinical situation end points are much less precisely defined,

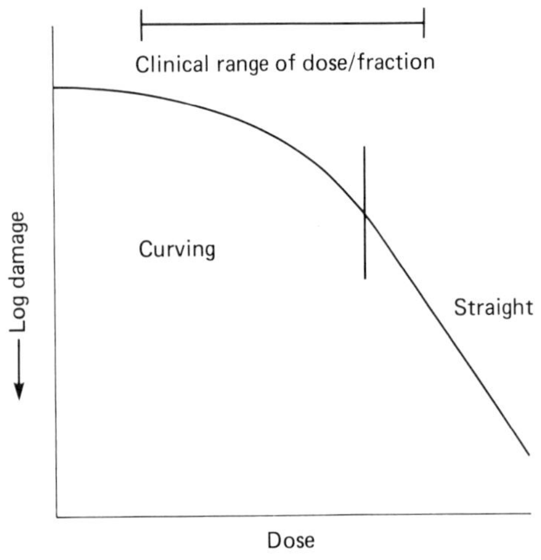

Figure 1.6 Early radiobiological thinking was much concerned with predictable but clinically irrelevant linear portion of the single dose iso-effect curve

and individual perceptions of acceptability (of early and late normal tissue effects) are subjective.

Clinical radiobiologists are accustomed to considering the late effects on normal tissues as the relevant end points; practising radiotherapists commonly modify their treatment on the basis of acute effects. The cellular basis of both these types of decisions is similar, that is to say, both are consciously or unconsciously based on knowledge or speculation about cell death. Established and effective treatment regimens have generally been based on careful assessment of clinical effectiveness, and have thus been empirically derived. To date radiobiology has contributed nothing of note in terms of effective innovation. Nevertheless, increasingly precise knowledge of the way in which individual cells, and the tissues of which they are components, react to irradiation aids the understanding of currently employed treatment regimens. Novel stratagems must be designed in a fashion which acknowledges that laboratory derived data can prevent dangerously inappropriate experimentation.

Acute reacting tissues

Having due regard to the wide variety of clinical practice throughout the world, it is clear that the desired aims of radiation therapy can be achieved in many different ways. It is the responsibility of the clinical radiobiologist to identify the common features that successful regimens share. Briefly stated, the imperative is to irradiate one cell population while leaving other cell populations, if not intact, then at least capable of self-regeneration. Normal tissues have an intrinsic capacity for self-repair; as far as is known malignant tumours lack this orderly capacity for self-regulation, indeed this is a feature of malignancy. Radiation kills cells, and that it can be exploited as an effective therapeutic modality depends entirely upon the recuperative capabilities of normal tissues. There is apparently no consistent difference in the radiovulnerability of normal and malignant cells; the ability of radiation to eradicate abberant clones of cells is due to the replicative ability of the tissues which surround and have given rise to the malignancy. Accordingly, knowledge of the responses of normal tissues is central to the safe practice of radiotherapy.

The metabolic processes of cells are virtually uninfluenced by radiation but the disruptive effect of ionization on the genetic apparatus of the cell determines the future reproductive career of that cell, and it determines the behaviour of the tissue involved. Immediate and late tissue responses are determined by the same mechanisms, but the rate at which different tissues express radiation induced effects differs widely. Characteristically, epithelial elements express radiation damage early, whereas stromal and parenchymal elements are slow to do so. It used to be considered appropriate to regard normal tissues as naturally falling into three catergories. Operationally, there are only two categories of tissues:

(1) Those in which the mature cells have a limited life span, and in which the tissue's regular and sizeable anticipated natural cell loss is normally compensated for by regular and predictable cell division in a stem cell compartment. The finely-responsive progenitor cells usually form a small proportion of the tissue cell population, but this proportion can be increased in response to demand, for example towards the end of a course of fractionated irradiation, when repeated episodes of damage induce maximal regenerative efforts. The relatively small progenitor cell population sustains a much larger population of mature cells by a cascade of amplifying cell divisions, with progressive differentiation at each intermediate stage, exemplified in epithelia and the haemopoietic system.

(2) Those in which the mature cells have a long life span, and in which no specific progenitor cells can be identified. In these tissues, it seems that many or all of the constituent cells can respond to a reparative stimulus, each cell apparently undergoing one division in response to the loss of another. During maturation and differentiation, many cells lose the ability to divide, but equally, many differentiated and apparently specialized tissues retain the capacity to divide, making good cellular depletion by sporadic, but perhaps not random, division of cells which form a major constituent of the tissue; examples are found in the thyroid, the liver, and skeletal muscle.

Classical radiobiology was dominated by the

notions that the only practical definition of cell death was loss of clonogenic potential, and that (in the clinically relevant dose range) cells expressed the lethality of received radiation damage only when they or their immediate progeny attempted mitosis. The latter concept remains appropriate, but the cells which divide to maintain the functional complement in this type of tissue are probably not clonogenic in the sense that they have almost limitless replicative ability. In this type of tissue, reparative cell division can be considered as arithmetical in Malthusian terms, whereas cell division in rapidly renewing tissues is geometrical.

The functional consequences of cellular death in a tissue will not become apparent until attempts at division unmask the lethality of previously administered irradiation, and accordingly, mitotically inert tissues composed of long-lived cells are slow (months or years) to demonstrate radiation damage, whereas mitotically active tissues respond early, often within a matter of days, the time taken to manifest damage depending on the normal time taken for the sequence: (clonogenic cell to mature functioning cells). Mucosal reactions appear several days before skin reactions, and whole body irradiation not quite sufficient to cause gut death may cause haemopoietic death several days after the peak of the gastrointestinal reaction.

Late reacting tissues

Thyroid failure after radioiodine treatment for thyrotoxicosis illustrates well the behaviour of late-responding tissues; although there is a gradual and progressive increase in the incidence of hypothyroidism with time, patients who have remained euthyroid for many years may rapidly become myxoedematous, evidenced by a swift rise in the serum TSH levels over a relatively short period of weeks or a very few months. The natural longevity of the follicular cells generates little demand for replacement, and following modest doses of radioiodine, many of the mitoses that do take place will be successful, i.e. the daughter cells will be viable. Following larger doses of radioiodine, a bigger proportion of the mitoses will be unsuccessful, leading to continued stimulus for mitosis in as yet quiescent cells. When the functioning complement of cells is just inadequate to maintain normal circulating levels of the thyroid hormones, the TSH level rises above the normal range, imposing an accelerated proliferative stimulus, and hence accelerated cell loss, with even higher levels of TSH; in this way, the ultimate failure of the organ appears rapidly. Clearly the latent period to organ failure will be reduced with higher radiation doses, whereas in rapidly reacting tissues, the latency is determined by the proliferative dynamics of the tissues in question, provided the radiation dose is large enough to induce a perceptible effect. Larger doses will produce more complete tissue failure, but do not shorten the time for its expression.

Vascular and stromal tissues

The manifestations of late radiation injury are tissue-dependent, and at the dose levels commonly employed in therapeutic regimens, develop at different rates in different tissues. Irrespective of the latency, which reflects most of all the natural lifespan of long-lived cells, different tissues vary considerably in respect of the radiation doses which generate given probabilities of injury, reflecting intrinsic differences in radiosensitivity in various cell types. With few exceptions (cartilage, lens) all tissues share a very similar vascular supply, which is itself radiovulnerable, and the time course of the vascular changes appears to vary little between different normal tissues. To some extent therefore, the late effects of radiation are an admixture of tissue-specific response, expressed on a background of commonality of vascular response. Novel therapies may alter the relationship between these two types of response, and since clinical radiotherapy invariably involves the simultaneous irradiation of several different types of tissue, it is again clear that radical departures from conventional practice must be assessed at two-dose levels for the experimental treatment.

Human skin is very similar to pig skin in its vasculature, morphology and response to irradiation. Capillary perfusion of skin can be estimated by the clearance of intradermally injected radioactive pertecnetate ions. Approximately 3 months after fractionated irradiation, dermal blood flow is reduced, but returns to normal over the succeeding 3 months (Hopewell, 1980). (Radiosodium clearance studies in 37 previously irradiated patients (Roswit, Wishaven and Sorrentino, 1953) indicated that effective blood flow in densely fibrotic, scarred, atrophied tissues is functionally unimpaired for up to 10 years. These results seem to have been disregarded, possibly because they did not fit in with then current notions of late effects as being due to 'ischaemia'.) The time when the perfusion is most reduced in pig skin corresponds to a period when the irradiated supplying arterioles are nearly occluded by proliferation of endothelial cells. Although considerable reduction of the arteriolar lumen persists indefinitely, perfusion and vascular density return to normal. When endothelial proliferation is maximal, and perfusion minimal, 3 months after irradiation, the inadequacy of the circulation can be estimated by the degree to which it is unable to support a single-pedicle skin flap; the more inadequate the circulation, the shorter is the length of the flap that remains viable, (Wiernick, Patterson and Berry, 1974). Although the circulation apparently returns to normal 6 months after irradiation, its ability to support subsequently raised skin flaps is no better than at 3 months post-irradiation (Hopewell, 1980). Nuclear swelling and giant cell formation may be seen within 2 weeks of the completion of fractionated irradiation, and these changes can be seen after many years if there is a proliferative stimulus, such as surgical trauma (Zollinger, 1970). In this sense, the vasculature is behaving as a late responding tissue, such as thyroid.

The experimental findings in pig skin are consistent with clinical experience in that wound healing is normal provided that surgery is performed immediately or shortly after irradiation, but the incidence of complications can rise steeply if surgery follows irradiation by several months or years. An implication is that when preoperative irradiation is part of a planned dual approach, then surgery should be performed within a very few weeks of the end of the irradiation, rather than as is commonly the case, deferred for 6–8 weeks. Another implication is that since surgical complications may be expected (and are observed to be) higher when irradiated tissues require surgery months or years after treatment, patients requiring such surgery should be referred to specialist units with concentrated experience of the problems.

Changes in vascular permeability

Early endothelial damage may be the cause of the insudation of plasma constituents into the blood-vessel wall that is observed following irradiation especially in arterioles and capillaries (Zollinger, 1970). Chief among the plasma constituents that transude into the blood-vessel walls and interstitial tissues is fibrinogen which, following conversion to fibrin, may be organized, causing respectively arteriolar narrowing and interstitial fibrosis (Law and Thomlinson, 1978). Hypertension and diabetes are said to reduce radiation tolerance in patients, and if transendothelial leakage of plasma constituents is enhanced by high intra-arteriolar pressures, hypertension would result in acceleration and enhancement of arteriolar narrowing; this has been shown in mesenteric arteries (Asscher, Wilson and Ausan, 1961) and in brain (Hopewell and Wright, 1970). Also hypercholesterolaemia causes atheromatosis at lower radiation doses than in normocholesterolaemic rats (Gold, 1961).

Novel fractionation schemes

In the best major radiotherapy institutions in the world, strikingly similar cure and complication rates are obtained from numerous teletherapy regimens, but they differ widely in respect of total dose given, number of fractions, fraction size, and overall treatment time. This suggests that prospective comparisons of regimens which themselves fall within the limits of conventional practice are unlikely to lead to improvements in the therapeutic ratio. This point is well illustrated by the two British Institute of Radiology (BIR) fractionation trials, in which three fractions per week were compared with five, and 20 fractions were compared with 30, over 4 and 6 weeks respectively (Wiernick *et al.*, 1982). These well-designed trials have failed to demonstrate significant superiority for any one approach. It is fashionable to stress the experimentally derived notion (for which there is now some clinical support), that smaller fraction sizes spare rapidly renewing tissues more than they spare slowly renewing tissues (Fowler, Joiner and Williams, 1983). Astute choice of treatment parameters led to the different treatment regimens of the BIR trials resulting in very similar incidences of morbidity, yet local control rates were equally similar; it appears that in regimens generating equivalent morbidity, smaller fraction sizes reduce the intensity of early transient normal tissue effects, but do not increase the therapeutic ratio in terms of late normal tissue effects.

Apparently equivalent radiotherapy regimens employ fraction sizes ranging from 180 cGy (many North American centres) to 350 cGy (several northern English centres). In this context ‘equivalent’ means that very similar local control rates and late normal tissue effects are obtained: the qualification ‘apparently’ is used because treatment volumes in North America are generally appreciably larger than those in UK departments, an important factor fre-

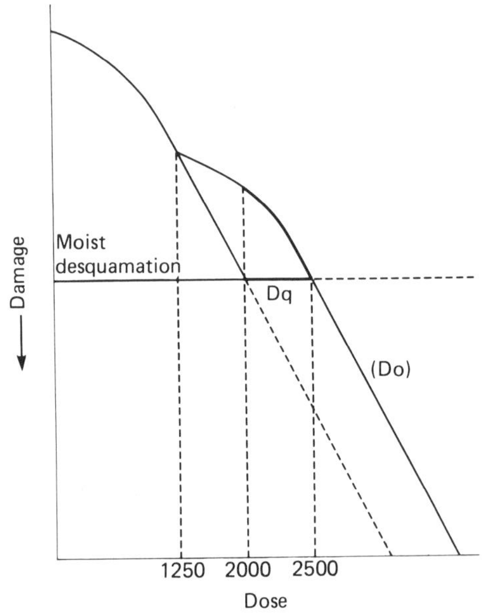

Figure 1.7 Split dose data for skin illustrating that Dq corresponds to the last part only of the shoulder

quently not acknowledged when fractionation data are compared internationally. Irrespective of the true 'equivalence' of regimens employing fraction sizes at the extremes of the range, each individual fraction is eitherwholly (180 cGy per fraction) or very largely (350 cGy per fraction) on the shoulder region of the single-dose cell survival curve, so that the initial slopes of the dose-response curve are clinically much more important than the final (exponential) slope. Accordingly, radiobiological interest has swung away from consideration of Dq and Do values (defined in *Figure 1.7*) and is now more concerned with the shapes of the initial slopes of dose-response curves, which are different for early and late responding tissues.

The initial slopes of the dose-response curve make up the shoulder, which is a reflection of rapid intracellular repair of sublethal damage.

Split-dose experiments

Familiar split-dose experiments involving two separate exposures give an indication of the extent to which a tissue can repair sublethal damage, and also the time-course of such repair. For example, to produce an acute effect in skin identical to that produced by a single high dose rate exposure of 2000 cGy, two 1250 cGy exposures are required when given 24 hours apart. In previously unperturbed skin, repopulation plays a negligible role in producing the observed requirement for an extra 500 cGy to produce an equal effect; 500 cGy is an approximation to the value of Dq if repair does not occur following each of the two exposures, but only after the first. The 2000/2 × 1250 cGy split dose skin data are illustrated in *Figure 1.8*. However, to estimate the value of Dq accurately from split-dose experiments, it is clearly necessary that the doses used should be on the exponential portion of the curve, otherwise less than the maximum repair capacity will be demonstrated. When more than two fractions of number N are used to achieve an isoeffect, the number of occasions on which repair can take place is:

$$(N-1);\text{ i.e. } \mathrm{Dq} = \frac{\mathrm{Df} - \mathrm{Ds}}{N-1}$$

where Df is the total fractionated dose and Ds the isoeffect single dose. Accordingly, if an acute response identical to that resulting from a single 2000 cGy exposure is to be achieved in eight fractions, then:

$$500 = \frac{\mathrm{Df} - 2000}{7},\text{ i.e. } \mathrm{Df} = 5500.$$

In clinical practice, the areas of skin which are given single doses of 2000 cGy are circles of 2 cm diameter or less and, in the present author's institute, such small areas are never given eight-fraction treatments. However, areas of skin up to 4 cm diameter (three times the area of a 2 cm circle) proceed to moist desquamation when 4500 cGy are delivered in eight fractions (dose per fraction approximately 560 cGy), which is not inconsistent with the smaller area tolerating 5500 cGy in eight fractions (dose per fraction approximately 690 cGy). In this simple situation at least, uncomplicated by repopulation in the irradiated tissues, radiobiologically derived predictions about fractionation from *in vitro* studies do not seem to be seriously misleading.

Since the shoulder of the dose-response curve becomes progressivley more curved, it is clear that at lower doses the repair mechanisms are more efficient than at higher doses, and that repair is most efficient in the region of the initial slope of the shoulder. The initial slopes for early and late reacting normal tissues are now thought to be consistently different, and if this is true, it has considerable impact on current investigations into novel regimens involving multiple fractions per day (*see below*).

Eclipse of the concept of the nominal standard dose (NSD)

The expression $D = \mathrm{NSD} \times N^{0.24} \times T^{0.11}$ describes the relationship between total dose (D), number of fractions (N) and overall time (T), where NSD is a constant, the nominal single dose. The relationship holds quite well for skin between four and 30 fractions administered 5 days per week. From the first, Ellis (1969), the originator of the expression, stressed that his suggestions were strictly applicable to skin only, but for many years NSD equivalents became almost obligatory statements for publications, particularly in American journals. The limitations of the NSD concept were slow to emerge, but the relationship does usefully stress the fact that (for 'daily') fractions, the number of fractions is much more important than the time over which they are delivered, a factor of great importance in experimental fractionation patterns involving increasing of the number of fractions (*see below*).

The limitations of the NSD concept are now perceived as:

(1) The N exponent is 0.24 for skin, but may be different for other tissues; in particular a value of 0.4 is suggested for spinal cord (van der Kogel, 1979), but this suggestion is based on non-human data
(2) The time exponent is fixed at 0.11, which fails to account for the fact that during fractionated radiotherapy repopulation begins after some delay, and then proceeds at an increasing rate with further time. The proliferative response to irradiation in many late-reacting tissues does not begin until after the course of treatment is

over, and since the NSD formula refers to late (skin) effects, the disadvantage of a fixed time exponent may in practice be minimal.

Multiple fractions per day

Frustration with the inability of multiple daily fractions to control many of the more advanced tumours generated experiments involving multiple fractions per day several years before the rationale for them was suggested by newer radiobiological concepts. It was soon recognized that repair of sublethal damage is complete in under 8 hours, so that two or even three fractions could be administered daily. For practical reasons, most studies have and continue to be limited to two fractions per day. Development has proceeded along two dissimilar lines:

(1) Hyperfractionation, in which an increased number of fractions is given over 'conventional' overall time
(2) Accelerated fraction, in which a 'conventional' number of fractions is given over a shorter time.

Accelerated fractionation seemed to have potential relevance to the clinical use of hypoxic cell radiosensitizers, since the early compounds were dose limited by their cumulative neurotoxicity; the shortened overall treatment time would reduce the 'area under the curve' and permit more fractions to be given simultaneously with effective levels of sensitizer. On the other hand, hyperfractionation was expected to result in relative sparing of the late effects on normal tissues, permitting an increase in effective dosage to bring the normal tissue late effects back up to the conventionally accepted level, with concomitant increase in tumour control.

The differences between hyperfractionation and accelerated fractionation are summarized in *Table 1.1*. It will be seen that in both cases, an alteration in total dose is required. A small reduction in total dose may be necessary for accelerated fractionation, for although the number of fractions is unchanged, and hence the same number of episodes of repair of sublethal damage can take place, the shorter overall time permits less repopulation, and accordingly the total dose may need to be reduced if morbidity is not to rise. However, the effects of proliferation in late reacting tissues are small until several weeks after the start of 'daily' irradiation, so that enhanced effects are only likely in acutely reacting tissues. In the case of hyperfractionation, the increased number of fractions increases the occasions on which sublethal damage repair can occur; and an increase in total dose is necessary to restore the equivalence of the response in acutely reacting tissues, but this may not necessarily lead to increased late tissue effects. No study published to date has been carried out at two doses in the novel fractionation arm of the trial, and equivalence of morbidity (late effects) between the novel and conventional treatments has only been very loosely established so that, not surprisingly, neither of these approaches has yet emerged as superior to conventional approaches.

α/β Ratios

If the initial slope of the shoulder is compared to the rest of the shoulder (*Figure 1.8*), a value (in cGy) can be found at which the damage attributable to the processes responsible for the linear initial slope is equal

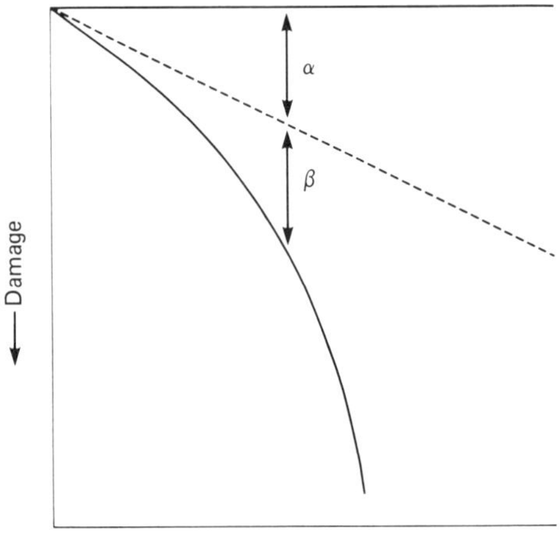

Figure 1.8 The derivation of the α/β 'ratio', a dose which describes the 'curviness' of dose-effect relationships

Table 1.1 Accelerated fractionation versus hyperfractionation

	Accelerated fractionation	*Hyperfractionation*
Fractions/day	2–3	2–3
Fraction number	Conventional	Two to three times conventional
Overall time	½ – ⅓ Conventional	Conventional
Dose/fraction	? Very small reduction	Appreciable reduction
Total dose	? Small reduction	Appreciable increase

to the damage attributable to the processes responsible for the increasingly curving shoulder. This dose is referred to as the α/β ratio, α and β being algebraic terms in the linear quadratic relationship:

$$\text{Damage} = n(\alpha d + \beta d^2)$$

where n = number of fractions, of size d. Many such experimentally derived dose-response curves happen to fit the linear–quadratic description, a circumstance which has generated models of radiation action involving notions of 'α cell kill' ('one-hit', irreparable) and 'β cell kill' ('multi-hit', reparable). Whatever the merits or relevance of such notions, the ratio α/β (in cGy) can be experimentally derived for a wide variety of tissues and end points. The values for early-reacting tissues range from 600–1300 cGy, whereas for late-reacting tissues, the range is 100-500 cGy. In general, α/β values are three to four times greater for early-reacting than for late-reacting tissues, which means that the dose-response curve for the former is less 'curvy' than that for the latter, as illustrated in *Figure 1.9*. α/β values for tumours are difficult to determine, but appear to be even larger than for acutely reacting tissues. *Figure 1.9* shows in exaggerated form the differences between the shapes of the single-dose response curves for early-and late-responding tissues. Such representations are now increasingly widely canvassed, and notions derived from them seem likely to become the radiobiological preoccupation of the mid 1980s. Before the implications of this latest fashion are too enthusiastically accepted, it should be noted that:

(1) In the interests of clarity the depiction exaggerates the differences between early and late reacting tissues
(2) The point at which early and late tissue effects become equal (d_1) is not known with certainty for any human tissue, nor is

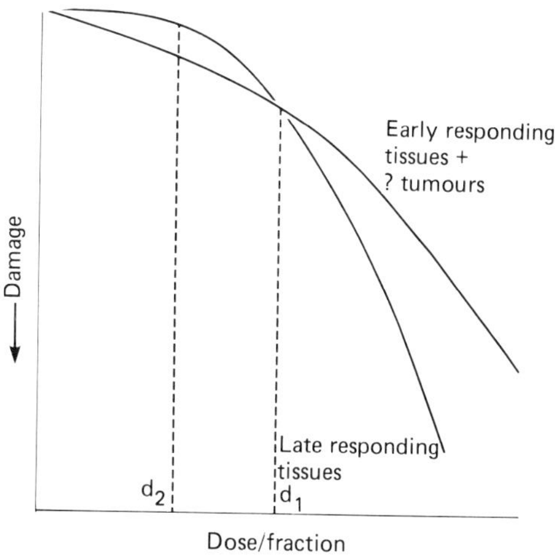

Figure 1.9 Most late-responding tissues have less 'curvy' dose-response relationships than do most early-responding tissues, possibly including tumours

(3) That dose at which separation of the acute and late curves is maximal (d_2).

It seems to be widely assumed that hyperfractionation (small doses per fraction) will be operative early on the curves, whereas accelerated fractionation (large doses per fraction) is assumed to be relevant to the later portions of the curves. There is at present little justification for these assumptions, which may prove to be expensively misleading.

Standquist (1944), better known for his parallel (and inaccurate) log–log plots of normal tissue reactions and tumour cure, was the first to display human data on tumour control and skin necrosis in the form of sigmoid dose-response curves, and to subtract the latter from the former, yielding a complication-free curve (*Figure 1.10*). As these data were derived from clinical experience, only the later part of the curve for

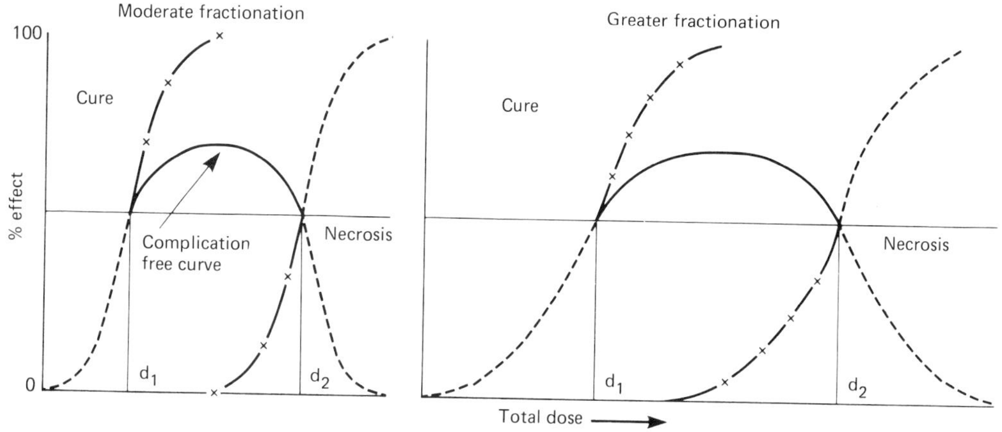

Figure 1.10 Unless the ratio between d_1 and d_2 increases, no therapeutic gain is obtained by increasing fractionation, i.e. an effective new fractionation scheme will incline the necrosis curve more to the right than the cure curve. In this depiction greater fractionation has inclined equally both cure and necrosis curves to the right, so that no therapeutic gain results.

tumour contol, and the early part of necrosis, are shown. Increased fractionation itself leads to less steep dose-response curves (*see above*), but if both curves incline to the right equally, no therapeutic gain is achieved: what is required is an increase in the ratio of the two doses that results in 50% complication-free cure, that is, a true separation of the cure and necrosis curves. Fractionation regimens designed to exploit the apparent differences in the dose-response curves for early- and late-reacting tissues could achieve separation in normal tissues, but it remains to be demonstrated that tumours will behave like acutely-reacting tissues.

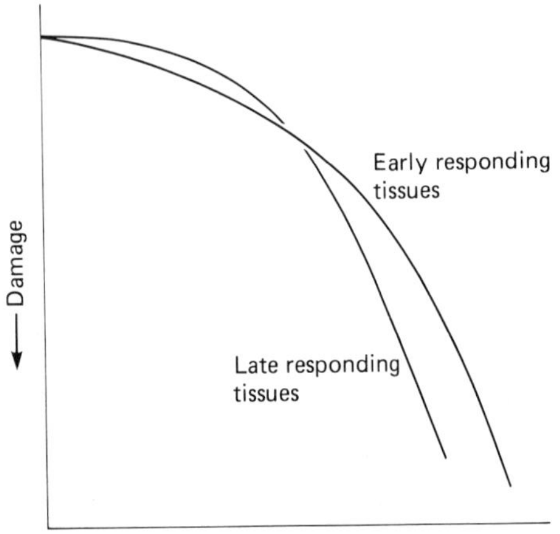

Figure 1.11 Human tissues (including possibly many tumours) may have as above early- and late- responding curves less separated than in *Figure 1.9*

If reality is closer to *Figure 1.11* than to *Figure 1.9* little gain is to be expected from either hyperfractionation or accelerated fractionation, unless other mechanisms play an important part. (For example, bulk disease in Burkitt's lymphoma frequently requires two or three fractions daily to induce regression; the proliferative kinetics of Burkitt's tumour are so far removed from those of most commonly encountered tumours that it is extremely doubtful that this situation demonstrates a general advantage of hyperfractionation.)

It remains true that when acute (human skin) reactions are matched, late effects are worse when small numbers of large fractions are used than when larger numbers of smaller fractions are used (Singh, 1978). Most European, all Third World, and many North American radiotherapists will be seeking significant gains from regimens involving two or more fractions per day. Expressed bluntly, advantages of less than 10% in local tumour control are unlikely to be regarded as economically justified; the present author is unaware of any leading radiobiological theoretician who has committed to paper estimates or predictions of what advantages are expected to accrue from hyperfractionation or accelerated fractionation. Some industrious radiotherapists are combining two or three fractions per day with other agents such as heat and hypoxic radiosensitizers, and if past experience is a guide, there will be early claims of superior results. Few if any of these studies are likely to be designed to ensure equivalence of late morbidity with conventional treatments, and accordingly it may take as long to evaluate adequately multiple fractions per day as it did to evaluate the supposed benefits of fast neutrons.

Dose-rate effects

Any specified dose of radiation produces the same number of ionizing events irrespective of the rate at which that dose is administered, but at the extremes, the biological consequences may differ widely, lower dose rates being associated with lesser effects. For example, a conventionally fractionated course of radiation for an oral cancer requires 6 or 7 weeks to administer a dose of 6500 cGy, whereas a low dose-rate interstitial treatment can safely deliver even larger doses within 1 week, with if anything, more desirable late normal tissue consequences.

The effects of very low dose-rates may be considered as resulting from uninterrupted reduplication of the initial slope of the single-dose cell survival curve; the higher the dose rate, the steeper the resultant curve will be (*Figure 1.12*). Note that low-dose rate curves have no shoulder, being themselves an infinite overlapping series of greater or lesser parts of the single dose curve shoulder at very low dose.

Clinical importance of dose rates

The presence of an initial shoulder on single-dose survival curves reflects the capacity of individual cells to repair sublethal damage, and densely-ionizing radiations such as fast neutrons which have very little shoulder show very little dose-rate effect. Similarly, cells that inherently show small shoulders, for example haemopoietic stem cells, show dose-rate effects much less striking than do cells whose inherent properties result in large shoulders, for example intestinal epithelial stem cells.

Advantage is taken of these phenomena when whole-body treatments are given with the intention of ablating the bone marrow in preparation for bone marrow transplantation. The classical mode of death for acute large whole-body radiation exposure is the gastrointestinal syndrome, since the transit-time of gut epithelium from progenitor cell to the loss of the mature cell at the tip of a villus, is shorter than the transit time of the haemopoietic cells. Doses not quite sufficiently high to cause death from the gas-

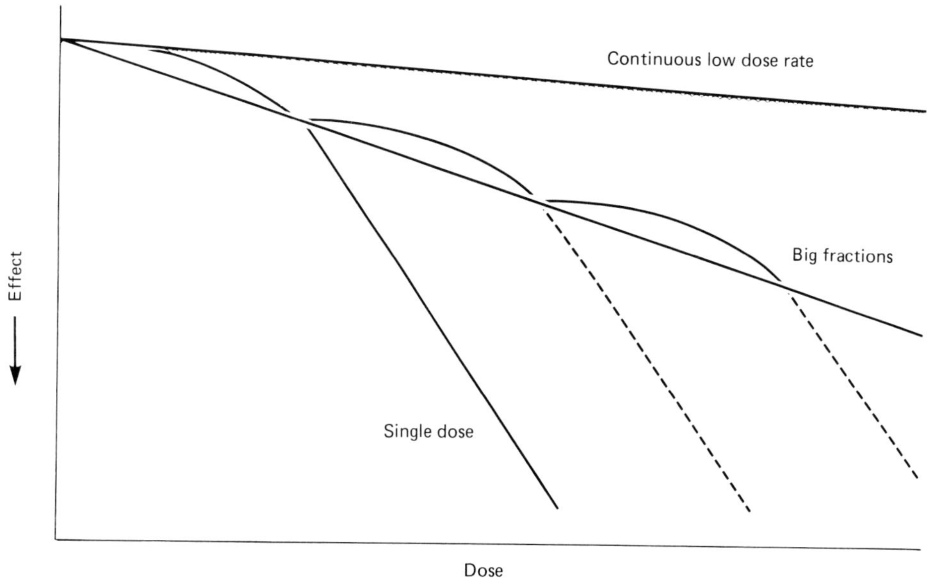

Figure 1.12 Both fractionated and continuous low dose rate dose-response curves have no 'shoulder' as they can be considered the resultants of reduplication of the single dose-response curve shoulder

trointestinal syndrome commonly result in death a few days later from the haematological syndrome; in other words the haemopoietic system is inherently more radiovulnerable than the intestinal epithelium renewal system, but does not have sufficient time to express this vulnerability at high doses. Haemopoietic vulnerability is partly the consequence of the relative inability of the constituent cells to sustain reparable injury. Consequently, at high dose rates, doses sufficient to produce therapeutic marrow ablation are certain to cause earlier gastrointestinal death. However, at low dose-rates, (for example 1000 cGy over 24 hours at approximately 40 cGy/hour, haemopoietic stem cells retain most of their radiovulnerability, whereas the intestinal stem cells are sustaining damage at a rate only slightly higher than their capacity to repair it. Dose-rate effects are principally notable over the range between 1 and 100 cGy/minute, a range which is of clinical significance in two situations. The first is when protracted intracavitary treatments are replaced by treatments giving either modestly or greatly increased dose rates, as in remote afterloading systems such as the Selectron and Cathetron. The second is when interstitial treatments result in calculated treatment times different from those originally intended for the dose specified. In practice this most commonly occurs when the 'volume' of a volume needle implant is found to be less than that from which the amount and distribution of the sealed sources were originally calculated. Radiotherapy centres adhering to the Manchester radium system apply a correction for the altered dose rate, the time of the interstitial treatment being adjusted to result in the actual dose administered being either increased (dose rate lower than intended) or more commonly decreased (dose rate higher than intended). These corrections were derived empirically when interstitial treatments were more commonly employed than they are today. Since subsequent experimental data indicate that dose-rate effects change rapidly in the same range as encountered clinically, it is interesting that Pierquin (1973) found no difference in the incidence of necrosis, irrespective of whether a standard dose of 7000 cGy is given in 3, 5 or 8 days, corresponding to dose rates of 97, 58, and 36 cGy/hour. The reasons for this conflict of experience are not known, but the following are suggested as possible explanations:

(1) The data on which the Manchester corrections are based came from experience with relatively early and therefore curable lesions; consequently there was a high proportion of long-term survivors in whom the true incidence of late normal tissue damage could be assessed
(2) The French data came from later cases, in whom there would be a higher (and probably irreducible) incidence of tumour-related 'necroses' and the smaller numbers of long-term survivors would obscure differences in the incidence of treatment-related late damage in the three groups.

Radiotherapists with wide experience of low dose rate interstitial and external mould treatments are convinced of the superiority of such treatments in terms of the late normal tissue effects which result from them.

Why tumours are vulnerable to slowly delivered doses which relatively spare the surrounding normal tissues is not known, but the following mechanisms have been suggested:

(1) It may be that reoxygenation occurs in tumours during continuous irradiation over an interval of up to 7 days (Hall, 1975) and that in consequence, hypoxic and radioresistant tumour cells become progressively more radiosensitive as the protracted exposure proceeds. As very little corresponding reoxygenation can occur in the normal tissues, an increase in therapeutic ratio results, so that a specified dose given slowly causes proportionately more tumour damage than when given rapidly. As reoxygenation also occurs during the course of fractionated treatments at high dose rates (Kallman, 1972), this explanation fails to explain convincingly the superiority of low-dose rate interstitial treatments over conventionally fractionated X-ray treatments.

(2) Radiation-induced mitotic delay may so lengthen the cell-cycle time that partial synchrony occurs in the clonogenic cells of the tumour, such that they accumulate at the late G2-mitosis interphase, with depletion of cells present in the late S-phase; in some normal tissues, late S-phase is known to be relatively radioresistant, hence depletion or disappearance of cells in this phase would inevitably result in increased radiosensitivity of the tissue as a whole. If, as is likely, the depletion of late S-phase cells is common to both normal and malignant tissues, there may be no therapeutic gain, unless the longer cell-cycle times of the normal tissues limit the increase in sensitivity during the exposure. Also, normal tissues may contain a higher proportion of non-cycling potentially clonogenic cells which, in the duration of the exposure, would not be expected to accumulate in the radiosensitive late G2-phase.

Interstitial treatments

Interstitial treatments are characterized by highly localized volumes and low dose rates. For a given lesion, modern linear accelerators and accurate beam direction can result in high dose volumes only a little larger than would have resulted if the lesion had been treated by implantation of radioactive sources, and the intensity and time-course of the resolution of the two resultant acute normal tissue reactions is very similar. The notion that it is low dose rate *per se* which confers the special advantages of interstitial treaments has been explored, most notably by Pierquin (1985) using teletherapy regimens compressed into intervals comparable with the duration of conventional interstitial treatments, delivered at dose rates of between 100 – 200 cGy/hour. (This would appear to be the ultimate test of the hypothesis that multiple fractions per day may be superior to multiple daily fractions.) The modest, perhaps illusory, gains achieved by low dose rate teletherapy appear to bode ill for the many current trials of accelerated fractionation (*see above*), but the relative or absolute failure of the low dose rate approach may have resulted from factors not shared by accelerated fractionation treatments.

Brachyteletherapy

Low dose rate teletherapy differs from the interstitial therapy which it is intended to mimic in two possibly important respects:

(1) The treatment is discontinuous, treatment times exceeding 8 hours/day being impractical or unsupportable. The discontinuity of the teletherapy treatments may have allowed some crucial factor, for instance radiation-induced synchrony, to escape from control during the major part of 24 hours when the tumour and its normal environs were unirradiated

(2) The dose rate was actually 2.5–5.0 times higher than that attained by interstitial treatments, or rather those interstitial treatments practised in the UK, typically 35–40 cGy/hour.

Dose-rate effects themselves alter rapidly over the range 1–100 cGy/hour, and the dose rates in the teletherapy experiments may have exceeded an as yet undetermined but critical limit above which clinically significant advantages of brachytherapy are no longer present. Another, disagreeable, explanation for the failure of brachytherapy is that the tumours treated were simply too advanced to be curable by radiotherapy in any circumstances; very few treatments in medicine are totally effective, and it could be that radiation therapy is already close to its horizons.

Intracavitary therapy

Alteration of dose rates

Increasingly stringent recommendations concerning radiation protection have led to the widespread adoption of remote afterloading equipment. Some types of this equipment are capable of providing conventional dose rates, whereas others are specifically designed to increase modestly (by three or four times) or markedly (100 times) the delivered dose rate. If the expression $T = A.R^{-1.35}$ (Orton and

Webber, 1977), relating irradiation time (T) and dose rate (R), where A is a constant, is rearranged to express D as a power of T, an exponent of T of 0.26 is obtained from human data. This suggests that dose rate is more important than overall treatment time, at least for normal tissue damage. *Figure 1.13* relates

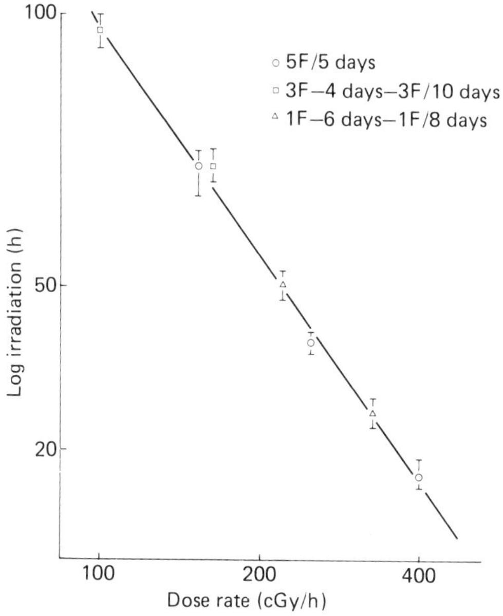

Figure 1.13 Irradiation time necessary to produce 50% necrosis in mouse-tails related to different dose rates (after Wilkinson, Hendry and Hunter, 1980)

dose rate to irradiation time for a late tissue end point, in this case the production of necrosis in 50% of irradiated mouse tails. This experiment was designed to be relevant to the adoption of Selectron afterloading equipment with source strength such that the dose rate at point A is increased by a factor of 3.5 over that conventionally attained in the Manchester radium system (*see* Chapter 9). Three fractionation schedules were employed, each at dose rates varying from 95 to 365 cGy/hour:

(1) Three daily fractions, a gap of 4 days, followed by three more daily fractions (roughly equivalent to the Manchester radium system)
(2) A single exposure, a gap of 6 days, and a second single exposure (roughly equivalent to the proposed Selectron treatment)
(3) Daily fractions over 5 days.

All data points fall on the same curve, which can be described by the relationship: Irradiation time = Constant × (Dose rate)$^{-1.33}$. The dose-rate exponent of −1.33 is remarkably close to that derived for human skin by Orton and Webber (1977), that is, −1.35.

A dose-rate exponent of −1.33 indicates that an increase in dose rate of 3.5 above the conventional Manchester point A dose rate requires a reduction in total dose of 33%, from 7500 cGy to 5000 cGy. Clinicians involved in the evaluation of the Selectron in Manchester found such a large reduction in absolute dose unacceptable, fearing that it would lead to serious failure of local control in early-stage disease, which might not become apparent until 2–3 years after the adoption of the new treatment technique. Accordingly, it was decided to initiate a prospective randomized trial of the conventional Manchester radium system versus the Selectron system, at two-dose levels; the upper absolute dose level was set with some misgivings, at 7500 cGy, identical to the radium dose, while the lower dose level was at 7000 cGy, a difference of approximately 7%. It was thought that Selectron overdosage would declare itself swiftly, permitting an early readjustment of the absolute dose range. The expectation of early declaration of overdose was realized, initially in the form of bowel damage, which was caused in 19% of 26 patients in the 7500 cGy group. This was taken to indicate system overdosage, and the dose range was revised to 6500–7000 cGy, it being assumed that the 'overdosage' resulted solely from a reduction in absolute dose insufficient to compensate for the effect of increased dose rate. It was not until later (Sherrah-Davies, 1985) that it was recognized that factors other than dose-rate effect could be responsible (*see* Chapter 9). The first anomaly to emerge was that bowel morbidity in the lower (7000 cGy) arm of the first Selectron trial was less than in the 7000 cGy arm of the antecedent pilot study — 3% as against 25%. The second anomaly is that if the radiobiological recommendation for dose reduction is correct, a Selectron dose of 7500 cGy would be equivalent to a radium dose of $7500 \times \frac{7500}{5000}$ cGy = 11 250 cGy at point A. Such a dose in the Manchester radium system would virtually ensure damage in all patients who received it, whereas it was observed in (only) 19% of patients who received 7500 cGy from the Selectron. This supports the argument that effects other than dose rate change are responsible, at least in part, for the enhanced morbidity seen in the early Selectron patients.

The current range of dose in the Manchester Selectron trial is 6000–6500 cGy, at which levels morbidity seems equivalent to that seen in the conventional arm of the trial; when adequate numbers of patients have been entered into this trial, its two-dose level design should permit a precise statement about the conversion factor for the absolute dose which is required when intracavitary treatments are performed at 3.5 times the dose rate of conventional Manchester radium treatments. The value of the exponent in the relationship T = Constant × (Dose rate)^{exponent} will lie between −1.0 and −1.3. Unfortunately, this study will add only one datum point to the knowledge of dose-rate effects in radiotherapy, as in the three phases of the trial (7500/7000, 7000/6500, 6500/6000 cGy), it has been the absolute dose, and not the dose-rate, which has been varied.

When very high activity cobalt-60 sources are substituted for radium in intracavitary treatments, as in the Cathetron, the dose rate at point A is increased by up to 100 times. A fractionated high dose rate regimen of N fractions should be equivalent in terms of absolute dose to a continous low dose rate treatment of duration t hours when $N = t/4$ (Liversedge, 1967), provided that no less than 12 fractions are given. For the radical treatment of early-stage disease, the equivalent of a 72-hour radium insertion would require 18 acute fractions over 72 hours, each of 214 cGy. The impracticalities of such a regimen are overcome in practice by reducing the number of fractions, extending the overall time, and increasing the dose per fraction. This effectively results in the simultaneous alteration of three independent variables which makes prediction of the likely effects on both tumour and normal tissues difficult. Accordingly, the development of acceptable treatment regimens using high dose rate equipment has been somewhat iterative, and has proceeded in diverse directions. Six fractions of 500–550 cGy over 12 days (point A dose) have been judged equivalent to 4000 cGy at point A from a 48-hour radium insertion (Howard, 1973), but this equivalence was based on observation of acute reactions occurring in the vault mucosa, and not on observation of late reactions in the clinically more relevant bowel, and furthermore, the observations were in the context of preoperative treatment, when no significant late effects are to be anticipated. In the more critical context of radical intracavitary treatment for early stage disease, five weekly fractions of 850 cGy at point A (total dose 4250 cGy) are considered equivalent to a Manchester radium system dose of 7500 cGy (Joslin and Peel, 1982).

Dose-modifying chemical adjuvants

The oxygen effect

Agents that are dose modifying are defined as those that alter the response to radiation throughout the whole of the dose-response curve (Alper and Howard-Flanders, 1956). The first such agent to be identified was oxygen. Following the demonstration of the presence of hypoxic zones in many tumours, (zones which were thought to contain relatively resistant cells capable of surviving radiation doses close to tolerance for normally oxygenated tissues, Gray, Conger and Ebert, 1953), several attempts were made to improve the oxygen supply to tumours undergoing irradiation (Hall, 1975). Most, if not all, of these early attempts failed because of underperfusion in all or parts of the tumour. Although many tumours are luxuriantly vascular, the almost invariable presence of zones of necrosis indicates that *blood flow* is seriously inadequate in some regions of all but the smallest tumours. Hypoxic cells that already have an oxygen debt utilize an increased oxygen supply within microseconds, so that small increments in the oxygen supply to hypoxic zones of tumours are swiftly consumed by those cells nearest to perfused capillaries, and the extra oxygen fails to penetrate deeply into the hypoxic microenvironments of tumours. Oxygen exerts its dose-enhancing effects by virtue of its ability, in the molecular state, to prolong the extremely short-life of the free radicals which are believed to cause the ultimately lethal damage to the reproductive integrity of cells, by consuming momentarily displaced electrons and thereby preventing their recombination with highly energized parent moeities (Adams and Dewey, 1963) (*see* Chapter 2).

For some time, radiotherapists attempted to improve their results by using hyperbaric chambers. Superficially this was a very attractive idea. Atmospheric air is 20% oxygen, and therefore at 100% compressed to 3 bars, it delivers 15 times the oxygen to the patient. Patients receive 15 times their normal supply of oxygen, but their tumours receive only a fraction of this, since the oxygen–haemoglobin association/dissociation curve is sigmoid. At normal temperature and pressure, haemoglobin is 96% saturated, so that most of the extra oxygen is carried in simple solution in the blood; the deliverance to hypoxic tumour cells is much less than would be expected by the times 15 factor imagined above. It was recognized (Adams and Dewey, 1963) that oxygen enhanced radiation effects by virtue of its affinity for electrons, but that its clinical potential was either marginal or negligible because it is so rapidly consumed. Accordingly, attention was directed to the development of electron-avid compounds that were only slowly metabolized, and which, given a sufficiently powerful concentration gradient down which to perfuse, might be expected to penetrate hypoxic zones in tumours which oxygen could not reach.

The failure of hyperbaric oxygen is widely acknowledged by the fact that many hyperbaric tanks still exist, but few are in use. Such hyperbaric tanks that are operational are used by radiotherapists convinced of the advantage, all of whom have failed to demonstrate the method's equal morbidity with that of in-air treatments at higher dose. There may be a genuine benefit from the use of hyperbaric oxygen in some circumstances, when for example, the oxygen-transporting capability of the blood is reduced by anaemia (Dische, Sealy and Watson 1983), but in the context of the treatment of chronically anaemic women with advanced cervical cancer, the general applicability of the superiority of hyperbaric oxygen treatments is not convincingly established.

When Urtasun *et al.* (1976) published a study of high-dose metronidazole and radiation in high grade supratentorial adult gliomas, it was at first widely accepted that an important biological principle had been established. This study prospectively compared radiation alone with identical radiation given in concert with metronidazole, an established antimicrobial and a relatively feeble electron-affinic drug. The radiation treatment was such that all patients in both treatment groups were dead within 20 months, although the metronidazole-treated patients had a better survival curve. High grade gliomas almost invariably contain necrotic zones, rarely metastasize, and the majority are rapidly lethal. Nearly all deaths in this study were due to failure of local control, and the superior survival of the metronidazole-treated patients was assumed to be an unequivocal demonstration of hypoxic cell radiosensitization.

When a new treatment is compared to a conventional treatment, poor performance in the control (conventional) arm of the trial always casts doubt on the validity of apparent superiority of the new treatment. The surprising feature of the Urtasun study was that patients in *both* treatment arms died so swiftly; the radiation regimen used is compared with two regimens in regular use at the Christie Hospital, Manchester (*Table 1.2*). The important features of this *Table* are that:

(1) Both Christie Hospital regimens yield 20% survival rates in adults under the age of 50 years
(2) The Urtasun regimen most resembles Christie treatment (a) in respect of number and size of fractions, and (b) in respect of overall time.

The time exponent of 0.11 in the Ellis formula $D = \text{NSD} \times N^{0.24} \times T^{0.11}$ is fixed, strictly applicable only to normal skin, and fails to take account of the progressive nature of the increase in repopulation that begins to occur some time after the commencement of 'daily' irradiation; in mammalian central nervous tissue, such repopulation is believed to be neglible under 'daily' irradiation periods of less than 6 weeks (Fowler, 1984 a,b). Therefore the effect of Urtasun's nine fractions being delivered over 20 days, instead of the Christie Hospital's 11, should be minimal, (at least in terms of normal tissue effects). Furthermore, the N exponent of 0.24 in the Ellis formula for skin may be replaced by one of 0.4 (van der Kogel, 1979) — the 'neuro-ret' — a very operative difference, and one which swamps the T exponent 0.11, which is itself probably irrelevant to central nervous tissue treatments that are complete in under 3 weeks. Urtasun's regimen should therefore be very similar in its late effects on the normal central nervous system to the first of the Christie Hospital treatments, but its effects on tumour control are inferior to both of the Christie Hospital regimens. The reasons for this are obscure, but whatever the explanation, the poor performance of both treatment arms seriously undermines the conclusion that a radiosensitizer had worked in a clinical situation.

Failure of misonidazole

Hypoxic cells are characteristic of malignant tumours, but not of most normal tissues, the exceptions being avascular tissues such as cartilage, and parts of the eye. Treatment in hyperbaric oxygen increases radiation damage in normal cartilage (Henk, Kunkler and Smith, 1977). The central nervous system is generally regarded as being very well perfused, but enhanced damage to the spinal cord is also seen in hyperbaric treatment for advanced head and neck malignancy. Misonidazole is a poor radiosensitizer (*see below*), but even this drug is capable of enhancing the radiation response of some normal human tissues (Arcangeli, Nervi and Munroe, 1980). Many animal experiments also demonstrate radiosensitization of a wide range of normal tissues (oesophagus, spinal cord, cartilage, testis) by this rather inefficient drug (Stewart, Denekamp and Randhawa, 1982). Rapid development is taking place of drugs which, compared to misonidazole, are up to seven times more electron-affinic, and less dependent for their electron-affinity on the presence of nitro-groupings, which appear to be neurotoxic. Misonidazole failed clinically (Dishe, Sealy and Watson, 1983), probably due to poor electron affinity as

Table 1.2 Treatment schedules for high grade gliomas

	Total dose (cGy)	*Fraction number*	*Fraction size (cGy)*	*Overall time (h)*
CHHRI (1)	3000	8	375	11
Urtasun	3200	9	355	20
CHHRI (2)	3750	16	235	20

CHHRI: Christie Hospital and Holt Radium Institute

demonstrated *in vitro*, and dose-limiting, insupportable neurotoxicity *in vivo*. Alternatively, hypoxic cells may be of little consequence in determining the outcome of fractionated treatments (*see* Chapter 2).

Development of sensitizers is occurring simultaneously in several directions:

(1) Increase or decrease in lipophilicity. Lipophilic drugs may be less neurotoxic to humans, but the one agent clinically tested, desmethylmisonidazole, was twice as rapidly excreted by the kidneys because of its polarity. It penetrated the central nervous system less than misonidazole, and had approximately half its plasma half-life. However, tissue exposure, judged by the area under the curve of plasma concentration versus time, showed desmethylmisonidazole to be twice as neurotoxic as misonidazole

(2) The introduction of more than one electron-affinity moeity in the nitroimidazole nucleus. 4-Nitroimidazoles so substituted at position 5 are much more powerful sensitizers than would be expected from their electron-affinic properties alone, partly because of their ability to neutralize radioprotective sulphydryl groups within the cell

(3) The combination of sensitizers with drugs that deplete intracellular glutathione, such as diethylmaleate: potentiation occurs by removal of — SH groups.

Malignant tumours contain hypoxic cells, and larger tumours contain more such cells than do smaller ones. The hypothesis that these cells contribute materially to the failure of conventional radiotherapy regimens has been canvassed for over 30 years, but is still to be validated, and probably will not be proven or disproven until much more efficient, powerful and selective radiosensitizers are available.

The most convincing demonstration that sensitizers can affect the response to irradiation of human tumours is the significant prolongation of the time-to-regrowth of intradermal metastases given large single radiation doses (Thomlinson *et al.*, 1976). This effect has not been translated into identifiable improvement in local tumour control when fractionated treatments are employed (Dische, Sealy and Watson, 1983). The reoxygenation that occurs during fractionated treatment may be sufficiently great to swamp the effects of weakly-sensitizing misonidazole, and more efficient drugs may be required to demonstrate an effect greater than that achieved by reoxygenation alone (Danekamp and Joiner, 1982).

Reduced sensitizer toxicity would permit higher doses of drugs to be given which are themselves powerful sensitizers, with the obvious danger that normal tissue damage may be worsened, even though sensitization of normal tissues (by misonidazole) is less at small radiation doses per fraction than at high radiation doses. It is not yet known whether radiosensitization for early normal tissue effects and late effects is similar or different.

Future possibilities and pitfalls

In future trials of hypoxic sensitizers, three approaches may be adopted:

(1) Two identical radiation treatments may be given, one with sensitizer, and one without. This approach was adopted in the three MRC-sponsored trials (1983, 1984, 1984) of misonidazole in advanced cervical cancer, supratentorial gliomas, and advanced head and neck cancer (*see* Chapter 2).

The above decision with regard to the MRC trials reflected either a lack of confidence in misonidazole as an effective sensitizer, or forgetfulness about enhanced normal tissue effects widely reported in studies of hyperbaric oxygen. Animal experiments designed to estimate the magnitude of enhancement of normal tissue effects at the radiation fraction sizes used clinically, indicate that total radiation dose should be reduced by 3% to compensate for the concurrent administration of misonidazole (Hendry and Sutton, 1984). Radiation regimens of up to 30 fractions given over 6 weeks generate less steep dose-response curves than do 15 or 16 fraction regimens given over 3 weeks, which exploit higher doses per fraction (*see Figures 1.4 and 1.5*). The steep curve shows a higher criticality of total dose in determining outcome, and a dose-effect enhancement of only 3% could result in a 5% increase in laryngeal cartilage necrosis; such an effect would be unlikely in the less steep curve; if more potent radiosensitizers are developed, dose reduction factors (DRFs) are likely to be higher, and will be of major concern to radiotherapists exploiting regimens resulting in steep dose-response curves of high criticality.

If two identical radiation schedules, one with sensitizer, one without, are compared, and the results indicate worse late normal tissue responses with modest gains in local tumour control, once again large amounts of time, effort, and money will have been squandered due to poor trial design. It could be argued that such a trial *might* result in clear advantage in tumour control for only a modest increase in late normal effects, clearly establishing the clinical usefulness of radiosensitizers; this is the Micawber approach to trial design and has no place in scientific clinical investigation. (Also, such an outcome, greatly favourable to sensitizers, looks rather unlikely, in view of the failures of hyperbaric oxygen, fast neutrons, and misonidazole, to confer even modest gains in local tumour control.)

(2) A second approach to the problem is to derive an estimate of the DRF required for the new sensitizer, and apply this reduction to the dose given on the sensitizer arm of the trial, in the hope that late effects of sensitizer plus reduced radiation dose will equal those of the unreduced conventional radiation treatment alone. The chief disadvantage of this approach is that the estimated DRF will be based on animal studies; laboratory-derived predictions of the behaviour of human tissues are less wildly inaccurate than they once were, but can only be regarded as a rough guide. Estimates of DRF derived from data on acute normal human tissue reactions are likely to be very misleading (Withers, Thames and Peters, 1982), and reliable data on late normal human tissue responses will be slow to accumulate, especially if for instance the necrosis rate increased from only 4% to 10%.

(3) The third option is to accept the best available estimate of DRF, and carry out a study of two dose levels, one significantly higher and the other lower than the estimate equivalent dose (*see* introductory section); this dispenses with both guesswork and Micawberism, and the resulting data are almost guaranteed to indicate whether or not the new sensitizer has improved the therapeutic ratio.

It has been argued (*see* (2) *above*), that if seriously inconvenient regimens involving two or more fractions per day are to be financially acceptable, they must demonstrate a clear superiority over conventional treatments. However, even modest gains from sensitizers would be worthwhile, since it should, in time, prove possible to develop cheap, orally administered, non-toxic and effective compounds. The demonstration of modest gains is easily obscured if the trial design does not permit comparison of tumour control rates achieved by different drugs which generate equal levels of morbidity. (The radiosensitizers thus far tested clinically are present in higher concentrations in normal than in malignant tissues: if that gradient could be reversed, the above argument for two-dose level studies may become less powerful. If basic side chains are substituted into the nitroimidazole molecule, the resultant compounds accumulate in zones of high acidity, such as are found in the hypoxic areas (Saunders *et al.*, 1982).

Certain compounds, for example thiosulphates, are powerfully radioprotective, with a large differential effect noted between normal tissues (relatively great protection) and malignant tissues (less protection because already partly hypoxic); also some radioprotectors hardly penetrate tumours. Radioprotectors are the pharmacological equivalent of the limb tourniquet (Suit and Lindberg, 1968). Attempts to exploit these compounds clinically will necessarily require higher radiation doses to bring acute and late normal tissue effects back up to the levels found acceptable in convential treatment schedules. Early and late effects may be affected differently, and the need for two-dose level studies is again obvious.

One hopes that radiosensitizers of hypoxic cells will not ultimately prove to be another as Matthew Fenner once said, 'elegant, but expensive way, of saving electricity'.

References

ADAMS, G. E: and DEWEY, D. L. (1963) Hydrated electrons and radiobiological sensitisation. *Biochemical and Biophysical Research Communications*, **12**, 473–477

ALPER, T. and HOWARD-FLANDERS, P. (1956) Role of oxygen in modifying the radiosensitivity of *E. coli* B. *Nature*, **178**, 978–979

ARCANGELI, G., NERVI, C. and MUNROE, F. (1980) Misonidazole also sensitises some normal tissue. *British Journal of Radiology*, **53**, 780–792

ASSCHER, A.W., WILSON, C. and AUSAN, S. G. (1961) Sensitisation of blood vessels to hypertensive damage by X-irradiation. *Lancet*, **1**, 580–583

CATTERALL, M. and BEWLEY, D. K. (1979) *Fast Neutrons in the Treatment of Cancer*. London: Academic Press; New York: Grune and Stratton

DANEKAMP, J. and JOINER, M. C. (1982) The potential benefit from a perfect radiosensitiser and its dependence on reoxygenation. *British Journal of Radiology*, **55**, 657–663

DISCHE, S., SEALY, R. and WATSON, E. R. (1983) Carcinoma of the cervix — anaemia, radiotherapy and hyperbaric oxygen. *British Journal of Radiology*, **56**, 255

DUNCAN, W., ARNOTT, S. J., BATTERMAN, J. J., ORR, J. A., SCHMITT, G. and KERR, G. R. (1984) Fast neutrons in the treatment of head and neck cancer: the results of a multi-centre randomly controlled trial. *Radiotherapy and Oncology*, **2**, 293–300

DUNCAN, W., ARNOTT, S. J., JACK, W. J. L. *et al.* (1985) A report of a randomised trial of d(15)+Be neutrons compared with megavoltage X-ray therapy of bladder cancer. *International Journal of Radiation Oncology, Biology and Physics*, (in press)

EASSON, E. C. and POINTON, R. C. S. (1985) *The Radiotherapy of Malignant Disease*. Berlin: Springer-Verlag

ELLIS, F. (1969) Dose, time and fractionation: a clinical hypothesis. *Clinical Radiology*, **20**, 1–7

FOWLER, J. F. (1984a) What next in fractionated radiotherapy? *British Journal of Cancer*, **49**, (Suppl VI), 285–300

FOWLER, J. F. (1984b) Review: total doses in fractionated radiotherapy — implications of new radiobiological data. *International Journal of Radiation Biology*, **46**, 103–120

FOWLER, J. F., JOINER, M. C. and WILLIAMS, M. V. (1983) Low doses per fraction in radiotherapy: a definition for 'flexure dose'. *British Journal of Radiology*, **56**, 599–601

GOLD, H. (1961) Production of arteriosclerosis in the rat: effect of X-ray and a high-fat diet. *Archives of Pathology*, **71**, 268–281

GRAY, L. H., CONGER, A. O. and EBERT, M. (1953) The concentration of oxygen dissolved in tissues at the time of irradiation as a factor in radiotherapy. *British Journal of Radiology*, **26**, 638–648

HALL, E. J. (1975) *Radiobiology for the Radiotherapist*, 2nd edn, p.152. Hangerstown, Maryland: Harper and Row

HENDRY, J. H. and SUTTON, M. L. (1984) On the sensitisation of skin radionecrosis in mice by misonidazole at low doses. *British Journal of Radiology*, **57**, 507–514

HENK, J. M., KUNKLER, P. B. and SMITH, C. W. (1977) Radiotherapy and hyperbaric oxygen in head and neck cancer. Final report of the first controlled clinical trial. *Lancet*, **2**, 101–103

HOPEWELL, J. W. (1980) The importance of vascular damage in the development of late radiation effects in normal tissue. In *Radiation Biology in Cancer Research*, edited by R. E. Meyn and R. H. Withers, pp. 449–459. New York: Raven Press

HOPEWELL, J. W. and WRIGHT, E. A. (1970) The nature of latent cerebral irradiation damage and its modification by hypertension. *British Journal of Radiology*, **43**, 161–167

JOSLIN, C. A. F. and PEEL, K. R. (1982) In *Treatment of Cancer*, edited by K. E. Halnan, p.561 London: Chapman and Hall

KALLMAN, R. F. (1972) The phenomenon of reoxygenation and its implications for fractionated radiotherapy. *Radiology*, **105**, 135–142

LAW, M. P. and THOMLINSON, R. H. (1978) Vascular permeability in the ears of rats after X-irradiation. *British Journal of Radiology*, **51**, 895–904

MEDICAL RESEARCH COUNCIL (1983) A study of the effect of misonidazole in conjunction with radiotherapy for the treatment of grades 3 and 4 astrocytomas. *British Journal of Radiology*, **56**, 673–682

MEDICAL RESEARCH COUNCIL (1984) The Medical Research Council trial of misonidazole in carcinoma of the uterine cervix. *British Journal of Radiology*, **57**, 491–499

ORTON, C. G. and WEBBER, B. M. (1977) Time-dose factor (TDF) analysis of dose-rate effects in permanent implant therapy. *International Journal of Radiation Oncology, Biology and Physics*, **2**, 55–60

PIERQUIN, B. and BAILLET, F. (1971) La téléradiothérapie continué à faible debit. *Annals of Radiology,* **14**, 617–629

POINTON, R. S., READ, G. and GREENE, D. (1985) A randomised comparison of photons and 15 MeV neutrons for the treatment of carcinoma of the bladder. *British Journal of Radiology*, **58**, 219–224

ROSWIT, B., WISHAM, L. H. and SORRENTINO, J. (1953) The circulation of radiation-damaged skin. Radiosodium clearance studies. *American Journal of Roentgenology,* **69**, 980–990

SAUNDERS, M. I., DISCHE, S., FERMONT, D. *et al.* (1982) The radiosensitiser Ro 03-8799 and the concentration which may be achieved in human tumours — a preliminary study. *British Journal of Cancer*, **46**, 706–719

SHERRAH-DAVIES, E. (1985) Morbidity following low-dose-rate Selectron therapy for cervical cancer. *Clinical Radiology*, **36**, 131–139

SINGH, K. (1978) Two regimens with the same TDF but differing morbidity used in the treatment of stage III carcinoma of the cervix. *British Journal of Radiology*, **51**, 357–362

STEWART, F. A., DENEKAMP, J. and RANDHAWA, V. (1982) Radiosensitisation of normal mouse skin by misonidazole: single and fractionated dose studies. *British Journal of Cancer*, **45**, 869–877

STOPPARD, T. (1972) *Jumpers*. London and Boston: Faber and Faber

STANDQUIST, M. (1944) Studien über die kumulative Wirkung der Roëntgenstrahlen bei Fractionierung. *Acta Radiologica (Stockholm)*, **55**, (Suppl 1)

SUIT, H. and LINDBERG, R. (1968) Radiation therapy administered under conditions of tourniquet-induced local tissue hypoxia. *American Journal of Roentgenology, Radium Therapy and Nuclear Medicine*, **102**, 27–37

SUTTON, M. L. and HENDRY, J. H. (1984) Applied radiobiology. In *The Radiotherapy of Malignant Disease*, edited by E. C. Easson and R. C. S. Pointon, ch.2, Berlin: Springer-Verlag

THOMLINSON, R. H., DISCHE, S., GRAY, A. J. and ERRINGTON, L. M. (1976) Clinical testing of the radiosensitiser Ro 07-0582. III Responses of tumours. *Clinical Radiology*, **27**, 167–270

URTASUN, R. C., BAND, P., CHAPMAN, J. D., FELDSTEIN, M. L., MIELKE, B. and FRYER, C. (1976) Radiation and high-dose metronidazole in supratentorial glioblastomas. *New England Journal of Medicine*, **294**, 1364–1367

VAN DER KOGEL, A. J. (1979) Mechanisms of late radiation injury in the spinal cord. In *Radiation Biology in Cancer Research*, edited by E. R. Meyn and R. H. Withers, New York: Raven Press

WIERNICK, G., BATES, T. D., BERRY, R. J. *et al.* (1982) Seventh interim progress report of the British Institute of Radiology fractionation study of 3F/week versus 5F/week in radiotherapy of the laryngo-pharynx. *British Journal of Radiology*, **55**, 505–510

WIERNICK, G., PATTERSON, T. J. S. and BERRY, R. J. (1974) The effect of fractionated dose-patterns of X-irradiation on the survival of experimental skin flaps in the pig. *British Journal of Radiology*, **47**, 343–345

WILKINSON, J. M., HENDRY, J. H. and HUNTER, R. D. (1980) Dose-rate consideration in the introduction of low dose-rate afterloading intracavitary technique for radiotherapy. *British Journal of Radiology,* **53**, 890–893

WITHERS, H. R., THAMES, H. D. and PETERS, L. J. (1982) Differences in the fractionation response of acutely and late-reacting tissues. In *Progress in Radio-oncology*, Vol II, edited by Karcher *et al.*, New York: Raven Press

ZOLLINGER, H. U. (1970) Structural changes in blood vessels. *Current Topics in Radiation Research Quarterly,* **10**, 58–74

2

The role of radiosensitizers

J. M. Henk

Attempts have been made for over 40 years to improve the effectiveness of radiotherapy by the addition of chemical agents. So far none has been demonstrated to be sufficiently effective to be accepted for widespread clinical use, and the quest for a useful radiosensitizing drug continues.

Definition of radiosensitizers

Strictly speaking the term radiosensitizer should be applied to a drug which enhances the effect of radiotherapy on tumours, but when administered alone has no effect on tumour growth. However, the term is often also applied to an agent which has an antitumour effect in its own right, but when used in combination with radiotherapy produces a greater response than would be expected from the sum of the responses to each used alone.

Therapeutic index

A drug which enhances the action of radiation equally on both tumours and normal tissues is of no clinical value, it has the same effect as merely increasing the dose of radiotherapy. In order to be useful clinically a radiosensitizer must improve the differential effect of radiotherapy on tumours compared to normal tissues. In this context, the distinction between acute and late effects of radiation on normal tissues is important.

Acute effects occur early in a course of radiotherapy and are due to the death of cells in rapidly replicating tissues, e.g. mucosa, skin and intestinal epithelium. Such effects are responsible for the acute morbidity which occurs during and immediately after a course of radiotherapy and which in some cases may limit the amount of radiotherapy that can be given. However, these effects are reversible and the tissues rapidly regenerate after radiotherapy leaving little or no long-term sequelae.

Late effects occur months or years after radiotherapy and are due to the death of cells in slowly replicating tissues, for example vascular endothelium. Such changes are usually irreversible. In most patients treated by radiotherapy the dose of radiation administered to the tumour volume is limited to that which can safely be given without causing unacceptable late damage.

A radiosensitizer may enhance both early and late effects of radiotherapy on normal tissues. Enhancement of early effects may increase acute morbidity but not necessarily reduce the total dose of radiotherapy which can safely be given, whereas enhancement of late damage can be catastrophic unless the dose of radiotherapy is proportionately reduced. In assessing the radiosensitizing capabilities of a drug, it is therefore important to assess its effect on late normal tissue damage as well as on tumour control probability. Unfortunately, late effects are much more difficult to measure experimentally than acute effects and in a clinical trial take a long time to become manifest.

In order to sensitize tumours more than normal tissues it is necessary to exploit differences in radiation response between the two. So far in practice only two such differences are known for certain, cell proliferation kinetics and oxygenation. A third possibility is that normal tissues have a greater capacity than tumours to repair sublethal and potentially lethal damage; if so, an agent which inhibits repair is likely to exert an adverse effect on therapeutic ratio.

Cell kinetics

Tumours contain a heterogeneous population of cells. In most tumours a significant proportion of the viable cells are actively multiplying, so that at any given moment there will be many cells which are at some point in the mitotic cycle. On the other hand, the normal tissues which show dose-limiting late damage have a very slow cell turnover, and at any one time very few or no cells are in the mitotic cycle. The radiosensitivity of a cell varies during the mitotic cycle; it is lowest during the S phase when the cell is synthesizing DNA. A chemical agent which increases the radiosensitivity of cycling cells, especially in S phase, but does not affect resting (G0) cells may be expected to enhance the effect of radiotherapy on tumours without increasing the risk of late damage. It will, however, increase the acute normal tissue effects of radiotherapy. A number of such agents, for example, methotrexate and bromouracildeoxyriboside (BUdR) have been tried as radiosensitizers on this rationale, (*see below*).

Oxygenation

The studies of Gray *et al.* (1953) and Thomlinson and Gray (1955) demonstrated that hypoxia was unlikely to have any effect on the radiation response of normal tissues, but might well be a cause of radioresistance in tumours. The relative radioprotection of tumour cells by physiological hypoxia represents the one large radiobiological difference between tumours and normal tissues which is potentially exploitable; not surprisingly, current interest centres mainly on hypoxic cell radiosensitizers.

The importance of the oxygen effect in clinical radiotherapy remains controversial. During a course of fractionated radiotherapy 're-oxygenation' occurs, i.e. the oxygen supply to hypoxic tumour cells improves as the tumour shrinks. It is not known to what extent human tumours re-oxygenate during radiotherapy; probably they all do to some extent but with considerable variation between different tumours. Radiobiological calculations (Denekamp, 1983) suggest that re-oxygenation should be greater with multiple small fractions of radiotherapy, e.g. 30 fractions of 200 cGy, than with larger fractions, e.g. six fractions of 600 cGy, and that there may be little to be gained from the use of a hypoxic cell sensitizer with conventionally fractionated radiotherapy. Nevertheless, the results of trials of hyperbaric oxygen (*see below*) strongly suggest that tumour cell hypoxia remains an important cause of radiotherapy failure, at least in the case of many squamous cell carcinomas, even with conventionally fractionated radiotherapy, and that there probably is a benefit to be gained from an effective chemical hypoxic-cell sensitizer.

Radiosensitization of hypoxic cells

Hyperbaric oxygen

The curve relating radiosensitivity to the concentration of oxygen present at the instant of irradiation rises steeply as the oxygen tension increases from zero to physiological levels, i.e. 40–100 mmHg. Increasing oxygen tension above physiological levels produces only a very small increase in radiosensitivity (Alper and Howard-Flanders, 1956). This finding led to the first attempt to sensitize hypoxic tumour cells to radiotherapy, which was to irradiate while the patient was breathing oxygen at raised pressure in a hyperbaric chamber. By raising the partial pressure of oxygen dissolved in plasma, oxygen can be made to diffuse further from capillaries into hypoxic areas of tumours thereby improving their radiosensitivity; at the same time there should be scarcely any radiosensitizing effect on fully-oxygenated normal tissues.

Gray *et al.* (1953) demonstrated the benefit of hyperbaric oxygen in the radiotherapy of a mouse tumour, and shortly afterwards the technique was introduced into clinical radiotherapy (Churchill-Davidson, Sanger and Thomlinson, 1955). Early clinical results were promising, but unfortunately adequate controlled trials did not begin until nearly 10 years later, by which time many of the early workers in this field were expressing disillusionment.

A number of controlled trials were conducted between 1964 and 1979, but most contained too few patients for meaningful conclusions to be drawn. Carcinomas at four sites were studied: head and neck, uterine cervix, bladder, and lung. The following conclusions can be drawn from an overall assessment of the results of the trials.

(1) Hyperbaric oxygen improved local control in head and neck cancer; a small effect was seen in carcinoma of the cervix and bronchus. No benefit was demonstrated in carcinoma of the bladder.
(2) When equal dosage with the same fractionation was given in hyperbaric oxygen and in air, there was an increase in late normal tissue damage in the former.
(3) The greatest improvement in local tumour control occurred when large dose fractions were used.
(4) The improvement in local tumour control from hyperbaric oxygen was most marked in the case of smaller tumours, especially squamous carcinomas of the head and neck less than 5 cm in diameter.
(5) Many patients proved unfit to enter a compression chamber because of other medical problems, while some failed to complete the course of treatment because of claustrophobia or convulsions.

(6) Irradiation in high pressure oxygen is a complex and time-consuming technique which became disliked by the staff of radiotherapy departments.

Many radiotherapists consider that these trials show that hyperbaric oxygen is of no clinical value, on the grounds that there is no improvement in therapeutic ratio and that the effect of tumour cell hypoxia is negligible with daily radiotherapy using small fractions of 200 cGy or less because re-oxygenation occurs. One trial set out to test this point of view – the second Cardiff head and neck trial (Henk and Smith, 1977) which compared a 10-fraction scheme in hyperbaric oxygen with a conventional 30-fraction scheme in air. The total radiation doses were chosen so that the same incidence of late normal tissue damage would be expected in the two groups, based on previous experience with these two treatment schedules. Five-year follow-up of the 106 patients in this trial (Henk, 1984) revealed significantly higher survival and local tumour control rates in the group treated in hyperbaric oxygen; the greatest advantage was seen with lesions less than 5 cm diameter. No difference in late normal tissue effects between the two groups could be detected. This trial strongly suggests that the oxygen effect does exist, even with fractions of 200 cGy per day, and that sensitization of the hypoxic tumour cell can improve the therapeutic ratio. Nevertheless, hyperbaric oxygen as an approach to the problem of the hypoxic tumour cell has now virtually been discarded, mainly because of the technical complexity of the procedure in relation to the very small overall benefits observed.

Access of oxygen to tumour cells depends on blood flow. High pressure oxygen may induce vasoconstriction and therefore be largely self-defeating. Its relative failure with larger tumours may be due to lack of penetration of the oxygen to hypoxic areas because of inadequate blood flow. Little is known of the physiological mechanisms of tumour vasculature, so it is not possible to know how to use hyperbaric oxygen in the optimum manner with regard to fractionation, pressure, anaesthesia, other drugs, and soak times. Hence the best has probably not yet been obtained from hyperbaric oxygen; if more could be learned about the factors influencing the temporal and spatial distribution of oxygen in tumours, greater benefit may yet become possible. However, for the present, hyperbaric oxygen has been overtaken by other methods of attacking the problem of hypoxic tumour cells. Its contribution so far has been to demonstrate the existence of the oxygen effect, and to encourage further research into hypoxic-cell sensitizing drugs.

Menadiol

The vitamin K analogue menadiol diphosphate (Synkavit) was the first substance tried as a radiosensitizer for clinical use. In the early 1940s it was thought worthy of investigation as a radiosensitizer because of its ability to block nucleic acid synthesis, and it was shown to potentiate the cell-killing effects of X-rays on tissue cultures. More recently, Gronow (1965) demonstrated that it lowered the concentration of sulphydryl groups in cells. It is also an electron-affinic agent, and its effect may be to sensitize hypoxic cells in a similar manner to nitroimidazole compounds such as misonidazole (*see below*).

Most of the early clinical trials of menadiol as a radiosensitizer were performed with carcinoma of the lung. Mitchell (1953) gave 100 mg of the drug intravenously 30 minutes before each fraction of radiotherapy and claimed that it had a small but useful effect. In a random prospective trial at the Christie Hospital, Manchester from 1959 to 1963 involving 504 patients with carcinoma of the bronchus, the survival rate from radiotherapy with menadiol, given as recommended by Mitchell, was no different from that of radiotherapy alone (Evans and Todd, 1969). However, the patients admitted to this trial had advanced disease; only 3% lived 3 years and local control was not studied. In these circumstances quite a large sensitizing effect could have been missed.

Krishnamurthi, Shanta and Nair (1967) studied the effect of menadiol and radiotherapy on carcinoma of the buccal mucosa in South India. In India buccal mucosa carcinoma is frequently associated with submucosal fibrosis, and it had previously been shown that patients in whom there was an advanced fibrotic reaction in the tumour bed responded poorly to radiotherapy. One hundred and thirty-one such patients were admitted to a controlled trial; they were randomly allocated to receive menadiol or placebo 30 minutes before each fraction of radiotherapy; a daily tumour dose of 200 cGy was given up to a total dose of 6500 – 7000 cGy. The 3-year recurrence-free survival rate was 35.4% in the patients who received menadiol and 18.1% in the patients who received placebo ($P = 0.04$). This result suggests that menadiol had a real effect and may have been acting as a hypoxic cell sensitizer. Despite the results of this trial the use of menadiol as a radiosensitizer has not been pursued. This is partly because of the disappointing results in carcinoma of the bronchus, but mainly because by the time Krishnamurthi's results appeared interest had switched to the use of concomitant cytotoxic agents as radiosensitizers, and newer electron-affinic compounds were being investigated.

Nitroimidazoles

Most radiosensitizers under investigation at present

are agents aimed at increasing the sensitivity of hypoxic cells. The property of oxygen which affects radiosensitivity is its electron affinity, or reduction potential. Compounds which mimic the radiobiological properties of oxygen all have a high electron affinity and selectively sensitize hypoxic cells.

The search for a suitable 'oxygen mimic' began in the 1960s. Many compounds were found which sensitized anoxic microorganisms to radiation, and the relationship between electron affinity and sensitizing efficiency was recognized. One of the earlier compounds to show sensitizing activity in mammalian cells was PNAP (para-nitroacetophenone) which directed attention to other heterocyclic nitro-compounds as potential radiosensitizers. One such compound tested which was already in clinical use was the antibiotic metronizadole, a 5-nitroimidazole. This was tested as a radiosensitizer in the treatment of glioblastoma multiforme (Urtasun *et al.*, 1976) and found to have a slight effect. However, the dose required for hypoxic cell sensitization is very much higher than that normally administered when the drug is used as an antibiotic, and thus causes nausea, vomiting and some risk of cerebral toxicity. Theoretical considerations indicated that 2-nitroimidazoles should be more effective than 5-nitroimidazoles; this was confirmed by experiments both *in vitro* and *in vivo*. One such compound, misonidazole, proved particularly effective.

For a hypoxic sensitizer to be of value it must meet the following criteria.

(1) A high sensitizing efficiency of hypoxic tumour cells with no sensitization of well-oxygenated normal tissue.
(2) Free distribution throughout the body to reach tumours.
(3) Diffusability, so that it can penetrate poorly vascularized tumours and can reach hypoxic cells distant from capillaries.
(4) Ability to penetrate within cells.
(5) A sufficiently slow rate of metabolism so that it reaches hypoxic cells and remains there during the time of irradiation.
(6) Sensitization present at the dose levels given with a fractionated course of radiotherapy.
(7) The drug must be non-toxic at dose levels sufficient to give effective radiosensitization.

In animal radiobiology, misonidazole met all these criteria. Initial studies showed that it was widely distributed, with high tumour levels and a long retention time in man. In animal tumours non-toxic concentrations gave gain factors of about two with large single doses, and about 1.5 for fractionated courses of radiation. Radiosensitization was confirmed in man; patients with multiple metastases of the skin (Thomlinson *et al.*, 1976) and the lung (Ash, Peckham and Steel, 1979) were treated with varying doses of radiation with and without misonidazole. Enhancement ratios were found to be rather less than in experimental animal tumours, varying between 1.2 and 1.5 for single doses, with a slightly lower range for 10 fractions.

Sensitization of hypoxic normal tissues was demonstrated by Dische, Gray and Zanelli (1976) by observing the skin reaction after radiation with a strontium-90 plaque; patients' arms were irradiated with and without temporary occlusion of the circulation by a sphygmomanometer cuff. Misonidazole enhanced the acute skin reaction only when the blood supply was occluded during radiation.

Unfortunately, misonidazole is neurotoxic. High total doses cause a peripheral sensory neuropathy which can be distressing and long-lasting in severe cases. The incidence of neurotoxicity depends mainly on the total dose administered, the maximum safe level being 12 g/m^2 when used with a fractionated course of radiation. The pharmacokinetics vary from patient to patient. The higher the peak blood level and the longer the serum half-life, the greater is the risk of neurotoxicity; drugs which reduce the serum half-life, e.g. anticonvulsants, reduce the incidence of neurotoxicity.

Pilot studies of misonidazole in clinical radiotherapy showed some promising results. For example, Paterson *et al.* (1981) treated 29 patients with advanced head and neck cancer using the same dose and fractionation scheme which had previously been used with hyperbaric oxygen, i.e. 4000–4500 cGy in 10 fractions in 3 weeks, giving 1.2 g/m^2 of misonidazole before each treatment. After 9 months the local control rate was 60%, similar to that which had been achieved with hyperbaric oxygen. These promising early results led to a number of controlled clinical trials. Worldwide over 5000 patients have been included in such trials. A wide variety of fractionation schedules has been tested in an attempt to use the maximum dose of 12 g/m^2 to the greatest advantage.

Misonidazole with every fraction

In the majority of clinical trials with misonidazole, the drug has been given before each fraction of radiotherapy to a total dose of 12 g/m^2. The smaller the number of fractions the larger is the dose of drug administered on each occasion and the greater the expected radiosensitization. For example, if six fractions are administered the dose of misonidazole will be 2 g/m^2, which has been estimated to give a probable level in hypoxic tumour cells of 40 μg/g and a sensitizing efficiency of 1.50. At the other extreme only 0.4 g/m^2 can be given with each of 30 fractions of radiotherapy, achieving a probable drug level in the hypoxic tumour cells of 8 μg/g and a sensitizing efficiency of 1.15.

Most radiotherapists believe that without a sensitizer radiotherapy yields a better therapeutic ratio when given in many small fractions than when given in a few large fractions. Trials in carcinoma of the cervix tend to confirm the advantage of smaller fractions (Bennett, 1978), but not in the head and neck where 10 or 12 fractions appear to give the same results as 30 or more fractions (Henk and James, 1978). The influence of fractionation probably depends more on the critical normal tissue irradiated than on properties of the tumour itself. It is debatable whether the greater sensitization of hypoxic cells by larger doses of sensitizer will more than compensate for any disadvantages of larger fractions of radiotherapy. Misonidazole has been used with fractionation regimens from as few as six fractions to as many as 30 fractions, but no clear pattern has emerged.

Misonidazole at the beginning or end of a course of radiotherapy

There are theoretical reasons for believing that the effect of a hypoxic cell sensitizer will be greatest either at the beginning of a course of radiotherapy when the total number of hypoxic cells is largest, or at the end of the course of radiotherapy where the few tumour cells surviving are likely to have been derived from an initially hypoxic population and some may still be hypoxic. An example of misonidazole used in this way is the trial of Kogelnik *et al.* (1982) in malignant glioma. A total dose of 6650 cGy was administered in 31 fractions over 7.5 weeks; in the first, second and eighth week 400 cGy were given twice a week with misonidazole or placebo. In the intervening third to seventh weeks a daily tumour dose of 170 cGy was administered. This trial shows the most significant improvement in survival yet achieved with misonidazole ($P < 0.02$). Unfortunately, the number of patients in the trial is small, and with so many trials in progress chance can lead to at least one showing some benefit. Hence, on the basis of this trial alone, it is not possible to say whether this is the best way to use a sensitizer.

Misonidazole with multiple small fractions

Another way of attempting to make the best possible use of misonidazole is to take advantage of the relatively long plasma half-life in man, which is between 10 and 17 hours after a single oral dose of the drug. A dose of misonidazole is followed by three fractions of radiotherapy within this period, either three on the same day or two on the same day and another the following morning. So far no advantage has been reported from using misonidazole this way.

Results with misonidazole to date

Clinical trials have been performed in head and neck cancer, carcinoma of the cervix, carcinoma of the bladder, malignant glioma and carcinoma of the bronchus.

Approximately 15 controlled clinical trials have been started worldwide in head and neck cancer. To date most of them show a small advantage to misonidazole which does not reach statistical significance, at the expense of an incidence of neuropathy varying from 20 to 60%. For example, the Medical Research Council trial on head and neck cancer (1984) was abandoned because of the high neuropathy rate and lack of a significant benefit, i.e. only a 4% improvement in local tumour control in a trial involving 267 patients. However, the largest trial performed to date, that of the DAHANCA group in Denmark shows a statistically significant advantage to misonidazole for local control of pharyngeal cancer.

Several trials involving tumours at each of the other four sites have been started, none show an advantage to misonidazole with the exception of the glioma trial by Kogelnik *et al.* (1982) mentioned above.

In contrast to the promise shown by misonidazole in the laboratory, the clinical results have been disappointing. This is probably mainly because the toxicity of the drug in man has limited dosage to a level below that which has been effective in the laboratory. As a result, the degree of sensitization of hypoxic cells has been insufficient to improve significantly tumour control by radiotherapy.

Other nitroimidazoles

Currently newer electron-affinic compounds are being tested which may offer greater sensitization of hypoxic cells with lower toxicity. For example, the 2-nitroimidazole compound SR 2508 (Brown *et al.*, 1981) has the same radiosensitizing effect as misonidazole at equivalent concentrations, but investigations of its toxicity and diffusability suggest that levels in human tumours 7.5 times those obtained with misonidazole can be achieved without toxicity, and hence a greater effect may be possible. Compounds consisting of a sensitizer with an alkylating group are also under investigation, in the hope that they may act more specifically on the DNA target within the hypoxic tumour cell (Stratford, Sheldon and Adams, 1983).

Cytotoxic drugs as radiosensitizers

Many cytotoxic drugs used in cancer therapy are radiosensitizers in the sense that their cell-killing effect in combination with radiotherapy *in vitro* is greater than that expected from the sum of the effects of the agents used alone. In particular, the S-phase specific drugs show considerable radiosensitization when tested on mammalian cells in culture.

Several antimetabolites, e.g. methotrexate and hydroxyurea, are lethal to cells only during the S phase of the mitotic cycle, i.e. during synthesis of DNA, which is the phase of greatest radioresistance (Berry and Asquith, 1973). Simultaneous use of one of these drugs with radiation may therefore be expected to give an enhanced antitumour effect.

In practice it has not been possible to exploit the radiosensitizing potential of S-phase specific drugs. This is because radiotherapy in general gives the best therapeutic advantage when administered daily over several weeks. Phase-specific drugs on the other hand, are best given intermittently in large widely-spaced doses; when given daily the toxicity on the bone marrow and gastrointestinal epithelium is prohibitive. Although such agents, especially methotrexate, are often given in combination with radiotherapy, they are used more for their additive cytotoxic effect than as true radiosensitizers (*see* Chapter 20).

Halogenated pyrimidines

Pyrimidine analogues labelled with chlorine, bromine or iodine have the property of being incorporated into DNA in place of the natural base. Cells which have a halogenated pyrimidine incorporated into their DNA have an increased radiosensitivity, but only if the DNA is replicated more than once in the presence of the drug. Djordjevic and Szybalski (1960) suggested that there may be a selective effect on tumour cells, because more tumour cells than critical normal cells would be cycling during radiotherapy.

BUdR was tried as a radiosensitizer in head and neck cancer (Doggett, Bagshaw and Kaplan, 1967). In common with all halogenated pyrimidines this compound has a very short half-life in the body if administered systemically, and so has to be given by arterial infusion. A considerable enhancement of radiation effects on normal skin and mucosa and on the tumour was observed. Epilation and desquamation of normal skin occurred in the infused but unirradiated areas and, in addition, there was a remote effect on the skin of the hands and feet. It was concluded that BUdR was such a potent normal tissue sensitizer that it was not of clinical value.

Razoxane

Razoxane (ICRF 159) is an antitumour agent originally investigated for its capacity to inhibit the formation of metastases. In several animal systems it was found to enhance the antitumour effects of radiation (Hellman, Grimshaw and Hutchinson, 1978). The mechanism of radiosensitization is not clear. The drug increases oxygen tension in tumours, either by an effect on tumour vascular growth or by diminishing oxygen utilization. However, the sensitizing effect is seen regardless of whether the drug is given before or after irradiation, suggesting that it is not acting as a hypoxic cell sensitizer. An alternative explanation is the capacity of the drug to arrest cells in the radiosensitive phase of the cell cycle, i.e. G2 and M.

Razoxane was initially tried as a radiosensitizer in the treatment of soft tissue sarcoma (Ryall, 1978). Early results appeared promising, but no adequate controlled trial could be done because of the heterogeneous nature of this type of tumour. Double-blind placebo controlled trials in squamous cell carcinoma of the head and neck (Bakowski, MacDonald and Mould, 1978) and uterine cervix (Belloni, Mangioni and Bortolozzi, 1983) showed no benefit of razoxane over placebo. At the same time, the drug was shown to enhance late normal tissue damage in the lung (Bates, 1978).

Clinical evidence to date has failed to demonstrate that razoxane can differentially sensitize tumours compared to normal tissues and it is now no longer used as a radiosensitizer.

Platinum

The cytotoxic drug cisplatin potentiates the effect of radiation on living cells. Experiments by Douple and Richmond (1978) showed that cisplatin sensitized hypoxic but not fully oxygenated mammalian cells in tissue culture. However, further experiments (Nias, Bocian and Laverick, 1979; Carde and Laval, 1981) have shown that platinum complexes sensitize both oxic and hypoxic cells, with a greater effect on the latter. There is also a sensitizing effect on plateau-phase cells. In exponentially growing cells, the slope of the cell survival curve is unaffected, but there is inhibition of repair of sublethal and potentially lethal damage. The nature of the interaction of platinum compounds and radiation is complex and not thoroughly understood; it seems similar to that of the bifunctional alkylating agents. A sensitizing effect on normal tissue has also been demonstrated on the gastrointestinal tract crypt cells (Burholt *et al.*, 1979) and on the skin (Douple, Eaton and Tulloch, 1979).

Cisplatin is a difficult drug to use because of its renal and gastric toxicity and so far there are few clinical studies of its use as a radiosensitizer. Liepzig (1983) reported a small pilot study of 14 patients with advanced head and neck cancer treated by conventionally fractionated radiotherapy with cisplatin given on each day of the first and fourth weeks of treatment. Tumour regressions were said to be impressive but there were four cases of renal toxicity, one fatal. As less nephrotoxic platinum compounds are developed as chemotherapeutic agents it may be worthwhile investigating their radiosensitizing properties. However, the enhancement of normal tissue effects seen experimentally suggests that there may be very little improvement in therapeutic ratio, and that combinations of platinum compounds and radiotherapy should be used with extreme caution.

References

ALPER, T. and HOWARD-FLANDERS, P. (1956) The role of oxygen in modifying the radiosensitivity of *E. coli*. *Nature*, **178**, 978–979

ASH, D. V., PECKHAM, M. J. and STEEL, G. G. (1979) The quantitative response of human tumours to radiation and misonidazole. *British Journal of Cancer*, **40**, 883–892

BAKOWSKI, M. T., MACDONALD, E. and MOULD, R. F. (1978) Double-blind controlled clinical trial of radiation plus razoxane (ICRF 159) versus radiation plus placebo in the treatment of head and neck cancer. *International Journal of Radiation Oncology, Biology and Physics*, **4**, 115–119

BATES, T. (1978) A clinical evaluation of ICRF 159 as a radiosensitising agent. *International Journal of Radiation Oncology, Biology and Physics*, **4**, 127–131

BELLONI, C., MANGIONI, C. and BORTOLOZZI, G. (1983) ICRF 159 plus radiation versus radiation therapy alone in cervical carcinoma. A double-blind study. *Oncology*, **40**, 181–185

BENNETT, M. B. (1978) The treatment of stage III squamous carcinoma of the cervix in air and hyperbaric oxygen. *British Journal of Radiology*, **51**, 68

BERRY, R. J. and ASQUITH, J. C. (1973) Cell-cycle dependent and hypoxic radiosensitisers. In *Advances in Chemical Radiosensitisation*. Vienna: IAEA pp. 52–58

BROWN, J. M., YU, N. Y., BROWN, D. M. and LEE, W. (1981) SR 2508: A 2-nitroimidazole amide which should be superior to misonidazole as a radiosensitiser for clinical use. *International Journal of Radiation, Oncology, Biology and Physics*, **7**, 695–703

BURHOLT, D. R., SCHENKEN, L. L., KOVACS, C. J. and HAGEMANN, R. F. (1979) Response of the murine gastrointestinal epithelium to cis-dischlorodiammine-platinum II radiation combinations. *International Journal of Radiation Oncology, Biology and Physics*, **5**, 1377–1381

CARDE, P. and LAVAL, F. (1981) Effect of cis-dichlorodiammine platinum II and X-rays on mammalian cell survival. *International Journal of Radiation Oncology, Biology and Physics*, **7**, 929–933

CHURCHILL-DAVIDSON, I., SANGER, C. and THOMLINSON, R. H. (1955) High pressure oxygen and radiotherapy. *Lancet*, **1**, 1091–1095

DENEKAMP, J. (1983) Does physiological hypoxia matter in cancer therapy? In *The Biological Basis of Radiotherapy*, edited by G. G. Steel, G. E. Adams and M. J. Peckham, pp. 139–156. Amsterdam: Elsevier

DISCHE, S., GRAY, A. J. and ZANELLI, G. D. (1976) Clinical testing of the radiosensitiser RO-07-0582. Radiosensitisation of normal and hypoxic skin. *Clinical Radiology*, **27**, 159–166

DJORDJEVIC, B. and SZYBALSKI, W. (1960) Incorporation of 5-bromo and 5-iododeoxyuridine into the deoxyribonucleic acid of human cells and its effect on radiation sensitivity. *Journal of Experimental Medicine*, **112**, 509–531

DOGGETT, R. L. S., BAGSHAW, M. A. and KAPLAN, H. S. (1967) Combined therapy using chemotherapeutic agents and radiotherapy. In *Modern Trends in Radiotherapy*, edited by T. J. Deeley and C. A. P. Wood, pp. 107–131. London: Butterworths

DOUPLE, E. B., EATON, W. L. and TULLOCH, M. E. (1979) Skin radiosensitisation studies using combined cis-dichlorodiammineplatinum II and radiation. *International Journal of Radiation Oncology, Biology and Physics*, **5**, 1383–1385

DOUPLE, E. B. and RICHMOND, R. C. (1978) Platinum complexes as radiosensitisers of hypoxic mammalian cells. *British Journal of Cancer*, **37**, (Suppl. 3), 98–101

EVANS, C. M. and TODD, I. D. H. (1969) Synkavit and radiotherapy in the treatment of bronchial carcinoma A random trial. *Clinical Radiology*, **20**, 228–230

GRAY, L. H., CONGER, A. D., EBERT, M., HORNSEY, S. and SCOTT, O. C. A. (1953) The concentration of oxygen dissolved in tissues at the time of irradiation as a factor in radiotherapy. *British Journal of Radiology*, **26**, 638–648

GRONOW, M. (1965) The effect of a radiosensitiser and its tritiated analogue on the sulphydryl levels of mouse ascites tumour *in vivo*. *International Journal of Radiation Biology*, **9**, 123–132

HELLMAN, K., GRIMSHAW, M. B. and HUTCHINSON, G. E. (1978) Combination of radiation and razoxane (ICRF 159) *in vivo*. *International Journal of Radiation Oncology, Biology and Physics*, **4**, 109–113

HENK, J. M. (1984) Update of clinical trials of fractionation and hyperbaric oxygen in radiotherapy of head and neck cancer. *British Journal of Radiology*, **57**, 675

HENK, J. M. and JAMES, K. W. (1978) Comparative trial of large and small fractions in the radiotherapy of head and neck cancer. *Clinical Radiology*, **29**, 611–616

HENK, J. M. and SMITH, C. W. (1977) Radiotherapy and hyperbaric oxygen in head and neck cancer. Interim report of second clinical trial. *Lancet*, **2**, 104–105

KOGELNIK, H. D., KÄRCHER, K. H., SZEPESI, T. and SCHRATTER-SEHN, A. V. (1982) High dose irradiation and misonidazole in the treatment of malignant gliomas. In *Progress in Radio-Oncology II*, edited by K. H. Kärcher, H. D. Kogelnik and G. Reinartz, 189–195. New York: Raven Press

KRISHNAMURTHI, S., SHANTA, V. and NAIR, M. K. (1967) Studies of chemical sensitisation in the radiotherapy of oral and cervical carcinomas. *Cancer*, **20**, 822–825

LIEPZIG, B. (1983) Cisplatin sensitisation to radiotherapy of squamous cell carcinomas of the head and neck. *American Journal of Surgery*, **146**, 462–465

MEDICAL RESEARCH COUNCIL WORKING PARTY ON MISONIDAZOLE IN HEAD AND NECK CANCER (1984) A study of the effect of misonidazole in conjunction with radiotherapy for the treatment of head and neck cancer. *British Journal of Radiology*, **57**, 585–595

MITCHELL, J. S. (1953) Clinical assessment of tetra-sodium 2-methyl 1:4 naphthoquinone disphosphate as a radiosensitiser in the radiotherapy of malignant tumours. *British Journal of Cancer*, **7**, 313–328

NIAS, A. H. W., BOCIAN, E. and LAVERICK, M. (1979) The mechanisms of action of cis-dichlorobis (isopropylamine) trans dihydroxyplatinum IV on Chinese hamster and C_3H mouse tumour cells and its interaction with x-irradiation. *International Journal of Radiation Oncology, Biology and Physics*, **5**, 1341–1344

PATERSON, I. C. M., DAWES, P. J. D. K., HENK, J. M. and

MOORE, J. L. (1981) Pilot study of radiotherapy with misonidazole in head and neck cancers. *Clinical Radiology,* **32**, 225–229

RYALL, R. D. H. (1978) Radiotherapy and ICRF 159 in the treatment of soft tissue sarcomas. *International Journal of Radiation Oncology, Biology and Physics,* **4**, 133–134

STRATFORD, I. J., SHELDON, P. W. and ADAMS, G. E. (1983) Hypoxic cell radiosensitisers. In *The Biological Basis of Radiotherapy*, edited by G. G. Steel, G. E. Adams and M. J. Peckham, pp. 211–224. Amsterdam: Elsevier

THOMLINSON, R. H., DISCHE, S., GRAY, A. J. and ERRINGTON, L. M. (1976) Clinical testing of the radiosensitiser RO 07-0582, III. Response of tumours. *Clinical Radiology,* **27**, 167–173

THOMLINSON, R. H. and GRAY, L. H. (1955) The histological structure of some human lung cancers and the possible implication for radiotherapy. *British Journal of Cancer,* **9**, 539–549

URTASUN, R. C., BAND, P., CHAPMAN, J. D., FELDSTEIN, M. L., MIELKE, B. and FRYER, C. (1976) Radiation and high dose metronidazole (Flagyl) in supratentorial glioblastoma. *New England Journal of Medicine,* **293**, 1364–1367

3

Urological malignancies

H. F. Hope-Stone

Neoplasms of the bladder

This disease is increasing both in the Western hemisphere (possibly related to smoking habits) and in the Middle East and Africa (due to the rising incidence of schistosomiasis). The incidence in the UK is 6% of all malignancies.

Classification

Histologically there are four main groups, with transitional cell carcinoma predominate in the UK, but squamous cell carcinoma more common in the Middle East (*Table 3.1*).

Table 3.1 Histological classification of neoplasms of the bladder

Histological classification	*Incidence in the London Hospital series (%)*
Transitional cell	84
Squamous cell	10
Adenocarcinoma	5
Lymphoma	< 1

Staging

The system most commonly used is that of the International Union Against Cancer (UICC) 1978 (*Table 3.2*).

Table 3.2 International Union Against Cancer (UICC) T staging (abbreviated)

TIS	*In situ* flat tumour
T0	Non-invasive carcinoma
T1	Mobile mass absent after TUR
T2	Superficial muscle invasion
T3	(a) Deep muscle involvement (b) In perivesical fat
T4	Fixed extension to neighbouring organs

Grading

The modern system of grading G1–G3 takes into account the degree of differentiation of the neoplastic cells and the pathological stage. P1s to P4b describes the detailed involvement of the bladder structure. Unfortunately, most of the quoted earlier series do not use such detailed systems which makes comparison difficult.

Methods of staging

Ideally all patients should be staged by cystoscopy and deep transurethral resection of the tumour (TUR) under a general anaesthetic, preferably with a radiotherapist present. A bimanual examination of the organ can also be carried out — a much disclaimed simple technique but which, combined with

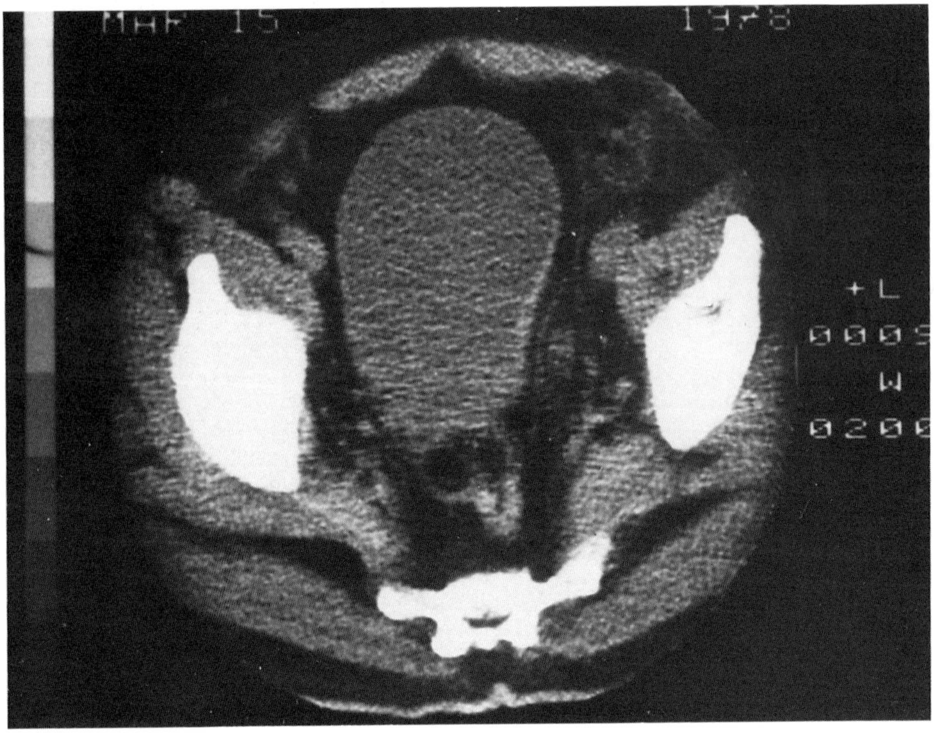

Figure 3.1 CT scanning for invasive bladder cancer

the more sophisticated methods now available, will give the best possible assessment. An intravenous pyelogram (IVP) is mandatory, as it will show ureteric obstruction if present and will also give an idea of the bladder outline. Routine chest X-ray will exclude gross lung metastases (which are very rare in this condition). Ultrasound is an excellent non-invasive imaging technique but does require an experienced radiologist to interpret the results (Husband and Hodson, 1981); it is however cheaper than CT scanning, but the latter method is probably more effective (Kellet *et al.*, 1980) and certainly easier to interpret (*Figure 3.1*). Unfortunately, although the para-aortic lymph nodes are readily recognized if grossly infiltrated with tumour, this is not so in the pelvic nodes. Lymphangiography might theoretically solve this problem but has not been proven to do so, as it has a high false positive and false negative rate. Surgical staging would be the final arbiter, but this means at least a retroperitoneal lymph node dissection, and radical irradiation after this might be quite hazardous due to subsequent bowel adhesions (*see below*). Attempts to demonstrate the presence of generalized disease are probably fruitless; a pilot study of pre-treatment bone marrow biopsy was carried out at The London Hospital but this failed to produce more than a 5% positive yield.

Radiosensitivity of bladder tumours

The normal bladder mucosa is relatively tolerant of irradiation. Doses of 5000–6000 cGy in 4 – 6 weeks (or its radiobiological equivalent) will not produce lasting damage (Moss, 1965), although this presumes that the mucosa was normal before starting. Previous chronic infection, and in particular schistosomiasis, will lower this tolerance. The sensitivity of the tumour varies from being very high in the rare lymphoma to moderately so in the transitional cell lesion, and relatively resistant in the adenocarcinoma.

Indications for treatment

T1s, T1 (P1, G1) tumours are now best treated with closed cystodiathermy (CCD), although in the past very good results were obtained by interstitial irradiation for single tumours (Dix *et al.*, 1970). If multiple lesions cannot be controlled with CCD, intravesical chemotherapy can be very effective, and should be used immediately or possibly prophylactically after the initial TUR.

T2, G1 tumours can be treated with CCD, but if the grade is 2 or 3 then irradiation should be considered first. For T3 of any grade, irradiation with or without subsequent surgery is the treatment of choice. In T4 either palliative irradiation or chemotherapy should be considered except in those cases where the only spread is into the prostate — here radical irradiation should be considered. Adenocarcinoma is best treated surgically.

Treatment techniques

Interstitial irradiation

This method, using small radioactive seeds or wire, is now only of historical interest although is still practised occasionally (Williams *et al.*, 1981), but very few radiotherapists will be called upon to use it. The technique involved opening the bladder, removing the tumour by diathermy snare and then implanting the base with radon seeds, ^{198}Au seeds or tantalum-182 wire. The results were remarkably good considering that even T3 cases were treated (Dix *et al.*, 1970). Implantation by radium needles is still favoured as part of the management of T3 tumours (<5 cm) (Werf-Messing, 1982a), although this does mean two operations — one to open the bladder and another to remove the needles. Local irradiation to the scar is required to prevent implant metastases (3 × 350 cGy) (Werf-Messing *et al.*, 1981).

External beam irradiation and salvage cystectomy

Orthovoltage irradiation has no place in the management of this condition as the beam penetration is so poor that multiple fields are required, and this leads to very high doses to all the pelvic contents and may cause small and large bowel damage.

Megavoltage irradiation, 3–8 MeV, is perfectly adequate for most patients although an exceptionally large person might benefit from treatment with a 12–14 MeV accelerator. Thus cobalt irradiation is quite satisfactory unless the anteroposterior diameter of the pelvis is greater than 22 cm, when a linear accelerator would be an advantage.

The London Hospital technique

This was first started in 1957 using a fixed head Picker cobalt unit. Beam direction was achieved with a pin and arc technique using one anterior and two posterior oblique fields, each angled at 120° from each other. This machine had a John's Collimator which produced a very well-defined beam of irradiation. Today one can use an isocentric unit which has the advantage of allowing the patient to lie either prone or supine (thus not requiring him to turn over) and therefore increasing the accuracy of the treatment.

Localization of the bladder is carried out with a cystogram using a Foley catheter to instil 20 ml of Conray 40 into the bladder. Skin marks, with or without tattooing, can be used and films taken preferably on a simulator (in the absence of such equipment a diagnostic X-ray machine can be used if the source-skin distance (SSD) is the same as that of the treating machine). Magnification factors can be worked out either with a ladder or metal rings (*Figures 3.2a,b*). Anterior, posterior and lateral films are required, although if the patient has to be turned over they must be taken both in the prone and supine positions.

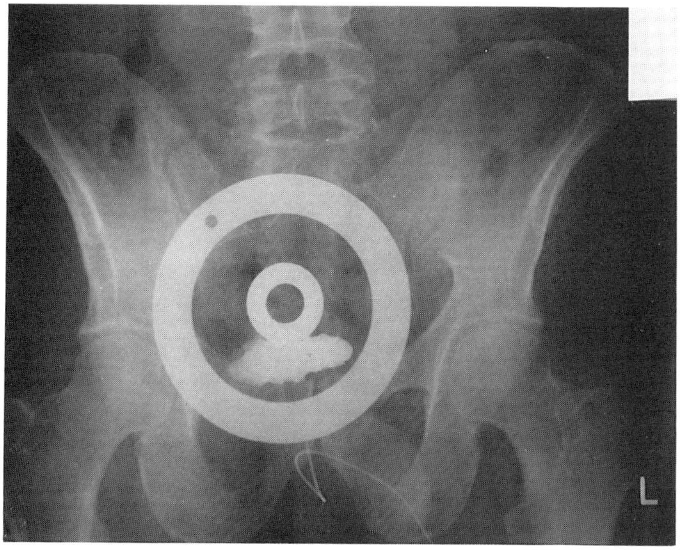

Figure 3.2 Localization films for three fields fixed head telecobalt unit. *(a)* Anteroposterior

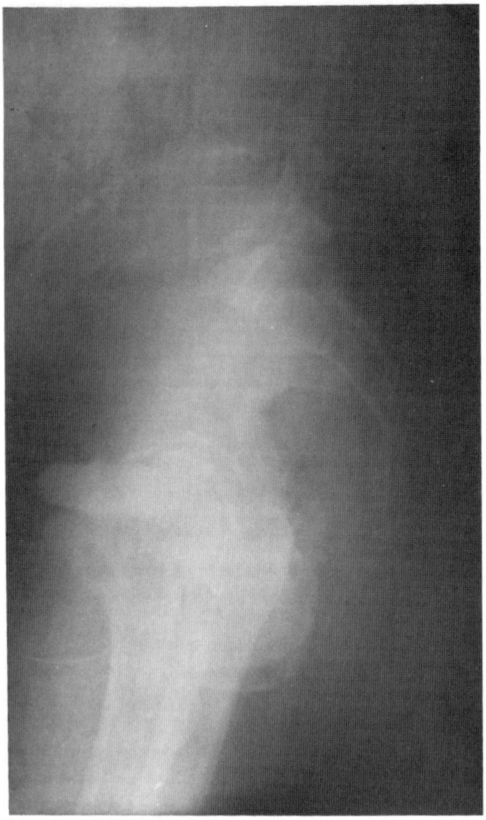

Figure 3.2 Localization films for three fields fixed head telecobalt unit. *(b)* Lateral

The aim is to treat the whole bladder and its associated tumour with a 1–2 cm margin: field sizes are in the order of 8 × 8 to 10 × 12 cm. The bladder is emptied prior to irradiation and all three fields are treated daily 5 days a week for 20 fractions. A tumour dose of 5000–5500 cGy is given (the lower dose being used for the larger field sizes). The rectum should not receive more than 4000 cGy (*Figure 3.3*). Most patients can be treated on an outpatient basis providing they are not too old, or have long distances to travel or suffer from physical difficulties that make travelling difficult (in such cases hostel accommodation is ideal).

The above tumour dose may not always be achieved, and this was so in 15% of The London Hospital series (Hope-Stone, 1984), the reasons usually being the development of metastases, deterioration of general physical condition, and occasionally urinary or bowel upsets which require a rest from treatment. If possible, when treatment time is prolonged for the latter reason or because of machine failure, an appropriate addition to the final tumour dose should be made. Although the normal standard dose (NSD) formula (Ellis, 1968) may be used, it is not necessarily accurate and this author prefers a rule of thumb method which usually works out at about 500 cGy to be added for each week's gap.

If a linear accelerator is available the extra penetration and sharper beam will be useful in larger patients, and all will benefit from the shorter treatment time. Another advantage is the fact that the maximum dose will be 1.5–2.0 cm below the skin which will reduce late subcutaneous oedema and

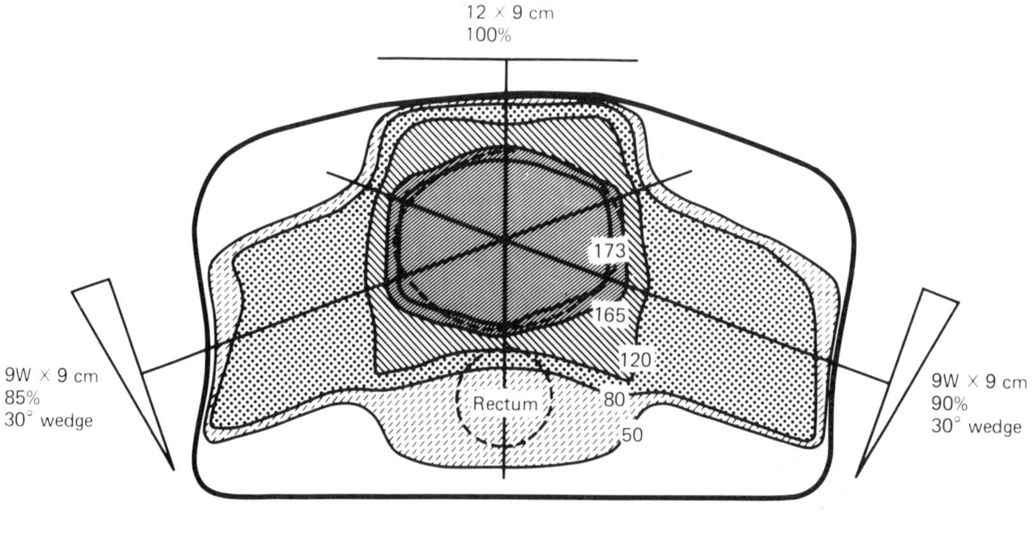

Figure 3.3 Isodose curves for isocentric three field technique on Gammatron (cobalt 60). ▨ >165; ▧ 120–165; ░ 80–120; ⬚ 50–80; □ <50

fibrosis and make salvage cystectomy an easier operation. Used isocentrically with the patient usually in the supine position, simulator localization can be performed, either screening the patient when the dye is in the bladder or using standard films (*Figures 3.4a,b*). It has been suggested that as the patient is treated with an empty bladder a cystogram does not accurately outline the extent of the bladder tumour and a CT therapy planning technique is to be preferred (Ash, Andrews and Stubbs, 1983). An improvement of 20% in the accuracy of localization is claimed and in those departments where such equipment is available this may well be the ideal method.

Treating the patient in the prone position is only usually required in those who are very fat and have a floppy abdomen, which makes accurate marking dif-

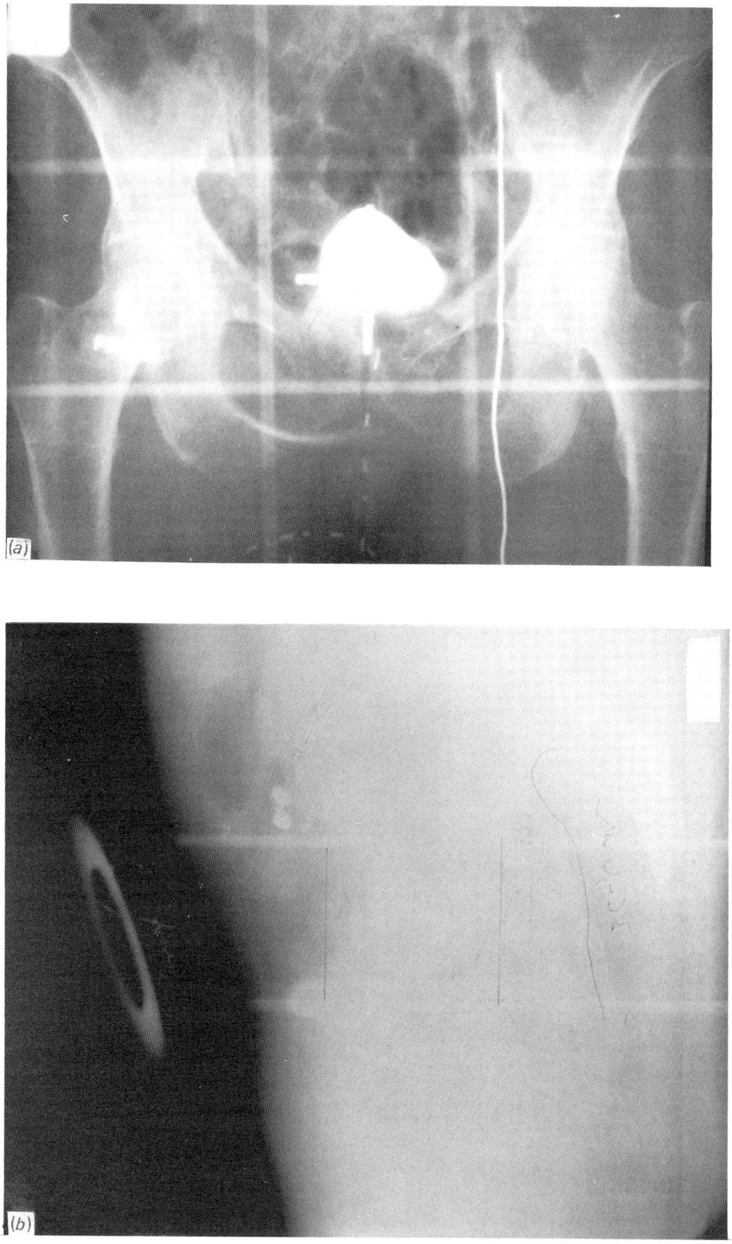

Figure 3.4 Localization films taken on Ximitron simulator. *(a)* Anteroposterior, *(b)* lateral

ficult to achieve and allows the bladder to move into different positions day by day. The prone position will help to alleviate this situation, although it is more uncomfortable.

The final isodose curves are very similar to those of a cobalt unit (*Figure 3.5*), but check films can be taken on the accelerator itself (*Figure 3.6*) to confirm the exact treatment position and if necessary can be repeated weekly. The dose/time fractionation is the same. It is interesting to note that the immediate

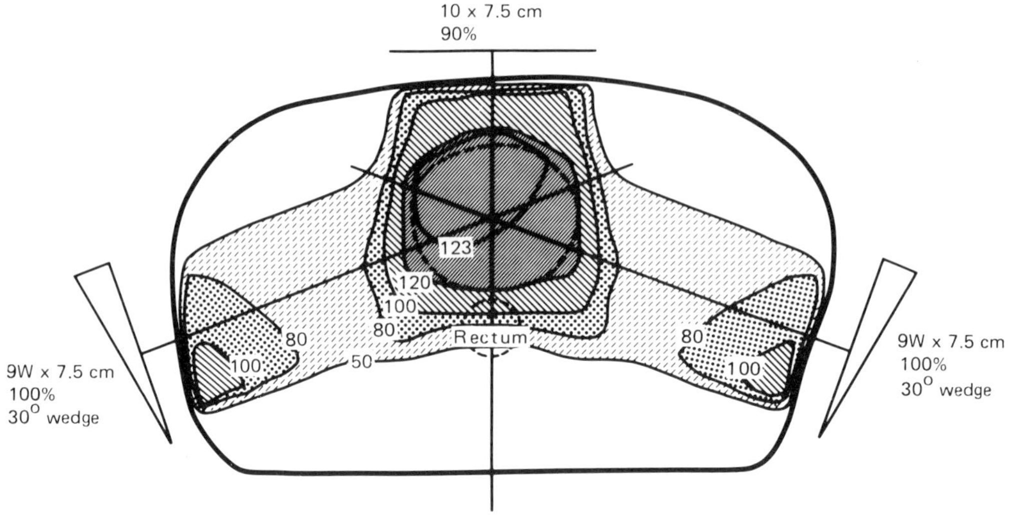

Figure 3.5 Isodose curves for three field isocentric set-up.
8 MV linear accelerator ▨ >120; ▧ 100–120; ▦ 80–100; ▤ 50–80; ☐ <50

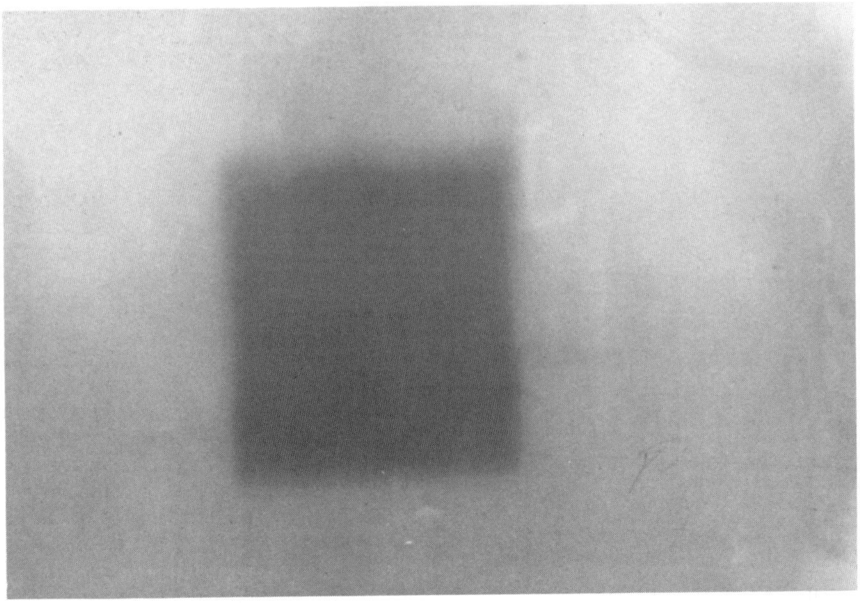

Figure 3.6 Confirmation films taken on 8 MV linear accelerator

lymph nodes will receive a dose of about 4500 cGy (*Figure 3.7a*) and this may be relevant in subsequent discussion of the merits of salvage versus elective cystectomy.

Stage IV (prostate only involved) may also be treated radically in the above fashion, although larger fields will be required and some of the rectum will receive the maximum tumour dose — leading to increased morbidity from bowel upset.

Alternative methods of external beam irradiation

Rotation

This method is favoured by many radiotherapists on the grounds that it produces a more homogeneous dose to the bladder and possibly the lymph nodes as well, the disadvantage being that the integral dose to the pelvis will be higher, thus producing increased morbidity from bowel upset. Using a 300° arc (missing out the posterior 60° to avoid the rectum) a dose of 6000 cGy in 6 weeks is advocated by Backhouse (1979) although his reported results are not very satisfactory.

Multiple fields

A four field technique — two anterior oblique and two posterior oblique fields — was described by Morrison (1975). A tumour dose of 4250–5000 cGy in 20 daily fractions was prescribed. Unfortunately, the higher dose, although slightly improving the results, also increased the morbidity to such an extent that it could not be given in many cases.

A three field technique using one anterior and two lateral wedge fields giving 6000–7000 cGy in 6–7 weeks has been advocated by Werf-Messing, Heal and Ledehorr (1978), but these results are disappointing and again the morbidity is relatively high.

The four field brick technique (one anterior, one posterior and two lateral fields) has the same disadvantage as rotation — namely treating too much of the pelvic contents to a high dose and irradiating the heads of both femora (*Figure 3.7b*).

Preoperative irradiation

As surgery alone produced such poor results it was thought that a lower preoperative irradiation dose should be combined with elective cystectomy. The usual technique has been to use a pair of parallel and opposed fields to treat the whole pelvis to a tumour dose of 4000 cGy in 20 daily fractions (Wallace and Bloom, 1976). A shorter course of 2000 cGy in 5 days ('flash' irradiation) has been advocated by Whitmore (1981), who claims that subsequent elective cystectomy is just as easy after this method, which saves patients time and is less expensive. Surgery can be carried out almost immediately in the latter case and within a month of the former.

If elective cystectomy is not to be carried out (as in one-half of the patients in the Institute of Urology Bladder Trial), then after completion of irradiation to the whole pelvis (4000 cGy), the bladder alone is given a further dose of 2000 cGy in 10 daily fractions (using a three field technique as outlined above). It should be noted, however, that the total tumour dose of 6000 cGy in 6 weeks is a lower radiobiological dose than the 5500 cGy in 4 weeks used in The London Hospital technique. If tumour doses are increased to 8000 cGy in 6 weeks the complication rate is very high indeed and this method had to be discontinued by Laing and Dickinson (1965).

Methods of improving radiosensitivity

Oxygenation

Henk (*see* Chapter 2) discusses the rationale of this method. In bladder cancer Kirk, Wingate and Watson (1976) reported a trial of hyperbaric oxygen therapy giving a dose of 6000 cGy in 5 weeks, but the complication rate was high — nine out of 27 cases requiring a cystectomy to relieve symptoms, and survival was not improved. The MRC trial (Cade *et al.*, 1978) again showed no difference in survival in 128 cases so treated.

Neutrons

Trials of this method using fast neutrons are currently being assessed in Edinburgh (Arnott, personal communication 1982) and Manchester (Pointon, personal communication 1982), but the results so far do not seem to indicate any real benefits.

Hypoxic cell sensitizers

Misonidazole has been tried in the UK for advanced carcinoma of the cervix and the head and neck, but with little evidence of improved results (*see* Chapter 2).

Hyperfractionation

Edsmyr (1981) suggested that the problem of anoxic tumour cells could be overcome by increasing the standard fractionation to three times daily. In a controlled trial 71 patients were treated with daily fractionation of 240 cGy to give a tumour dose of 6400 cGy over 8.5 weeks. The other 71 patients were treated three times a day (100 cGy every 4 hours) to a total tumour dose of 8400 cGy over 7.5 weeks (with a two-week gap in the middle of the course). The results showed better tumour control for the latter method at 6 weeks, but at 3 years the survival figures were identical.

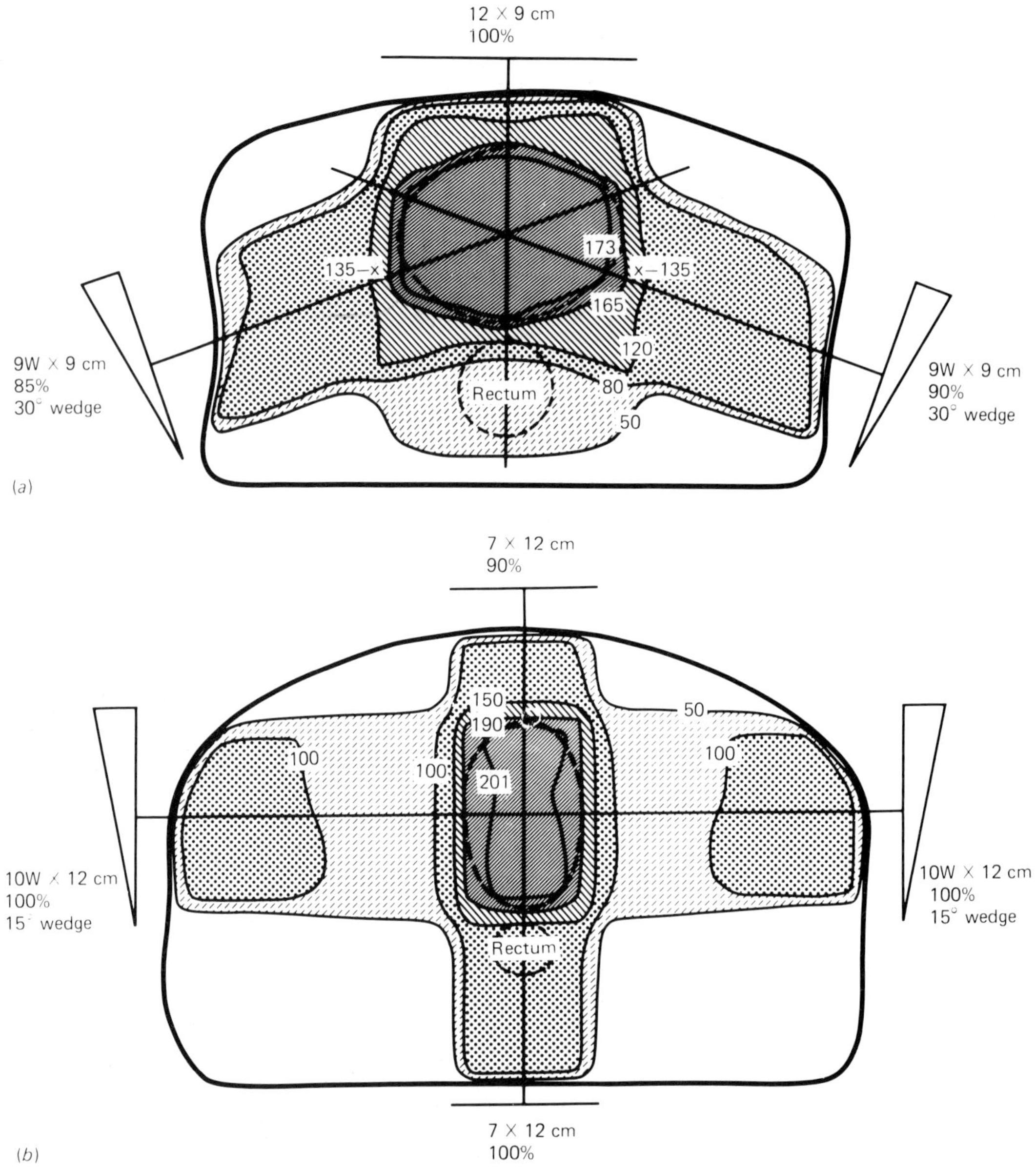

Figure 3.7 *(a)* Isodose curves for three field technique to show dosage to first lymph node chain. X = 135% >190; 150–190; 100–150; 50–100; <50.
(b) Isodose curves four field brick technique. Linear accelerator 5 MV >165; 120–165; 80–120; 50-80; <50

Lymphoma

If entirely confined to the bladder this rare condition is well worth treating with radical irradiation. It is best to treat the whole pelvis and include the inguinal nodes, giving a dose of 4000 cGy in 4 weeks with a pair of parallel and opposed fields.

Palliation

In more extensive carcinoma of the bladder (stage T4) good relief of the urinary symptoms can be achieved by treating the whole pelvis with a pair of parallel and opposed fields to a tumour dose of 3000 cGy in 2 weeks. If there is no evidence of generalized

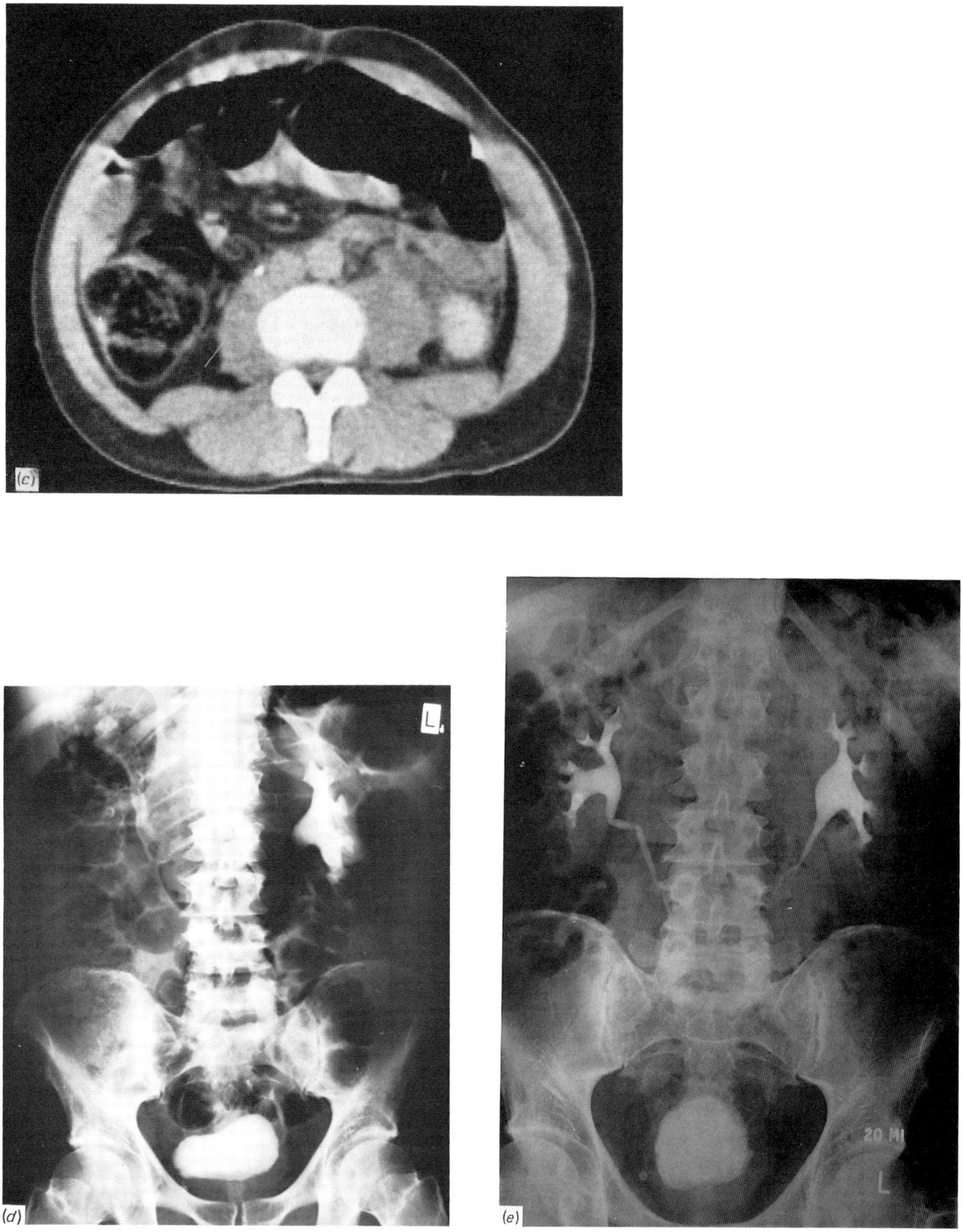

Figure 3.7 *(c)* Para-aortic nodes positive on CT scan. *(d)* IVP before radiotherapy. *(e)* IVP after radiotherapy

metastases this dose can be increased to 4000 cGy in 4 weeks. Lymph node metastases or skeletal involvement can be treated with single fields giving an incident dose of 3000 cGy in 2 weeks. Occasionally patients with only para-aortic node involvement (*see Figure 3.7c*) may be worth treating if the bladder is clear. *Figure 3.7d* shows the IVP of a patient with uraemia. After 4000 cGy tumour dose the kidney function returned to normal (*Figure 3.7e*).

Morbidity of irradiation

Bladder

Severe frequency or dysuria are the main problems. To help avoid this the urine should be kept sterile if at all possible by simple antibiotics and alkalinization of the urine with mist. potassium citrate or Effercitrate tablets (potentially toxic antibiotics such as gentamycin should not be used). All patients should keep up a high fluid intake and reduce their alcohol consumption as much as possible. If urinary symptoms persist they may be relieved with antispasmodics such as Cetiprin or Pyridium. Treatment is rarely interrupted unless doses above 7000 cGy are prescribed (Laing and Dickinson, 1965).

Bowel

The rectum is fairly tolerant of doses below 4500 cGy (Moss, 1965). However, tenesmus and diarrhoea do occur and may be relieved with simple means as outlined below. In patients who have had previous surgery to the lower abdomen (including staging laparotomy) or who have previous bowel disease (such as ulcerative colitis or diverticulitis), adhesions may occur so that loops of small bowel are tethered into the pelvis and will remain constantly in the radiation field, instead of moving in and out of the pelvis as would normally occur, thus not receiving the maximum dose of irradiation. The symptoms so produced usually respond to simple measures such as kaolin, Kaolin and Morphine mixture or codeine phosphate. More serious symptoms will probably require Lomotil or Imodium and, if necessary, a few days rest from treatment.

Long-term side-effects

The bladder should not develop severe irradiation cystitis leading to a contracted or bleeding organ if the dose of 5500 cGy in 4 weeks (or its radiobiological equivalent) is not exceeded, providing schistosomiasis or gross chronic infection was not previously present. With increased doses (7000–8000 cGy in 6–7 weeks) this form of morbidity is very high (Laing and Dickinson, 1965).

Follow-up

The first cystoscopy should not be carried out for 3 months after the end of irradiation. Before this time it is not only unpleasant for the patient, but the tumour regression will not be marked. If at 3 months regression has occurred, a further cystoscopy is carried out at 6 months. Providing regression continues this examination should subsequently be performed at 3-monthly intervals for 2 years, then 6 monthly for 2.5 years and finally at yearly intervals. The indications for salvage cystectomy are shown in *Table 3.3*. The operation is a standard radical cystectomy with removal of the pelvic lymph nodes, and an ileal conduit is constructed. The ureter is only removed *en bloc* in patients with multifocal tumours (Blandy, 1978b). Since a linear accelerator has been available a straight paramedian incision can be used instead of a modified Phamelstein loop and healing takes place more rapidly (Blandy, personal communication 1984).

Table 3.3 Indications for salvage cystectomy for invasive bladder tumour

(1)	Failure of regression at 3 months
(2)	Residual tumour at 6 months
(3)	Recurrence of tumour after complete clearance at any time

Results

The majority of reported results from radical irradiation are poor (*Table 3.4*), with a range of 20–28% (average 24%). The combination of preoperative irradiation and elective cystectomy are better, with a range of 33–51% (average 36%) (Whitmore, 1979).

There are only three reported clinical trials comparing preoperative irradiation and routine cystectomy versus radical irradiation and salvage cystectomy (*Table 3.5*). It will be seen that only Miller showed an improvement with the former technique. In the Institute of Urology trial, although the results appear to be better, there is still no significant difference between the two methods at 8 years (Bloom *et al.*, 1982). The mortality rate for elective cystectomy ranges between 8–12%.

In The London Hospital series of 279 cases a 37% crude actuarial survival rate was reported by Hope-Stone (1984) in patients treated by radical irradiation and salvage cystectomy. It is interesting to note that if the squamous cell carcinomas (with a survival rate of 23%) are removed from the total, the survival rate is increased to 39%. More important, however, one should examine the results by age groups. Whichever

Table 3.4 Radical radiotherapy in invasive (T3) bladder cancer

	Number of patients	*Dose (cGy)/ time ratio*	*5-year survival, uncorrected, actuarial (%)*
Morrison (1975)	128	4250–5000/4 weeks	27.6
Goffinet, Schneider and Glastein (1975)	218	7000/7 weeks	28
Backhouse (1979)	124	6000/6 weeks	23
Institute of Urology Cooperative Trial, Wallace and Bloom (1976)	91	6000/6 weeks	25
Edsmyr (1981)	283	6000/7 weeks	20

Table 3.5 Controlled trials of radical radiotherapy alone versus preoperative radiotherapy and elective cystectomy in T3 bladder carcinoma

	Radiotherapy alone		*Preoperative radiotherapy and cystectomy*	
	Number of patients	*Survival*	*Number of patients*	*Survival*
Blackard and Byar (1972)	22	40% (3 years)	27	40% (3 years)
Miller (1977)	34	22% (5 years)	35	46% (5 years)
Institute of Urology Bloom *et al.* (1982)	85	31% (5 years)	77	44% (5 years $P > 0.05$)

Table 3.6 Effect of age on survival in invasive bladder carcinoma

	Age	*5-year survival (%)*
Institute of Urology series radiation and elective cystectomy	< 60 years	40
The London Hospital series radical radiation and salvage cystectomy	< 55 years	51

method of treatment is used, patients aged over 70 fare badly — only 23% surviving 3 years. The younger patients have a much better outlook — and probably better in the radically irradiated group than those having elective cystectomy (*Table 3.6*). The mortality rate for those having salvage cystectomy is also falling, being now only 4% (Blandy, personal communication 1984). The serious morbidity in The London Hospital patients having radical irradiation is very low. Only two patients required cystectomy for a contracted bladder and one for a bleeding bladder (Hope-Stone *et al.*, 1984).

Importance of correct dose levels

In The London Hospital series it has been shown that a dose of 5000–5500 cGy in 4 weeks gives the

Table 3.7 The effect of downstaging after radiotherapy in T3 bladder cancer

	5-year survival no downstaging (%)	*5-year survival with downstaging (%)*	
Werf-Messing, Heal and Ledehorr (1978)	20	70	Preoperative 4000 cGy
Bloom (1981)	27	64	
Hope-Stone (1984)	18	69	Radiotherapy only 5–5500 cGy

optimum results (Hope-Stone, 1984). This dose is radiobiologically higher than in any other of the reported series using radical radiotherapy (*see Table 3.4*). With this dose and the techniques outlined previously, the immediate lymph nodes will receive 4500 cGy, which is higher than that received by those patients having preoperative irradiation and elective cystectomy (*see Figure 3.7*).

Downstaging effect

In those patients treated by elective cystectomy after irradiation it has been shown that downstaging is a good prognostic sign (Bloom, 1981). Similarly, in The London Hospital series the same effect was demonstrated. When no response occurred after irradiation only 18% of cases survived for 5 years, whereas if a complete response was demonstrated at 6 months, 69% survived for 5 years (Hope-Stone, 1984) (*Table 3.7*). It is possible that 'flow cytometry' may be able to predict this response before surgery is carried out (Klein *et al.*, 1983).

Impact of salvage cystectomy

In The London Hospital series only 10% required salvage cystectomy. If the tumour recurred after complete response to irradiation, there was a 74% 5-year survival figure after salvage cystectomy. The partial responders had a 42% survival rate; if surgery was not performed only 12% survived for 5 years.

Causes of failure

Failure to control the local disease occurs in about 23% of patients, although in the The London Hospital series the percentage was much higher if the histology was of squamous carcinoma. Distant metastases occurred in 20% of all cases.

Conclusions

Since the older patients do badly with cystectomy, and in those under 60, the morbidity (total impotence in the male, a shortened vagina in the female, and a permanent urinary diversion in both sexes) is so unpleasant, there seems little point in carrying out routine elective cystectomy if there is no improvement in the overall results. A watching policy after radical irradiation, followed by salvage cystectomy if the tumour fails to respond or if it relapses later, will spare patients the problems of radical surgery but will not jeopardize their overall lifespan.

Future prospects

All the above quoted results are poor, and even in the younger age group over 50% of patients will die from their cancer. It is doubtful whether changes in radiotherapeutic techniques will improve this result, even if the new radiosensitizers prove to be more effective than those presently available. Two possible improvements can be considered: first earlier salvage cystectomy can be carried out in those patients in whom there is no or very little response to irradiation after 6 months; second adjuvant chemotherapy could be considered, either given before irradiation or immediately afterwards. In the former case, this may be dangerous if not immediately effective, as the tumour may enlarge before irradiation is commenced. Post-irradiation chemotherapy might prove to be better, but the single agents such as methotrexate, hydroxydaunorubicin, cisplatin and bleomycin have not proved to be very useful. At present, the Yorkshire Urological Cancer Research Group is trying a combination adjuvant trial of hydroxydaunorubicin and 5-fluorouracil. The London and Oxford Co-operative Urological Cancer Group (1981) is carrying out a trial using methotrexate alone as adjuvant therapy.

Prostatic cancer

This is the third most common malignancy in males with an incidence of 8% in the UK. It is usually found over the age of 55, although in older men its slow growth produces a relatively high morbidity compared to its mortality.

Histologically more than 95% are adenocarcinomas, varying in degrees of differentiation and usually multifocal in origin (Byar and Mostofi, 1972). The other 5% include transitional and squamous cell carcinomas. Spread is by the lymphatic system and by the blood stream, but local spread particularly to the seminal vesicles (17.8% in Byar and Mostofi series) is important from a radiation treatment point of view.

Staging

The UICC classification (1978) of T stage is the most useful (*Table 3.8*), although the lymph node aspect of this staging is somewhat academic in view of the difficulties in diagnosis.

Biochemical staging should always be carried out, because if the acid phosphatase is very much raised, it suggests the presence of metastatic disease even if the latter is difficult to prove. Skeletal surveys will only demonstrate gross disease, but gamma camera scanning should pick up earlier signs of bone involvement. The role of lymphography is doubtful, as interpretation of the results is difficult. If, however, this is combined with CT scanning its value might increase. Ray and Bagshaw (1975) advocated routine surgical staging with retroperitoneal lymph node biopsy of as many glands as possible, having abandoned the transperitoneal approach. The latter led to a high incidence of small bowel obstruction after radical irradiation, and even the former method causes high morbidity from lymphoedema (Pistenma, Bagshaw and Freiha, 1979).

CT scanning of the prostate itself will certainly give some indication of local spread — particularly to the seminal vesicles (*Figure 3.8b*), but also to the bladder (*Figure 3.8a*) (although the latter organ will need to be examined by routine cystoscopy as well).

Table 3.8 T stage carcinoma of the prostate (UICC)

T0	Incidental carcinoma
T1	Intracapsular carcinoma — surrounded by normal gland
T2	Intracapsular carcinoma causing deformity of the gland
T3	Extension beyond the capsule
T4	Extension and/or fixation to normal organs

Abbreviated Buenos Aires 1978

Radiosensitivity

In the past these tumours were thought to be radioresistant, but this is a relative term as, given a sufficiently high dose, 5500 – 7000 cGy in 4 – 6 weeks, it should theoretically be possible to eradicate all malignant cells. Certainly in the past, when low doses of irradiation (2500–3000 cGy) were given to the pelvis (in the management of metastatic disease), it was noted that the primary tumour would also respond. Megavoltage equipment should be used in order to obtain enough deep penetration and to produce a sharply defined beam which will not damage the surrounding organs.

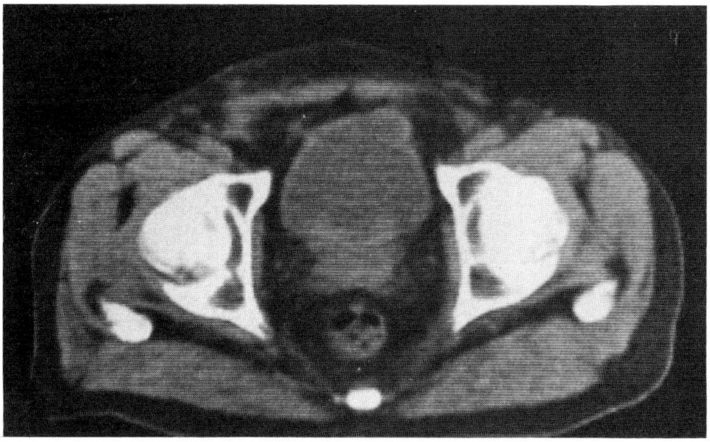

Figure 3.8 (*a*) CT scanning of the prostate. Bladder involved

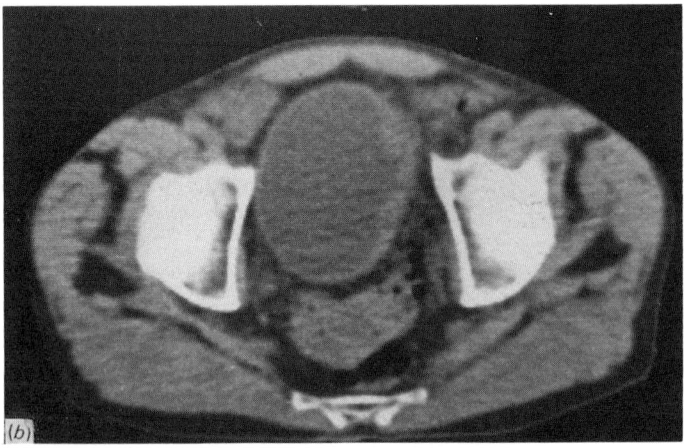

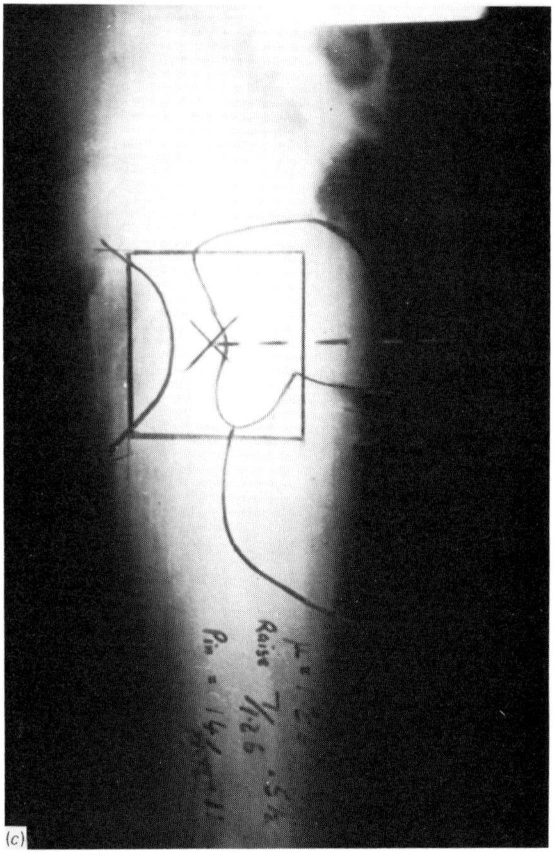

Figure 3.8 *(b)* CT scanning of the prostate. Seminal vesicles involved. *(c)* Localization films for carcinoma of the prostate taken on conventional diagnostic set

Techniques

Radical irradiation

The Stanford group were among the first radiotherapists to treat these tumours in a radical fashion (Bagshaw *et al.*, 1965). They used a 4.8 MeV linear accelerator with a 360° rotation field; the patient was treated standing and supported in a special jig. The volume of tissue included the prostate and the seminal vesicles with fields of 6 × 6 cm. Localization was carried out using a Foley catheter in the bladder (the balloon being distended by 5 ml of mercury): 10 ml Gastrograffin were instilled into the bladder and 60 ml of barium into the rectum. A tumour dose of 7000 cGy in 6 weeks was given. At the same time in the UK somewhat lower doses were being used; Budhraja and Anderson (1964) described a three field cobalt technique giving 5000 cGy in 5 weeks and Lloyd Davies, Vinnicombe and Collins (1971) gave 3750 cGy in six fractions over 18 days.

A recent Stanford technique (Bagshaw, personal communication 1981) consists of treating the whole pelvis with a four field technique — one anterior, one posterior and two lateral fields giving a tumour dose of 2600 cGy in 13 fractions over 2.5 weeks. This is followed by a booster dose to the prostate only, using the rotation method described above, giving 2000 cGy in 2 weeks. Subsequently the pelvis receives a further 2400 cGy in 12 fractions over 2.5 weeks. The para-aortic nodes (as part of a trial in irradiating this site) are given a dose of 5000 cGy over 7 weeks with two parallel opposed fields supplemented by opposed lateral or oblique fields.

The London Hospital technique

Telecobalt irradiation was used originally because no

linear accelerator was available, and it is still acceptable providing the patient is not too large (anterior/posterior diameter of the pelvis less than 22 cm). The tumour is localized with a cystogram — 50 ml of Conray 50 are instilled into the bladder (the Foley catheter is pulled down hard so that the balloon lodges against the internal urethral orifice); 60 ml of barium are put into the rectum, skin marks and tattooing are used to define the entry point and ideally films taken on a simulator, although if not available a diagnostic X-ray machine can be used (*Figure 3.8c*). A four field isocentric technique is usually required, and will give quite a good dose distribution (two anterior oblique wedge fields at 45° from the vertical and two posterior oblique fields at 60°) (*Figure 3.9*). The aim is to treat the prostate and seminal vesicles with field sizes of the order of 5 × 5 × 5 cm to 7 × 7 × 7 cm. A dose of 5500 cGy is given in 20 daily fractions over 4 weeks, all fields being treated daily. It should be noted that at least one-third of the rectum will receive the maximum tumour dose.

If a linear accelerator (5–8 MeV) is available this is preferable, particularly in the larger patient. Here a three field isocentric technique can be used (one anterior and two posterior oblique — usually wedged and angled at 120° from each other) (*Figure 3.10*). Simulator films should be taken (*Figure 3.11*). The patient lies supine, and because of the small size of the fields a check film should be taken on the accelerator (*Figure 3.12*). The same dose/time fractionation is used. If the patient cannot be treated in 4 weeks due to illness or machine failure, an increased dose will be required (as described in carcinoma of the bladder).

Interstitial irradiation

This is described in detail by Ash (*see* Chapter 16). The aim is to give a very high dose to the prostate only, using permanent implants of ^{198}Au grains (Flocks 1973), ^{125}I seeds or by iridium-192 wire (the latter can be removed and in theory gives a more accurate dose). The disadvantages of these methods are that an open operation is required to implant the seeds or wire, and the dose distribution may not be homogeneous. It is also unlikely that the seminal vesicles would be adequately treated although this might be overcome if external irradiation is given as well, as described by Chan and Gutierrez (1977) who gave 4000 cGy by implant and a further 4000 cGy by megavoltage irradiation.

Irradiation for T3 tumours

Here, with the tumour extending beyond the prostatic capsule, one must assume that the regional lymph nodes are involved, and therefore it would be logical to treat the whole pelvis. A pair of parallel and opposed fields is used, treating from the level of the fourth lumbar vertebra down to the obturator foramen and out to the side wall of the pelvis (*Figure 3.13a*). A dose of 4000–4500 cGy in 20 daily fractions is reasonably well tolerated.

Bagshaw (1979) would then top up the prostate

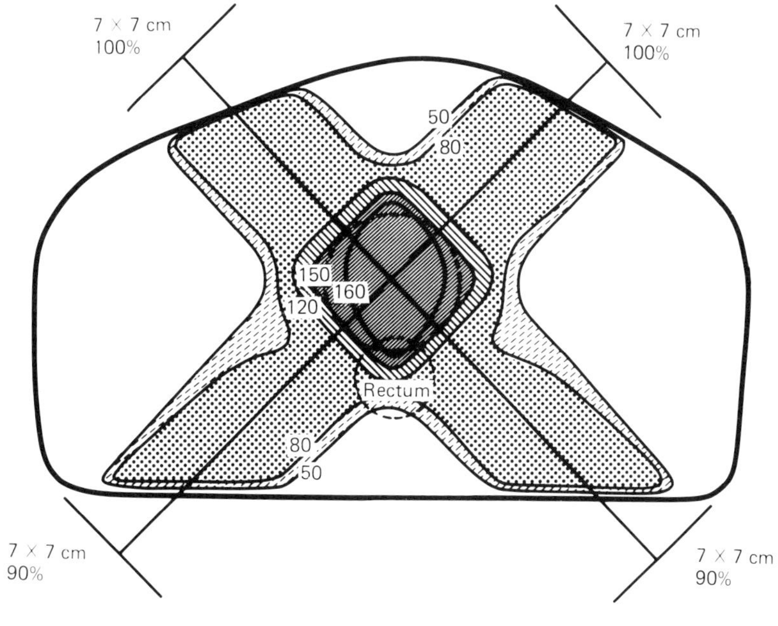

Figure 3.9 Isodose curves for four field isocentric technique using a Gammatron
>150; 120–150; 80–120; 50–80; <50

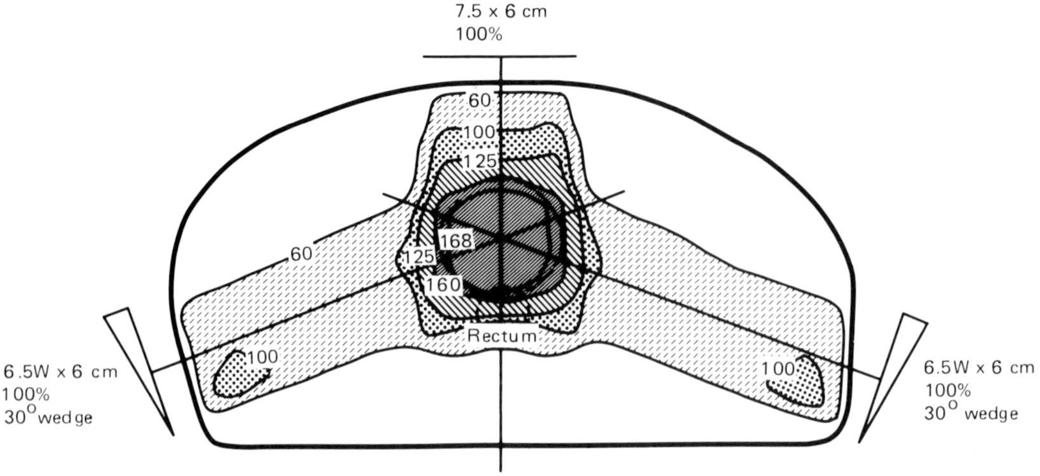

Figure 3.10 Isodose curves for three field isocentric technique on 8 MV linear accelerator

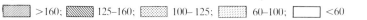

>160; 125–160; 100–125; 60–100; <60

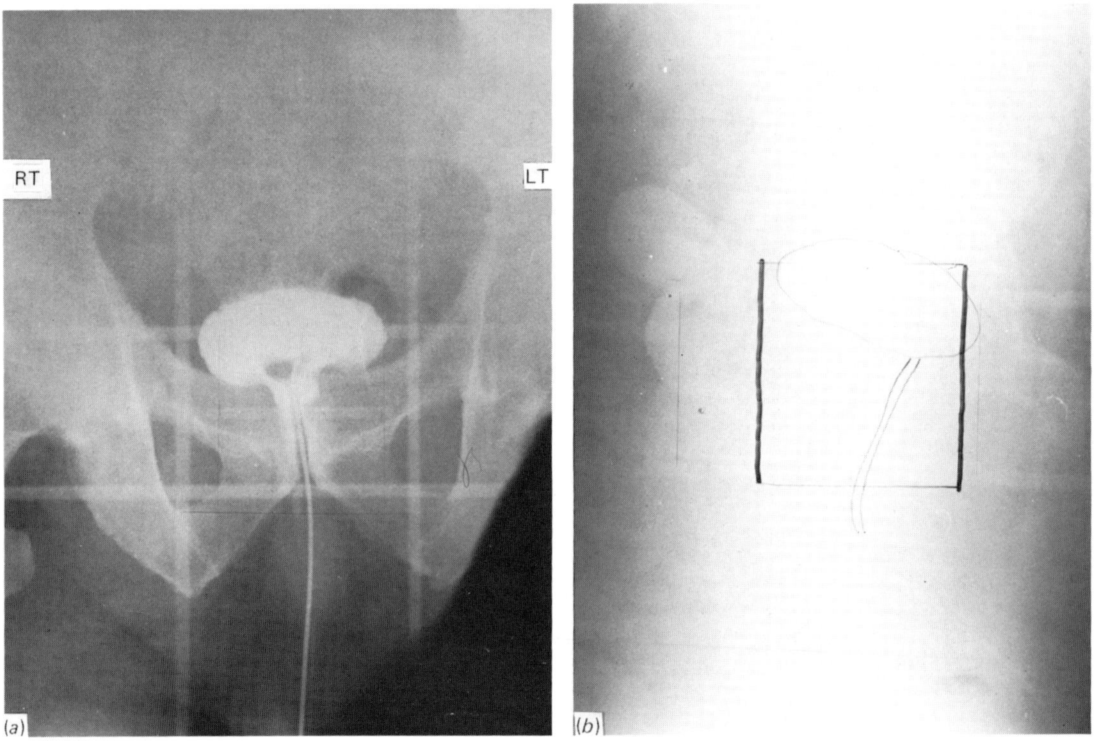

Figure 3.11 Localization films for three field technique — Ximitron simulator. *(a)* Anteroposterior, *(b)* lateral

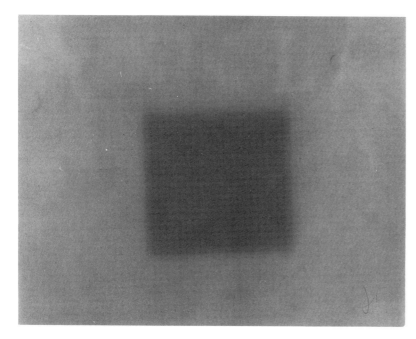

Figure 3.12 Check films taken on linear accelerator

with a further dose of 1500–2000 cGy in 10 treatments (using the rotation technique described above). Whether or not this is necessary is open to debate. If there is gross involvement of the pelvic nodes (which will only receive 4500 cGy) a booster dose to the prostate alone would not appear to be of value.

If, on the other hand, only micro-metastases are present in the lymph nodes, these might be sterilized by the lower dose, and a booster to the prostate might well be worth giving even though the morbidity may be greater.

Palliation

With generalized skeletal metastases it is customary to start treatment with hormone therapy (low dose oestrogens or orchidectomy). If, however, the primary tumour is very large, and particularly if the tumour is undifferentiated, a hormone response may well not occur. In this group of patients irradiation to the whole pelvis will serve two purposes: first to relieve the pain from the bony metastases, and second to shrink the primary tumour. A dose of 3000 cGy in 10 fractions will suffice for the former, and will certainly deal with the latter if increased to 4000 cGy over 20 fractions. Chemotherapy has very little to offer at the present time.

Localized skeletal metastases

These are often painful, and unless hormone therapy rapidly relieves the pain some form of irradiation should be tried. The commonest site is the vertebrae, and here a direct field to the affected area may be treated with megavoltage irradiation, giving a dose of 2500 cGy at the calculated depth of the involved bone in 10 daily fractions, or alternatively 2100 cGy in seven fractions on alternate days. If the patient is very ill a single dose of 1000 cGy can be given and appears to be effective (Penn, 1976). In all cases a field size large enough to cover the vertebrae above and below those involved should be used as more than one is usually affected. Orthovoltage can be used; an incident dose of 3000 cGy in 10 daily treatments or 2800 cGy in seven treatments (alternate days) is very effective and probably produces less nausea when given to the lumbar region and fewer sore throats when treating the cervical spine (Hope-Stone, 1980). The disadvantage of this method, and of single treatments generally, is that if the treatment has to be repeated subcutaneous fibrosis may occur.

The ribs are a common site for painful metastases. A direct field using orthovoltage is very effective for treating these and produces less systemic upset than megavoltage (Hope-Stone, 1980). Dose levels are described above.

Involvement of a weight-bearing bone such as the femur can usually be treated with irradiation alone, using a pair of parallel and opposed fields to give a tumour dose of 2500 cGy in 10 treatments. Internal fixation is not required unless there is a pathological fracture.

Generalized painful bone metastases

These can be treated in the same way as in breast

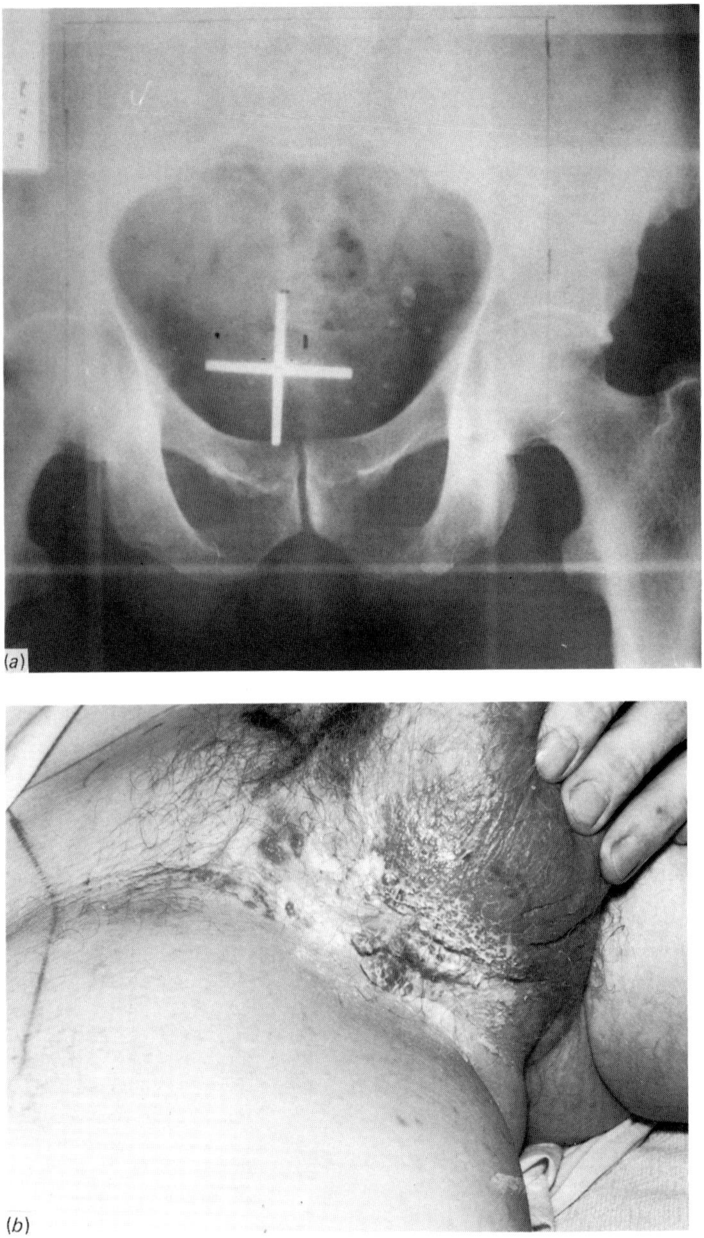

Figure 3.13 *(a)* Whole pelvis irradiation for T3 prostate carcinoma. *(b)* Skin infiltration after open prostatectomy

carcinoma with a pelvic bath or hemibody irradiation, the latter method being described by Fitzpatrick and Rider (1976). The most painful part of the body is treated first (which is usually the lower half). A single dose of 800 cGy is given by a pair of lateral opposed fields from the umbilicus down to the knees (or lower if metastases are present). The patient is treated supine with bolus to compensate for air gaps. If given suitable antiemetics and steroids and admitted overnight he will suffer no major upset, and the pain maybe relieved within 48 hours. After a month's gap the upper half from the umbilicus to just below the eyes (unless there is evidence of brain or cranial bone involvement in which case the whole skull is treated) is given a lower dose of 600 cGy as this will reduce the risk of irradiation pneumonitis.

Skin infiltration

This may occur after open prostatectomy (*Figure 3.13b*). Palliation may be achieved with local irradiation to a dose of 3000 cGy (with orthovoltage) in 2 – 3 weeks.

General side-effects of irradiation

Bowel

The predisposing factors are the same as in treating the bladder. The commonest upset is diarrhoea occurring in varying degrees depending on the volume of tissue irradiated. If the prostate alone is treated it occurs in about 10–15% of cases, but if the whole pelvis is irradiated then a figure of 40% is probably more realistic (Ray and Bagshaw, 1975). Treatment is by the simple methods outlined in the management of bladder cancer.

The rectum can receive the maximum tumour dose to at least one-third of its volume which leads to proctitis, tenesmus, and the passage of bloody stools. Prednisol suppositories will relieve the symptoms, but occasionally irradiation needs to be curtailed for a few days.

The long-term effects are mainly from small bowel obstruction which occurs most often if a transperitoneal staging laparotomy has been performed (Pistenma, Bagshaw and Freiha, 1979). Many such cases will require at least a temporary colostomy.

Urinary tract

As described in bladder complications these should be minimal if the urine is kept sterile. Urethral stricture is unlikely to be due to irradiation and is more probably associated with repeated cystoscopies before irradiation was commenced. In the Stanford series it occurred in 16 out of 430 cases. Urinary incontinence should not occur at all.

Lymphoedema

This is not seen unless previous retroperitoneal staging laparotomy has been performed. In the Stanford series it was present in 55% of cases and affected the penis, scrotum, suprapubic region and the lower limbs (Pistenma, Bagshaw and Freiha, 1979).

Impotence

Irradiation itself is unlikely to cause impotence, yet in the Stanford series it was described in 40% of 110 patients who could be assessed — their mean age was 59 years before treatment (Ray and Bagshaw, 1975). Possibly the staging laparotomy was responsible for some of these cases, although most authors agree that an accurate estimation of this symptom is difficult to achieve.

Results

Interpretation of published figures is difficult owing to the varying methods of staging used and the fact that, in some series, cases were treated with hormones as well. Even the natural history of this disease when untreated is not well documented.

Table 3.9 describes some of the larger reported series treated by irradiation alone. A smaller series treated at The London Hospital showed a 4-year survival figure of 69% in stage 1 and 2 (Hope-Stone, 1985). Similar results are also reported by Flocks (1973) using a combination of pelvic lymphadenectomy and ^{198}Au implant to the prostate.

Pistenma, Bagshaw and Freiha (1979) describe an interesting trial at Stanford where 55 T1, T2 patients (nodes negative by surgical staging) were treated by radical irradiation, either to the prostate alone, or to the prostate and pelvic lymph nodes. There was no significant difference in survival 15 months to 7 years later. At the same time, patients with positive pelvic nodes were treated either by whole pelvic irradiation or the latter plus para-aortic irradiation, but again

Table 3.9 Radical radiotherapy in the management of carcinoma of the prostate

	No. of cases	*Stage*	*Survival (%)*	*No. of years on follow-up*
Resnick (1977)	31	3	29	5
McGowan (1977)	86	1 and 2	83	5
		3	39	
Stanford group } (1975)	230	1 and 2	71	5
Ray and Bagshaw } (1975)	200	3	41	5

there was no difference in survival. The author stressed that in those patients with positive pelvic nodes there was a 56% incidence of bony metastases within 15 months.

Bagshaw (personal communication) updated the latest results from Stanford: in 351 cases (T1, T2) there was a 78% 5-year survival and in 310 cases (T3) a 59% survival. The 10 to 15 year figures for the early stages were 57% and 39%, and for the more advanced groups 39% and 30% respectively.

Future management

Radiosensitization by oxygenation, neutron therapy, or chemical sensitizers seems no more likely to alter the prognosis than it has done in bladder cancer.

Proton irradiation might help to increase the dose to the prostate by means of a perineal boost. A trial of this method has been undertaken at the Massachusetts General Hospital but with no obvious advantage (Shipley, 1983). This form of irradiation is very expensive and not readily available.

Radical surgery and hormone therapy do not produce better survival figures than radical irradiation, but will always produce impotence and other side-effects, so that there is good reason for abandoning this latter method of treatment. Byar (1973) states that there is no evidence that any active treatment will alter the prognosis and therefore all treatment should be deferred until symptoms arise. A trial to compare a no-treatment group with a group receiving radical irradiation would seem to be indicated.

Such a trial has been started in the UK by the MRC. Patients under 75 years with histologically proven carcinoma of the prostate localized to the gland only (UICC classification T0–T1 M0) can be entered. Patients will only be included if the acid phosphatase and an isotope bone scan are normal. Radical irradiation will be to a high dose (5500 cGy in 4 weeks) to the prostate only, or 4000 cGy in 4 weeks to the whole pelvis, followed by a booster dose to the prostate of 2000 cGy over a further 2 weeks.

A second trial has also been set up to look at the management of T2, T3 and T4 tumours without metastases. Here immediate orchidectomy will be compared with radical irradiation alone or a combination of both. The staging criteria will be the same, but a positive lymphangiogram will not exclude the patient. Surgery will be a supracapsular orchidectomy, and radical irradiation (either 4250 cGy to the whole pelvis in 4 weeks, or this dose plus a booster to the prostate gland of 1500–2000 cGy in 2 weeks) will be given.

It would seem logical for these and other randomized trials to be carried out as soon as possible, in order to determine finally the correct management of this disease, as otherwise various factions — surgical, radiological and oncological — will continue to proclaim the superiority of their own particular techniques, and the patient will remain without benefit or even made worse by the treatment he has undergone.

Testicular tumours

These are uncommon tumours in the UK, occurring in 2.3 per 100000 men and comprising about 1.2% of all neoplasms in males; recently there has been an increase in its reported incidence. Its major importance lies in the ability of radiotherapists, surgeons and oncologists to cure a high proportion of cases.

Classification

Table 3.10 compares the accepted British classification with that used in the USA.

It should be noted that the age incidence for teratomas (20–30 years) is lower than for seminomas (30–40 years) (Hope-Stone, Blandy and Dayan, 1963).

Surgery

Removal of the whole testis and spermatic cord should be carried out through an inguinal incision, as scrotal operation leads to a high local recurrence rate (Hope-Stone, 1979) and if carried out will result in the necessity to irradiate the inguinal nodes and the opposite testis.

Staging

When Blandy, Hope-Stone and Dayan (1970) advocated their staging classification the methods available — both clinical and radiological — were very simple. Today we have the advantage of lymphangiography, ultrasound, CT scanning and tumour markers. Peckham (1982) has updated this classification to take this into account. An abbreviated version is shown in *Table 3.11*.

Investigations

Tumour markers

Beta human chorionic gonadotrophin and α-fetoprotein should be estimated before any treatment is undertaken and preferably prior to orchidectomy. Routine clinical examination should be combined with abdominal palpation whilst under anaesthesia at the time of surgery.

Radiological

A chest X-ray should be taken first to exclude gross

Table 3.10 Classification of testicular tumours

UK	*USA*
Seminoma	Seminoma
Teratoma	Teratoma
Teratoma differentiated (TD)	Teratoma
Malignant teratoma intermediate (MT1)	Terato-carcinoma
Malignant teratoma undifferentiated (MTU)	Embryonal-carcinoma
Malignant teratoma trophoblastic	Chorion carcinoma
Combined seminoma/teratoma	Embryonal carcinoma
Yolk sac tumours	
Sertoli cell tumours	
Interstitial cell tumours	
Malignant lymphomas	

Table 3.11 Staging of testicular tumours (after Peckham, 1982 abbreviated)

Stage 1	Disease confined to testis
Stage 2	Infradiaphragmatic lymph node involvement (a) Maximum diameter of any lymph node < 2 cm (b) Maximum diameter of any lymph node 2–5 cm (c) Maximum diameter of any lymph node > 5 cm
Stage 3	Mediastinal and neck node involvement ± subdiaphragmatic nodes
Stage 4	Extension of tumour to extralymphatic sites

metastases, then a lymphangiogram performed combined with an IVP. Until recently the lymphangiogram was thought to be mandatory as moderate lymph node enlargement can easily be identified. CT scanning may make it superfluous but for the moment a combination of the two methods is to be preferred. The false negative rate of lymphangiography alone is 24.7% in the Royal Marsden series (Peckham, 1982). An IVP will be helpful in those cases with the nodes sufficiently enlarged to produce deviation of the ureter (*Figure 3.14a*) and the CT scan will usually confirm this (*Figure 3.14b*).

CT scanning

Although whole lung tomography will pick up some small metastases, CT is more accurate and no more time consuming. Small abdominal and pelvic nodes may be shown and even measured. This will prove useful in radiation treatment planning, and can be used to monitor the response of radiotherapy and chemotherapy as well as to recognize signs of recurrence (Husband, 1979). It should be remembered that even with CT there will be a proportion of false positive and false negative cases.

Ultrasound

This is probably less effective in the diagnosis of lymph node involvement, but more useful than CT scanning in the detection of early liver involvement. It is also useful in the initial differential diagnosis of difficult testicular swellings.

Routine blood tests should include a full blood count, liver function tests, blood urea and renal function tests (if chemotherapy is indicated).

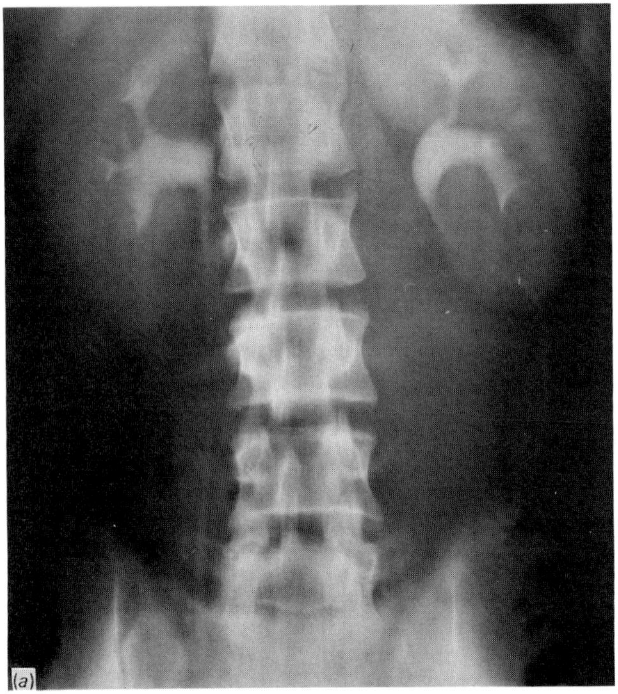

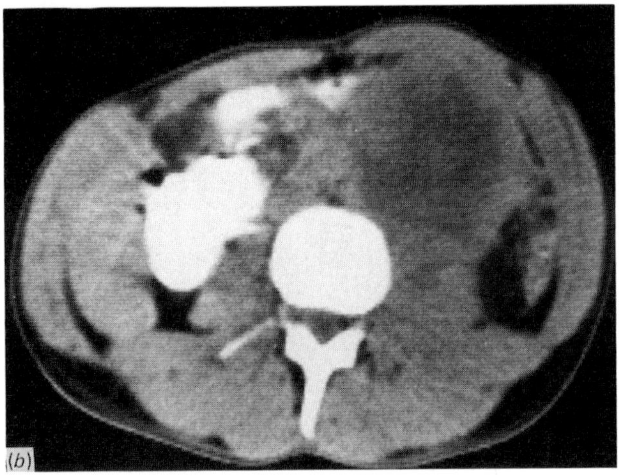

Figure 3.14 *(a)* IVP to show deviation of ureter by (L) para-aortic gland. *(b)* CT scan confirming cystic mass of glands

Treatment policy

Seminoma

Stage 1

After orchidectomy irradiation should be given to the pelvic and para-aortic lymph nodes.

Stage 2a

Treatment is given as in stage 1. In the past this was often followed after a month's gap by irradiation of the mediastinal and supraclavicular lymph nodes. Unfortunately, if chemotherapy is subsequently required the extra dose of irradiation might reduce bone marrow tolerance, so a watching policy is now preferred.

Stage 2b

Owing to the likelihood of spread beyond the known lymph node involvement, chemotherapy should be used first (possibly with cisplatin alone). CT scanning will show the presence of any residual disease which could subsequently be irradiated. Routine irradiation to the site of previous bulk disease is probably not necessary unless the toxicity of chemotherapy is such that it cannot be continued and irradiation should be used instead.

Stages 3 and 4

Here chemotherapy should be the first line of treatment and irradiation only used for failure of response. Whole lung irradiation can be very successful if the tumour is confined to these organs.

Teratoma

Stage 1

MT1 and MTU

For the past three decades in the UK radical irradiation to the pelvis and para-aortic nodes was the treatment of choice. Retroperitoneal node dissection was not considered to be of value (*see below*).

Stage 2a

MT1

The results from irradiation alone, as with seminoma, have been very good and, if confined to below the diaphragm, subsequent chemotherapy will not be comprised.

MTU

The results from irradiation alone are poor (Hope-Stone, 1981). Chemotherapy should be the first line of treatment probably using cisplatin, vinblastine and bleomycin (Einhorn and Donohue, 1977). Irradiation is only used for residual tumour or possibly the site of bulk disease.

Stage 2b and 2c

MT1 and MTU

Chemotherapy is the treatment of choice, possibly with irradiation later to the site of bulk disease.

Stages 3 and 4

Chemotherapy is used first as above but with etoposide replacing vinblastine. Residual tumour can be treated subsequently with irradiation, but it should be remembered that what appears to be residual tumour in the lymph nodes may well turn out to be a well differentiated benign teratoma. Surgery may be required to prove this, but removal of such masses may be highly dangerous and it may be safer to leave well alone. However, in the future it may well be that nuclear magnetic resonance will be able to differentiate between tumour and fibrous mass, and this will become increasingly important if these so-called benign teratomas do contain some malignant cells.

Lymphoma of testes

If the tumour is confined to the testis, irradiation to the pelvic lymph nodes and the scrotum will suffice. Over 53% will show signs of widespread disease, and in these cases treatment should be started with chemotherapy, and irradiation then given to the site of bulk disease. Read (1981) suggests that even early cases should receive adjuvant chemotherapy.

Surgical management

Radical retroperitoneal node dissection has been widely advocated, particularly in the USA, in the treatment of teratomas (stage 1 and 2), and more recently as a staging procedure as well. This is a major surgical operation with a complication rate of 12% (Staubitz, 1974) and ejaculatory impotence in the majority (Kedia, Markland and Frayley, 1977). It necessitates a large abdominal incision, possible intestinal adhesions and some morbidity from wound infection, lower limb oedema and pulmonary embolism (McLorie and Skinner, 1980). The results of series treated by this method compared with irradiation alone are similar (Hope-Stone, 1979; Peckham, 1982). It is interesting to note that in a randomized trial comparing orchidectomy and routine irradiation with a similar group treated by node dissection and irradiation, the results were the same (Maier, 1977).

The advocates of surgery as a staging procedure ignore the morbidity associated with this operation, which is no more accurate than the modern staging methods described above. However, when the tumour markers return to normal after chemotherapy in advanced disease, residual masses may still be seen on the CT scan and it may well be necessary to excise them (*see above*).

Radiotherapy technique

Prophylactic irradiation should be given with megavoltage equipment. An IVP is required to localize the kidneys, then skin marks can be placed on the anterior abdominal wall (*Figure 3.15*), and with the patient lying supine localization films are taken on the simulator. If both lymphogram and CT scan are avail-

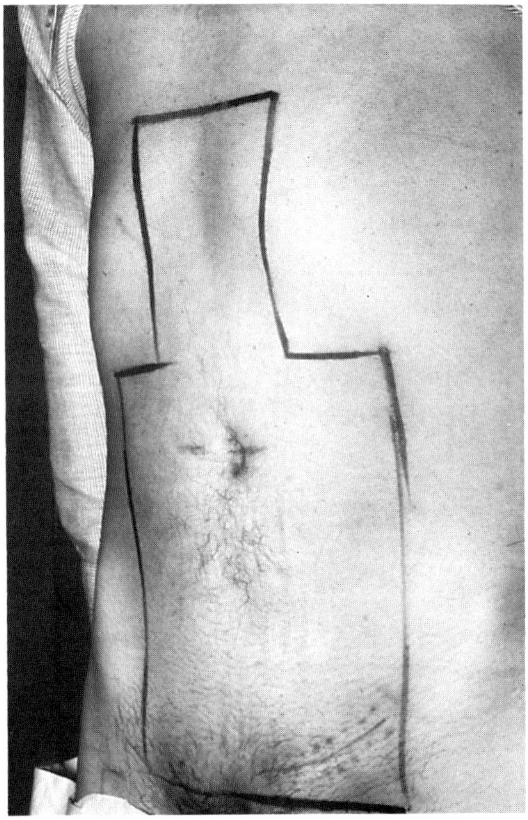

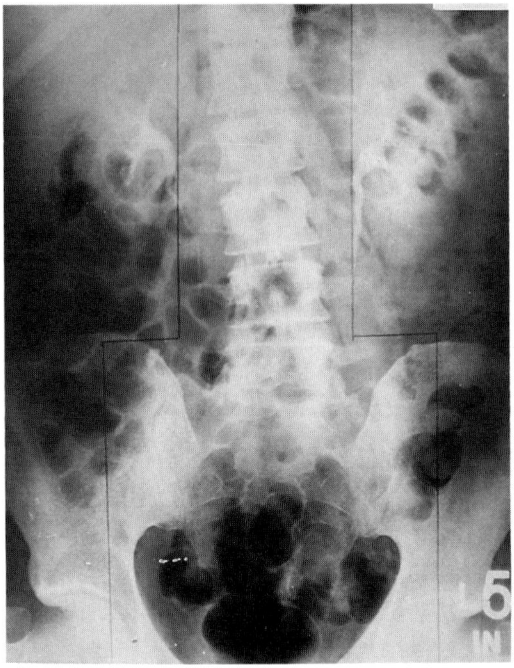

Figure 3.16 Standard inverted T-shaped fields to para-aortic and pelvic lymph nodes

Figure 3.15 Skin marks on patient

able these may be used to decide on the volume to be treated, which will include the para-aortic nodes from the level of the tenth thoracic vertebra down to the obturator foramen. An inverted 'T'-shaped field is used to include all the pelvic nodes (*Figure 3.16*), although in some centres only the ipsilateral pelvic nodes are included (Peckham, 1982). As retrograde spread may occur to either side of the pelvis it would seem more logical to treat all the nodes. Films are taken in the prone and supine position as it is not possible to treat very long fields with an isocentric set up. When the fields have been accepted as correctly marked on the X-ray films a template can be constructed which will allow accurate set up from day to day (*Figure 3.17a,b*) without any alteration of skin marks (a central cross can be tattooed on the skin, both front and back, and this will act as a reference point throughout the treatment). Accelerator check films will confirm the correct position (*Figure 3.18*).

The kidneys are shielded with lead blocks (*Figure 3.19*) on the anterior and posterior fields. The normal testis is always shielded (indirectly with lead blocks and directly by not allowing the lower edge of the field to be within more than 3–4 cm from the organ). Thermo Luminescent dosmeter measurements should be taken on the normal side of the scrotum for future reference with regard to fertility. The normal testis will only need to be irradiated if the scrotum has been incised or a trans-scrotal biopsy performed. In these unfortunate cases, the whole of the scrotum and the inguinal node drainage area will have to be included in the field.

For seminoma a tumour dose of 3000 cGy is given, using a pair of parallel and opposed fields in 20 daily treatments over 4 weeks (both fields treated daily). Teratoma will require a dose of 4000 cGy over the same time. Occasionally para-aortic lymph node involvement is so extensive that it is not possible to shield the kidney completely. In seminoma, if chemotherapy is not used it would be safe to treat the whole of one kidney to a dose of 2000 cGy and then protect the kidney while the rest of the volume is brought up to a dose of 3000 cGy.

Prophylactic mediastinal irradiation

A 'T'-shaped field, to include the mediastinum and supraclavicular nodes, is matched with the upper end of the original para-aortic fields (*Figure 3.20*). A previous skin tattoo combined with the original template and localization films will ensure a good match, but a gap of 1 cm should be left between the two fields to prevent overlap. This technique is rarely used today because it may compromise subsequent

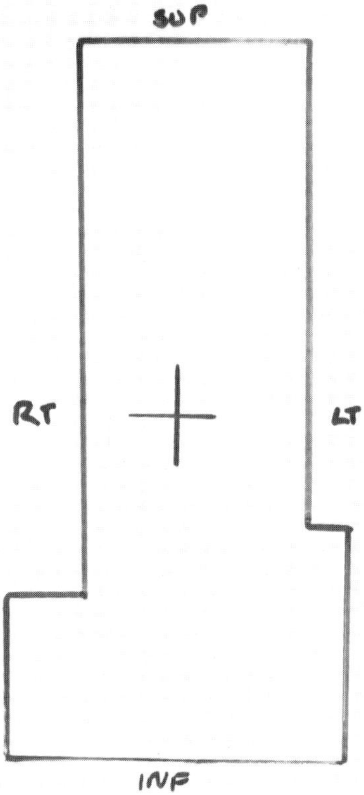

(a)

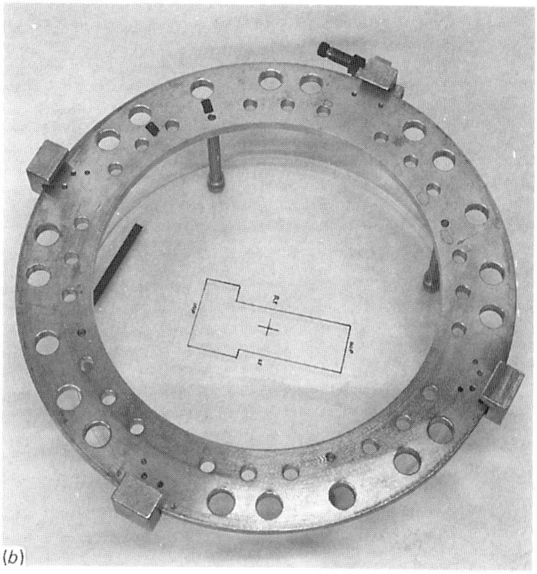

(b)

Figure 3.17 *(a)* Template for accurate setting up procedure. *(b)* Template mounted on shadow tray

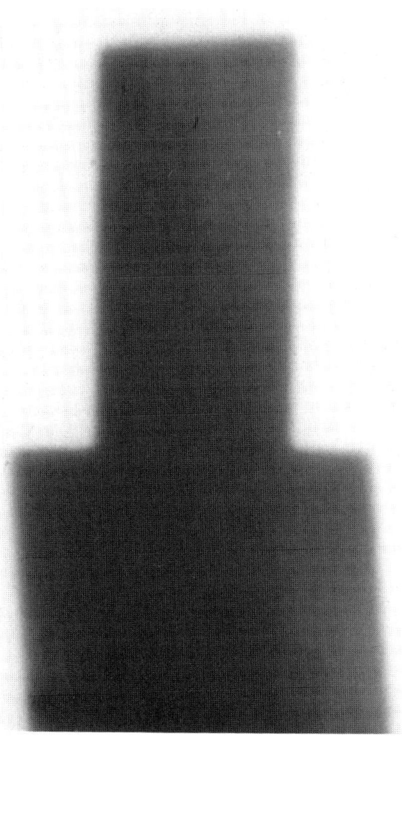

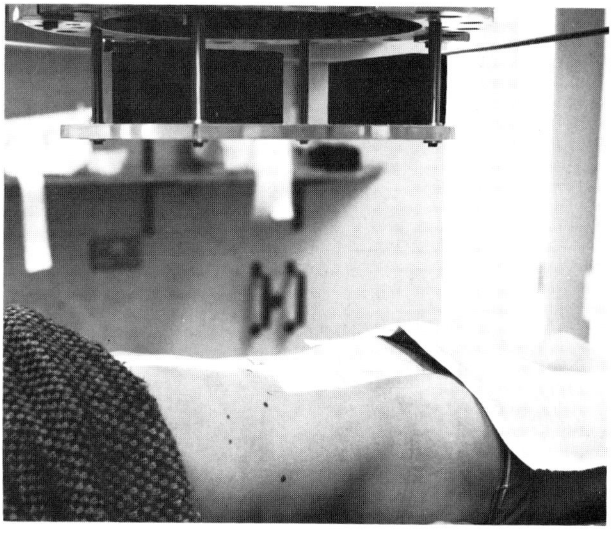

Figure 3.19 Indirect shielding of kidneys and testes with lead alloy blocks. Light mark to show fields. Central tattoo

Figure 3.18 Film taken on linear accelerator to confirm the template position

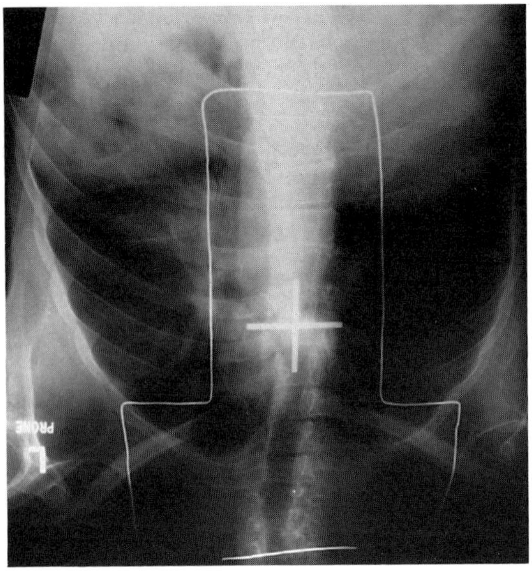

Figure 3.20 T-shaped fields mediastinal and supraclavicular nodes

chemotherapy, but if required a dose of 3000 cGy can be safely given to the mediastinal and supraclavicular nodes providing a month's gap is allowed before the second course of treatment is commenced.

Whole lung irradiation

Occasionally, in seminomas with intrapulmonary metastases where chemotherapy is not indicated, it is possible to treat both lung fields to a tumour dose of 2250 cGy. Localization films are taken on the simulator and accuracy is ensured by the use of a template.

Palliative irradiation

If chemotherapy fails to relieve the symptoms from metastases to lymph nodes or even to bones, then palliative irradiation by simple direct fields should be given. In one of The London Hospital patients with seminoma, bone pain was successfully relieved in the humerus (*Figure 3.21*).

Immediate morbidity

Treatment can be given on an outpatient basis. Nausea and vomiting should not occur, but if they do, they can be relieved with standard antiemetics such as Torecan, Maxolon and Motilium. Occasional mild bowel upsets can be treated by kaolin. Blood counts should be taken twice weekly; if the white blood cell count falls below $3 \times 10^9/\ell$ or the platelets below $100 \times 10^9/\ell$, treatment can be temporarily discontinued, (although this rarely happens with tumour dose levels below 4000 cGy). If the level of platelets continues to fall, an intramuscular injection of Deca-Durabolin 50 mg will prevent any haemorrhagic tendency and will often produce an increase in the count so that irradiation may continue.

Long-term side-effects

Radiation myelitis

This has been reported by Lewis (1948), in patients given doses above 4500 cGy. As only the lower part of the cord is irradiated and since dose levels are in the region of 4000 cGy in 4 weeks, it is perhaps not surprising that no cases have been seen in The

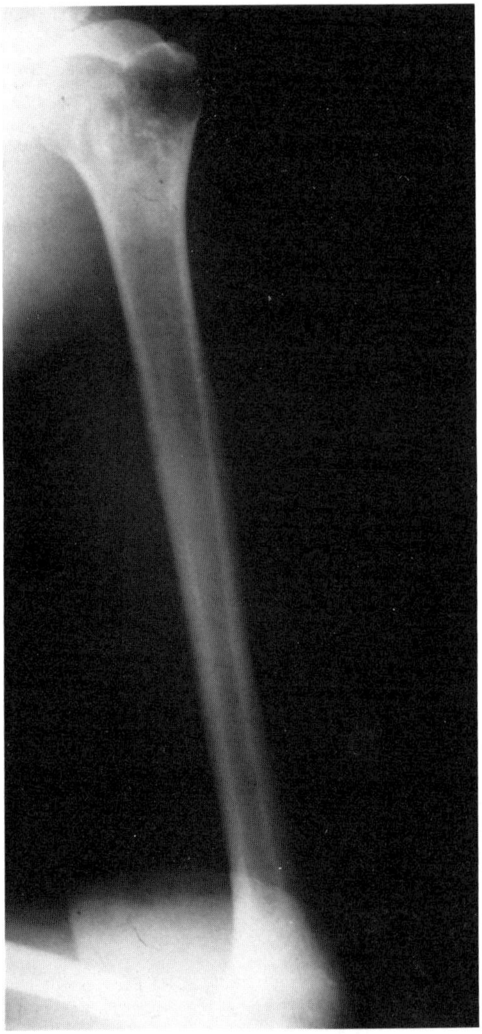

Figure 3.21 Bone metastases in head of humerus in seminoma of testis

London Hospital series (Blandy, Hope-Stone and Dayan, 1970). The most likely chance of this happening would be in those patients who had irradiation above and below the diaphragm — an overlap of the fields at the junction point would be the cause, but again in The London Hospital series no myelitis occurred although a number of cases were treated in this way. L'Hermitte's syndrome of transient irradiation myelopathy is not likely to occur unless the cervical or dorsal spinal cord is irradiated to a dose above 3500 cGy, and may be avoided with the use of spinal cord shielding.

Gastrointestinal upset

Neither gastric perforation nor duodenal ulceration have been seen in any of the UK series although again they were reported by Lewis (1948) and the higher dose of 4500 cGy given in those cases was probably responsible. Small bowel damage is rarely seen although a protein losing enteropathy might occur if very high doses to a large volume of tissue are given.

Lung

Fibrosis should not occur even if the mediastinum has to be irradiated, as the field width is rarely greater than 8 cm. Radiation pneumonitis will not occur even when the whole lung is treated if the dose is kept below 2250 cGy in 4 weeks.

Kidney

Fatal radiation nephritis presenting as albuminuria, anaemia, leg oedema and hypertension 6–9 months after finishing radiotherapy was first reported by Kunkler, Farr and Luxton (1952) but only when the whole kidney received a dose greater than 2250 cGy. Shielding of the kidney throughout the course of treatment has eliminated this problem, but even if part of the kidneys are treated above this dose it is unlikely that nephritis will occur (Hope-Stone, 1981).

Marrow

Bone marrow apalsia should not occur. The possibility of inducing leukaemia should always be considered; it was reported in one case in The London Hospital series (Hope-Stone, 1981) but as it occurred only 2 years after irradiation it was probably not related to the treatment.

Carcinogenesis

It would be difficult to prove whether irradiation is a causative factor as even younger patients can develop more than one primary carcinoma without receiving any irradiation. A far more likely cause is a combination of chemotherapy and subsequent irradiation, but as this is only used in the more advanced tumours it may be considered to be an acceptable risk. The problem was recently reviewed by Hay, Duncan and Kerr (1984) who showed that second malignancies were twice as common in the irradiated patients than in the normal population, but they occurred just as often outside the high dose volume as inside.

Sexual function

Potency should not be affected by irradiation. Infertility is a potential problem but 20–30% of patients are sub-fertile on presentation of their disease (Barrett *et al.*, 1981). The remaining normal testis can be shielded, as described above, and a dose of the order of 25–150 cGy will be received. This will certainly produce temporary infertility and indeed one should advise patients not to attempt to produce children for at least 12 to 18 months after treatment has finished. Subsequently normal children will be produced in many cases (Blandy, Hope-Stone and Dayan, 1970). In the present author's opinion there is absolutely no indication for irradiating the opposite normal testis; the incidence of a second primary is less than 1% and even if it occurs, further irradiation can be given. This occurred in two patients in The London Hospital series both of whom are alive and well 10 and 16 years respectively, after the second course of radiotherapy.

Sperm storage

In view of the present generation's attitude towards irradiation and fertility it would be wise for every patient to have a sperm count before starting treatment. If the patient so wishes he could consider putting the sperm into a bank for future use — providing of course the sperm is of sufficiently good quality to be worthwhile (Barrett *et al.*, 1981).

Results

Seminoma

Treatment by postoperative irradiation alone has shown a steady improvement in survival.

Stage 1

In The London Hospital series from 65% before 1960 to 98% in 1976 (Hope-Stone, 1979); in the Royal Marsden series Peckham (1982) gave a very similar 5-year survial.

Stage 2

Here the outcome has not been so favourable but is continuing to improve (*Table 3.12*).

Table 3.12 Results of treatment in stage 2 seminoma of testes

	Number of cases	*5-year survival (%)*
The London Hospital		
1960–1976	26	57 (crude)
1970–1978	16	88 (crude)
The Royal Marsden Hospital		
1963–1975	54	92 (corrected)
The Massachusetts General Hospital		
1950–1976	35	91 (corrected)

Table 3.13 Improvement in survival of teratoma of the testes, MTU, MT1 stage 2a

	No. of cases	*5-year survival (%)*
The London Hospital		
1960–1969	10	50
1970–1978	17	76
1974–1978	8	100
The Royal Marsden Hospital		
1962–1975	55	41
1976–1978	3	66

Stages 3 and 4

The numbers are small in most series, but two out of eight survived 5 years in The London Hospital series and five out of 52 in the Royal Marsden series. More radical chemotherapy regimens may well show an improvement in these results by the next decade.

Teratoma

One of the most important features of the last decade has been the effect of modern staging methods on the results of treatment. Thus, in The London Hospital series, upstaging of MT1 cases occurred in 26% before 1977 and 33% between 1977 and 1980. This was more marked in the MTU group where the figures were 42% and 60% respectively. This has affected the survival figures of the early stages, particularly in the MTU group whose 2-year figures have improved from 50% to 79% (Hope-Stone, 1981). The Royal Marsden series shows a similar trend (*Table 3.13*). In the MT1 stage 1 the 5-year survival figures have reached 90% at The London Hospital and 95% in Edinburgh (W. Duncan, personal communication). Nevertheless, the results in the more advanced cases with irradiation alone in Stages 2b, 3 and 4 have been poor: 25%, 31% and 10% respectively. Improvement on these results is only likely to be achieved by better chemotherapy, probably using bleomycin, etoposide and cisplatin (BEP). Peckham *et al.* (1983) have reported a 78.9% survival (8–38 months) in 19 cases treated in this way.

Future

In seminoma of the testis with survival figures from orchidectomy and irradiation nearly 100%, it is doubtful if any change in the form of treatment should be considered. Nevertheless, it must be accepted that even if an orchidectomy alone was performed and patients put on a careful watching policy, then a relapse when it occurred could be successfully treated with chemotherapy. As the side-effects of irradiation are so minimal and those of chemotherapy so great, including nausea and vomiting, nephrotoxicity, ototoxicity, infertility and carcinogenesis, it would seem reasonable to stick to the well established methods which give such good results. A good tumour marker such as placental alkaline phosphatase (which is now being developed) might alter this view.

In a stage 1 MT1 teratoma, as the results from irradiation are just as good, this author would advocate prophylactic irradiation only. For stage 1 MTU, as the results are not quite so good, a different argument could be used. As it is likely that 80% of cases will not require irradiation, and the 20% that subsequently do so can be successfully treated by chemotherapy and irradiation, a watching policy could be followed. This policy could prove to be dangerous unless it is carried out in specialist centres where a 100% follow-up can be guaranteed. This must include monthly estimations of tumour markers and CT scanning. Pilot studies to evaluate this method have been started at The London Hospital, the Royal Marsden Hospital, and the Christie Hospital and Holt Radium Institute, and the results so far suggest this is not decreasing the survival of these patients. On the other hand, if prophylactic irradiation is used, only 5–10% of stage 1 patients will require chemotherapy, instead of the 20% with a surveillance policy: and the physiological disadvantages of a watching policy cannot be ignored. In the meantime in the other centres it would certainly be wrong to alter the successful irradiation treatment for stage 1 MT1 and MTU teratomas. It should be remembered that if chemotherapy does have to be used it has a high morbidity rate, as described above, nor is the treatment itself (often prolonged over many months) particularly pleasant for the patients or even accepted by them (some patients will certainly not complete the full course).

Neoplasms of the kidney

The three main types of tumours are Wilms (*see* Chapter 10), renal cell carcinoma (hypernephroma) and renal pelvic tumours (transitional cell carcinoma). They are all uncommon, comprising about 2% of all malignant disease.

Renal cell carcinoma

Surgery is the mainstay of treatment, with preoperative embolization playing an increasingly important role. Irradiation has been used although its effectiveness is in doubt.

Preoperative irradiation

Theoretically this might work by shrinking the tumour and rendering it more operable by reducing the viability of any cells which might be spread by surgical manipulation. Two large controlled trials have been reported. A dose of 3000–4000 cGy is given in 3–4 weeks but no survival benefit has been shown (Hubener and Eibach, 1977; Werf-Messing, Heal and Ledehorr, 1978).

Postoperative irradiation

The rationale here is that irradiation might kill off cells which have spilled at the time of operation. Riches, Griffiths and Thackeray (1951) were keen advocates of this method, but Peeling, Mantell and Shepherd (1969) suggested that such treatment worsened the prognosis; unfortunately their selection of cases was poor — only the more advanced cases were given irradiation. One controlled trial has been reported (Finney, 1973) — there was no significant difference in the results, and because of the extremely high dose used (5000 cGy in 5 weeks) some liver damage occurred.

Indications for irradiation

If the capsule has been invaded and definite spill of tumour cells has occurred, there might be a case for postoperative irradiation providing the renal vein was not involved.

Inoperable primary tumours, often massive in size, can cause distressing haematuria and pain. Alleviation of these symptoms can be simply achieved with doses of 3000 cGy in 2–3 weeks.

Bony metastases are well worth treating, with direct fields to 3000 cGy in 2 weeks. Pathological fractures will require internal fixation and irradiation. Solitary brain metastases (as defined by CT scanning) can be excised, but they are often multiple, and irradiation can be given with a dose of 4000 cGy in 4 weeks to the whole brain. A solitary lung metastasis can be excised, but if multiple, irradiation can be given treating one lung only to a maximum dose of 3000 cGy in 3 weeks. In all cases of metastatic disease progesterone should be considered (Bloom, 1971). Whether the response to hormone therapy is genuine or due to spontaneous regression of tumour remains in doubt.

Irradiation technique for primary tumours

A pair of parallel and opposed fields can be used to give a tumour dose of 3500–4000 cGy in 3–4 weeks (20 daily fractions). At this dose the liver is unlikely to be damaged and the opposite kidney can be shielded after appropriate IVP localization (*Figure 3.22*). For right-sided lesions if a higher dose seems indicated, one posterior and one lateral field would suffice to avoid damaging the liver. The advantage of

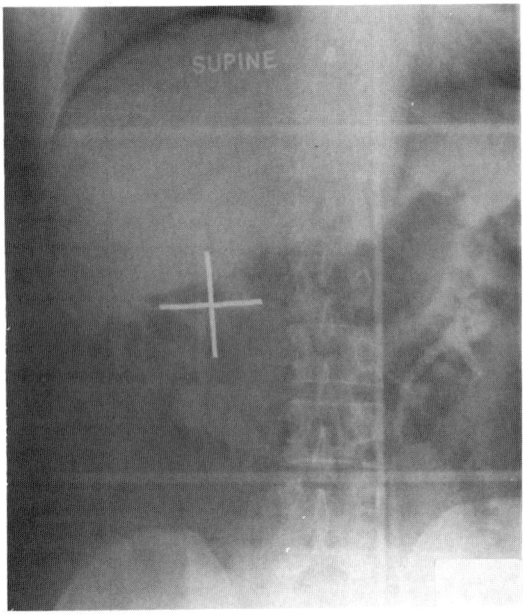

Figure 3.22 IVP localization for treating kidney bed

a lower dose, apart from reducing possible liver damage, is that side-effects, particularly to the small bowel, are minimized, and subsequent stricture formation does not occur; and if the midline region has to be treated there will be no danger of radiation myelitis.

Transitional cell carcinoma of the renal pelvis and ureter

These tumours, which may be multifocal as part of a generalized urothelial disease, are best treated by surgery in the first instance (usually nephro-ureterectomy). If there is evidence of peri-ureteral lymphatic invasion, postoperative irradiation to the renal bed and the line of the ureter down to the bladder might be given. A pair of parallel opposed fields to give a tumour dose of 4000 cGy in 4 weeks is well tolerated.

Preoperative irradiation

It has been suggested that the prognosis might be improved if this is used. Histological diagnosis is made by ureteral brushings. The kidney and upper ureter are treated by a pair of parallel and opposed fields (*Figure 3.23*). The normal kidney is localized

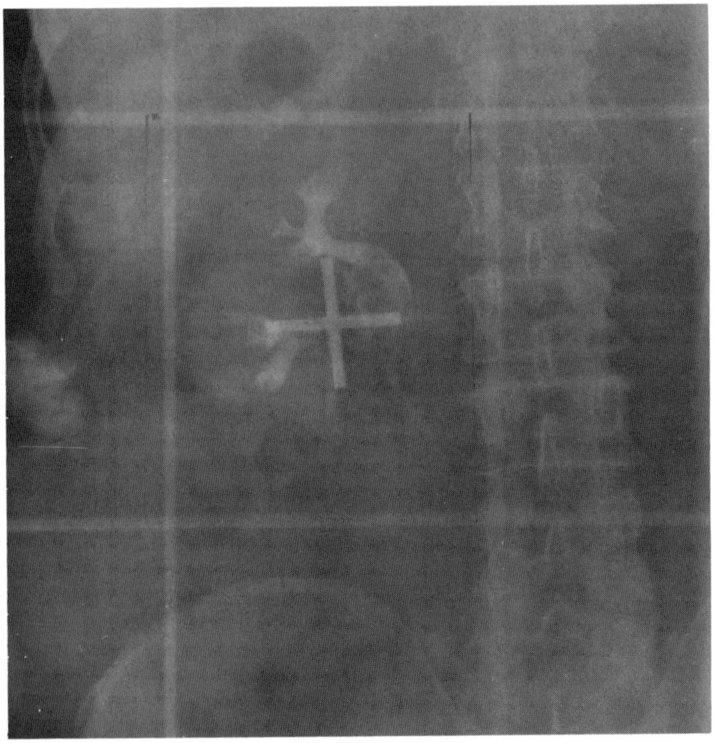

Figure 3.23 Transitional cell carcinoma of the renal pelvis—pre-operative irradiation

on the simulator with an IVP. Johnson (1982) recommends a dose of 5000 cGy in 25 daily fractions. At The London Hospital, in order to eliminate the risk of irradiation myelitis, we have reduced this dose to 4000 cGy in 20 fractions.

Urethral carcinoma

Both squamous cell and transitional cell carcinomas may be found. In males, surgery is the treatment of choice unless the tumour is inoperable, when palliative irradiation might be considered for a distal lesion using external irradiation as described for carcinoma of the penis. For a proximal lesion a radical three field technique as used in carcinoma of the prostate may be tried, but the skin of the perineum will be severely affected if doses of 5000–5500 cGy are given, and treatment may have to be curtailed.

In the female there may be a role for radiotherapy, as radical surgery may be too mutilating for the patient to accept. For localized superficial tumours at the external urethral orifice (squamous cell carcinoma) (*Figure 3.24*) interstitial irradiation may be curative. A permanent ^{198}Au seed implant, to give a dose of 6500 cGy at 0.5 cm treating distance, is well tolerated (*Figure 3.25*), and if successful a urinary diversion can be avoided. If irradiation fails salvage surgery can still be carried out.

An alternative method is described by Werf-Messing (1982) using a radium needle implant, but unless one is very experienced at this method it should not be attempted.

For more penetrating lesions or those which involve most of the urethra, external beam irradiation should be considered. Three fields (one anterior, and two lateral wedged megavoltage fields) will give only slight skin reaction and not damage the rectum. A tumour dose of 5500 cGy in 4 weeks (20 daily fractions) can be given (*Figure 3.26*). Alternatively, electron therapy (10 MeV) can be used with a single direct field and giving a tumour dose of 5500 cGy at 3 cm. If the tumour is thicker than this, higher electron energies will be required. The disadvantage of this latter method is that the skin will receive the maximum tumour dose.

Werf-Messing (1982) advocates a combination of preoperative irradiation with anterior wedge fields to give 4000 to 4500 cGy in 4–5 weeks followed by radical surgery.

Results

There are no large reported series. Surgery appears to cure about 50% of cases. Radiotherapy in selected cases appears to produce similar results (Werf-Messing, 1982).

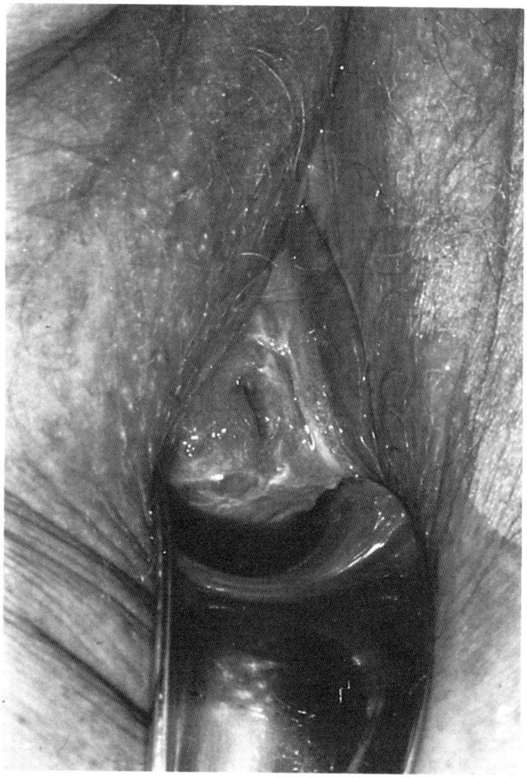

Figure 3.24 Carcinoma of the urethra

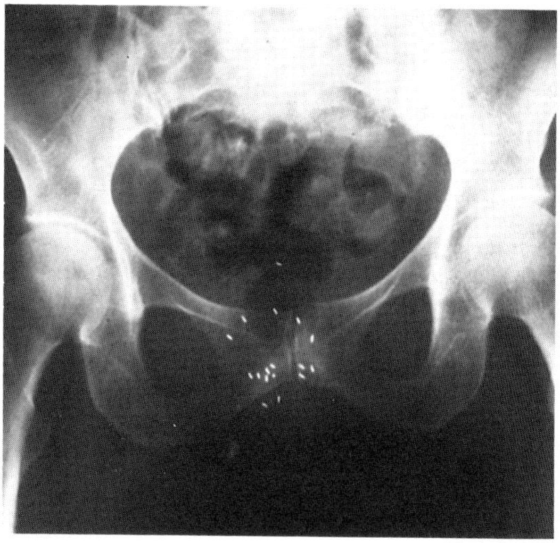

Figure 3.25 ^{198}Au implant for carcinoma of the urethra

Carcinoma of the penis

This is a rare condition in the UK with an incidence of 2% of all malignant diseases. Eastern countries have a higher incidence, 15% in India and 17.5% in parts of China. The primary lesions are all squamous cell

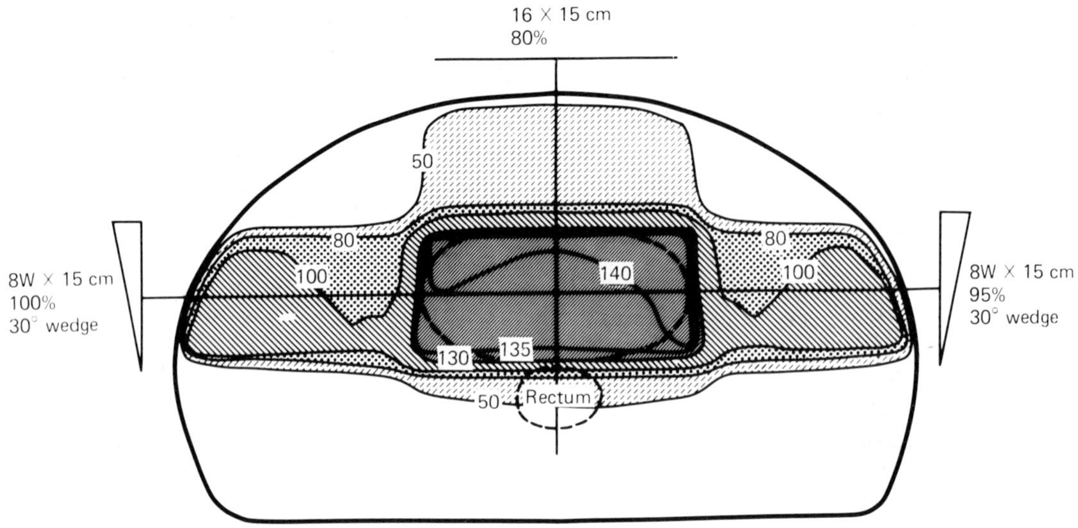

Figure 3.26 Urethra-wedge technique megavoltage 3 fields
▨ >130; ▧ 100–130; ▦ 80–100;
▤ 50–80; ☐ <50

carcinomas but secondary carcinomas may be seen from direct spread, the primary arising in the bladder (15%), prostate (19%) and rectum (14%); rarely, a lymphomatous deposit may be found.

Staging

At The London Hospital we have used a modified version of the clinical staging proposed by Jackson (1966) (*Table 3.14; Figure 3.27*). In stage 1 the tumour is limited to the glans or prepuce — the TNM system subdivides these according to diameter, but the real consideration is whether an iridium mould can be fitted (all our stage 1 would fall in the T1 or T2 category). Stage 2 tumours are those which involve the shaft proximal to the glans (equivalent to T3). Stage 3 includes cases where the primary tumour is so

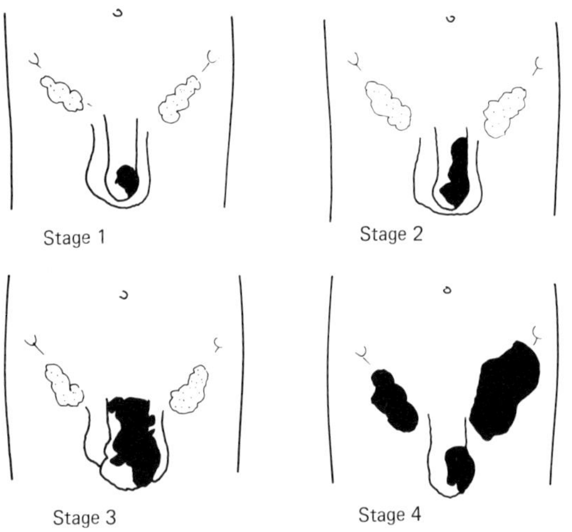

Figure 3.27 The London Hospital staging of carcinoma of the penis

Table 3.14 The London Hospital staging of carcinoma of the penis (modified from Jackson, 1966)

		Equivalent
Stage 1	Tumour limited to the glans or prepuce	T1 and T2
Stage 2	Invasion of the shaft proximal to the glans	T3
Stage 3	Primary tumour so large partial amputation not possible or iridium mould cannot be fitted	T4
Stage 4	Inguinal nodes are fixed — histologically positive. Primary tumour encroaches onto the abdominal wall or perineum	T4

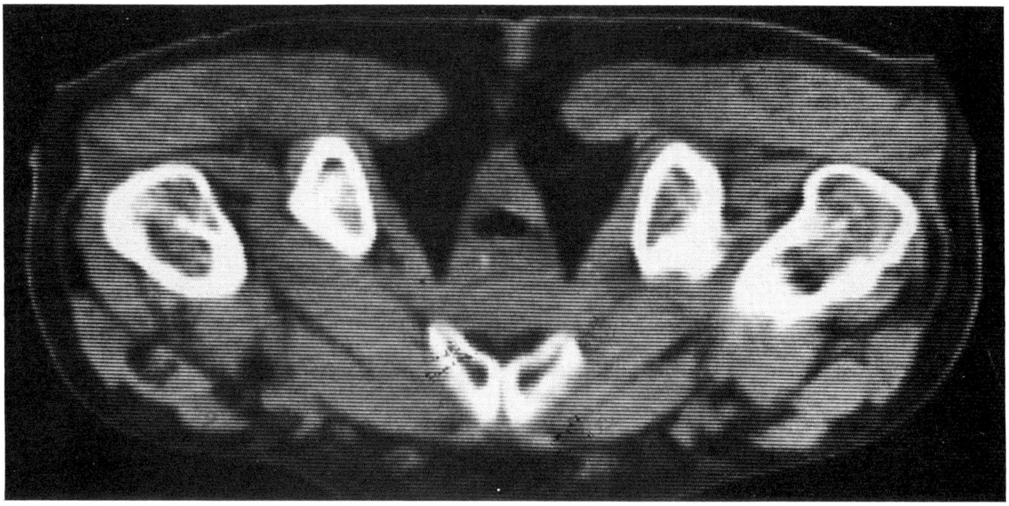

Figure 3.28 CT scan stage 3 carcinoma of the penis — inguinal glands only involved

large that no partial amputation can reasonably clear the growth and no iridium mould can be fitted (equivalent to T4). In stage 4 the primary tumour has spread locally beyond the penis, or has metastasized to nodes or to distant sites. Lymph node staging is not relevant when the patient is first seen, as it is well known that 50% of all palpable inguinal nodes will prove to be due to infection. Only fixed hard nodes would be considered significant. Some information can be gained concerning node involvement by the use of lymphangiography, CT scanning (*Figure 3.28*) and aspiration cytology after the primary has been successfully treated.

Treatment — mould technique

Stage 1

After biopsy and a formal complete circumcision, any infection should be vigorously treated and the postoperative oedema allowed to settle down. Irradiation should not be started until this is achieved (*Figure 3.29*).

In The London Hospital technique, fully described by Hope-Stone (1975), a perspex mould of cylindrical form is required to be fitted by the patient himself. He attends the mould room as an outpatient and the mould is made individually for each patient (modification of previously used moulds are often satisfactory). The primary tumour and a margin proximal to this of at least 2 cm needs to be irradiated, and a margin of 1 cm is taken distal to the tip of the penis. The patient must learn to fix the mould himself (practising with it unloaded). It is made in two parts which can be fitted together, the penis being held up by a ridge on the plastic cylinder (*Figure 3.30a,b*). The radiation source carrier (which is loaded with concentric rings of iridium-192 wire) is placed over the inner cylinder and twist-locked into position (*Figure 3.30c*) (before 1969 radium needles were used to load the carrier).

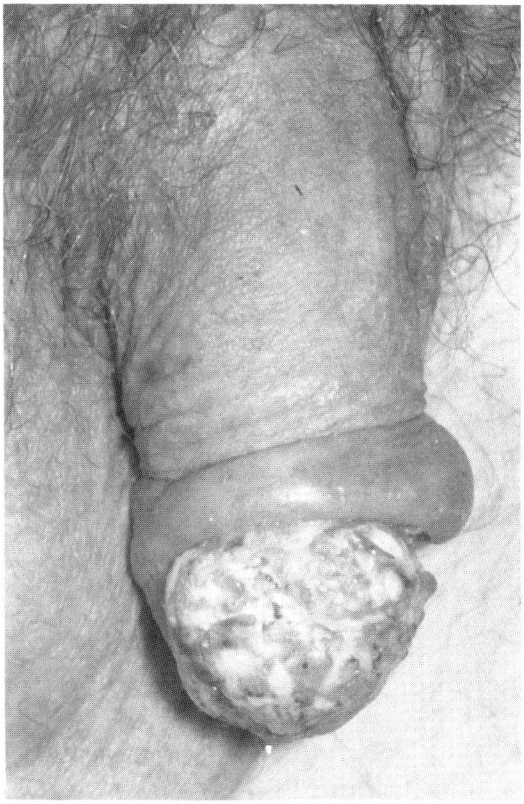

Figure 3.29 Primary tumour stage 1

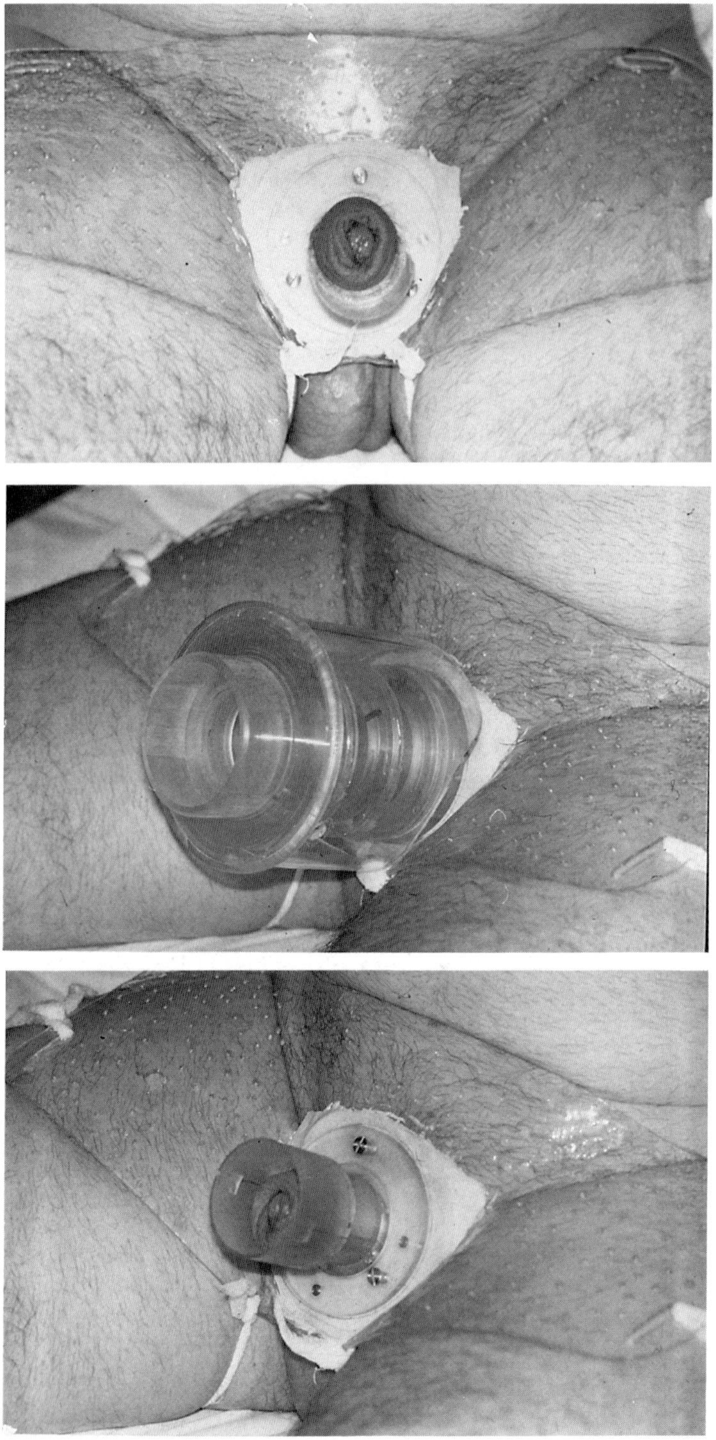

(a)

(b)

(c)

Figure 3.30 *(a)* Half of mould in position. *(b)* Full mould in position. *(c)* Radiation source carrier locked in position. (From Hope-Stone 1975, courtesy of the Editor and Publisher *Proceedings of the Royal Society of Medicine*)

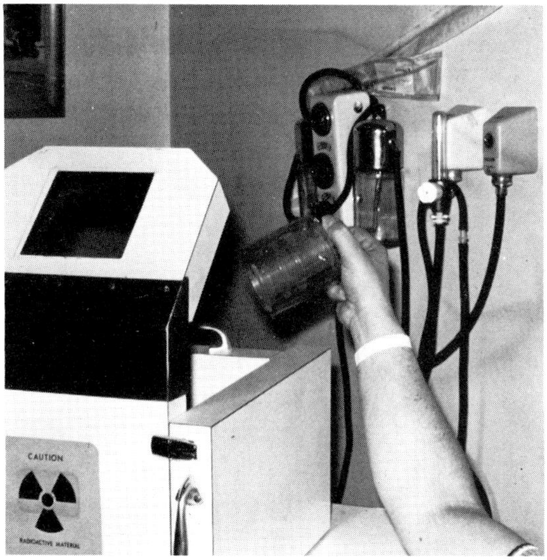

Figure 3.31 Lead safe for temporary storage of loaded mould

The aim is to give a dose of 6000 R (5560 cGy) to the surface of the tumour, but not to exceed 5000 R (4630 cGy) on the urethra. The mould is worn for 12 hours a day (usually 3 hours at a time) for about 7 days. It can be removed for micturition, and when not in use can be placed in a mobile protected safe in the single room in which the patient resides (*Figure 3.31*), thus eliminating nearly all radiation hazard to the nursing and other staff.

Radiation problems

If using an iridium wire cutter, a well-trained mould room technician will receive very little dose while loading the apparatus — less than 20–30 milliroentgen (Hope-Stone, 1975). The nursing staff are protected as described above.

The main hazard is to the patient's own gonads which may receive a dose of 600 – 800 cGy. This will not cause impotence but may well produce permanent infertility, although fortunately the majority of patients are too old for this to be a problem.

Radiation reaction

The week's treatment is usually well tolerated. A moist fibrous reaction (*Figure 3.32*) will develop 1–2 weeks later. This is best treated with local cleansing solution (Eusol), and 1% hydrocortisone cream can be applied if there is severe irritation. Micturition is seldom interfered with, but sexual intercourse should not be resumed for about 6 months (after which it should be painless and satisfactory) (**Figure 3.33**). Occasionally mild superficial crusting of the skin will occur and this can be treated with Flamazine, hydro-

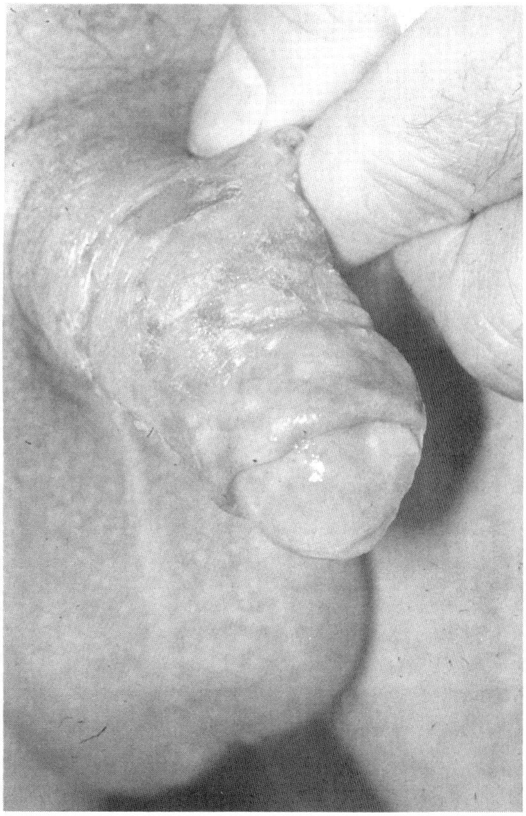

Figure 3.32 Moist reaction at 2 weeks after treatment

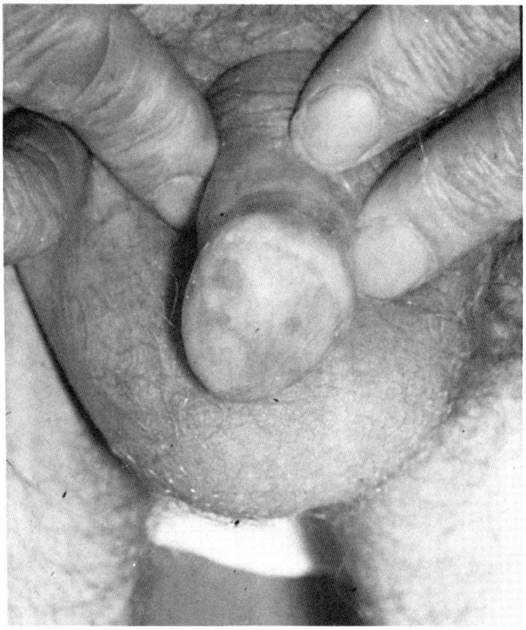

Figure 3.33 Penis healed at 6 months

cortisone cream and temporary sexual abstinence (Hope-Stone, 1977).

External radiation

An alternative to the above method is described by Newaishy and Deeley (1968) and Duncan and Jackson (1972), the main advantage being the absence of any radiation hazard to hospital staff. A wax block technique is used with the penis sandwiched between the two halves (*Figure 3.34a,b*). Either 300 Kv or cobalt irradiation can be used to treat a pair of parallel and opposed fields giving a central tumour dose of 5000–5750 cGy in 4 weeks (20 daily treatments) or three times a week over 22 days. The latter method is likely to increase the skin reaction (Duncan and Jackson, 1972). The problem with this technique is that it is much more difficult for the patient and the radiographer, since the radiation reaction will occur in the third to fourth week and will make the fitting of the wax block both difficult and unpleasant. The urethra will receive the same dose as the tumour and is more likely to develop a stricture. In this author's opinion the technique should only be used in the occasional stage 1 and 2 patient in whom the iridium mould method cannot be used (due to poor cooperation of the patient and/or a very small penis). It may need to be used preoperatively in stage 3. Interstitial implantation has also been described with good results (*see* Chapter 16).

Stage 2

If the urethra is not involved and the shaft only par-

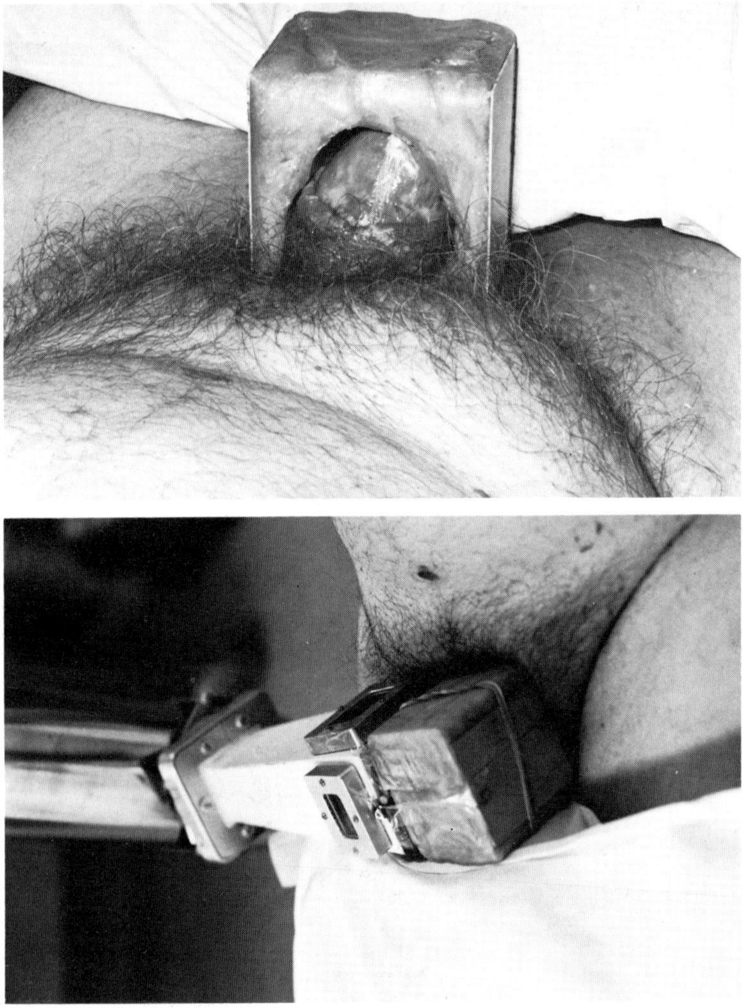

(*a*)

(*b*)

Figure 3.34 Wax block technique for external radiation technique. (*a*) Half of block in position, (*b*) two halves joined together. Application of 300 kV machine

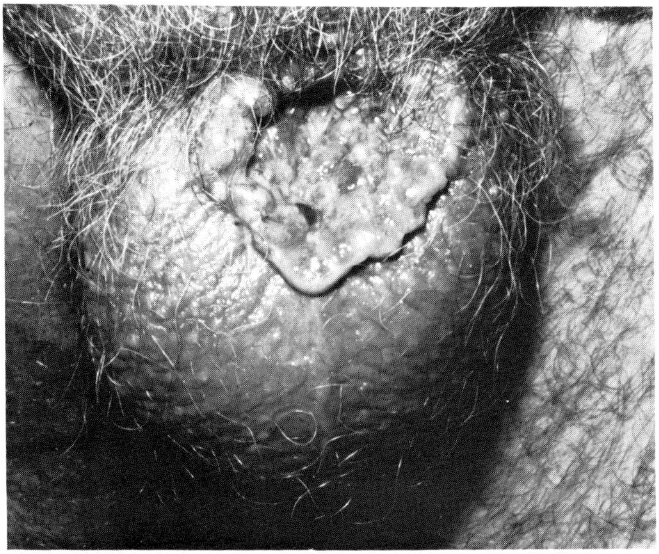

Figure 3.35 Auto-amputation of penis

tially infiltrated, an iridium mould can be used. If the tumour is more advanced it may be possible to use the mould or external irradiation, and follow this with a partial amputation.

Stage 3

Here a radical amputation as described by Blandy (1978a) is required. Occasional preoperative irradiation with external irradiation can be used to shrink the tumour (Salaverria *et al.*, 1979).

Stage 4 — nodes involved

If the nodes disappear 1 month after treatment of the primary tumour, a watching policy can be pursued.

One month after completion of the primary treatment, if the nodes are histologically positive (preferably proven by aspiration cytology), and the lymphogram and CT scan show no evidence of spread to the para-aortic and iliac nodes, a radical approach should be considered. An immediate bilateral inguinal node dissection can be performed. Unfortunately this is not always very successful and an alternative approach would be to give a full preoperative course of irradiation using a pair of parallel and opposed fields to include all the inguinal, internal and external iliac nodes. If a small central lead block is used to shield the rectum a dose of 4500 cGy in 20 daily fractions will be well tolerated. If the glands completely disappear a further watching policy can be followed and a block dissection carried out only if they recur. If the glands do not disappear then immediate surgery is required.

Stage 4 — tumour spread locally beyond the penis

Palliative irradiation may be attempted with tumour doses of the order of 3000 cGy given in 2 weeks. *Figure 3.35* shows a patient who had an auto-amputation of the penis and who had to be given palliative irradiation, but unfortunately the tumour spread rapidly up the abdominal wall.

Chemotherapy may be tried — bleomycin given as an intramuscular injection of 15 mg in 3 ml of 1% lignocaine. This can be used either alone or combined with irradiation (given 1 hour before treatment). In one patient this produced quite marked shrinkage of the primary tumour and the lymph nodes (only the latter received irradiation) (*Figure 3.36a,b*).

Results

Stage 1

Most series report at least 75% 5-year survival figures *Table 3.15*. In The London Hospital series 14 cases were treated by the mould technique using radium needles and a 77% 5-year survival was achieved, but four cases required salvage surgery. With the iridium wire technique 13 cases were treated with a 100% survival (only one required subsequent surgery). There were no cases of stricture or necrosis. An update of this series is reported by El Demiry *et al.* (1985).

Although the 5-year survival figures were equally good in Newaishy and Deeley's series (1968), four cases developed urethral stricture. Similarly in the series reported by Duncan and Jackson (1972) there was a stricture and necrosis rate of 30%, most of whom required salvage surgery.

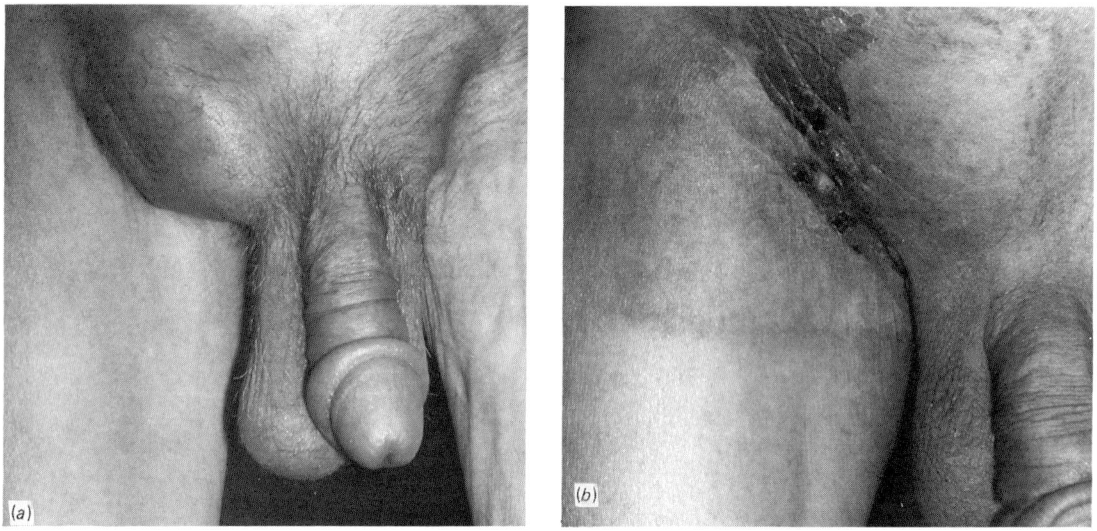

Figure 3.36 External irradiation and bleomycin for stage 4 carcinoma of the penis. *(a)* Before treatment, *(b)* after treatment

Table 3.15 Results of treating stage 1 carcinoma of the penis

		No. of cases	*5-year survival (%)*
Newaishy and Deeley (1968)	External irradiation	11	80
Duncan and Jackson (1972)	External irradiation	20	90 (3 years)
Hope-Stone (1975)	Mould radium and iridium	23	83
Salaverria **et al**. (1979)	Mould iridium only	13	100
Demiry **et al**. (1984)	Mould iridium only	23	84

Stage 2

In The London Hospital series there were nine cases — six treated by iridium mould and three by partial amputation, the 5-year survival figures being 83% (Salaverria *et al*., 1979).

Stage 3

In The London Hospital series, 10 patients were treated by radical amputation and three by irradiation and surgery — 80% survived 5 years.

In conclusion it would seem that the best results in early cases can be achieved with the iridium mould technique; this should be the treatment of choice and will still allow salvage surgery if failure occurs.

Queyrat's erythroplasia

This condition, which includes carcinomas *in situ* and Bowen's disease, is potentially malignant and should be treated as such. Mantell and Morgan (1969) described an elegant technique using a ^{90}Yt mould giving 1500 cGy in two treatments (separated by 1 week's gap). Unfortunately, this form of irradiation is not now available, therefore the iridium mould method should be considered, but giving a slightly lower dose (5000 cGy on the surface of the tumour).

Palliation for secondary carcinomas

If the penis if infiltrated by direct spread from the

bladder, rectum or prostate (*Figure 3.37*) deep X-ray therapy can be given with external irradiation and a wax block to give a dose of 4000 cGy in 3 weeks. The skin reaction is minimal and the result can be quite reasonable.

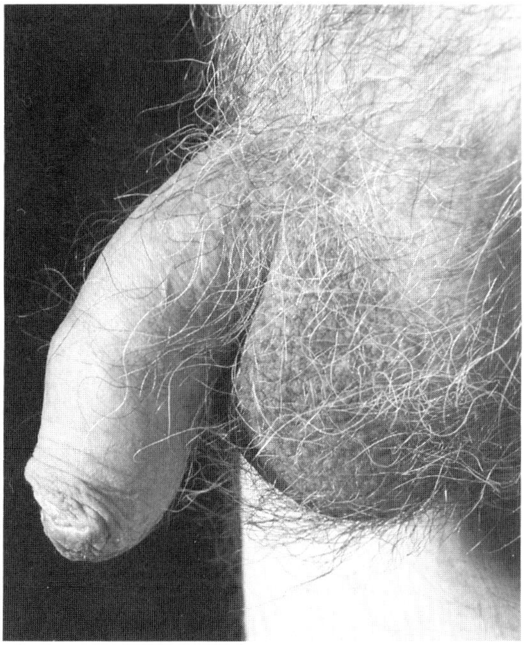

Figure 3.37 Secondary carcinoma of penile shaft — primary in the prostate

References

ASH, D.V., ANDREWS, B. and STUBBS, B. (1983) A method for intergrating computed tomography into radiotherapy planning and treatment. *Clinical Radiology*, **34**, 103–112

BACKHOUSE, T.W. (1979) A rotation technique for irradiation of the bladder and results obtained. *Clinical Radiology*, **30**, 259–262

BAGSHAW, M.A. (1979) External radiation therapy of carcinoma of the prostate. *Cancer*, **45**, 1912–1921

BAGSHAW, M.A., HENRY, M.D., KAPLAN, S. and SAGERMAN R.H. (1965) Linear accelerator supervoltage radiotherapy for carcinoma of the prostate. *Radiology*, **85**, 121–129

BARRETT, A., STREDONSKA, J., HENDRY, W.F. and PECKHAM, M.J. (1981) Fertility of patients with testicular tumours and the effects of treatment in germ cell tumours. In *Germ Cell Tumours*, edited by C.K. Anderson and W.G. Jones, pp. 395–398 London: Taylor and Francis

BLACKARD, C.E. and BYAR, D.P. (1972) Results of a clinical trial of surgery and radiotherapy in stage I of carcinoma of the bladder. *Journal of Urology*, **108**, 875–887

BLANDY, J.P. (1978a) *Operative Urology*. pp. 188–191. Oxford: Blackwell Scientific Publications

BLANDY, J.P. (1978b) *Operative Urology*. pp. 124–141. Oxford: Blackwell Scientific Publications

BLANDY, J.P., HOPE-STONE, H.F. and DAYAN, A.D. (1970) *Tumours of the Testicle*. London: Heinemann

BLOOM, H.J.G. (1971) Medroxyprogesterone acetate (Provera) in the treatment of metastatic renal cell carcinoma. *Cancer*, **25**, 250–265

BLOOM, H.J.G., (1981) Pre-operative immediate dose radiotherapy and cystectomy for deeply invasive carcinoma of the bladder: rationale and results. In *Bladder Cancer: Principles of Combination Therapy*, edited by R.T.S. Oliver, W.F. Hendry and H.J.G. Bloom, pp. 151–176. London: Butterworths

BLOOM, H.J.G., HENDRY, W.F., WALLACE, B.M. and STREET, R.G. (1982) Treatment of T3 bladder cancer — controlled trial of pre-operative radiotherapy and radical cystectomy versus radical radiotherapy. *British Journal of Urology* **54**, 136–151

BUDHRAJA, S.N. and ANDERSON, J.C. (1964) An assessment of the value of radiotherapy in the management of carcinoma of the prostate. *British Journal of Urology*, **36**, 535–540

BYAR, W.P. (1973) The Veterans Administration Cooperative Urological Research Group's studies of cancer of the prostate. *Cancer*, **22**, 1126–1131

BYAR, D.P. and MOSTOFI, F.K. (1972) Carcinoma of the prostate — prognostic evaluation of certain pathological features in 268 radical prostatectomies. *Cancer*, **30**, 5–13

CADE, I.S., MCEWEN, J.B., DISCHE, S. *et al.* (1978) Hyperbaric oxygen and radiotherapy: a Medical Research Council trial in carcinoma of the bladder. *British Journal of Radiology*, **51**, 876–878

CHAN, R.C. and GUTIERREZ A.E. (1977) Carcinoma of the prostate — its treatment by a combination of radioactive gold grains implant and external irradiation. *Cancer*, **37**, 2449–2454

DIX, V.W., SHANKS, W., TRESIDDER, G.C., BLANDY, J.P., HOPE-STONE, H.F. and SHEPHEARD R.G.F. (1970) Carcinoma of the bladder: treatment by diathermy snare incision and interstitial irradiation. *British Journal of Urology*, **42**, 213–228

DUNCAN, W. and JACKSON, S.M. (1972) The treatment of early cancer of the penis with megavoltage X-rays. *Clinical Radiology*, **23**, 246–248

EDSMYR, F. (1981) Radiotherapy in the management of bladder carcinoma. In *Bladder Cancer: Principles of Combination Therapy*, edited by R.T.D. Oliver, W.F. Hendry and H.J.G. Bloom, pp. 139–149. London: Butterworth

EINHORN, L.H. and DONOHUE, J.P. (1977) Improved chemotherapy in disseminated testicular cancer. *Journal of Urology*, **117**, 65–69

EL DEMIRY, M., OLIVER, R.T.S., HOPE-STONE, H.F. and BLANDY, J.P. (1985) A re-appraisal of the role of radiotherapy and surgery in the management of carcinoma of the penis. *Journal of Urology*, (in press)

ELLIS, F. (1968) The relationship of biological effect to dose time fractionation factors in radiotherapy. *Current Topics in Radiation Research*, **4**, 357–397

FINNEY, B. (1973) An evaluation of post-operative radiotherapy in hypernephroma treatment — a clinical trial. *Cancer*, **32**, 1332–1340

FITZPATRICK, R.J. and RIDER, W.D. (1976) Half body radiotherapy of advanced cancer. *Journal of Canadian*

Association of Radiologists, **272**, 75–79

FLOCKS, R.H. (1973) The treatment of stage C prostatic cancer with special reference to combined surgical and radiation therapy. *Journal of Urology*, **109**, 461–463

GOFFINET, D.R., SCHNEIDER, K.J. and GLASTEIN, E.S. (1975) Bladder cancer: results of radiation therapy in 384 patients. *Radiology*, **117**, 149-153

HAY, J.H., DUNCAN, W. and KERR, G.R. (1984) Subsequent malignancies in patients irradiated for testicular tumours. *British Journal of Radiology*, **57**, 597–602

HOPE-STONE, H.F. (1975) Carcinoma of the penis. *Proceedings of the Royal Society of Medicine*, **68**, 777–779

HOPE-STONE, H.F. (1977) Carcinoma of the penis. *British Journal of Sexual Medicine*, **3**, 13–17

HOPE-STONE, H.F. (1979) *Recent Results of Cancer Research*, edited by C. Bonadonna, C. Mathe and S.E. Salmon, Ch. 68, pp. 178–183. Berlin, Heidleberg, New York: Springer Verlag

HOPE-STONE, H.F. (1980) Clinical application of the R.T. 305. *Medicamundi*, **25**, 113–117

HOPE-STONE, H.F. (1981) The case for radiotherapy in early cases of malignant teratoma In *Germ Cell Tumours* edited by C.H. Anderson, W.G. Jones and A. Milford Ward, pp. 271–290. London: Taylor and Francis

HOPE-STONE, H.F. (1984) Radiotherapy for invasive bladder cancer. In *Bladder Cancer*, edited by P. Smith and G.R. Prout, pp. 203–222. London: Butterworth

HOPE-STONE, H.F. (1985) External radiation therapy for prostatic cancer. In *The Prostate*, edited by J.P. Blandy and B. Lytton. London: Butterworth

HOPE-STONE, H.F., BLANDY, J.P. and DAYAN, A.D. (1963) Treatment of tumours of the testicle. *British Medical Journal*, **1**, 984–989

HOPE-STONE, H.F., OLIVER, R.T.S., ENGLAND, H.R. and BLANDY, J.P. (1984) T3 bladder cancer. Salvage rather than elective cystectomy after radiotherapy. *Urology*, **24**, 315–320

HUBENER, K.H. and EIBACH, E. (1977) Strablentherapie des Nierenkarzinous—Untersuchungen und Ergenheisse. *Strablentherapie*, **153**, 726–732

HUSBAND, J.E. (1979) The role of CT in the management of testicular teratoma. *Clinical Radiology*, **30**, 243–252

HUSBAND, J.E. and HODSON, N.J. (1981) CT for staging and assessing response of bladder cancer to treatment. In *Bladder Cancer: Principles of Combination Therapy*, edited by R.T.D. Oliver, W.F. Hendry and H.J.G. Bloom, pp. 27–36. London: Butterworth

JACKSON, S.M. (1966) The treatment of carcinoma of the penis. *British Journal of Surgery*, **53**, 33–35

JOHNSON, D.E. (1982) Renal pelvis and ureteral tumours: an overview. In *GU tumours, fundamental principles and surgical techniques*, edited by D. Johnson and M. Boileau, pp. 353–370. New York: Grune and Stratton

KEDIA, K.D., MARKLAND, C. and FRAYLEY, E.E. (1977) Sexual function after high retroperitoneal lymphadenectomy. *Urology Clinics of North America*, **4**, 523–527

KELLET, M.J., OLIVER, R.T.A., HUSBAND, J.E. and KELSEY, F. (1980) CT as an adjunct to bimanual examination for staging bladder tumours. *British Journal of Urology*, **52**, 101–106

KIRK, J., WINGATE, G.W.H. and WATSON, E.R. (1976) High dose effects in the treatment of carcinoma of the bladder under air and hyperbaric oxygen conditions. *Clinical Radiology*, **27**, 137–144

KLEIN, F.H., WHITMORE, W.F., WOLF, R.M. *et al.* (1983) Presumptive downstaging from pre-operative irradiation for bladder cancer as determined by flow cytometry. *International Journal of Radiation Oncology, Biology and Physics*, **9**, 487-494

KUNKLER, F.B., FARR, N.F. and LUXTON, N.W. (1952) The limit of renal tolerance of X-rays. *British Journal of Radiology*, **25**, 190–200

LAING, A.H. and DICKINSON, K.M. (1965) Carcinoma of the bladder treated by supervoltage irradiation. *Clinical Radiology*, **16**, 154–164

LEWIS, L.G. (1948) Testes tumours — report on 250 cases. *Journal of Urology (Baltimore)*, **59**, 763–772

LLOYD-DAVIES, R.W., VINNICOMBE, J. and COLLINS, C.D. (1971) The treatment of localized prostatic carcinoma. *Clinical Radiology*, **22**, 230–236

LONDON AND OXFORD COOPERATIVE UROLOGICAL CANCER GROUP (1981) A clinical trial of methotrexate combined with radiotherapy in deep infiltrating T3 carcinoma of the bladder. In *Bladder Cancer: Principles of Combination Therapy*, edited by R.T.D. Oliver, W.F. Hendry and H.J.G. Bloom, pp. 239. London: Butterworth

McGOWAN, D.G. (1977) Radiation therapy in the management of localised carcinoma of the prostate. *Cancer*, **39**, 98–103

McLORIE, G.A. and SKINNER, D.G. (1980) Metastatic non-sarcomatous testis tumours — morbidity of treatment. *Journal of Urology*, **124**, 479–481

MAIER, J.G. (1977) Management of testicular carcinoma. Reported at *14th International Congress of Radiology*. Rio de Janeiro: Abstract no. 50243

MANTELL, B.S. and MORGAN, W.Y. (1969) Queyrat's erythroplasia of the penis treated by beta particles of irradiation. *British Journal of Radiology*, **42**, 855–857

MILLER, L.S. (1977) Bladder cancer. Superiority of pre-operative radiation and cystectomy in clinical stages B2 and C. *Cancer*, **39**, 973–980

MORRISON, R. (1975) The results of treatment of cancer of the bladder — a clinical contribution to radiobiology. *Clinical Radiology*, **26**, 67-75

MOSS, W.T. (1965) *The Urinary Bladder in Therapeutic Radiology*, p. 277. St Louis: C.V. Mosby Co.

NEWAISHY. G.A. and DEELEY, T.J. (1968) Radiotherapy in the treatment of carcinoma of the penis. *British Journal of Radiology*, **41**, 519–552

PECKHAM, M.J. (1982) Testes and epididymis. In *Treatment of Cancer*, edited by K. Halnan, pp. 501–527. London: Chapman and Hall

PECKHAM, M.J., BARRATT, K.H., LIEW, A. *et al.* (1983) The treatment of metastatic germ cell tumours with BEP. *British Journal of Cancer*, **47**, 613–619

PEELING, W.B., MANTELL, B.S. and SHEPHERD, B.G.F. (1969) Post-operative irradiation in the treatment of renal cell carcinomas. *British Journal of Urology*, **41**, 23–31

PENN, C. (1976) Single dose and fractionated palliative irradiation for osseous metastases. *Clinical Radiology*, **27**, 405–408

PISTENMA, D.A., BAGSHAW, M.A. and FREIHA, F.S. (1979) Extended field radiation therapy for prostatic carcinoma — status report of a limited prospective trial. *Cancer of the GU Tract*, edited by D.E. Johnson and M.L. Samuels, pp. 229–247. New York: Raven Press

RAY, G.R. and BAGSHAW, M.A. (1975) The role of radiation therapy in the definitive treatment of adenocarcinoma of the prostate. *Annual Review of Medicine*,

26, 567

READ, G. (1981) Lymphoma of the testis. Results of treatment 1960–1977. *Clinical Radiology*, **32**, 687–692

RESNICK, M.I., KAPUTSKA, E., HOLLAND, J.M. and GRAYHACK, J.T. (1977) Radiation therapy for carcinoma of the prostate: 5-year follow up. *Journal of Urology*, **117**, 214–215

RICHES, E.W., GRIFFITHS, I.H. and THACKERAY, A.C. (1951) New growths of the kidney and ureter. *British Journal of Urology*, **23**, 297–338

SALAVERRIA, J.C., HOPE-STONE, H.F., PARIS, A.M., MULLAND, E.A. and BLANDY, J.P. (1979) Conservative treatment of carcinoma of the penis. *British Journal of Urology*, **51**, 32–37

SHIPLEY, W. (1983) Radiation therapy for patients with testicular and extra gonadal seminoma. In *Testis Tumours*, edited by J.R. Donohue, pp. 224–231. Baltimore and London: William and Wilkins

SHIPLEY, W., DUTTENHAYER, J.R., PERONET VERHEY, L.J. *et al.* (1983) Protons or megavoltage X-rays as boost therapy for patients irradiated for localized prostatic carcinoma. *Cancer*, **51**, 1599–1604

STAUBITZ, W.J. (1974) Surgical management of testis tumour. *Journal of Urology*, **111**, 205-209

UICC (INTERNATIONAL UNION AGAINST CANCER) (1978) *TNM Classification of Malignant Tumours*, edited by M.H. Harmer. Geneva: UICC

WALLACE, D.M. and BLOOM, H.J.G. (1976) The management of deeply infiltrating (T3) bladder carcinoma: controlled trial of radical radiotherapy versus pre-operative radiotherapy and radical cystectomy. *British Journal of Urology*, **48**, 587–594

WERF-MESSING, B. VAN DER (1982a) Bladder. In **Treatment of Cancer**, edited by K. Halnan, p. 465. London: Chapman and Hall

WERF-MESSING, B. VAN DER (1982b) Kidney. In *Treatment of Cancer*, edited by K. Halnan, pp. 496–499. London: Chapman and Hall

WERF-MESSING, B. VAN DER, FRIEDELL, G.H., MENON, R.S. and HOP, W.C.J. (1981) The contribution of radiation therapy to the treatment of bladder cancer in Rotterdam. In **Proceedings of the 15th International Congress of Radiology**, Brussels

WERF-MESSING, B. VAN DER, HEAL, N.O. VAN DER, LEDEHORR, R.C. (1978) Renal cell carcinoma trials. *Cancer Clinical Trials*, **1**, 13–21

WHITMORE, W.F. (1979) Management of bladder cancer. In *Current Problems of Cancer*, edited by D. Hickey, pp. 3–48. Chicago: Year Book Medical Publications

WHITMORE, W.F. (1981) Pre-operative low dose radiotherapy and cystectomy. In *Bladder Cancer: Principles of Combination Therapy*, edited by R.T.D. Oliver, W.F. Hendry and H.J.G. Bloom, pp. 175–182. London: Butterworth

WILLIAMS, G., JONES, M.A., TROTT, P.A. and BLOOM, H.J.G. (1981) Carcinoma of the bladder treated by local interstitial irradiation. In *Bladder Cancer: Principles of Combination Therapy*, edited by R.T.D. Oliver, W.F. Hendry and H.J.G. Bloom, pp. 117-126. London: Butterworth

4

Breast Cancer

J. S. Tobias

Introduction

Breast cancer is the commonest cancer in women, and has an annual mortality rate in the UK of over 12 000. It is the major cause of death in middle-aged women of 35–55 years, and the average woman has a one in 14 chance of developing this illness. A number of aetiological agents have now been identified. Those with mothers or sisters affected by breast cancer are more likely to develop the disease. The disease varies geographically, and is commonest in North American and Northern European women with lower death rates in Eastern Europe, Japan and the Far East. In Japanese immigrants to the USA, the incidence gradually rises, suggesting environmental as well as genetic factors, although even after several generations, Japanese women still have a lower incidence than Caucasians (Kalache and Vessey, 1982). In the UK, there are marked variations in the mortality rate from breast cancer, with a lower death rate in the North of England and high rates in the Midlands and South-East (Gardner *et al.*, 1983). Nulliparous women, or those whose age of first pregnancy is over 20 years, also have a higher incidence. Previous radiation exposure has now been documented as an unequivocal factor since survivors of the Hiroshima bomb have an increase in the incidence rate which is dose-related, and grossly elevated when the incident dose was greater than 125 cGy (Tokunaga *et al.*, 1982). It has recently been claimed that prolonged use of some types of contraceptive pill (particularly those containing high levels of progestogen) may result in an increased incidence (Pike *et al.*, 1983), although other studies have refuted this suggestion. Reduction in indigenous oestrogen levels appears to protect against breast cancer as oophorectomy at an early age lowers its incidence. Interestingly, when breast cancer occurs in daughters of women who themselves suffered from the same illness, it characteristically appears at an earlier age than in the mother. Finally, although the possible protective role of breast feeding remains uncertain, there seems little doubt that in societies where infants are routinely breast fed, the incidence of breast cancer is lower than in more 'developed' countries. Screening methods, including mammography, thermography, or clinical examination by a doctor, nurse or the patient herself have so far failed to make any real impact on the incidence of invasive carcinoma or overall survival figures.

Pathology

The wide variability in histological appearance has led to a number of attempts at classifying these tumours according to their microscopic appearance (recently with the help of histochemical stains). Descriptive terms are often used, including *polygonal* cell carcinoma, *scirrhous* carcinoma (in which there is a marked fibrous stromal reaction), *comedo* carcinoma (with microscopic appearances suggestive of a small skin papule or blackhead), and *mucoid* carcinoma (with pronounced mucus formation). These terms are generally unhelpful since they have little bearing on prognosis. Important exceptions are first *inflammatory carcinoma* of the breast, which has a distinct microscopic and clinical appearance, with infiltration of subdermal lymphatics, and erythema and tenderness of the whole breast — this is a particularly aggressive form of disease, characterized by early local invasion and lymphatic involvement; and second, *medullary* carcinoma, a slow-growing tumour with intensive lymphocytic infiltration and a good prognosis.

Far more important is the histological *grade* of the

tumour, which is an important determinant of the ultimate outcome. Increase in cell size, pleomorphism, nuclear-cytoplasmic ratio and cellular pyknosis are all indications of a more malignant tumour. Other features, such as lymphocytic and histiocytic cell reaction to the tumour may also be important.

Staging

There have been a number of attempts to devise a simple staging system, and most of these classifications are based on the size of the primary tumour, the presence or absence of axillary node metastases by palpation and subsequently at operation, and the presence or absence of distant metastases. The Manchester classification was successful to the extent that it classified patients into three groups which had significantly different survival probabilities. However, this classification is proving increasingly limited because more detailed information has now been obtained, showing the prognostic importance of variables such as the size of primary tumour and the number of involved axillary lymph nodes. The TNM staging system proposed by the International Union Against Cancer (UICC) has become widely accepted for classifying tumours more accurately. Further modifications are likely, in order to take account of more detailed information regarding the pathological grade of the tumour, and its endocrine receptor status.

Hormone receptors in breast cancer

It is now well recognized that a proportion of breast cancers carry cellular receptors for oestrogen and other steroid hormones (including progestogen) both in their cell nuclei and also in the cytoplasm (McGuire, 1980). These are present in 65% of postmenopausal and 30% of premenopausal women. Hormone dependence of some breast cancers can be demonstrated clinically by alteration of the hormonal environment, and it now seems likely that a response to hormonal manipulation occurs only in patients whose tumours are receptor positive. It is not entirely clear whether oestrogen receptor (ER) status is a reflection of a genuine and fundamental difference between 'negative' and 'positive' breast cancers or whether there is a continuous distribution from ER-rich tumours to those with no detectable ERs whatever. The evidence at present favours the latter view, and ER 'positivity' is normally used to describe tumours in which the level of ER is greater than a certain defined figure, usually 5 fmole/mg cytoplasmic protein or 25 fmole/mg nuclear DNA. It seems that ER positivity is associated with well-differentiated and often slow-growing tumours. Both primary tumours and metastases show similar ER content, although ER-negative metastases are sometimes encountered from an ER-positive primary tumour. The reverse is rarely true.

Surgical operations for breast cancer

A good deal of controversy surrounds the choice of operation in patients with 'early' breast cancer (Fisher and Gebhardt, 1978). The classical operation of radical mastectomy, introduced by Halsted over 80 years ago, was designed to ensure local control by removing the breast, and as far as possible, all of the primary lymphatic routes of spread (Halsted, 1907) — an entirely logical approach at a time when lymphatic spread was thought to be of critical importance and dissemination via the blood stream largely unrecognized. In this procedure, the whole breast is removed, with division of the pectoralis minor muscle and complete dissection of the axillary contents. In order to achieve a complete clearance, the surgical incision is large, and the loss of contour very considerable, involving loss of far more soft tissue then the breast itself. There is no doubt that an excellent probability of local control is achieved by radical mastectomy, even in patients with axillary node involvement. However, with increased understanding that patients with breast cancer die not from uncontrolled local disease but from distant blood-borne metastases, there has been an increasing tendency to offer less mutilating procedures, although radical operation still has many proponents. Indeed, radical mastectomy has been performed with increasing frequency over the past decade as a means of obtaining detailed information as to the degree of local invasion and axillary lymph node involvement.

Although Urban and Castro (1971) and others have claimed high survival rates from radical operations in patients with small tumours without axillary node involvement, many British surgeons now favour a more conservative approach, using the 'total mastectomy' (essentially a simple mastectomy plus axillary dissection, with preservation of the pectoralis minor), which was originally described by Patey. The advantage of this operation is that there is less surgical mutilation with better preservation of contour and often better mobility of the shoulder. More conservative still was the approach favoured by McWhirter in Edinburgh (McWhirter, 1955), in which simple mastectomy without full axillary dissection was followed by postoperative radiotherapy to local nodal drainage areas (*see below*). All of these procedures give comparable survival rates (*Table 4.1*), and there is little if any evidence that survival rates depend on the operation itself, providing that local control is ensured. Inflammatory carcinoma should never be treated by mastectomy alone because of its locally advanced nature and poor prognosis.

Table 4.1 Randomized studies of simple or radical mastectomy with or without postoperative radiotherapy (modified from Henderson and Canellos, 1980)

Study centre	*Treatment*	*Survival (%)* *Radiotherapy*	*No radiotherapy*
Oslo	RM + oophorectomy	72 86*	70
Stockholm	RM	77	73
Manchester	RM SM oophorectomy	44 70 38	46 68+ 53‡
NSABP	RM SM	56 81	62 78+
CRC	SM	77	72‡

NSABP: National Surgical Adjuvant Breast Project (USA)
RM: radical mastectomy
SM: simple mastectomy
+: Stage I patients
‡: Stage II patients
* Patients treated with megavoltage postoperative radiotherapy

Role of radiotherapy in the management of breast cancer

Although breast cancer was one of the earliest malignant diseases to be treated by radium (Pfahler, 1932), the precise role of radiotherapy in the management of carcinoma of the breast has emerged slowly, and continues to evolve. Despite the undoubted radiosensitivity of breast cancer as typified by the common clinical observation of regression of large locally extensive tumours, the exact role of radiotherapy remains highly contentious, particularly since the increasing use of radiotherapy as an alternative to mastectomy. It is fair to say that the management of 'early', i.e. operable, carcinoma of the breast has become one of the most controversial issues in cancer medicine today.

It seems scarcely possible that despite the use of both radical surgery and radiotherapy stretching back almost a century, the claims of these two quite different methods of local treatment for breast cancer are still so vigorously argued. Part of the explanation lies in the complex history of these treatments (*Figure 4.1*) which reflects both the current surgical and biological philosophies of the day and also the technical limitations of radiotherapy equipment. Even now, the importance of technical details such as the radiation tolerance of the breast (both early and late), optimal fractionation and dose, avoidance of overdosing at matchlines, and integration of radiotherapy, conservative surgical procedures, chemotherapy and hormone therapy remain poorly explored.

Broadly speaking, radiotherapy has been used in three distinct clinical situations. First and most frequently, as an addition to surgical treatment (usually some form of mastectomy), particularly where lymph node sampling has confirmed the presence of metastatic axillary lymph nodes but formal axillary lymph node dissection has not been undertaken; second, as the definitive local procedure in patients who undergo conservative surgery, or where there is extensive local tumour felt to be inoperable; and third, for recurrent disease either at the primary site or elsewhere, particularly if bone or brain metastases are causing disabling symptoms.

Postoperative radiotherapy following mastectomy

The philosophy underlying choice of local therapy has altered gradually over the past 50 years. Attitudes are now very different from those which prevailed at the time when Halsted designed his radical mastectomy operation (Tobias and Peckham, 1985). Radical mastectomy rapidly gained acceptance because of the relatively low rate of local recurrence (Halsted, 1907) and also as a result of wide acceptance of the hypothesis of tumour dissemination first suggested by Handley. His view was that breast cancer, in general, spread contiguously and in a centrifugal fashion, chiefly by direct and lymphatic invasion, involving axillary, internal mammary and

	Developments in radiotherapy	*Developments in surgery*
c 1895	Discovery of X-rays by Röntgen and radium by Curie	Radical mastectomy designed by Halsted
1910	Early development of diagnostic radiology and orthovoltage irradiation	Publication of results of radical mastectomy
1920	Interstitial therapy with radium needles starting to be practised	Increasing tendency to less radical surgical procedures
1930	Publication of early results and comparisons with surgical series	
1940	Development of megavoltage beams (^{60}Co)	McWhirter's approachy recognized and results of combinations of surgical and radio-therapeutic treatments
1950	Further technical developments including introduction of linear accelerators and combinations of	starting to be published. Patey mastectomy assessed.
1960	external and interstitial irradiation	
1970–80	Increasing use of combinations of simple mastectomy and postoperative irradiation with tendency to more conservative surgery	

Figure 4.1 History of radiotherapy and surgery of breast cancer

supraclavicular lymph nodes at a relatively early stage. Wide surgical excision of the whole of these lymph node groups, in continuity with removal of the primary cancer, would therefore be expected to eradicate the disease far more commonly than a less aggressive surgical procedure. It was not until the Second World War that this concept was seriously challenged, in favour of the now well established view that blood-borne metastases occur independently of lymphatic invasion and are usually present (although frequently undectable) at the time of diagnosis. It is also accepted that patients with obvious axillary lymph node involvement are particularly likely to be harbouring haematogenous metastases in other parts of the body. Most would agree that the more recent 'systemic' concept of breast cancer fits the observed facts more closely than the Halsted/Handley hypothesis, although it remains possible that occult metastases result from tumour cells dislodged into the circulation at the time of the initial surgery, rather than developing at the earliest stage of the disease.

It is not surprising that the question of whether or not patients with early breast cancer should be offered routine postoperative radiotherapy has become more contentious in recent years. Surgical techniques have themselves been evolving over the same period, quite apart from an increasing interest in the possible roles of early ('adjuvant') chemotherapy and hormone treatment as part of the initial treatment of the tumour. Patients in whom local irradiation after mastectomy might be beneficial clearly include those in whom residual loco-regional disease has been left postoperatively, although without evidence of more widespread metastatic disease. This group would include patients in whom primary resection was complete (usually a straightforward surgical task), but in whom the local lymph node chains had not been fully excised. Since microscopic involvement of internal mammary, supraclavicular and axillary nodes is common but surgical removal of all of these node groups is impossible, this group of patients might not be as uncommon as has usually been believed. For these patients, the addition of a further local therapy such as radiotherapy might offer a better chance of local control and thereby perhaps an improved chance of survival. The difficulty of course is that since positive axillary nodes are closely associated with the risk of distant metastases (Nemoto *et al.*, 1980), additional local treatment is unlikely to affect survival in the majority of patients. However, to attack the use of postoperative irradiation on these grounds is to misunderstand the purpose of the treatment since it is neither the intention nor expectation of the radiotherapist that survival will be prolonged by a further local procedure. The realistic but more modest aim is to increase the chance of local control in a group of patients with a high risk of local recurrence following surgery alone.

There is no longer any doubt that postoperative irradiation will substantially reduce the incidence of local recurrence in patients who have undergone any type of mastectomy other than radical mastectomy with formal axillary dissection, and in whom positive axillary lymph nodes have been identified. Patients who have undergone a radical mastectomy have an extremely low risk of local recurrence even without postoperative irradiation (Haagensen *et al.*, 1969) and this low risk, coupled with the high incidence of lymphoedema when radical surgery is followed by radical radiotherapy, makes radiotherapy inadvisable under these circumstances. The situation is very different in patients who have undergone less radical surgical procedures. McWhirter, in a large series of patients treated in Edinburgh, demonstrated that simple mastectomy with local radiotherapy to lymph node drainage areas was as effective a means of local control as the routine use of more radical surgery (McWhirter, 1955). A prospective controlled study of over 500 patients with operable breast cancer was performed by Kaae and Johansen (1977), who offered their patients either extended radical mastectomy or simple mastectomy with postoperative irradiation. After 15 years of follow-up there were no discernable differences either in local recurrence rate, likelihood of distant metastases, or crude survival rate (*Figure 4.2*), although the probability of lymphoedema and weakness of the arm was substantially greater in the patients undergoing radical mastectomy.

Two other important prospectively randomized studies have confirmed the value of postoperative irradiation in patients undergoing mastectomy, as well as clarifying the indications for its use. In the first of these, over 1000 patients were treated at a single centre, either by radical mastectomy alone, or by the same operative procedure followed by local irradiation (Host and Brennhovd, 1977). As expected, the number of local recurrences was low in both groups (39 local chest wall recurrences out of 542 patients undergoing surgery alone, and 23 recurrences out of 548 patients undergoing combined treatment) so there was no discernable improvement in local control with irradiation. However, there was a clear difference in regional node recurrence in the axilla or supraclavicular fossa, particularly evident in patients with stage II disease. The authors also noted a small increase in survival when radical surgery was routinely followed by *megavoltage* irradiation, as was practised in the second half of the study, suggesting that there might be a small group of patients with loco-regional disease, without distant metastases, who could be cured by radical postoperative radiotherapy. This slight survival advantage was not, however, observed in a prospective study of similar design carried out in Manchester (Lythgoe, Leck and Swindell, 1978), although once again there was a clear-cut reduction in the incidence of local recurrence.

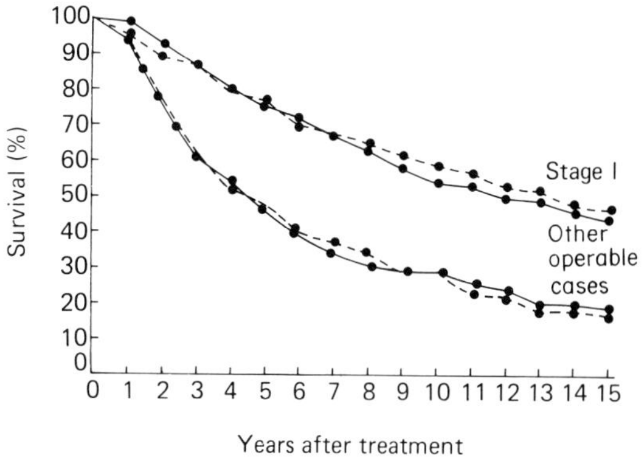

Figure 4.2 Crude survival ratios. NB— Other operable cases includes patients with axillary node-positive disease deemed suitable for mastectomy. (---) Extended radical mastectomy; (—) simple mastectomy. (From Kaae and Johansen, 1977 courtesy of the Editor and Publisher *International Journal of Radiation Oncology, Biology and Physics*)

With the increasing popularity of simple or Patey mastectomy as the initial surgical procedure, doubts began to emerge regarding the desirability of routine postoperative irradiation. It was felt that it might perhaps be unnecessary for local control, and also that it might possibly be harmful since regional lymph nodes which had successfully destroyed cancer cells could be playing an important part in maintaining systemic immunity. For these reasons, a prospective study was carried out in the UK, in which patients were randomized to undergo treatment either by simple mastectomy alone or by the same operation with immediate postoperative irradiation (Cancer Research Campaign Working Party, 1980). Of the 2800 patients with 'early' breast cancer (clinical stages I or II), over 2200 were evaluable. A modest dose of postoperative irradiation was employed — 3250 cGy in 15 fractions in 3 weeks to 4600 cGy in 30 fractions in 6 weeks for orthovoltage treatment, with a 10% increase in dose for megavoltage. At the tenth year of follow-up, there were no major differences either in the likelihood of metastases or in crude survival although there was an impressive difference (11% vs 30% at 10 years) in the risk of local recurrence (*Figure 4.3a, b*). At both 5 and 10 years after mastectomy, the likelihood of local recurrence was some three times greater in patients undergoing surgery alone, and an analysis of the small number of patients in the irradiated group who developed a local recurrence revealed no evidence of an increased risk even if the radiation dose was relatively low. This suggested that the recommended dose regimen was more than adequate, and that nothing more was to be gained by increasing the radiation dosage still further — a welcome result since radiation-induced side-effects are closely related to dose. The study also provided data on the probability of local recurrence in axillary node-negative patients who are generally assumed to be at low risk and therefore unsuitable for radiotherapy. In these node-negative patients, the risk of local recurrence was relatively high if the tumour was large or of a high grade, making post-operative irradiation a worthwhile consideration (Elston *et al.*, 1982).

Although a difference in local recurrence rate might have been predicted from previous uncontrolled studies and from the Manchester analysis of radical mastectomy with and without irradiation, the magnitude of the difference at 10 years was surprising, and the results of this study have aroused considerable debate. One view has been that, despite the obvious improvement in local control, radiotherapy should not be routinely offered to patients who have undergone simple mastectomy, as local irradiation is usually effective for local recurrence, and to delay such treatment until necessary does not appear to jeopardize survival. On the other hand, this approach places considerable reliance on radiotherapy as a locally curative procedure in patients who do develop overt local recurrence — about 30% in the first 10 years of the Cancer Research Campaign trial (CRC). Moreover, local recurrence is always unpleasant, often highly offensive to the patient and her family, often difficult to disguise and responsive to radiotherapy in no more than three-quarters of cases (Zimmerman, Montague and Fletcher, 1966). If routine postoperative irradiation in axillary node-positive patients were to be discontinued, this would leave a substantial group in whom local recurrence — only partly responsive to radiation treament — might become a dominant and sometimes untreatable problem.

Only the Oslo study (Host and Brennhovd, 1977) has shown a *survival* advantage from postoperative irradiation (the 5-year survival was increased from 70% to 86%) although further follow-up data are clearly required since this should be regarded as a

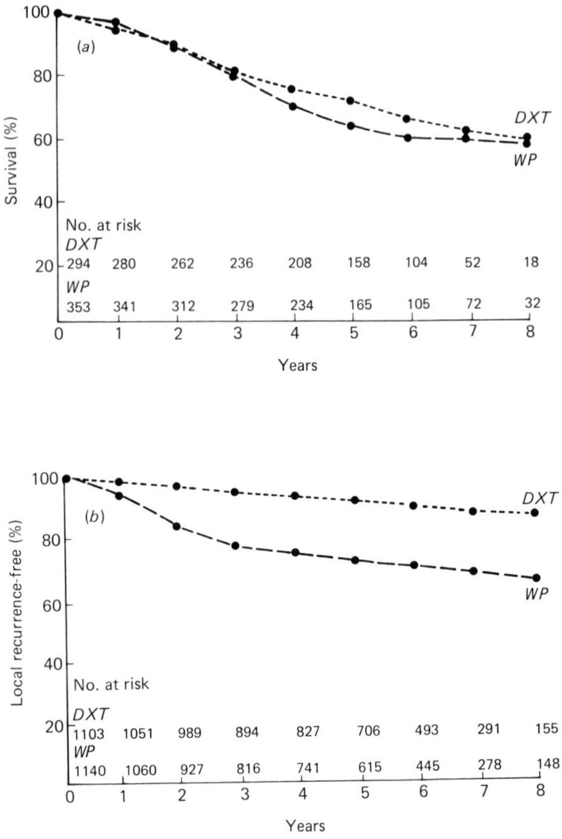

Figure 4.3 (*a*) Survival (*b*) local recurrence in patients undergoing simple mastectomy alone (WP) or with local irradiation (DXT) in patients with early breast cancer. (From Cancer Research Campaign Working Party, 1980 courtesy of the Editor and Publisher *The Lancet*)

relatively short-term result. In the remainder of the randomized trials, no survival advantage or disdvantage from adjuvant postoperative irradiation has yet been demonstrated (*see Table 4.1*), although a bold attempt was made by Stjernsward (1974) to suggest that when all these data were pooled together, a statistically significant *reduction* in survival became evident in the irradiated group — a claim later shown to be unfounded because of serious flaws in his statistical technique (Levitt and McHugh, 1975). The general view at present is that the major competing local methods of treatment for 'operable' breast cancer all give a similar survival figure, with 60–70% of all patients alive at 5 years (*Table 4.2*) and without any obvious advantage for the most radical forms of mastectomy. Now that simple mastectomy with partial axillary dissection has become the most commonly performed operation in the UK, the proportion of patients referred for radiotherapy is rising, as this operation cannot be expected to give such low

Table 4.2 Five-year survival rates following surgical and radiotherapeutic approaches in breast cancer. (From Pierquin, Baillet and Wilson (1976), *American Journal of Roentgenology*, **127**, 645–648, **with kind permission)**

Treatment	*Five-year survival*
Extended radical surgery (Handley)	67
Radical surgery (Halsted)	69
Mastectomy plus axillary dissection (Patey)	67
Simple mastectomy plus irradiation (McWhirter)	66
Radiotherapy alone (or after tumourectomy)	74

local recurrence rate as a radical mastectomy. It follows that simple mastectomy has become more acceptable to many surgeons because of an increasing confidence in postoperative radiotherapy as a means of sterilizing loco-regional disease.

Despite this broad agreement, the position is by no means clear, particularly since the emergence of adjuvant chemotherapy (*see below*). This has paradoxically led to a resurgence of interest in radical mastectomy as detailed information on the state of the axillary contents is often considered essential for deciding whether or not such treatment should be given. Since radical surgery offers good local control for most patients, radiotherapy is not usually recommended in these cases, particularly as the combined use of both radical surgery and intensive radiotherapy leads to an unacceptably high complication rate, in particular from lymphoedema of the arm. The degree of disagreement surrounding the possible contribution of local irradiation as an adjuvant to mastectomy is best illustrated by two recent leading articles in authoritative British and American Journals.

> 'Until chemotherapy has proved itself in the treatment of regional disease and until (and indeed, if) radiotherapy can be shown to be harmful, the complete radical and regional treatment for patients with breast cancer and affected axillary lymph nodes still requires postoperative radiotherapy'
>
> (*British Medical Journal*, 1981).

> 'Ethical considerations require that physicians be willing at some point to call a halt to a procedure (i.e. postoperative irradiation for breast cancer) that has shown little or no benefit in well conducted clinical trials, that will be almost impossible to test adequately even if new techniques for delivery of radiation therapy become available, that will be predicted to fail according to common theory, and in which new risks have become apparent'
>
> (Lipsett, 1981).

In summary, postoperative radiotherapy is of proven value as a means of preventing local recurrence in patients with positive axillary lymph nodes, who have undergone simple or extended mastectomy but without full axillary dissection. This group of patients is known to be at high risk from local recurrence, approaching 30% at 10 years for patients who have undergone simple mastectomy alone. Postoperative irradiation is also indicated in patients with clinical stage II disease in whom there has been no attempt to clear or even sample the axilla. In patients where the axilla is clinically normal, or in those who have undergone axillary sampling with negative results, routine adjuvant irradiation is not usually recommended. Although unnecessary in the majority of these patients, those with large or high grade primary tumours appear to be at increased risk of local recurrence (Elston *et al.*, 1982), and should perhaps be considered for such treatment. Although a major re-evaluation of postoperative irradiation has become necessary because of the increasing use of adjuvant chemotherapy and/or hormone therapy, most clinicians would regard such approaches as a means of attempting control of distant micrometastases rather than part of the local treatment. Despite the general view that survival is unaltered by the addition of local irradiation, a single study (Host and Brennhovd, 1977) has suggested that there may be a survival advantage providing a high dose of megavoltage irradiation is employed.

Radiation technique

For irradiation of the chest wall and axilla following mastectomy, most radiotherapists prefer to use megavoltage rather than orthovoltage treatment, employing telecobalt apparatus or a linear accelerator of 4–10 MeV energy. Although treatment to ipsilateral internal mammary and supraclavicular node chains is widely practised, there are few data to justify routine treatment of these areas, and some authors limit the postoperative treatment to the skin

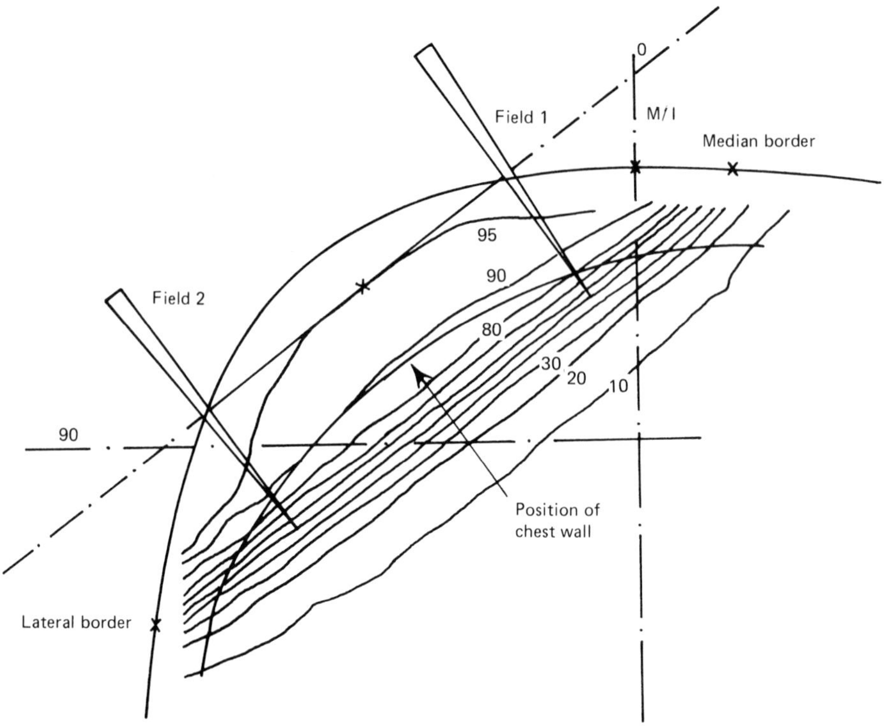

Figure 4.4 (*a*) Use of two wedged fields to irradiate chest wall, axilla and internal mammary node chain in patients who have undergone mastectomy

flaps (including of course the whole of the mastectomy scar) and axilla. With megavoltage equipment the skin reaction is much less intense than with orthovoltage apparatus and treatment to a dose of 4600–5000 cGy modal chest wall dose in 23–25 daily fractions of 200 cGy (i.e. total treatment period 4–5 weeks) can usually be achieved without difficulty, although doses are conventionally 10% lower when orthovoltage equipment is employed. Bolus has often been used routinely, to ensure an adequate dose to the skin, but it is nowadays not generally recommended although some authorities prefer to use bolus over the mastectomy scar, where local recurrence is so frequent. Use of bolus certainly leads to a higher incidence of late skin change, particularly telangiectasia.

The chest wall can usually be encompassed adequately by two tangential wedged fields (*Figure 4.4*) positioned obliquely with respect to the chest wall. Although a good distribution can often be achieved with a parallel opposed pair of fields, it is sometimes necessary to alter the angle slightly, in order to avoid overtreatment of underlying lung. Typical fields sizes are 20–22 cm long × 15 cm wide, and care must be taken to treat the whole of the mastectomy scar and chest wall down to the level of the inframammary fold of the opposite breast. The posterior border of the treatment volume is situated at the level of the posterior axillary fold, and medially the fields cross the midline by 2–3 cm if the ipsilateral internal mammary nodes are to be included in the treatment volume. Superiorly, the volume is limited by the clavicle.

Using two large obliquely situated wedged fields, the whole of the axilla can be encompassed provided the patient abducts the arm in either a horizontal or vertical direction, using an arm support for comfort. In order to ensure precision in treatment planning, the patient's body contour must be obtained at the central axis midpoint, enabling the radiotherapist to choose an adequate treatment volume in the usual way. Ideally, both fields should be treated each day. If the supraclavicular fossa is to be routinely treated (as is the practice of the present author), the simplest approach is to use a direct anterior field whose inferior border abuts onto the superior border of the tangential chest wall field, extending superiorly as far as the level of the hyoid bone in order to treat the whole of the supraclavicular contents and lower cervical nodes. Medially, the field should be limited by the sternomastoid muscle in order to avoid irradiation of the larynx and pharynx, and a gantry twist of

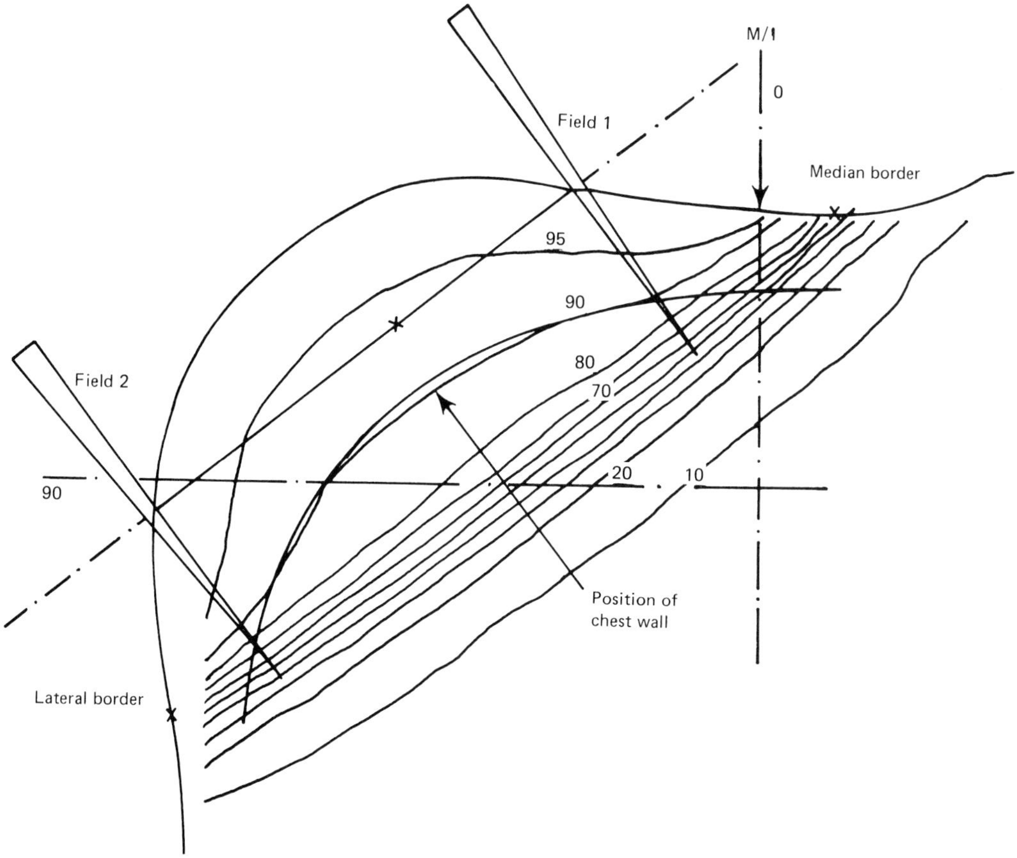

Figure 4.4 (*b*) In patients undergoing radical radiotherapy without mastectomy, a similar technique can be employed. In both instances a portion of lung is unavoidably irradiated. (M/l — midline)

15° contralaterally will prevent over-irradiation of the spinal cord. Using this technique, a dose of 4600–5000 cGy (applied dose) can be given without difficulty, in 23–25 daily fractions of 200 cGy.

If the patient has obvious palpable axillary lymphadenopathy, an additional boost can be given to the axilla applying a small direct field (typical field size 5 × 7 cm) using short distance cobalt apparatus, electron therapy or telecaesium, to an additional applied dose of 1000 cGy given over 1 week (five daily treatments). Where departmental pressures make daily fractionation difficult, a reasonable treatment alternative would be to offer 4000 cGy in 10 fractions over 4 weeks, treating either two or three times a week. Although a higher incidence of late skin changes are to be expected with non-daily fractionation, this is of less importance in a patient who has undergone mastectomy than in patients in whom radical irradiation (without mastectomy) is the primary approach to treatment (*see below*).

Radical radiotherapy: an alternative to mastectomy?

Until recently, the use of radical radiotherapy with minimal surgery (either wide local excision, 'tylectomy', excision biopsy or even no surgery whatever) was considered only when the tumour was so hopelessly advanced that surgery was felt to be unwise, or if there were obvious distant metastases at diagnosis, or where the patient adamantly refused a mastectomy. However, the possibility of treating breast cancer by radiation therapy rather than mastectomy has become one of the most hotly debated questions in cancer medicine today, creating considerable technical challenges for the radiotherapist. This increased interest in primary treatment with radiotherapy has been stimulated by the realization that patients with breast cancer have a similar survival expectancy regardless of the extensiveness of the initial operation, and that almost all deaths from breast cancer are due to distant metastases rather than recurrence in the breast itself. Assessing the results of mastectomy after a 25-year follow-up period, Brinkley and Haybittle (1975) came to the conclusion that over 70% of all women with so-called 'early' breast cancer died of their disease, despite an attempt at cure by mastectomy (*Figure 4.5*). In 704 cases, after 20 years there was an increased death rate (×16) compared to the normal population. These data reinforce the sparse information from studies of untreated patients with breast cancer (Bloom, Richardson and Harries, 1962) which suggests that the impact of treatment on survival is small (*Figure 4.6*).

Early pioneers in France, the UK and the USA were attempting to offer curative radiotherapy for breast cancer during the first years of this century. For the most part, these were patients with advanced local disease although it rapidly became apparent that durable local control could sometimes be obtained by fractionating a high dose of radiotherapy over a lengthy period (Baclesse, 1949). In 1924 Keynes began work at St Bartholomew's Hospital, London, using interstitial radium needles, and usually with no attempt at surgical removal of the tumour. In 1937 he published his results in a series of 250 patients, and demonstrated that there was no difference between the results of his treatment and the standard surgical approach (Keynes, 1937). He also pointed out, with considerable force, the potential advantages of breast conservation, realizing both the psychological advantages and also the fear of mastectomy which deterred women with breast cancer from seeking early advice.

He was intuitively disinclined to accept the hypothesis laid down by Halsted in 1907 and followed by most other leading surgeons as if it had been written on tablets of stone:

> 'We believe that cancer of the breast in spreading centrifugally preserves in the main continuity with the original growth and, before involving the viscera may become widely diffused along surface planes'
>
> (Halsted 1907).

Keynes later wrote:

> 'I had been brought up on a trust in radical surgery based on Halsted's work and Handley's theory of "centrifugal permeation", but when I read Handley's book carefully I was greatly relieved and excited by discovering that the theory had been formulated by a distinguished surgeon who was rather old-fashioned in his ideas ... his concept proved to be based entirely on fallacies and could be disregarded. I was excited because, although I had done the radical operation a number of times, I hated the practice of such barbarous mutilation of the female body and was delighted to find further evidence against its

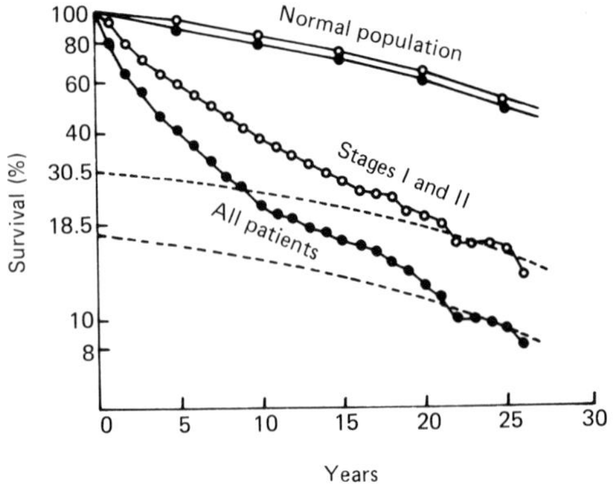

Figure 4.5 Actuarial survival rates in 704 cases of breast cancer compared with the expected survival of normal populations of the same age distribution. Logarithmic scale. Parallel lines indicate normal populations. Interrupted lines show extrapolation back to zero time of the portion of curves which are roughly parallel to the corresponding normal population. The intercepts on the vertical axis indicate the size of the cured group. (From Brinkley and Haybittle, 1975 courtesy of the Editor and Publisher *The Lancet*)

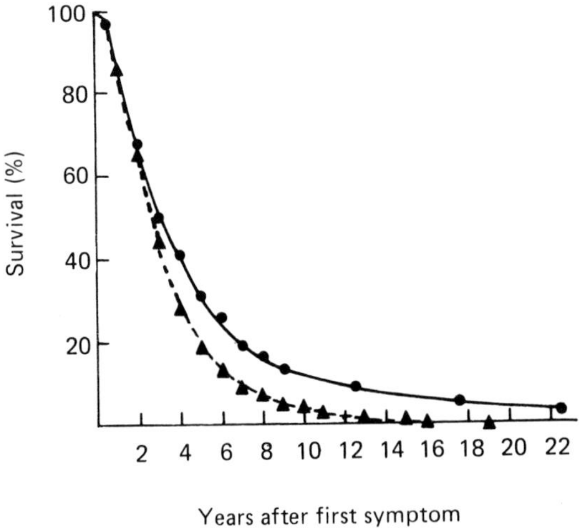

Figure 4.6 Life tables for patients with breast cancer. ▲ Untreated patients (Middlesex Hospital, 1805–1933); • patients treated with radical mastectomy (Johns Hopkins Hospital, 1889–1931). (Reprinted from Henderson and Canellos, *New England Journal of Medicine*, **302**, 17–30, 78–90, by permission)

performance ... I would tell my friends (not too seriously) that it was obvious that when the diagnosis was made the radical mastectomy was either too late or unnecessary, according to whether metastases had taken place or not; a deliberately foolish oversimplification, but nevertheless having some element of truth'

(Keynes, 1981).

By 1949, Baclesse had determined that the tumour size was a critically important determinant of radiosensitivity, and that advanced tumours with either ulceration or *peau d'orange* were much less likely to be controlled by radiation. These observations have now been extended (Timothy *et al.*, 1979) and the radiosensitivity of tumours of different sizes can now be predicted with considerable accuracy (*Figure 4.7*).

More recently, a number of additional studies, some with substantial periods of follow-up, have provided further evidence for the effectiveness of radical radiotherapy with minimal or no surgery. Peters (1975) reported a lifetime's experience of radical radiotherapy for breast cancer in which a study group of 145 patients treated by local excision and radiotherapy were retrospectively compared to a matched group of patients who had undergone mastectomy with postoperative irradiation, with careful selection for equivalence of prognostic features (age, stage and grade of tumour). In most cases the surgery performed had been a radical mastectomy. Careful 30-year follow-up showed no difference in survival between the two groups of patients. Pierquin, Baillet and Wilson (1976) reported results from six large cancer centres in France, all using radiotherapy alone (or with lumpectomy as the only surgical procedure) in the treatment of 'operable' breast cancer, and demonstrating that at 5 years after treatment, the local recurrence rate was low, although clearly (as predicted by Baclesse) related to the tumour size (*Table 4.3*). It was later shown that in patients who did suffer a local relapse, post-irradiation 'salvage' mastectomy could still be performed safely, thereby achieving local control. Unfortunately, when mastectomy was performed for suspected local recurrence, about one-third of the mastectomy specimens proved histologically negative — the 'recurrence' being due to a combination of scarring within the primary tumour coupled with irradiation fibrosis of the breat itself.

The largest series of patients so far reported has been that of Calle and his colleauges at the Institut Curie in Paris (Calle, 1985). Starting in 1960, this group has now treated over 1200 patients (268 by 'lumpectomy' (excision biopsy) followed by radical irradiation, and 1012 treated by radiotherapy alone). In general, small tumours (less than 3 cm) were treated by excision biopsy and external irradiation, larger tumours being treated by a higher dose of irradiation but without excision biopsy (*Figure 4.8*). Following a 'basal' dose of 5000 cGy given in 30 daily fractions over 6 weeks, the tumour bed and axilla were irradiated to a higher dose, the details depending on whether or not an excision biopsy had been performed (Calle *et al.*, 1978). The patients were treated almost entirely by external irradiation using telecolbalt apparatus, chiefly with a three field technique essentially similar to the approach described above (*see Figure 4.4*). Despite the fact that over 1000 of the 1280 patients had tumours measured at greater than 3 cm, the overall results were impressive (*Table 4.4*). In an interesting com-

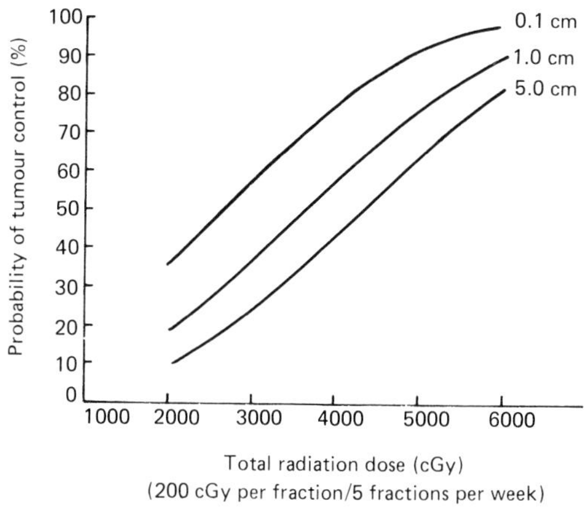

Figure 4.7 Dose–response curve for control of breast cancer in relation to tumour size. (From Timothy *et al.*, 1979 courtesy of the Editor and Publisher *The Lancet*)

Table 4.3 Pooled results for six European centres employing radical irradiation for operable breast cancer, showing local recurrences and survival rates.(From Pierquin, Baillet and Wilson (1976) *American Journal of Roentgenology* **127**, 645–648, **with kind permission)**

Clinical stage	*Three years*	*Five years*
Local recurrences		
T1	2/36	0/13
T2	1/72	0/21
T3	7/40	2/14
Total	10/148	2/48
Survival rates		
T1	34/36	12/13
T2	64/72	18/21
T3	31/40	7/14
Total	129/148	37/48

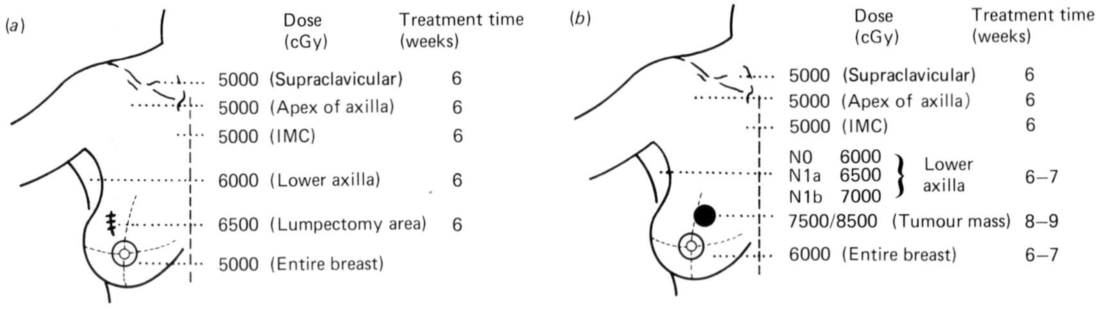

Figure 4.8 Radiation doses given by external cobalt beam therapy in patients treated by (*a*) lumpectomy followed by radiotherapy, for tumours less than 3 cm, or (*b*) radiation alone for tumours greater than 3 cm. IMC: internal mammary chain (From Calle *et al.*, 1978 courtesy of the Editor and Publisher *Cancer*)

parison with 10 year follow-up data from the Memorial Sloan Kettering Cancer Institute, New York, where treatment was chiefly by radical surgery, Calle demonstrated that his survival results at 10 years were identical (*Table 4.5*), although the approach to management could hardly have been more different. The major problem in interpreting Calle's data concerns the disparity between the results of lumpectomy plus irradiation for small tumours and irradiation *without* lumpectomy for larger tumours, with 10 year disease-free survival rates of 80% and 50% respectively. Is this difference due solely to the difference in size of the primary tumour, or were patients who were not subjected to any surgery whatever at an additional disadvantage because the primary tumour was left *in situ?*

This question has partly been answered by data from Hellman's group at Harvard, who have analysed their local failures following breast conserving radiotherapy (Harris, Levene and Hellman,

Table 4.4 Radical radiotherapy for breast cancer: results of treatment with external irradiation at the Curie Institute (From Calle, 1985)

	Number of cases	*Alive NED*	*Alive NED with breasts preserved*
Lumpectomy + radical radiotherapy, for small tumours (<3 cm)			
5 years	268	240/268 (90%)	226/240 (94%)
10 years	156	125/156 (80%)	111/125 (89%)
Radical radiotherapy alone, for tumours >3 cm			
5 years	1012	710/1012 (70%)	341/710 (48%)
10 years	511	257/511 (50%)	127/257 (49%)

NED: no evidence of disease

Table 4.5 Operable breast cancer – comparison of surgical and radiotherapeutic results at 10 years (From Calle *et al.* (1978) *Cancer*, **42**, 2045–2051, **with kind permission)**

	Memorial Hospital		*Fondation Curie*	
	Number of cases	*Alive NED*	*Number of cases*	*Alive NED*
T1, N0N1a	66	59 (89%)	40	36(90%)
T2N0, T1/T2, N1b	176	92(52%)	129	69(53%)
T3N0, T3N1b	62	18(29%)	89	27(30%)
Total	304	169(55%)	258	132(51%)

NED = No evidence of disease

Table 4.6 Local recurrence related to biopsy procedure and interstitial implantation.From Harris, Levene and Hellman (1978) The role of radiation therapy in the primary treatment of cancer of the breast. *Seminars in Oncology*, **5**, 403–416, **published by Grune & Stratton, by permission)**

	Implantation	*No implantation*	*Total*
Excisional biopsy	0/24	4/94	4/118
Less than excisional biopsy	0/8	3/9	3/17
Total	0/32	7/103	7/135

1978), showing a clear disadvantage if either the excisional biopsy or the interstitial boosting were omitted from treatment (*Table 4.6*). Equally impressive results have been obtained by Pierquin and colleagues (Pierquin and Huart, 1985), who have pioneered the use of combined treatment with lumpectomy followed by external irradiation (using telecobalt irradiation), electron beam boosting to the axilla and internal mammary chain, and finally an interstitial implant using afterloaded iridium-192 to the tumour bed (*Figure 4.9*) (*see* Chapter 16). Initial treatment is with external radiation using telecobalt to a dose of 4500 cGy in 5 weeks, generally employing large tangential chest wall fields with a directly applied anterior supraclavicular field and, in addition, a posterior axillary field which boosts the dose to the axilla. This is followed in all cases by electron beam irradiation to a direct axillary field and a separate internal mammary field, to an applied dose of 2400 cGy (axilla) and 1500 cGy (internal mammary nodes). Patients then undergo interstitial implantation using afterloaded iridium-192 wires, employing dosimetry described by the Paris group. A two-plane implant is generally necessary in order to encompass the tumour volume adequately. For T1 tumours the implant dose is taken to 2500 cGy, for T2 tumours, 3700 cGy (Pierquin *et al.*, 1980). As in Calle's series, tumours larger than 3 cm are not surgically removed. This highly sophisticated approach has produced excellent results at 5 years, both in terms of local control and also 5-year survival (*Table 4.7*). Of 134 patients with operable tumours (T1/2, N0 or N1a), 108 (81%) were alive and free of disease at 5 years and, in this group, 95% of the survivors had retained their breasts. Side-effects from this approach are very few. In an analysis of over 200 patients, rib fracture, radiologically evident pneumonitis and 'inflammatory sclerosis' of the breast were each seen in 2% of cases, with restriction of shoulder movement in a further 6%. Lymphoedema

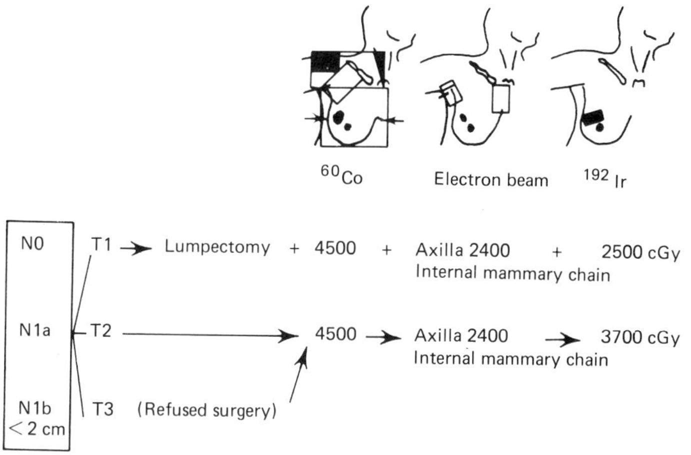

Figure 4.9 Schema of protocol of external and curietherapy irradiation (Paris technique). (From Pierquin *et al.*, 1980 courtesy of the Editor and Publisher *International Journal of Radiation Oncology, Biology and Physics*)

Table 4.7 Survival and recurrence rates at 5 years, following radical irradiation for breast cancer. (From Pierquin ***et al.*** **(1980), with kind permission of the author and editor of** ***International Journal of Radiation Oncology, Biology and Physics*****)**

	Survival (uncorrected)							
	Overall		Disease-free		Metastases		Loco-regional recurrences	
T stage	*No.*	*%*	*No.*	*%*	*No.*	*%*	*No.*	*%*
T1	40/43	(93)	36/45	(84)	7	(16)	2	(4.5)
T2	77/91	(84.5)	72/91	(79)	16	(18)	7	(7.5)
T3	30/43	(70)	24/43	(56)	16	(37)	10	(23)

of the arm occured in 14/228 patients treated by conservative surgery and radical irradiation, and in 46/121 patients treated at the same institution by mastectomy and radiotherapy (B. Pierquin, personal communication). Equally good results have been reported from Harvard (Harris, Levene and Hellman, 1978) and these authors have also stressed the great attention to detail which is necessary in order to achieve the very best cosmetic results. This includes, for example, careful simulation in every case (not routinely practised in many British centres), and particular care in placement of the supraclavicular field which abuts onto the tangential chest wall fields. By use of the 'hanging block' technique, in which the whole of the beam inferior to the central axis can be shielded, the edge of the beam can be made effectively vertical and without any divergence (*Figure 4.10*), allowing a close match without the danger of overtreatment and consequent telangiectasia.

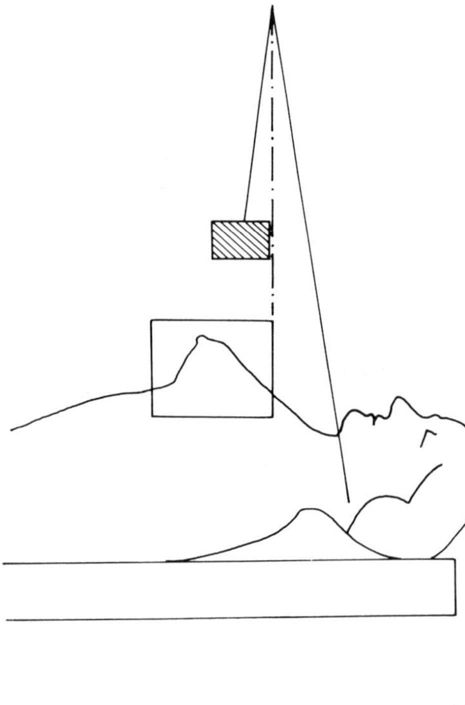

Figure 4.10 Use of a hanging block to avoid matchline over-irradiation by shielding out the lower portion of the supraclavicular field (*see text*)

Advocates of radical irradiation as an alternative to mastectomy have frequently faced the criticism that the cosmetic results are sometimes no better (and often worse) than a neatly performed simple mastectomy. However, the literature does not support this view, particulary since the publication of Pierquin's results (Pierquin *et al.*, 1980). These patients almost invariably had an 'excellent' or 'good' result and only four out of 128 cases were described as having a 'poor' cosmetic result (*Table 4.8*). Results from the Harvard group were broadly similar, the authors commenting that on the whole the patients seemed even more satisfied than their doctors, probably due, as one of the Harvard patients pointed out, to the fact that the physician was always comparing with the normal breast and looking for perfection, whereas the patient was more aware that a mastectomy would have been the inevitable alternative. A typical example of the cosmetic result following radical irradiation of the breast is shown in *Figure 4.11*.

There have been very few controlled studies comparing breast conservation to mastectomy. In the first of these, Atkins and colleagues at Guy's Hospital compared two groups of patients undergoing either wide local excision plus postoperative irradiation, or radical mastectomy also with postoperative irradiation (Atkins *et al.*, 1972). The study demonstrated a clear suvival advantage for radical mastectomy in patients with stage II disease (*Figure 4.12*), and a difference in local reccurence rate was also detectable in patients with both stage I and stage II disease. Although frequently quoted, this study was seriously flawed by the low dosage of radiotherapy throughout. Orthovoltage radiation was employed in the treatment of the axilla, which limited the dosage to a maximum of 2700 cGy in 18 days. The total dosage to

Table 4.8 Cosmetic results following radical irradiation for breast cancer (From Pierquin *et al.* (1980), with kind permission of the author and editor of *International Journal of Radiation Oncology, Biology and Physics*)

T stage	*Group 1*[a]	*Group 2i*[b]	*Group 2ii*[c]	*Group 3*[d]	*Not assessed*[e]	*Total assessed*
T1	24	9	7	0	3	40
T2	28	18	17	2	26	65
T3	6	10	5	2	20	23

[a]Group 1: excellent result; no sequelae visible at first glance.
[b] Group 2i: good result; sequelae only apparent on close inspection (e.g. scar slightly retracted, an occasional telangiectasis, etc.).
[c] Group 2ii: acceptable result; obvious sequelae but the breast retaining a normal contour (e.g. breast slightly elevated, plaque of telangiectasia limited to the high-dose area, a limited area of skin discolouration etc.). This result was considered preferable to a surgical mutilation.
[d] Group 3: mediocre or poor result; extensive sequelae both on the skin and the architecture of the breast. A surgical scar would have been preferable.
[e] Reasons for non-assessment: patients deceased, mastectomy, lost to aesthetic follow-up.

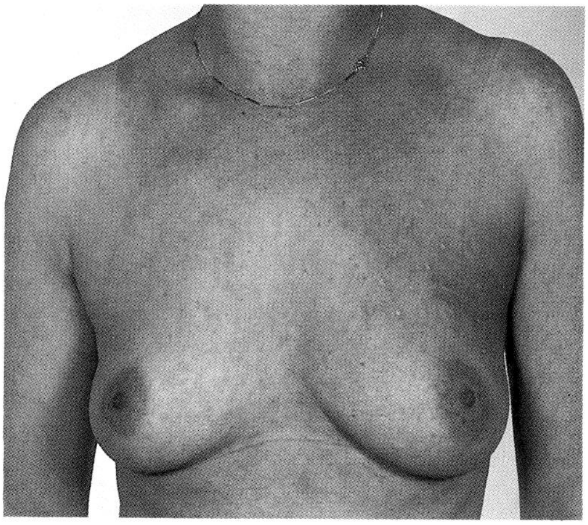

Figure 4.11 Typical cosmetic result following local excision (lumpectomy), external irradiation (5000 cGy in 25 fractions in 5 weeks, ^{60}Co) and boost to tumour bed with interstitial ^{192}Ir. Note barely detectable puncture marks either side of excision scar

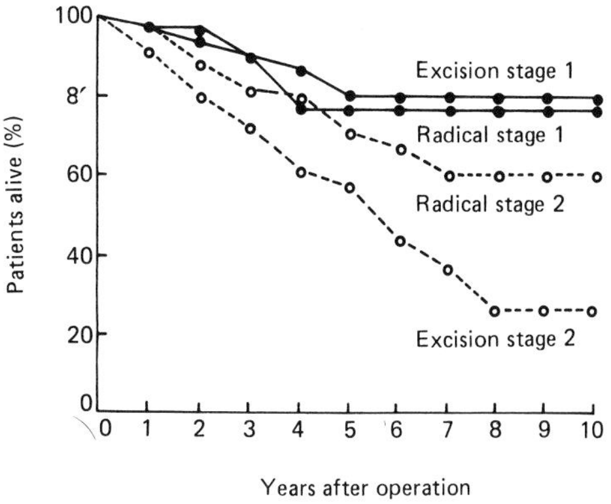

Figure 4.12 Survival proportions according to stage in patients treated by radical mastectomy plus local irradiation or by wide excision followed by local irradiation (Guy's Hospital trial). (From Atkins *et al.*, 1972 courtesy of the Editor and Publisher *British Medical Journal*)

the breast itself was also low (a maximum of 3800 cGy in 3 weeks), despite the fact that even when this study was commenced, Baclesse and others has already demonstrated that the likelihood of tumour control was clearly dose-related. An interesting result of the Guy's Hospital study was that in patients with stage I disease, wide excisional surgery plus postoperative irradiation with modest dosage as described above, gave survival rates at 10 years equal to those achieved by radical mastectomy.

In a more recent prospectively randomized study of radical mastectomy versus conservative surgery with postoperative irradiation to a total dose of 5000 cGy in 6 weeks, Veronesi and colleagues in Milan have failed to show any advantage for radical mastectomy in patients with small node-negative tumours in the outer half of the breast (Veronesi, 1985). In this study the conservative surgery performed was a 'quadrantectomry', with axillary node dissection, and over 700 patients were randomized, making it unlikely that there were any substantial differences between the two groups of patients.

It would represent a profound change in management policy if mastectomy were to be replaced by an alterntive approach which, despite many advantages, is less adequately documented and which might be appropriate only in certain subsets of patients with breast cancer. Moreover, the logistic implications of replacing a 45-minute operation by an extended period of radiotherapy (demanding both for the therapist and for the patient) are immense. However, a recent study from the NSABP (National Surgical Adjuvant Breast Project) has lent strong support to the breast-conserving approach (Fisher *et al.*, 1985). Over 1800 patients were prospectively randomized to undergo treatment either with simple mastectomy or local excision with or without radiation therapy. All node-positive patients received postoperative adjuvant chemotherapy. Not only was disease-free survival at 5 years after local excision plus radiotherapy better than with simple mastectomy, but also the overall survival following local excision (with or without radiotherapy) was slightly better than with mastectomy. Of the patients with positive axillary lymph nodes, 98% of those treated by radiotherapy remained free of local recurrence compared with only 64% of patients not given radiotherapy. Clearly, the next decade will see a major re-evaluation of the role of mastectomy. By the end of the century, mastectomy as a primary treatment for breast cancer could be a relatively uncommon procedure.

Radiotherapy for locally advanced breast cancer

Radiotherapy has long been recognized as the treatment of choice for patients with inoperable cancers. Patients with large lesions attached to skin or underlying muscle (T4), those with medial lesions or with obvious metastatic (M1) disease, and patients whose medical ill-health has precluded an operaion have frequently been managed in this way. In these circumstances, most radiotherapists treat the whole breast and axilla, usually including the internal mammary nodes and supraclavicular fossa. Even before the days of wide-field external beam irradiation, this could be achieved by careful placement of interstitial radium needles (Keynes, 1929), and 50 years ago Keynes used this technique to achieve a 5-year survival rate of 24% in patients with advanced inoperable tumours. More recently, Fletcher and Montague (1965) studied the role of radiotherapy in locally advanced disease, and demonstrated a local recurrence rate of only 11% even though many of these tumours measured over 5 cm across. Although surgery is sometimes used as an alternative, the results of radiotherapy appear to be as good (Mustakallio, 1972). In particular, the presence of fixed axillary lymph nodes (N2), supraclavicular nodes (N3) or local fixation of the tumour to skin or chest wall are all known to increase the likelihood of failure with surgical treatment (Harris, Levene and Hellman, 1978). The probability of local control with radiotherapy is closely related to the size of the primary tumour, and in one series the local recurrence rates were 20% for 5 cm tumours, but over 30% where the primary tumour was over 9 cm (Spratt and Donegan, 1967).

A high local dosage is required for successful control of large, fixed, or locally ulcerating tumours. Doses below 5000–6000 cGy in 5–6 weeks have repeatedly been shown to produce inferior local control rates (Rubens *et al.*, 1977; Karabali-Dalamaga *et al.*, 1978). Despite the high probability that most of these patients will rapidly develop blood-borne metastases, it is always a mistake to overlook the importance of local control. The Harvard group have recommended the use of limited surgery wherever possible, with removal of enlarged axillary nodes, followed by vigorous radiotherapy (5000–6000 cGy) to the beast and draining lymph node areas (Harris, Levene and Hellman, 1978). Where radical treatment (including in some cases an iridium implant) was possible, there were no local recurrences; if either excisional surgery or the interstitial implant were omitted, the local control rate fell to 77%. If neither of these procedures was possible (i.e. the patient was treated with external irradiation alone) the local control rate fell to 41%. Interestingly, patients receiving concomitant adjuvant chemotherapy also had a better overall local control rate (85%), although such treatment is often inappropriate for elderly or infirm patients for whom the side-effects would be unjustifiably severe. Morbidity of this intensive treatment includes fibrosis of the breast, rib fracture, pneumonitis and lymphoedema, in addition to the more acute reactions (myelosuppression, nausea, vomiting, neuropathy) resulting from the chemotherapy.

The use of hormone therapy, either alone or in combination with irradiation, is particularly valuable in this group of patients. Tamoxifen (20–40 mg daily by mouth) is now the most commonly used agent, with response rates, particularly in elderly patients, far greater than 30–40% one might expect from studies of endocrine-receptor status. Patients over the age of 80 years can usually be treated by tamoxifen alone, even where a local excision has not been performed, and radiotherapy is thereby avoided until there is progression of disease. If radiotherapy does become necessary in elderly patients, doses of 4000–5000 cGy (in daily fractions over 4–5 weeks) are usually sufficient to provide long-term control. In order to avoid unnecessary travelling it is sometimes acceptable to offer weekly treatment of 500 cGy in four or five treatments. In general, similar techniques to those described above (*see Figure 4.4*) can be employed. Elderly patients (over 75 years) with *operable* breast cancer can also be treated in this way since the disease is often indolent in this group.

Radiotherapy for metastatic disease

For decades, radiotherapy has been widely used as the treatment of choice for metastatic breast cancer at a variety of sites.

Bone metastases

For painful bone metastases, radiotherapy offers symptom relief in over 90% of cases, although objective radiological evidence of recalcification deposits is much less common. The treatment of these lesions forms a major part of the work of most radiotherapy departments as over one-half of all patients with disseminated breast cancer will require treatment for painful bone metastases. Several regimens have been used, with the object of delivering effective treatment as rapidly as possible. Since the median survival from time of diagnosis of metastases is over 1 year, a sufficient dose must always be prescribed to ensure durable pain relief. There have been few studies directly comparing one regimen with another, but it is widely accepted that painful rib deposits, for example, can be adequately treated with a single fraction of 800–1200 cGy, whereas deposits in the spine usually require fractionated treatment over 1 week or longer to avoid the danger of radiation myelitis — a particular problem in breast cancer since many patients survive long enough to require repeated courses of treatment in closely adjacent sites. Common treatment regimens include 3000 cGy in 10 fractions in 2 weeks; 2500 cGy in five fractions in 1 week; and 2400 cGy in six fractions in 1 week. Although the depth-dose characteristics of megavoltage irradiation permit simple techniques using direct fields to be effective, treatment to the femur or pelvis usually requires an opposed-field technique for satisfactory dose distribution. It is difficult to justify treatment times longer than 2 weeks (*see below*).

A lytic bone deposit will sometimes require treatment even if it is painless, most commonly where the site of the metastasis is a weight-bearing bone such as the femur and where there is a serious risk of fracture because of cortical erosion. In these circumstances a combination of prophylactic irradiation with internal orthopaedic fixation represents the best approach to treatment and ensures that the patient remains as mobile as possible. Ideally, the orthopaedic pinning should be performed first, followed by irradiation of the whole bone as there is a risk of tumour cells seeding in the path of the orthopaedic pin. A dose of 3000 cGy in 10 fractions in 2 weeks is commonly employed, using anterior and posterior (or, if necessary, lateral) opposed fields.

Even though the skeletal X-rays may not change, the bone scan frequently reverts to normal in the treated site. In patients with widespread pelvic metastases, the 'pelvic bath' technique is widely used, and the whole pelvis can be treated to a total dose of 2000 cGy in daily fractions over 1 week (five fractions), usually with satisfactory pain relief. Careful attention to the blood count is essential as such a large volume of marrow is necessarily treated. An alternative approach employs single fraction wide-field irradiation to the pelvis using doses in the region of 700–1000 cGy. Both of these treatments are best achieved using anteroposterior parallel opposed fields, treating with megavoltage equipment. With large treatment volumes such as these, prophylactic antiemetics are usually required. If marrow failure is a possibility treatment can be prolonged using a rising input technique, 25–50–75–100–150 cGy, the total dose then being given over 2 weeks or more.

A single dose of hemibody irradiation might prove to be quicker and simpler (*see* Chapter 3).

Spinal cord compression

This may occur either by direct extension from vertebral metastases or from soft tissue (epidural) deposits, although very rarely an intramedullary secondary deposit will cause a cord compression syndrome from within. The probability of successful treatment is inversely related to the duration of the clinical history, and spinal cord compression is rightly regarded as a radiotherapeutic emergency. Most patients will have back pain with tenderness at the site of the compression as there is usually direct metastatic involvement of the vertebra. Weakness or altered sensation in the legs is also common, sometimes with a sensory level though more often with less distinct or patchy sensory loss. There may be a history of increasing constipation and difficulties with micturition, particularly hesitancy. Incomplete cases of cord compression may occasionally present with a Brown-Sequard syndrome of ipsilateral motor paralysis and loss of proprioception, coupled with contralateral loss of pain and temperature sensation. If the compression takes place below the lower level of the cord (L2/3) the findings will be those of a 'cauda equina' syndrome, which is clinically distinct although often difficult to diagnose. Characteristically there is a sensory loss in sacral segments ('saddle anaesthesia') with weakness (and sometimes loss of sensation) of the lower limbs.

Investigation of the patient with spinal cord compression should include spinal X-rays, which may reveal single or multiple vertebral metastases, and a myelogram which is essential for detailed anatomy of the lesion (particularly its upper extent) unless full CT scanning of the spine is available. Myelography also demonstrates whether the block is complete or partial, and may also suggest a block at more than one site. In fit patients with a relatively short segment of cord affected, decompressive laminectomy is the quickest way of relieving the pressure and should always be considered, particularly if the block is complete. However, the poor general condition of many patients, and their unsuitability for transfer to a neurosurgical centre, often makes radiotherapy the preferred treatment (*see* Chapter 15). Even where surgical decompression has been performed, radiotherapy is almost always given since rapid decompression is the aim of most neurosurgeons, rather than excision of all local metastatic tumour — a point not always appreciated by radiotherapists. A total of 3000 cGy (applied dose) in 10 daily fractions (megavoltage) will be an adequate dose. Dexamethasone (1–4 mg twice to four times daily) is a useful addition to surgical and radiotherapeutic treatment as it may reduce local pressure and also radiation-induced oedema. The result of treatment depends largely on the duration of the compression. Where there is total paraplegia, less than 10% of patients recover the ability to walk (Gilbert, Kim and Posner, 1978).

In one recent series treated by radiotherapy alone, 50% of patients had a useful response to treatment, with a median survival from diagnosis of 6 months (Horwich, 1981). As there has been no direct comparison of treatment by laminectomy with post-operative irradiation or radiotherapy alone, it is uncertain whether the surgery is essential, although it clearly offers the most rapid means of decompression and few radiotherapists would deliberately withold it.

Brain metastases

Brain metastases are diagnosed in about 10% of patients with advanced metastatic breast cancer (*see* Chapter 15) although almost as many again are evident at post-mortem having produced no symptoms during life. Most patients with brain metastases have evidence of disease elsewhere, and it is unusual for the brain to be the first clinically evident metastatic site. Even in patients with proven brain metastases, over one-half will die of progressive disease outside the nervous system — uncontrolled brain metastases are the main cause of death in 45% (DiStefano *et al.*, 1979). The diagnosis should be suspected where there is a clinical history of raised intracranial pressure, focal cranial nerve palsy, epilepsy or cerebellar symptoms. Investigation should include isotope or CT scan of the brain, which may well demonstrate unsuspected multiple metastases, making the patient unsuitable for surgical removal.

Initial treatment with dexamethasone will rapidly reverse headache, nausea and diplopia if these symptoms are due to raised intracranial pressure. Failure of response to dexamethesone is often thought to imply that the response to radiotherapy will also be poor, although if the symptoms are disabling it may be difficult to withold such treatment. The whole brain is usually treated, common regimens including 3000 cGy as a midline dose in 10 fractions in 2 weeks or 4000 cGy as a midline dose in 15 fractions in 3 weeks. Successful treatment with radiotherapy should permit the dexamethasone dosage to be reduced rapidly, minimizing the likelihood of long-term steroid complications. Although the median survival of treated patients with brain metastases is only about 4–6 months, almost 30% of patients survive beyond 1 year, particularly where there has been a lengthy disease-free interval, where the brain metastasis was the first site of relapse, and where surgical resection of a single metastasis has been achieved. Untreated patients with brain metastases have a very short survival of the order of 6 weeks, although admittedly these patients are usually untreated because their general clinical condition is so poor. The management of *carcinomatous meningitis* is discussed in Chapter 15.

The Eye

The eye is an uncommon site for metastases, but carcinoma of the breast is much the commonest cause of choroidal deposits, which can result in blindness of the eye. Although choroidal metastases are usually unilateral, bilateral deposits are well documented. Despite the rarity of this metastatic site, this diagnosis constitutes a radiotherapeutic emergency as prompt irradiation can lead to complete resolution of the tumour and normal vision restored. The commonest approach is to treat with a single lateral megavoltage field, angled posteriorly to avoid the lens of the contralateral eye. A common dose regimen is 3000 cGy applied dose in 10 fractions in 2 weeks. Since irradiation cataract is not likely to be a long-term problem in these patients, a direct cobalt field can be used instead (giving the same dose).

Other sites

Mediastinal involvement from carcinoma of the breast is an unusual cause of superior vena caval obstruction (*see* Chapter 7) and should be treated promply by local irradiation. Skin and lymph node metastases (including local chest wall recurrences) are worrying to the patient, and easily treated by local irradiation using small direct fields. Electron beam irradiation can be useful for these superficial secondary deposits. Doses of the order of 2500 cGy in five fractions in 1 week are usually adequate. An alternative approach is the use of interstitial implants or iridium-192 (*see* Chapter 16), which can be particularly valuable in patients who have been previously treated. With re-treatment, however, there is always a risk of skin necrosis. Hepatic metastases, although usually treated by chemotherapy or hormone therapy, may cause capsular pain and, if the patient is no longer responsive to systemic treatment, local irradiation can provide effective symptom relieve (*see* Chapter 14). A dose of 2000–2500 cGy in 10–15 fractions in 2–3 weeks is usually well tolerated, using a single anterior direct field. Nausea and vomiting almost always occur during treatment, and prophylactic antiemetics should be given.

Hormone therapy in breast cancer

Patients with metastatic breast cancer cannot be cured with currently available agents, and treatment should therefore be regarded as palliative. Endocrine therapy has traditionally been the mainstay of such treatment since most patients tolerate treatment well, and responses can be very long lasting, often up to several years. In general, any patient who develops metastatic disease and is not known to be ER negative should be considered for hormone therapy. However, only a minority of patients (20–40%) are responsive to endocrine treatment (*Table 4.9*).

It is now fairly clear that the likelihood of an endocrine response is strongly related to the presence or absence of cytoplasmic and/or nuclear steroid receptors for oestrogen and progesterone in cells of the primary tumour (Jensen and de Sombre, 1973; Clark *et al.*, 1983). Patients who are ER negative have an insignificant chance of responding to hormone manipulation, whereas those with ER-positive tumours are usually (but by no means invariably) responsive.

Oophorectomy was first used before the end of the nineteenth century, and ablation endocrine approaches have a slightly higher response rate in patients with advanced disease than the administration of exogenous hormones (*Table 4.9*). The conventional 'first-line' appraoch with endocrine therapy was to offer ovarian ablation in premenopausal patients and additional oestrogen therapy (usually with ethinyl oestradiol) to post menopausal patients. However, over the past 10 years it has become apparent that for postmenopausal patients, tamoxifen is as effective as ethinyl oestradiol, and without the distressing side-effects of fluid retention and break-through bleeding (*see below*). In premenopausal patients, effective supression of oestrogen secretion can be equally achieved by surgical oophorectomy or by ovarian irradiation, but surgery has been traditionally preferred because there is a latent period of 3–6 months before radiation-induced ovarian failure is biochemically complete. However, ovarian irradiation ('artificial menopause') is often preferred in patients where

Table 4.9 Objective response rates to conventional forms of endocrine therapy. (Reprinted from Henderson and Canellos by permission of *The New England Journal of Medicine*, **302**, 17–30, 78–90 **(1980))**

Therapy	*No. of patients*	*Response rates (%)*	*Range of responses*
Hormones			
Oestrogens	1683	26	15-38
Androgens	2250	21	10-38
Progestogens	508	25	9-43
Corticosteroids	589	23	0-43
Ablation			
Oophorectomy	1674	33	21-41
Adrenalectomy	3739	32	23-46
Hypophysectomy	1174	36	22-58

there is no dire emergency making rapid response imperative, and particularly where the patient is a poor surgical risk. Various radiation dose schedules have been employed. The simplest is a single-fraction of 450 cGy which was widely used by the Manchester group (Cole, 1968), but which resulted in continued menstruation in up to 30% of cases. Fractionated treatment is now preferred, usually treating the whole pelvis (typical field size 15 × 15 cm) to a mid-line dose of the order of 1500–2000 cGy in five fractions in 8 days, after which continued menstruation does not occur. As with surgical oophorectomy, factors predictive of a probable response include a long tumour-free interval from mastectomy, known positive ER status, and metastatic bone disease rather than deposits in liver, soft tissues, or multiple sites. Ovarian irradiation has also been used as adjuvant or prophylactic treatment (*see below*).

Where 'first-line' hormone therapy has been unsuccessful, use of secondary hormonal agents is unlikely to be beneficial, although responses have been recorded, particularly with the use of progestational agents, in patients who have undergone oophorectomy, or been treated with exogenous oestrogens or tamoxifen. If there has been an initial hormone response, second-line hormone therapy should be employed when relapse occurs, although there is no agreement as to the sequence in which the agents should be preferred. The tradional second-line approach in oophorectomized premenopausal patients with an initial hormone response was by surgical adrenalectomy, but it has recently been shown that 'medical adrenalectomy' with oral aminoglutethimide (which suppresses corticosteroid synthesis) 250 mg two or three times daily is as effective (Santen *et al.*, 1981), and surgical adrenalectomy is now rarely performed. Side-effects of aminoglutethimide include nausea and skin rash, ataxia and lassitude, all usually transient; and additional treatment with hydrocortisone (20 mg in the morning and 10 mg in the evening) or other replacement therapy, e.g. cortisone acetate, is essential.

For postmenopausal patients, second-line hormone therapy includes androgens (e.g. nandrolone decanoate (Deca-Durabolin) 50–100 mg intramuscularly every 3–4 weeks), or progestational agents. Of the many progestogens currently available, medroxyprogesterone acetate (Provera) is one of the most widely used and may be more effective at high (e.g. 1 g/day) rather than low dosage. It is however usually prescribed at a lower dose, of the order of 100 mg three times daily by mouth. Oral corticosteroid therapy, usually with enteric prednisolone 10–40 mg daily, is sometimes used although there is little evidence that it is an active agent. Hypophysectomy is occasionally used for hormone responsive patients, and can be highly effective in selected cases. The transnasal or transethmoidal route makes craniotomy unnecessary.

Side-effects of endocrine therapy include virilization from androgens, fluid retention and breakthrough bleeding from oestrogens, and steroidal side-effects from corticosteroids. High doses of progestogens may also induce troublesome fluid retention and weight gain. All endocrine therapies may occasionally produce a 'flare'or rapid progression of disease, of which hypercalcaemia is the most dangerous manifestation. There is no convincing evidence that the use of combination hormone therapies is superior to single agent sequential hormone treatment. Median duration of responsiveness is 9–10 months after oestrogen therapy or oophorectomy, and 12–14 months after major endocrine ablation (Henderson and Canellos, 1980).

Of the more recently introduced endocrine treatments, both tamoxifen and aminoglutethimide rapidly established themselves as useful agents. Tamoxifen, an antioestrogen which blocks the uptake of oestradiol onto the oestrogen receptor present in some breast cancer cells, is now the most widely used endocrine treatment for recurrent disease in postmenopausal patients, and is well absorbed by mouth and remarkably free of side-effects. Nausea, hypercalcaemia, transient thrombocytopenia and fluid retention occur very occasionally. The usual dose is 10–20 mg twice daily, although the biological half-life is greater than 1 week, and a single oral daily dosage of 20 mg is probably as effective as twice daily treatment. Tamoxifen has also been employed as a form of adjuvant systemic therapy (*see below*).

Chemotherapy

A variety of agents has been shown to be active in metastatic breast cancer (*Table 4.10*). The most active drugs include hydroxydaunorubicin, cyclophosphamide, vincristine, methotrexate and 5-fluorouracil, and it is clear that breast cancer cells are sensitive to a number of biochemical disturbances since these agents are all from different classes. Unfortunately, response is usually obtained at the cost of some degree of drug-induced toxicity (*see* Chapter 20) and responses tend to be short-lived. As a general rule, chemotherapy-induced responses are less durable than those induced by endocrine therapy.

In view of the wide choice of partly effective cytotoxic drugs and the poor results of single agent chemotherapy, combination chemotherapy has been widely used. The first multi-drug regimen, reported by Cooper (1969), included cyclophosphamide, methotrexate, 5-fluorouracil, vincristine and prednisone (CMFVP), with a remarkable response rate of 90% which has never been repeated. The average response rate for this combination is in the region of 45%, although the complete response rate in most series is less than 20%. Because of uncertainty of the role of vincristine, coupled with its frequent neurotoxicity, the most commonly used regimen in recent years has been CMF(P), usually given as intermittent intravenous/oral treatment every 3 weeks. Despite the widespread acceptance of such treatment it is not entirely clear whether single agent therapy, using the most active agent until drug resistance emerges, then replacing it with another drug, may not be as effective. Hydroxydaunorubicin is currently the most active cytotoxic agent available and is sometimes given as a single agent, but more frequently included in combination with vincristine and prednisone (VAP), given as intravenous/oral therapy evey 3–4 weeks (*Table 4.11*). In general, chemotherapy is more effective for soft tissue, skin and lymph node deposits than for bone metastases. The overall response rate to CMF or VAP is of the order of 50–75%, but the complete response rate is much lower, around 10–20% (Henderson and Canellos, 1980).

The disappointing duration of response to chemotherapy, coupled with the high probability of troublesome side-effects, makes hormone manipulation the preferred first line treatment for most patients with disseminated disease, particularly with bone metastases, where the response to combination chemotherapy is usually disappointing. In addition, chemotherapy-related side-effects are often only slowly reversible, as with vincristine neuropathy, or indeed virtually irreversible, for example with hydroxydaunorubicin-induced cardiomyopathy. Nonetheless, the use of chemotherapy may be valuable in patients with widespread disease, including those with bone marrow metastases, lymphangitis carcinomatosa, massive hepatomegaly from diffuse hepatic involvment, and metastases at other soft tissue sites. It is often preferable in young patients with rapidly advancing disease where there may be insufficient time for a leisurely assessment of hormone responsiveness. Intrathecal chemotherapy with methotrexate or cytosine arabinoside is widely used for patients with carcinomatous meningitis (*see* Chapter 15).

It is not yet clear whether treatment of metastases with chemotherapy has made a major contribution to the survival of patients with advanced disease. Powles *et al.* (1980) in an analysis of patients treated at the Royal Marsden Hospital could show no convincing improvement in survival since the widespread use of chemotherapy.

Adjuvant chemotherapy

As cytotoxic drugs act by damaging or killing a constant fraction of cancer cells, it is widely thought that for their greatest effect, these agents should be given when the tumour burden is at its smallest, i.e. immediately following primary therapy with surgery or

Table 4.10 Activity of commonly used single agent therapy in breast cancer. (Modified from Henderson and Canellos, 1980)

Agent	*Class of drug*	*No. of patients*	*Objective response rate (%)*
Hydroxydaunorubicin	Antitumour antibiotic	193	35
Cyclophosphamide	Alkylating agent	529	34
Chlorambucil	Alkylating agent	54	20
Melphalan	Alkylating agent	177	22
Methotrexate	Antimetabolite	356	34
5-fluorouracil	Antimetabolite	1263	26
Vincristine	Mitotic inhibitor	226	21

Table 4.11 Combination chemotherapy for breast cancer

Study	*Regimen*	*No. of patients*	*Response rate (%)*		*Median duration (months)*	
			Complete plus partial responses†	*Complete responses*	*Response*	*Survival*
Swiss group for Clinical Cancer Research	CMP	78	43	4	7.3	15.4
	CMF-VP	91	49	7	8.0	16.0
Milan (1976)	CMF	53	57	11	8.0	17.5
Houston (1976)	FAC	44	73	14	8.0	15.0
Eastern Cooperative Oncology Group (1977)	CMF	90	48	15	5.3	14.8
	CMFP	88	63	25	8.5	18.0
	AV	178	53	18	8.0	13.0
Southwest Oncology Group (1978)	AF	105	42	10	5.5	16.0
	AFC	103	43	14	8.3	15.3
	AFCM	105	49	11	8.8	16.3
National Cancer Institute (1978)	CMF	40	62	7.5	6.0	17.0
	CAF	38	82	18	10.4	27.2

† Objective regressions of >50% of measurable tumour volume
C = cyclophosphamide; M = methotrexate; A = hydroxydaunorubicin; F = 5-fluorouracil; V = vincristine; P = prednisone.

radiation. Twenty years ago the first adjuvant chemotherapy trial was performed by Nissen-Meyer who gave a short course of cyclophosphamide immediately following mastectomy, showing a small but statistically significant improvement in the 10-year survival of treated patients (Nissen-Meyer *et al*, 1978). This study also demonstrated that for patients in whom chemotherapy was started more than 3 weeks after mastectomy, there seemed to be no survival advantage — suggesting perhaps that the value of such treatment related to the immediate treatment of metastases arising from tumour cells shed at the operation itself. More recent studies have given conflicting results. After preliminary reports of benefit from adjuvant therapy with intermittent melphalan, there appears to be no long-term survival advantage (Rubens *et al.*, 1983). The studies of Bonadonna and colleagues at Milan, chiefly using adjuvant combination chemotherapy with cyclophosphamide, methotrexate and 5-fluorouracil were initially hailed as a great advance despite the preliminary nature of the results (Bonadonna *et al.*, 1976). Later analyses of these data showed that the improvement in relapse-free survival appeared to be limited to the premenopausal group (Rossi *et al.*, 1981), and even this possible small advantage has been questioned since the randomization procedure of the Milan study appears dubious (Trask and Souhami, 1982).

The early acceptance of adjuvant chemotherapy for breast cancer has made further studies difficult, particularly in the USA where several authors have questioned the ethics of including a no-treatment group. In the UK, adjuvant chemotherapy is far less widely practised, and the morbidity of such treatment has been rightly stressed (Palmer *et al.*, 1980). Even more aggressive adjuvant chemotherapy regimens have been employed, but so far with disappointing results (Morrison, Howell and Grieve, 1981). In general, the most obvious advantage conferred by adjuvant chemotherapy appears to be in the improvement of disease-free survival, rather than overall survival, suggesting that patients who relapse following adjuvant chemotherapy are more difficult to treat effectively and that chemotherapy may be better withheld until relapse. Further criticism of the concept of adjuvant chemotherapy has come from the suggestion that its apparent activity may reflect no more than its effect on ovarian hormone production, i.e. that the cytotoxic effect is due to the chemical 'oophorectomy' which often occurs. This suggestion is certainly strengthened by the clear-cut ineffectiveness of chemotherapy in postmenopausal patients, although it seems unlikely to provide a complete explanation.

At present, the position remains unclear. Nissen-Meyer's short course, single agent postoperative treatment is the most mature (and so far the most fruitful) of the adjuvant chemotherapy studies, and this study is currently being repeated by the Cancer Research Campaign Adjuvant Chemotherapy Group. Combination adjuvant chemotherapy is unpleasant, but appears to lengthen disease-free survival and perhaps to have a marginal effect on overall survival in the premenopausal patient. Its effect may be no greater than that of adjuvant hormone therapy (*see below*) and it has not so far found an established role in the UK. There is clearly a pressing need for further prospective randomized trials of adjuvant chemotherapy, and at present the widespread administration of adjuvant combination chemotherapy outside clinical trials seems unwarranted (Smith, 1983). However, a recent and widely publicized 'overview' of major chemotherapy trials has suggested a real advantage for adjuvant treatment using combination chemotherapy in premenopausal women (Peto, 1984).

Adjuvant hormone therapy

Adjuvant ovarian irradiation was the first adjuvant hormone treatment to be evaluated and the largest study, from Manchester and Toronto, showed a delay in recurrence and an improvement in survival in premenopausal patients aged 45 years or more (the 'perimenopausal' group) (Meakin *et al.*, 1977). One drawback to such treatment is that it is both irreversible and of unpredictable value, although the increasing use of ER assays should allow earlier identification of patients who might benefit. In some women, the early cessation of ovarian function can cause psychological disturbances, including anxiety and/or depression which can be severe.

Preliminary results from a large UK multicentre study have suggested that administration of tamoxifen (20 mg daily by mouth) delays recurrence and may perhaps have some survival advantage (Baum *et al.*, 1983), but these early results need confirmation. This form of adjuvant systemic treatment has the advantage of minimal side-effects and very good patient compliance and is rapidly becoming popular in the UK, although it should be stressed that the long-term effects of continuous tamoxifen are still unknown.

Cancer of the breast in men

This is an unusual condition, 100 times less common than in women. Although little is known of the aetiology, a few family clusters have been reported and there may be an association with Klinefelter's syndrome, in which gonadotrophin levels are raised, and in patients with gynaecomastia or hyperoestrogenism following liver damage, for example with cirrhosis. Most patients present with a tender area close to the nipple, and there may also be crusting or discharge. The chest wall is usually involved early, and local and distant dissemination follows the usual pattern.

Mastectomy is the treatment of choice, many surgeons preferring a radical procedure because of the small size of the breast and the lesser importance of the final cosmetic result. As with women, there is a considerable risk of local recurrence when the axillary nodes are involved, and radiotherapy should be considered in such patients, although the high incidence of lymphoedema following radical mastectomy and intensive irradiation of the axilla should be borne in mind. For distant metastases, orchidectomy is usually considered to be the treatment of choice and responses have been reported in two-thirds of patients, reflecting a high incidence of hormone receptor positivity in males. Alternative hormone treatments include tamoxifen, progestogens, cyproterone, or hypophysectomy. If hormone treatment fails, chemotherapy may induce a short remission, although there have been few reports of durable response. In view of the paucity of information regarding the outcome in male cancer of the breast it is uncertain whether the disease has a different prognosis from female breast cancer. Although this issue remains contentious it is likely that stage for stage the outlook in men is no worse (Langlands, Maclean and Kerr, 1976).

References

ATKINS, H., HAYWARD, J. L., KLUGMAN, D. J. and WAYTE, A. B. (1972) Treatment for early breast cancer: a report after 10 years of a clinical trial. *British Medical Journal*, **2**, 423–429

BACLESSE, F. (1949) Roentgen therapy as the sole method

of treatment of cancer of the breast. *American Journal of Roentgenology, Radiotherapy and Nuclear Medicine*, **62**, 311–319

BAUM, M., BRINKLEY, D. M., DOSSETT, J. A. *et al.* (1983) Improved survival amongst patients treated with adjuvant tamoxifen after mastectomy for early breast cancer. *Lancet*, **2**, 450

BLOOM, H. J. G., RICHARDSON, W. W. and HARRIES, E. J. (1962) Natural history of untreated breast cancer (1805–1933): comparison of untreated and treated cases according to histological grade of malignancy. *British Medical Journal*, **2**, 213–221

BONADONNA, G., BRUSAMOLINO, E., VALAGUSSA, P. *et al.* (1976) Combination chemotherapy as an adjuvant treatment in operable breat cancer. *New England Journal of Medicine* **294**, 405–410

BRINKLEY, D. and HAYBITTLE, J. L. (1975) The curability of breast cancer. *Lancet*, **2**, 95-97

BRITISH MEDICAL JOURNAL (1981) Postoperative radiotherapy in breast cancer (leading article). *British Medical Journal*, **1**, 1498–1499

CALLE, R. (1985) Experience with conservation approaches in breast cancer at the Institut Curie. In *Primary Management of Breast Cancer: Alternatives to Mastectomy*, edited by J. S. Tobias and M. J. Peckham, pp.59–79. London: Edward Arnold & Co

CALLE, R., PILLERON, J. P., SCHLIENGER, P. and VILCOQ, J. R. (1978) Conservative management of operable breast cancer. Ten years' experience at the Foundation Curie. *Cancer*, **42**, 2045–2051

CANCER RESEARCH CAMPAIGN WORKING PARTY (King's/Cambridge) (1980) Trial for early breast cancer. A detailed update at the tenth year. *Lancet,* **2**, 55–60

CLARK, G. M., McGUIRE, W. L., HUBAY, C. A., PEARSON, O. H. and MARSHALL, J. S. (1983) Progesterone receptor as a prognostic factor in stage II breast cancer. *New England Journal of Medicine*, **309**, 1343–1347

COLE, M. P. (1968) In *Prognostic Factors in Breast Cancer*, edited by A. P. M. Forrest and P. B. Kunkler, pp.146-156. (From Proceedings of the 1st Tenovus Symposium, Cardiff.) Edinburgh: E. and S. Livingston

COOPER, R. G. (1969) Combination chemotherapy in hormone resistant breast cancer. *Proceedings of the American Association of Cancer Research and American Society of Clinical Oncology*, **10**, 15 (abstract)

DiSTEFANO, A., YAP, H. Y., HORTOBAGYI, G. N. and BLUMENSCHEIN, G. R. (1979) The natural history of breast cancer patients with brain metastases. *Cancer*, *44*, 1913–1918

ELSTON, C. W., GRESHAM, G. A., RAO, G. S. *et al.* (1982) (Cancer Research Campaign Working Party) The Cancer Research Campaign (King's/Cambridge) trial for early breast cancer: clinicopathological aspects. *British Journal of Cancer*, **45**, 655–669

FISHER, B., BAUER, M., MARGOLESE, R. *et al.* (1985) Five-year results of a randomised trial comparing total mastectomy and segmental mastectomy with or without radiation in the treatment of breast cancer. *New England Journal of Medicine*, **312**, 665–673

FISHER, B. and GEBHARDT, M. C. (1978) The evolution of breast cancer surgery: past, present and future, *Seminars in Oncology*, **5**, 385–394

FLETCHER, G. H. and MONTAGUE, E. D. (1965) Radical irradiation of advanced breast cancer. *American Journal of Roentgenology*, **93**, 573–584

GARDNER, M. J., WINTER, P. D., TAYLOR, C. P. and ACHESON, E. D. (1983) *Atlas of Cancer Mortality in England and Wales, 1968-1978*, p.4. Chichester, NewYork, Brisbane, Toronto and Singapore: John Wiley & Sons

GARMATIS, C. J. and CHU, F. C. H. (1978) The effectiveness of radiation therapy in the treatment of bone metastases from breast cancer. *Radiology*, **126**, 235–237

GILBERT, R. W., KIM, J. H. and POSNER, J. B. (1978) Epidural spinal cord compression from metastatic tumour: diagnosis and treatment. *Annals of Neurology*, **3**, 40–51

HAAGENSEN, C. D., MILLER, E., HANDLEY, R. S. *et al.* (1969) Treatment of early mammary carcinoma: a co-operative international study. *Annals of Surgery*, **170**, 875–899

HALSTED, W. S. (1907) The results of radical operations for the cure of cancer of the breast. *Annals of Surgery*, **1**,46

HARRIS, J. R., LEVENE, M. B. and HELLMAN, S. (1978) The role of radiation therapy in the primary treatment of carcinoma of the breast. *Seminars in Oncology*, **5**, 403–416

HENDERSON, I. C. and CANELLOS, G. P. (1980) Cancer of the breast — the past decade. *New England Journal of Medicine*, **302**, 17–30 and 78–90

HORWICH, A. (1981) The role of radiotherapy in locally advanced and metastatic breast cancer. In *Breast Cancer Management*, edited by R. C. Coombes, T. J. Powles, H. T. Ford and J. C. Gazet, pp.227–266. London, Toronto and Sydney: Academic Press, and New York and San Francisco: Grune & Stratton

HOST, H. and BRENNHOVD, I. O. (1977) The effect of post-operative radiotherapy in breast cancer. *International Journal of Radiation Oncology, Biology and Physics*, **2**, 1061–1067

JENSEN, E. V. and de SOMBRE, E. R. (1973) Estrogen-receptor interaction. *Science*, **182**, 126–134

KAAE, S. and JOHANSEN, H. (1977) Does simple mastectomy followed by irradition offer survival comparable to radical procedures? *International Journal of Radiation Oncology, Biology and Physics*, **2**, 1163–1166

KALACHE, A. and VESSEY, M. (1982) Risk factors for breast cancer. In *Breast Cancer* edited by M. Baum, pp. 661–678. London, Philadelphia and Toronto: W. B. Saunders Co Ltd

KARABALI-DALAMAGA, S., SOUHAMI, R. L., O'HIGGINS, N. J., SOUMILAS, A. and CLARK, C. G. (1978) Natural history and prognosis of recurrent breast cancer. *British Medical Journal*, **2**, 730–733

KEYNES, G. (1929) The treatment of primary carcinoma of the breast with radium. *Acta Radiologica Scandinavica,* **10**, 393–402

KEYNES, G. (1937) Conservative treatment of cancer of the breast. *British Medical Journal*, **2**, 643–647

KEYNES, G. (1981) Breast Cancer. In *The Gates of Memory*, pp.211-218. Oxford: Oxford University Press

LANGLANDS, A. O., MACLEAN, N. and KERR, G. R. (1976) Carcinoma of the male breast — report of a series of 88 cases. *Clinical Radiology*, **27**, 21-25

LEVITT S. H. and McHUGH, R. B. (1975) Early breast cancer and postoperative irradiation. *Lancet*, **2**, 1258–1259

LIPSETT, M. B. (1981) Postoperative radiation for women with cancer of the breast and positive axillary lymph nodes. Should it continue? *New England Journal of Medicine*, **304**, 112–114

LYTHGOE, J. P., LECK, I. and SWINDELL, R. (1978) Manchester regional breast study: preliminary results. *Lancet*, **1**, 744–747

McGUIRE W. L. (1980) The usefulness of steroid hormone receptors in the management of primary and advanced breast cancer. In *Breast Cancer Experimental and Clinical Aspects* edited by H. T. Mouridsen and T. Palshof, pp.39–43. New York: Pergamon Press

McWHIRTER, R. (1955) Simple mastectomy and radiotherapy in the treatment of breast cancer. *British Journal of Radiology*, **28**, 128–139

MEAKIN, J. W., ALLT, W. E. C., BEALE, F. A. *et al*. (1977) Ovarian irradiation and prednisone following surgery for carcinoma of the breast. In *Adjuvant Therapy of Cancer*, edited by S. E. Salmon and S. E. Jones, pp. 95–99. Amsterdam, Oxford and New York: North-Holland Publishing Co

MORRISON, J. M., HOWELL, A. and GRIEVE, R. J. (1981) The West Midlands Oncology Association trials of adjuvant chemotherapy for operable breast cancer. In *Adjuvant Therapy of Cancer III*, edited by S. Salmon and S. E. Jones, pp.403–410. New York: Grune & Stratton

MUSTAKALLIO, S. (1972) Conservative treatment of breast cancer — review of 25 years' follow-up. *Clinical Radiology* , **23**, 110–116

NEMOTO, T., VANA, J., BEDWANI, R. N., BAKER, H. W., McGREGOR, F. H. and MURPHY, G. P. (1980) Management and survival of female breast cancer: results of a national survey by the American College of Surgeons. *Cancer*, **45**, 2917–2924

PALMER, B. V., WALSH, G. A., McKINNA, J. A. and GREENING, W. P. (1980) Adjuvant chemotherapy for breast cancer: side-effects and quality of life. *British Medical Journal*, **281**, 1594–1597

PETERS, M. V. (1975) Cutting the Gordian Knot in early breast cancer. *Annals of the Royal College of Physicians and Surgeons of Canada*, **8**, 186–192

PETO, R. (1984) Review of mortality results in randomized trials in early breast cancer. *Lancet*, **2**, 1205

PFAHLER, G. E. (1932) Results of radiation therapy in 1022 private cases of carcinoma of the breast from 1902 to 1928. *American Journal of Roentgenology, Radium Therapy and Nuclear Medicine*, **27**, 497–508

PIERQUIN, B., BAILLET, F. and WILSON, J. F. (1976) Radiation therapy in the management of primary breast cancer. *American Journal of Roentgenology*, **127**, 645–648

PIERQUIN, B. and HUART, J. (1985) Experience with breast conservation at the Institute Gustave Roussy and Hopital Henri Mondor. In *Primary Management of Breast Cancer: Alternatives to Mastectomy,* edited by J. S. Tobias and M. J. Peckham, pp.80–101. London: Edward Arnold & Co

PIERQUIN, B., OWEN, R., MAYLIN, C. *et al*. (1980) Radical radiation therapy of breast cancer. *International Journal of Radiation Oncology, Biology and Physics*, **6**, 17–24

PIKE, M. C., HENDERSON, B. E., KRAILO, M. D., DUKE, A. and ROY, S. (1983) Breast cancer in young women and use of oral contraceptives: possible modifying effect of formulation and age at use. *Lancet*, **2**, 926–930

POWLES, T. J., COOMBES, R. C., SMITH, I. E., JONES, J. M., FORD, H. T. and GAZET, J. C. (1980) Failure of chemotherapy to prolong survival in a group of patients with metastatic breast cancer. *Lancet*, **1**, 580–582

ROSSI, A., BONADONNA, G., VALAGUSSA, P. and VERONESI, U. (1981) Multimodal treatment in operable breast cancer. *British Medical Journal*, **282**, 1427–1431

RUBENS, R. D., ARMITAGE, P., WINTER, P. J., TONG, D. and HAYWARD, J. L. (1977) Prognosis in inoperable stage III carcinoma of the breast. *European Journal of Cancer*, **13**, 805–811

RUBENS, R. D. HAYWARD, J. L., KNIGHT, R. K. *et al*. (1983) Controlled trial of adjuvant chemotherapy with melphalan for breast cancer. *Lancet*, **1**, 839–843

SANTEN, R. J., WORGUL, T. J., SAMOJLIK, E. **et al**. (1981) A randomised trial comparing surgical adrenalectomy with aminoglutethimide plus hydrocortisone in women with advanced breast cancer. *New England Journal of Medicine*, **305**, 545–551

SMITH, I. E.(1983) Adjuvant chemotherapy for early breast cancer. *British Medical Journal*, **287**, 379–380

SPRATT, J. L. and DONEGAN, W. L. (1967) *Cancer of the Breast*. St. Louis: Mosby

STJERNSWARD, J.(1974) Decreased survival related to irradiation postoperatively in early operable breastcancer. *Lancet*, **2**, 1285–1286

TIMOTHY, A. R., OVERGAARD, J., OVERGAARD, M. and WANG, C. C. (1979) Treatment of early carcinoma of the breast. *Lancet*, **2**, 25–26

TOBIAS, J. S. and PECKHAM, M. J. (1985) Changing trends in the management of early breast cancer. In *Primary Management of Breast Cancer: Alternatives to Mastectomy* edited by J. S. Tobias and M. J. Peckham, pp.41–55. London: Edward Arnold & Co

TOKUNAGA, M., LAND, C. E., YAMAMOTO, T. *et al*. (1982) Breast cancer in Japanese A bomb survivors. *Lancet*, **2**, 924

TRASK, C. and SOUHAMI, R. L. (1982) Multimodal treatment in operable breast cancer. *British Medical Journal*, **285**, 1571–1572

URBAN, J. A. and CASTRO, E. B. (1971) Selecting variations in extent of surgical procedure for breast cancer. *Cancer*, **28**, 1618–1623

VERONESI, U. (1985) Randomised trials comparing breast conservation with conventional surgery. In *Primary Management of Breast Cancer: Alternatives to Mastectomy*, edited by J. S. Tobias and M. J. Peckham, pp.131–152 London: Edward Arnold & Co

VERONESI, U., SACCOZI, R., VECCHIO, M. *et al*. (1981) Comparing radical mastectomy with quadrantectomy, axillary dissection and radiotherapy in patients with small cancers of the breast. *New England Journal of Medicine*, **305**, 6–11

ZIMMERMAN, K. W., MONTAGUE, E. D. and FLETCHER, G. H. (1966) Frequency, anatomical distribution and management of local recurrences after definitive therapy for breast cancer. *Cancer*, **19**, 67–74

5

Cancer of the head and neck

J. M. Henk

The term 'head and neck cancer' embraces malignant tumours arising in all parts of the head and neck except for the skin and central nervous system. It therefore covers tumours of the upper respiratory and upper alimentary tracts, the salivary glands, the orbit, and associated structures. It is an area of complex anatomical structure, therefore tumours arising at different sites can behave in very different ways. Many histological types of tumour occur, but squamous carcinoma is by far the commonest.

Head and neck cancer provides a considerable challenge to the clinicians treating it. The local disease, i.e. the primary tumour and the regional lymph node metastases, dominates the clinical picture and gives rise to severe symptoms. Distant metastases are not infrequent but they usually occur late in the course of the disease; nearly all patients who die of head and neck cancer have uncontrolled local disease which often causes severe distress. The aim of treatment should therefore be the complete elimination of tumour from above the clavicles and if this can be achieved a cure is likely. Unfortunately, this is not always possible; heavy smokers, alcoholics and the elderly comprise the vast majority of patients with this disease. Therefore a high proportion still present at a late stage, while others have associated medical problems which make it difficult to perform radical surgery or radiotherapy.

The modern treatment of head and neck cancer requires close collaboration between a number of specialists in different fields. ENT, plastic and oral surgeons should work in close collaboration with radiotherapists and oncologists. Ideally, every patient with head and neck cancer should be assessed in a joint consultation clinic where a policy of management suited to that particular individual and his disease can be decided upon.

Choice of management policy

For a large proportion of patients with head and neck cancer, both surgery and radiotherapy hold out possibilities of cure. The major decision which needs to be made is between a policy of radical radiotherapy and one of elective surgery.

The aim of radical radiotherapy is to eradicate all the disease; surgery is reserved for those patients who have residual tumour or develop recurrence after radiotherapy. Operating on such patients after failure of radical radiotherapy, known as 'salvage surgery', is more difficult and carries a higher complication rate than elective surgery. However, many of the survivors of such a management policy will not need surgery and so be spared its deformities and disabilities. Assessment of whether or not salvage surgery is necessary should be delayed until at least 6 weeks have elapsed after the end of the course of radiotherapy to allow time for the normal tissues to heal and tumour cells killed by irradiation to disappear. Before this time, both clinical and histological assessment of residual disease may be misleading. Subsequently careful follow-up is essential and biopsy should be performed in the event of any suspicion of recurrence.

Elective surgery aims to remove the entire tumour. It may be combined with radiotherapy used as an adjuvant, either pre-or postoperatively. In laboratory animals the advantage of preoperative radiotherapy over postoperative radiotherapy is well established. Controlled clinical trials of preoperative radiotherapy have shown a significant reduction in local recurrence especially when a short low dose technique was used (Strong, 1969; Terz, King and Lawrence, 1981) but, nevertheless, preoperative radiotherapy has never become popular in head and neck cancer clinics. This is because of logistic difficulties and the fear among surgeons (largely unjustified) that it will increase the risk of postoperative complications. Consequently, postoperative radiotherapy is more popular despite its inherent biological disadvantages; it usually has a low morbidity and does seem to reduce the risk of local recurrence especially in cases where the resection margins are close to or involved with tumour. Vikram *et al.* (1984b), in a retrospective review of patients treated surgically for stage III and IV carcinoma of various head and neck sites at the Memorial Sloan-Kettering Cancer Center, reported recurrence at the primary site in 39% of patients in whom the resection margins were deemed satisfactory histologically, and in 73% when the margins were considered unsatisfactory. With the addition of postoperative radiotherapy the recurrence rates were 2% and 10.5% respectively. The sooner radiotherapy begins after surgery the less the chance of recurrence. Vikram and his colleagues reported that when radiotherapy was delayed for more than 6 weeks after surgery it had much less effect in diminishing the local recurrence rate.

Elective surgery has become increasingly popular in recent years. The development of new reconstructive techniques, especially free flaps with microvascular anastomosis, has made possible the removal of larger tumours with less deformity. However, even with new techniques, there is usually some disfigurement, and functional difficulties, e.g. with speech and swallowing, are common.

The choice between the two policies in the individual patient depends on a number of factors, including the site, size, histology and stage of tumour, the medical condition of the patient, the patient's personality and his ability or willingness to attend for follow-up. The decisions should always be made in a joint clinic with consideration of all factors in the individual patient. When the decision on the treatment strategy has been made it should be adhered to, and only be changed in exceptional circumstances. A 'change of horses midstream' often leads to disaster; for example a decision not to operate after a preoperative course of radiotherapy because of apparent good tumour regression will result in a patient not having a curative operation or an optimun dose of radiotherapy, and the chances of failure are much increased. Similarly, it is very rarely advisable to abandon a course of radical radiotherapy before it is completed on the grounds that the tumour does not seem to be regressing well; there is poor correlation between the early regression rates of tumours and ultimate radiocurability (Suit, Lindberg and Fletcher, 1965) and treatment decisions based on how fast a tumour seems to be shrinking are best avoided.

Getting the best results from radical radiotherapy

Fractionation

Most radiotherapists treat head and neck cancer with five fractions a week over periods from 3 to 8 weeks. Some treat three times per week. The most popular regimen is 200 cGy per day 5 days per week over 6–7 weeks to a total dose of 6000 to 6600 cGy in 30 to 33 fractions. It is widely believed that longer fractionation schemes give a better therapeutic ratio between tumour cure and late normal tissue damage. However, the few controlled trials which have been done to compare different fractionation schemes have failed to confirm this, there being little difference between the results of fractionation schemes over 3 weeks and 6 weeks (Henk and James, 1978; Wiernik and Gunn, 1984). There are, however, qualitative differences in normal tissue effects. Shorter treatment times tend to cause more severe mucositis; when the area of mucosa irradiated is large this may lead to greater difficulty in maintaining nutrition. Late normal tissue effects are related to fraction size; the central nervous system is especially vulnerable to large dose fractions, so it is advisable to use small fractions and therefore longer treatment times where the tumour is close to the optic nerve, brain stem, or spinal cord. Multiple fractions per day are now under investigation as a possible means of improving the therapeutic ratio between tumour control and late normal tissue damage (*see* Chapter 1). The present author's policy is to treat over 3 or 4 weeks using fraction sizes of 275–300 cGy where the treatment volume is small; 200 cGy fractions over 6–7 weeks are used where central nervous system tissue is at risk and also where a large area of mucosa is irradiated.

Hyperbaric oxygen and hypoxic cell sensitizers

These have both been used in head and neck cancer with some improvement in tumour control, but so far neither have made a major impact (*see* Chapter 2).

Neutron therapy

This was introduced as another approach to the problem of the oxygen effect. In addition to the lower oxygen enhancement ratio, a further advantage of neutron irradiation in head and neck cancer is the reduced absorption in bone compared with soft tissue and therefore a lower risk of osteonecrosis. Disadvantages are the relatively low penetration of the neutrons which have been available until very recently, and the reduced capacity for slowly-replicating tissues to repair the radiation damage which results in increased late normal tissue effects.

So far the trials of neutron therapy in head and neck cancer have failed to demonstrate any definite advantages over photon therapy. Catterall and Bewley (1979) reported improved local control but with some increase in morbidity, especially in the larynx. Duncan *et al.* (1982) also reported increased morbidity without improvement in local control. Dose response curves constructed by Cohen (1982) suggested no difference in therapeutic ratio between neutron and photon therapy for squamous carcinoma, but he claimed to show an advantage of neutrons for treatment of salivary gland carcinoma.

Chemotherapy

Chemotherapy as an adjuvant to radiotherapy has been used extensively in head and neck cancer. A number of cytotoxic drugs have activity against squamous carcinoma in the head and neck, of which methotrexate, bleomycin and cisplatin show the highest response rates. These and several others have been given synchronously with radiotherapy in a variety of regimens and some encouraging results have been claimed. Unfortunately many controlled trials have failed to show a significant increase in survival or local control rates compared with radiotherapy alone. An exception is the trial by Shanta and Krishnamurthi (1977) which compared radiotherapy and concomitant bleomycin with radiotherapy alone in the treatment of carcinoma of the buccal mucosa in South India; a large and significant increase in survival was seen in the patients receiving bleomycin. Other trials have failed to show any advantage from simultaneous use of bleomycin with radiotherapy, and it is probable that buccal carcinoma in India is more responsive to this drug than many other types of squamous carcinoma.

Reports of the use of combinations of cytotoxic drugs are conflicting. Combinations containing vincristine, bleomycin, methotrexate and fluorouracil have been given before radiotherapy by Price and Hill (1982) and during radiotherapy by O'Connor *et al.* (1979); both groups claimed improved survival compared with historical controls. Two small controlled trials of chemotherapy before radiotherapy gave opposite results, neither reaching statistical significance. The trial of Bezwoda, De Moor and Derman (1979) showed a small advantage to chemotherapy, while in the study by Stell *et al.* (1983) the patients given chemotherapy fared appreciably worse than those treated by radiotherapy alone.

When chemotherapy is given before radiotherapy there seems to be no enhancement of radiation effect on normal tissues, but when it is given concurrently with radiotherapy there is a marked increase in mucosal reaction which often necessitates interruption of treatment and there may also be some increase in late normal tissue damage, for example, to the optic nerve (Chan and Shukovsky, 1976). With the drugs currently available there is so far no evidence to justify the routine use of chemotherapy in combination with radiotherapy.

Irradiation techniques

Ideally, the maximum tolerable dose of radiation should be delivered homogeneously to the entire tumour, with no radiation to the normal tissues. Of course this cannot be achieved in practice, but to obtain the best possible results from radiotherapy the high does target volume must encompass the entire tumour to as uniform a dose as possible, while the surrounding normal tissues receive the minimum possible dose. The requirments for accurate delivery of radiotherapy to a head and neck tumour are as follows.

(1) Accurate assessment of the extent of the disease. This requires clinical examination, often under an anaesthetic with endoscopy and appropriate radiology
(2) Satisfactory immobilization fo the patient's head and neck. Treatment shells individually made for each patient from a material such as cellulose acetate are ideal for this purpose. Such shells also serve to carry indelible marks indicating the entry and exit points of the radiation beams and the position of any lead blocks
(3) A suitable treatment plan. The fields must be arranged to deliver a uniform high dose to the target volume while avoiding irradiating sensitive structures such as the lens of the eye. Wedge filters and compensators should be used where necessary to achieve homogeneity of dosage. Fields should be shaped with lead blocks where appropriate, so that the high dose volume is kept as small as possible
(4) Accurate beam direction. Entrance and exit pointers are ideal, but not always practicable especially for anterior fields. Where a back pointer cannot be used, an isocentric method of aligning should be used instead
(5) Check radiographs. The position of each field should be verified, preferably using a simulator to obtain diagnostic-quality films, or using the actual treatment machine.

Management of lymph nodes in the neck

Failure to control lymphatic spread is the most frequent cause of death from head and neck cancer, therefore, the management of lymph node metastases is extremely important.

Staging

There are several lymph node staging systems in current use which lead to confusion in presentation of results of treatment. The most commonly used staging system is that of the International Union Against Cancer (UICC, 1978), in which the four nodal stages are based on therapeutic possibilities rather than prognosis. In contrast, the American Joint Committee (AJC) system (1977), is based on nodal size and correlates better with prognosis. The UICC system is used here as it divides patients with lymph node metastases into groups in whom different therapeutic strategies should be followed (*Table 5.1*).

Table 5.1 Staging systems in current use

	UICC system	*AJC system*
N0	No evidence of regional node involvement	No evidence of regional node involvement
N1	Clinically positive moveable homolateral node or nodes	Single clinically positive homolateral node less than 3 cm in diameter
N2	Clinically positive moveable contralateral or bilateral regional nodes	N_2a A single clinically positive homolateral node, 3–6 cm in diameter N_2b Multiple clinically positive homolateral nodes, none over 6 cm in diameter
N3	Clinically positive fixed node	N_3a Clinically positive homolateral node or nodes, one over 6 cm in diameter N_3b Bilateral clinically positive nodes N_3c Contralateral clinically positive nodes only

Incidence

The incidence of nodal metastases depends on three main factors:

(1) The size of the primary; the larger the tumour, the more likely is nodal disease
(2) Site of primary; for example, the incidence of nodal metastases is high in carcinoma of the nasopharynx and low in carcinoma of the maxillary antrum; it is high in supraglottic carcinoma and low in glottic carcinoma
(3) Histology; the incidence is higher with anaplastic carcinoma compared with well differentiated squamous carcinoma.

N0: no evidence of regional node involvement

Many patients in this category will have microscopic lymph node metastases at presentation, undetectable by clinical examination.

The place of elective treatment of subclinical lymph node metastases has been controversial for many years. Elective block dissection was much advocated in the past, but it is now widely accepted that where the primary is treated by radiotherapy, operation on the neck is not indicated. Where the primary is treated surgically, block dissection is usually combined with the resection if the likelihood of lymph node metastases is high.

Elective nodal irradiation

The studies of Fletcher (1972) and others show that the incidence of overt nodal metastases can be considerably reduced by irradiation to 5000 cGy in 5 weeks, strongly suggesting that this dose can destroy microscopic foci of tumour in the nodes.

The morbidity of elective nodal irradiation is low compared with that of neck dissection, especially when anterior and posterior fields are used with shielding of midline structure.

Irradiation of nodal areas is standard practice with anaplastic carcinoma of the nasopharynx and oropharynx; it is advisable for squamous cell carcinoma of the hypopharynx and supraglottis, and also for larger primaries of the oral cavity. A controlled trial comparing elective nodal irradiation with a watch and wait policy showed a reduction in the incidence of overt nodal metastases, but no increase in survival (Gleave, 1980).

N1: mobile homolateral nodal metastases

A mobile lymph node metastasis may be suspected at the time of diagnosis of the primary tumour, or be found at follow-up after treatment of the primary. It is often difficult to be sure on clinical examination if a mobile swelling in the neck is a lymph node metastasis or merely a benign lesion, such as an enlarged reactive lymph node or a submandibular salivary gland. Aspiration cytology is a useful confirmatory test; in experienced hands false positive results are very rarely seen. A negative aspirate however does not exclude cancer, and if there is real doubt, histological confirmation is necessary before definitive treatment. In these circumstances open biopsy increases the risk of subsequent local recurrence and is best avoided (McGuirt and McCabe, 1978); it is preferable to prepare the patient for a block dissection and excise the lump for frozen section before proceeding to neck dissection.

Lymph node metastases have the same inherent radiosensitivity as the primaries from which they are derived (Henk, 1975). The high incidence of failure in the neck is accounted for by the biological aggressiveness of carcinomas which metastasize to nodes, and to the anatomical difficulties of locating and radically treating lymphatic spread.

The control rates of lymph node metastases by radiotherapy alone tend to be unsatisfactory except for small nodes, or larger metastases from anaplastic primaries in the oropharynx or nasopharynx. Schneider, Fletcher and Barkley (1975) reported a 2-year local control rate of 81% for nodes of 3 cm maximum diameter or smaller, and 64% for single nodes larger than 3 cm. These results are probably falsely high, as only patients with control of the primary tumour were considered; these represent a selected favourable group. The experience of most radiotherapists suggests that the true control rate overall is only about two-thirds of that reported by Schneider.

The recurrence rate after neck dissection is also high, especially if there is involvement of several nodes, or if there is spread of tumour through the capsule of an involved node (De-Croix and Ghossein, 1981; Johnson *et al.*, 1981). Combined treatment gives better results than either radiotherapy or surgery alone. The value of preoperative radiotherapy was confirmed by the trial reported by Strong (1969).

There is good evidence for the value of postoperative radiotherapy from retrospective surveys (Decroix and Ghossein, 1981; Vikram *et al*, 1984a). The policy recommended by the present author for operable nodal metastases is immediate block dissection, with postoperative radiotherapy wherever there is involvement of two or more nodes, or extracapsular extension. The entire lymphatic drainage of the neck should be covered by a single anterior field, shielding the midline structures (*Figure 5.1*). The dose to the operated side of the neck should be at least 6000 cGy in 6 weeks or its radiobiological equivalent.

N2: bilateral mobile nodes, and contralateral lymph node metastases appearing after treatment of primary

These are associated with a poor prognosis except

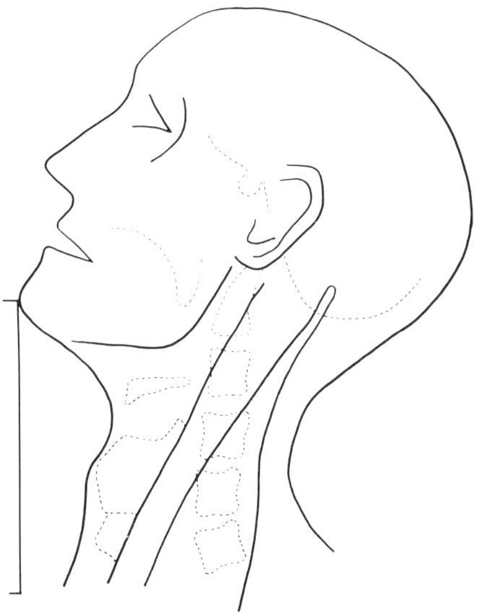

Figure 5.1 Lateral view of volume irradiated for postoperative or elective irradiation of the lymph nodes of the neck

possibly in the case of anaplastic carcinoma of the nasopharynx. Bilateral block dissection of the neck is not possible because of the risks associated with removal of both internal jugular veins; sometimes, however, a modified operation preserving the internal jugular vein is feasible on the second side, which should always be followed by radiotherapy. In practice, most patients with bilateral nodal metastases are treated by external radiotherapy alone.

N3: fixed nodal metastases

Fixity is a difficult sign to interpret and does not necessarily contraindicate surgery. A mass firmly attached to the base of the skull or the floor of the posterior triangle is unsuitable for resection. However, complete removal of a node which is apparently fixed to the mandible or carotid sheath is often possible, and such a case should be managed as described for stage N1 above.

Inoperable masses in the neck are most commonly treated by external irradiation but with generally poor results. In selected younger patients, it is worth trying to render a fixed mass operable by radiotherapy to a dose of 5000 cGy in 5 weeks as recommended by Jesse and Fletcher (1977). If the mass becomes mobile at the end of this course of treatment a block dissection can be attempted; if not a further 2000 cGy should be given by a smaller field to the residual mass.

Carcinoma of the lip

Carcinoma of the lip usually presents at an early stage and lymph node metastases occur in only about 10% of cases. Consequently, the prognosis is good; surgery and radiotherapy give equally successful results and the choice of treatment depends on convenience and the expected cosmetic result.

Diagnosis and staging

The diagnosis must be established by biopsy. The extent of the lesion can be ascertained in most cases by clinical examination. X-ray of the mandible is indicated if the tumour is attached to bone.

The UICC staging system for the primary tumour is as follows:

T1 tumour limited to the lip: 2 cm or less in its greatest dimension
T2 tumour limited to the lip: more than 2 cm but not more than 4 cm in its greatest dimension
T3 tumour limited to the lip: more than 4 cm in its greatest dimension
T4 tumour extending beyond lip to neighbouring structures. e.g. bone, tongue, skin of neck, etc.

Treatment

Surgery is preferable in most cases, lesions up to 2 cm in diameter can be resected with primary closure; this is a simple procedure, quicker and involving less discomfort for the patient than radiotherapy. If larger lesions are to be excised, a reconstructive procedure under general anaesthesia is necessary to achieve a good cosmetic and functional result. In such cases, the advantages and disadvantages of radiotherapy for the individual patient must be considered. In general, the early cosmetic results of radiotherapy are better, but after a few years atrophy and telangiectasia occur so that the long-term result may be no better or even worse than that of surgery.

Radiotherapy technique

The simplest method of radiotherapy is external beam using a single anterior field, with either orthovoltage X-rays or an electron beam of 8–10 MeV. The oral cavity is protected by a lead gum shield, and a lead cut out defines the area to be treated. The electron beam gives a more uniform distribution of dose through the thickness of the lip, and a better cosmetic result, than X-rays.

Using electrons, a dose of 5000 cGy in 10 fractions in 3 weeks is suitable. No benefit from more protracted fractionation has been established, although some radiotherapists claim that this results in less late radiation changes. Treatment over 4 or more weeks compares unfavourably with surgery in terms of cost and convenience.

Brachytherapy is now rarely used for carcinoma of the lip. The sandwich mould technique is obsolete. Interstitial irradiation using iridium wires afterloaded into steel tubes as described by Durrant and Ellis (1973) gives good results, but requires hospitalization for 1 week and a general anaesthetic (*see* Chapter 16). The advantages over electron beam therapy are minimal.

Elective irradiation of the nodal areas is not indicated for carcinoma of the lip. If lymph node metastases appear subsequent to treatment of the primary, they should be managed by neck dissection and radiotherapy as described above.

Adverse effects

Mucositis is inevitable regardless of fractionation. It appears at the end of the second week of treatment and persists until 2 or 3 weeks after the end of treatment. It is sore and uncomfortable. No local applications help very much. A barrier cream may prevent drying and cracking of the surface which can be very painful.

Results

The results of radiotherapy of carcinoma of the lip are generally good with an overall local control rate of about 90%. The success rate depends on tumour size, it is very rare to fail to cure a lesion less than 2 cm in diameter. There is a small mortality rate, due mainly to lymphatic spread.

Carcinoma of the oral cavity

Most malignant tumours in the mouth arise from the squamous epithelium. Mucus gland tumours are occasionally seen, of the same histological types that occur in the major salivary glands, and are treated according to similar principles. This section will discuss only squamous carcinoma.

Diagnosis and staging

The extent of a tumour in the mouth can usually be defined quite accurately by clinical examination. X-rays are needed if the lesion is close to the mandible or maxilla, to determine whether or not bone is invaded.

The diagnosis must be established by biopsy. If 'excision biopsy' of a very small lesion is performed, it must be accompanied by an accurate record of the position and limits of the lesion. Too often a radiotherapist is presented with a patient who has no visible or palpable abnormality, but is reported to have had a carcinoma in the mouth incompletely excised.

The UICC system for staging of the primary tumour is as follows:

- T1 tumour 2 cm or less in its greatest dimension
- T2 tumour more than 2 cm but not more than 4 cm in its greatest dimension
- T3 tumour more than 4 cm in its greatest dimension
- T4 tumour with extension to bone, muscle, skin, antrum, neck, etc.

This classification often proves unsatisfactory in practice. For example, a small tumour of the tongue with superficial infiltration into the muscle may be classified by one observer as T1, and by another as T4.

The AJC system is similar, but defines T4 less ambiguously as a 'massive tumour greater than 4 cm in diameter with deep invasion to involve antrum, pterygoid muscles, root of tongue or skin of neck'.

Treatment

Initial radical radiotherapy is preferable to elective surgery for most early and medium-size lesions, as cure rates are as high with radiotherapy and there is less deformity and disability than with surgery. Larger deeply-infiltrating tumours are not often cured by radiotherapy, so combined surgery and radiotherapy are better where feasible. Involvement of bone is also an indication for primary surgery; even if radiotherapy succeeds in eliminating tumour from bone, subsequent problems with osteoradionecrosis are almost inevitable.

Interstitial irradiation gives higher local control rates than external irradiation. It is the preferred method of treatment for suitable tumours, i.e. those where the lesion is clear of bone and can be encompassed in all dimensions by the implanted sources. Superficial tumours up to about 3 cm in diameter without nodal involvement in the tongue and cheek should be treated by implant alone. Larger lesions, especially those with infiltration of underlying muscle or with early nodal involvement, are best treated by a combination of external and interstitial radiotherapy. A dose of 5000 cGy in 5 weeks is given to the primary and nodal drainage areas, followed by a further 3000 cGy to the primary by an implant. If the nodes are involved, a block dissection of the neck should be performed after the implant.

For interstitial radiotherapy radium needles are now obsolete. The techniques using artificial radioisotopes described in Chapter 16 have the advantages of a lower radiation dose to the operator and less discomfort for the patient, and may lead to better results. Pierquin *et al.* (1970) reported a local recurrence rate of 33% using radium needles and 4% using iridium.

Radiotherapy techniques

Tongue

Carcinoma occurs most commonly on the lateral border of the mobile portion of the tongue. Small superficial lesions, especially on the anterior third are best treated with wide local excision. T1 and T2 tumours of the middle third and those where a more extensive surgical procedure would be necessary are best treated with interstitial irradiation as described in Chapter 16. For more advanced T2 tumours or where there is some deep infiltration confined to the lateral portion of the tongue and medial side of the floor of mouth, external beam irradiation should be used first, the fields covering the primary site and the first lymph node stations on both sides of the neck to a dose of 5000 cGy in 5 weeks or its radiobiological equivalent, followed by an implant.

Where the lesions are more extensive with involvement of the lower alveolus or deep infiltration into the tongue musculature the chance of local control is greater with elective surgery, but it must be borne in mind that extensive resection is necessary with associated disability; the alternative is external radiotherapy to maximum tissue tolerance dosage but this has a rather small chance of success.

Floor of the mouth

Carcinoma of the floor of the mouth has a similar aetiology and natural history to that of carcinoma of the tongue and is treated according to the same principles.

Radical radiotherapy is preferable to immediate surgery for lesions where there is at least 5 mm clearance between the edge of the tumour and the mandible, and where there is only minimal deep infiltration of the musculature of the tongue. A small tumour up to about 1.5 cm in diameter can be treated by interstitial therapy alone; a variety of techniques are in use, the simplest being the direct insertion of short iridium hairpins. A disadvantage of this technique is that the legs of the hairpins tend to splay apart after insertion and so some radiotherapists favour the use of more rigid sources inserted through a custom-made applicator as described by Marcus, Million and Mitchell (1980). Lesions more than 1.5 cm in diameter are best managed by a combination of external radiotherapy, giving 5000 cGy to the primary and the regional lymph nodes, followed by an implant (*Figure 5.2*).

Small tumours adjacent to the periosteum of the mandible are best managed by conservative surgery. The tumour is excised with partial thickness resection of the mandible; postoperative radiotherapy is not

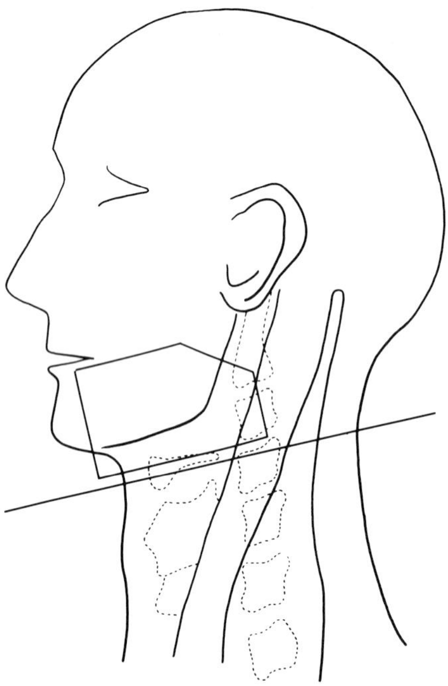

Figure 5.2 Fields of irradiation for carcinoma of the floor of the mouth

usually necessary unless the tumour is demonstrated histologically to be very close to the resection margins. Deeply infiltrating tumours and those recurring after radical radiotherapy require 'commando' resection.

Buccal mucosa

Carcinoma of the mucosa of the cheek in general tends to be less aggressive than carcinoma of the tongue or floor of the mouth, with a lower incidence of lymphatic spread. Provided there is a clear margin of at least 1 cm of mucosa between the lesion and the nearest bone, interstitial therapy is the treatment of choice. The simplest technique is insertion of rigid caesium needles percutaneously; a dose of 6500 cGy at 0.5 cm depth is given in 6 days. Where the tumour is close to the bone it cannot be encompassed adequately by an implant and so should be treated by external radiotherapy using a wedged pair technique. The primary tumour and first lymph node station can usually be covered by a target volume approximately 7 × 7 × 3 cm, so a dose of 5500 cGy in 4 weeks is suitable. If the treated volume is larger, 6500 cGy in 6.5 weeks is preferable, using daily fractionation.

Lower alveolus

Carcinoma of the lower alveolus invades bone at a very early stage and in general is best treated surgically. A possible exception is a very superficial early tumour which can be irradiated by iridium wires contained in plastic tubes looped over the alveolus, as described by Alcock, Paine and Weatherburn (1984). In a patient unfit for mandibular resection external radiotherapy using a wedged pair technique is used, but the chances of success are rather low and osteoradionecrosis is likely; 6500 cGy in 32 fractions in 6.5 weeks, or its radiobiological equivalent, is given.

Retromolar trigone and anterior faucial pillar

Carcinoma arising in this area tends to spread and infiltrate deeply at an early stage. Nevertheless, surgical clearance is difficult to obtain and the morbidity from resection is high. Consequently, external radiotherapy is the treatment of choice using a wedged pair technique to include the primary tumour and adjacent upper deep cervical nodes, similar to that used for carcinoma of the tonsillar fossa *(see below)*.

Adverse effects

The effects of interstitial therapy are confined to the tissues into which the sources have been introduced. Mucositis appears a few days after removal of the implant, and usually progresses to a thick confluent fibrinous membrane; it takes on average 4 weeks for re-epithelialization to occur. Small areas of necrosis of the mucous membrane are prone to occur most often during the first year after treatment; these normally heal readily with conservative measures.

External radiotherapy is associated with greater morbidity. Mucositis occurs within the irradiated volume; its severity depends on the dose and to some extent on the fractionation, the changes being more severe but shorter lasting when short courses of treatment are given. Most of the patients experience taste loss, the mechanism of which is not clear; it is more likely to be due to the effect of radiation on mucus and salivary glands than to a direct action on the taste receptor cells. Taste sensation generally recovers a few months after radiotherapy. Dryness of the mouth occurs at an early stage in the course of radiotherapy. Salivary gland function is permanently abolished by doses in excess of 2000 cGy. The severity of xerostomia depends on the volume of salivary tissue which receives this dose. Usually, when treating oral cavity carcinoma it is possible to avoid irradiating some of the parotid tissue, which can subsequently undergo compensatory hypertrophy, so that the xerostomia is not permanent.

Osteoradionecrosis may occur when any party of the mandible is in the high dose irradiated volume. It is caused by the action of radiation on both the osteoblasts and the vascular endothelium; the relatively poorly-vascularized mandible is at much greater risk than the well-vascularized maxilla. The incidence of this complication depends on the radiation dose absorbed in the bone, which in turn depends on the dose delivered and the type of radiation. Orthovoltage X-rays, with their high absorption in elements of higher atomic number, cause an appreciable incidence of osteoradionecrosis at therapeutic dose levels, whereas megavoltage X-rays at the same dose rarely cause it unless there is some other contributory factor. Neutron irradiation, where the absorption is dependent on the concentration of hydrogen atoms, in fact has a lower absorption in bone than in soft tissue.

The most important precipitating factor of osteoradionecrosis is trauma. There is normally very little mitotic activity in bone cells; they can therefore continue to function after a lethal dose of irradiation. However, trauma to the bone acts as a mitotic stimulus causing many of the irradiated cells to undergo mitotic death. Attempted re-modelling of the bone is therefore followed by necrosis. The commonest trauma is dental extraction; others are surgical operations and the entry of infection through periodontal disease or ulceration of the mucosa for any reason. Dental extractions should be avoided wherever possible in a patient receiving radiotherapy to the mouth; if they are necessary they are less likely to lead to osteoradionecrosis if performed before rather than after radiotherapy. In order to minimize the risk of osteoradionecrosis dental examination and treatment before radiotherapy is essential. Teeth should be conserved wherever possible, but any which seem unlikely to survive the lifetime of the patient or require very extensive restorative procedures, such as bridging or root filling, are best extracted atraumatically and the gums sutured so that healing is completed rapidly. Subsequent to radiotherapy scrupulous dental care and hygiene are necessary so that further extractions can be avoided. There is an especial risk of dental decay in patients with xerostomia and in such cases the teeth require extra care; methods which have been shown to preserve teeth under these circumstances include capping (Coffin, 1973) and topical application of fluoride gel (Daly, Drane and MacComb, 1972) (*see* Chapter 18).

Results

Survival depends on the stage of the disease at presentation, especially the presence or absence of lymph node metastases. It is also related to sex — females having a better prognosis than males, to histology — poorly differentiated and anaplastic carcinomas having a higher incidence of lymph node metastases (Langdon *et al.*, 1977), and to the site of the primary. Typical overall survival rates for oral cancer in the UK are shown in *Table 5.2*.

Local control by radiotherapy is related mainly to the size and degree of infiltration of the primary tumour. It does not correlate with the degree of differentiation of the tumour. Typical local control rates are shown in *Table 5.3*.

Table 5.2 Typical survival rates for squamous carcinoma of the oral cavity (from Langdon *et al.*, 1977)

Site	*5-year survival (%)*
Tongue	38
Floor of the mouth	29
Lower alveolus	26
Cheek	44

Table 5.3 Typical local control rates of radiotherapy for oral cavity carcinoma

Site	*Local control (%)*
Tongue	57 (T1–95)
Floor of the mouth	58
Lower alveolus	38
Cheek	75

Carcinoma of the oropharynx

The oropharynx is the central portion of the pharynx extending from the level of the palate above to the hyoid bone below. Its roof is formed by the soft palate; the lateral walls contain the tonsillar fossae and faucial pillars; the anterior wall consists of the base of the tongue, vallecula and anterior surface of the epiglottis. Most malignant tumours of this region are squamous carcinomas which tend to be less well-differentiated than in the oral cavity, with a tendency to more rapid growth and earlier involvement of lymph nodes.

Diagnosis and staging

General anaesthesia is advisable in order for an adequate piece of tissue to be obtained for biopsy. At the same time the pharynx can be examined by inspection and palpation to determine the exact extent of the tumour. If deep infiltration into the pterygoid fossa or parapharyngeal space is suspected a CT scan is helpful.

The UICC staging system for the primary tumour is as follows:

T1 tumour 2 cm or less in its greatest dimension
T2 tumour more than 2 cm but not more than 4 cm in its greatest dimension
T3 tumour more than 4 cm in its greatest dimension
T4 tumour with extension to bone, muscle, skin, antrum, neck, etc.

Treatment

Radiotherapy remains the most satisfactory treatment for carcinoma of the oropharynx. In recent years there has been increasing interest in surgical management with improved reconstructive techniques, but nevertheless, the morbidity of surgery remains high and most patients have severe difficulties with speech and swallowing after excision of oropharyngeal tumours. There is no evidence to date that survival rates are higher than those of radiotherapy alone. For example, Perez *et al.* (1982) compared the results of preoperative radiotherapy and surgery with those of radiotherapy alone in a retrospective study of 218 patients with carcinoma of the tonsillar fossa; no significant difference in survival or recurrence was detected and the authors concluded that radiotherapy remains the treatment of choice for carcinoma of the tonsillar fossa. In the case of tumours of the soft palate, posterior pharyngeal wall, and base of the tongue, the chances of successful surgical removal are low and the results of radiotherapy are usually better than those of surgery.

Radiotherapy technique

The incidence of lymphatic spread is high so lymph node drainage areas should be included in the treatment volume.

In the case of an early carcinoma of the tonsillar region without palpable lymph nodes it is only necessary to treat the primary site and the first station lymph nodes, i.e. the ipsilateral upper deep cervical and submandibular groups. Contralateral lymph node metastases are rare with disease of this stage; irradiation of the opposite side of the neck results in increased morbidity and is unnecessary (Murthy and Hendrickson, 1980). The required target volume can be easily encompassed using two oblique wedged fields from the same side (*Figure 5.3*). In all other cases, it is advisable to use parallel opposed lateral fields covering the whole oropharynx and first station lymph nodes, namely the retropharyngeal in the case of carcinoma of the soft palate, the upper deep cervical in the case of carcinoma of the tonsil, and the jugulo-omohyoid in the case of carcinoma of the base of the tongue (*Figure 5.4*). Where there is lymph node involvement the contralateral nodes and the lower part of the neck should also be irradiated using an anterior field with midline shielding; the upper border of the anterior field is matched to the lower borders of the lateral fields.

The primary site and any involved lymph nodes should receive a maximum tissue tolerance dosage, i.e. 6500 cGy in 32 fractions in 6.5 weeks or its radiobiological equivalent. Any clinically uninvolved nodal areas irradiated electively should receive 5000 cGy in 5 weeks. In the case of a carcinoma of the tonsil with unilateral nodal involvement the required dose distribution can be best achieved by parallel opposed lateral fields, weighting the field from the affected side 2:1 so that the contralateral upper deep cervical nodes receive approximately 85% of the maximum tumour dose.

Adverse effects

Mucositis occurs towards the end of a course of radiotherapy. The affected area of mucosa is greater when parallel opposed fields are used and in these cases there is often quite marked dysphagia. Patients should be encouraged to take adequate nourishment with a soft diet and liquid food supplements if necessary. Local analgesics such as aspirin mucilage help to ease the soreness and make swallowing easier. If the patient is not getting an adequate food intake or becoming dehydrated it is necessary to pass a fine

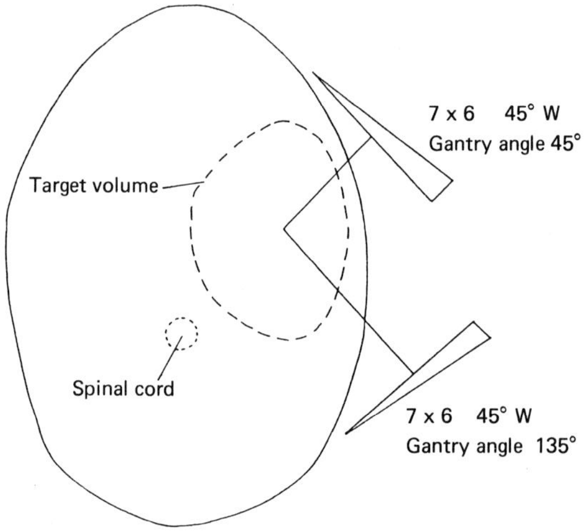

Figure 5.3 Field arrangement for treatment of early carcinoma of the tonsillar fossa, anterior faucial pillar or retromolar trigone. 6 MeV, 100 cm f.s.d.

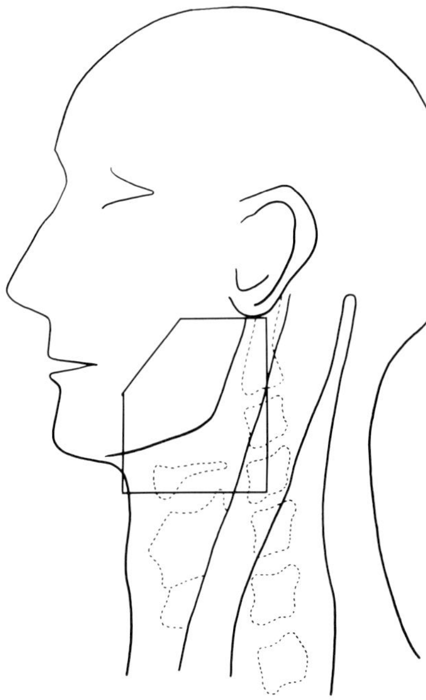

Figure 5.4 Lateral view of volume irradiated for carcinoma of the tonsil

nasogastric tube to maintain nutrition and hydration until the mucositis settles. Skin reaction occurs in the neck at the entry of the beams, but with megavoltage therapy this is usually mild.

Late morbidity from radiotherapy is uncommon. Osteoradionecrosis of the mandible, soft tissue necrosis, and pharyngeal fibrosis leading to permanent difficulty with swallowing have all been described, but provided the dose levels recommended are not exceeded, these complications are all rare in the absence of persistent tumour. If salvage surgery is attempted after radical radiotherapy there is an appreciable risk of postoperative complications including delayed healing, wound infection, fistulae and carotid artery rupture.

Results

The success rates of radiotherapy are higher than in the case of the oral cavity, with good local control rates for both primary tumours and lymph node metastases. This is probably because the more anaplastic tumours with lymphocytic infiltration are more radiosensitive. Nearly all local recurrences occur within 18 months of completing radiotherapy, and after 3 years the survival rate of patients with carcinoma of the oropharynx is the same as that of the normal population of the same age and sex. Distant metastases are a cause of death in some cases but only a relatively small proportion of patients die of distant metastases without residual or recurrent tumour in the head and neck.

The probability of local control and survival depends on the stage of disease at presentation. The 5-year survival ranges from over 80% for T1N0 carcinoma of the tonsil down to less than 20% for T4N3 carcinoma of the base of the tongue. Typical results for a regional radiotherapy centre in the UK were quoted by Henk (1978) (*Table 5.4*). Somewhat better results were quoted by Fletcher (1973) but it is difficult to compare treatment results because of different TNM staging systems and also the fact that in the USA the disease tends to occur in a younger age group.

Table 5.4 Results of treatment of all cases of carcinoma of the oropharynx seen in a regional radiotherapy centre between 1960 and 1971 (Henk, 1978)

Site	*Primary control at 2 years (%)*	*5-year survival (%)*
Tonsil	63 (T1–77)	33
Base of the tongue	45 (T1–67)	17
Soft palate	86	45
Posterior wall	50	10

Carcinoma of the nasopharynx

Carcinoma of the nasopharynx differs in many respects from other mucosal neoplasms in the head and neck. A greater proportion are anaplastic and occur in a younger age group compared with carcinoma at other head and neck sites. Anaplastic carcinoma at this site often has a lymphoid stroma, and was formerly known as 'lymphoepithelioma'; this term is now obsolete.

The incidence varies markedly in different parts of the world. In south-east China, it is the commonest malignancy; here the peak age incidence is in the fifth decade. In some parts of the world, for example North Africa, the tumour is common and the peak incidence occurs even earlier. In the Western World it is relatively rare. Where the disease is common the anaplastic type predominates; in those parts of the world where the disease is rarer, the well-differentiated squamous type is prevalent.

Presentation tends to be late because symptoms often do not occur until the disease has spread to adjacent structures, e.g. the Eustachian tube, base of the skull or regional lymph nodes. The incidence of lymph node metastases is high, in most series approximately 70% of patients have involved lymph nodes at presentation. Lymph node metastases are commoner in the anaplastic than in the well-differentiated type.

Routes of spread of the disease are important in planning target volumes for radiotherapy. Superiorly, the tumour may invade the base of the skull. The weakest barrier to upward spread is provided by the foramen lacerum immediately lateral to the basisphenoid bone through which tumour may enter the floor of the cavernous sinus. Hence a sixth nerve palsy may occur without radiological evidence of bone destruction. Laterally, the tumour may enter the parapharyngeal space by spread through the lateral wall of the nasopharynx where the cartilaginous portion of the Eustachian tube enters. Anteriorly, the tumour may spread via the sphenopalatine foramen to the pterygoid fossa and thence to the orbital apex through the inferior orbital fissure. The posterior part of the nasal fossa and the oropharynx may be involved by direct mucosal extension.

The nasopharynx has a rich lymphatic drainage. One of the first nodes which may be involved is the lateral pharyngeal, close to the root of the styloid process. Involvement of the node may result in lesions of the lower four cranial nerves. Lymphatics drain to the upper nodes in both the jugular and spinal accessory chains either directly or via the lateral pharyngeal node. The highest node in the spinal accessory chain in the submastoid region is often the first node to become palpable in the neck.

Diagnosis and staging

The diagnosis should be established by biopsy of the primary site wherever possible, only in cases of doubt should a lymph node be removed from the neck for histology. The extent of spread of the disease in the primary site and in the lymph nodes must be assessed by clinical examination, and by examination under anaesthesia, including the nasal fossa, the oropharynx and the cranial nerves. CT scanning is useful to assess the extent of disease, especially in the base of the skull. Distant metastases occur not infrequently especially with the anaplastic type and so clinical examination for metastases and a chest X-ray are essential. A bone scan is advisable in patients with extensive lymph node involvement.

The UICC staging system for the primary tumour is as follows:

- T1 tumour confined to one site (including tumour identified from positive biopsy)
- T2 tumour involving two sites
- T3 tumour with extension to nasal cavity and/or oropharynx
- T4 tumour with extension to base of skull and/or involving cranial nerves.

Treatment

Radiotherapy is well established as the sole curative treatment for this disease. The anaplastic type is chemosensitive but it is not yet clear whether the routine addition of chemotherapy to radiotherapy can improve the cure rate. A dose of 6000 cGy in 6 weeks is required for anaplastic carcinoma; a slightly higher dose is advisable for squamous carcinoma. These dose levels exceed the tolerance of many sensitive adjacent structures, especially the spinal cord, brain stem, optic nerve and retina, so an accurate radiotherapy technique is of paramount importance if patients are to be cured with a minimal incidence of complications.

There is some controversy regarding the value of prophylactic neck irradiation in a patient without involved nodes. Ho (1978) in a small controlled trial, demonstrated that in T1N0 lesions elective nodal irradiation conferred no survival benefit. However, most patients present at a later stage than this, and not many can be demonstrated with any certainty to be stage I. The present author's policy therefore is to irradiate the nodal areas in all cases, the whole neck in anaplastic carcinoma and the upper neck in squamous carcinoma.

Radiotherapy technique

The primary target volume should include the nasopharynx and the regions of potential spread of the disease. Structures to be irradiated must include the posterior half of the nasal fossa, the soft palate, the part of the base of the skull formed by the greater wing of sphenoid, and the parapharyngeal space. The posterior half of the orbit should also be irradiated but the dose should not exceed 5500 cGy; at the same time the dose to the spinal cord, brain stem and optic chiasma should not exceed 4000 cGy, on the basis of 200 cGy per fraction. As much as possible of the oral cavity should be avoided.

The majority of patients presenting for radiotherapy will have involved palpable lymph nodes in the neck. In these cases, it is advisable to treat the entire primary volume and the lymphatic drainage of the neck down to the clavicles with large lateral parallel opposed fields, to a dose of 3000 cGy in 3 weeks. The volume is the split into two parts, treating the primary area with small parallel opposed fields, covering the nasopharynx, parapharyngeal space, base of the skull and posterior half of the orbit, extending sufficiently far forward to cover any anterior extension into the nasal fossa and sufficiently far downwards to cover any extension into the oropharynx (*Figure 5.5*). The neck is treated at the same time by an anterior field with midline shielding. Treatment of the neck in this way is facilitated if the patient is positioned supine with the head well extended, when it is usually possible to position the junction between the lateral and anterior fields above the level of any palpable nodes. The fields should be reduced in size superiorly after 5500 cGy to avoid the optic nerve and retina.

Where there is no lymph node involvement the technique differs according to the histological type of the tumour. For a well-differentiated squamous cell carcinoma, a high dose is needed at the primary site. A dose of 5500 cGy is given in 5.5 weeks in 27 fractions with lateral fields, followed by a further 1500 cGy in eight fractions to a reduced volume covering the extent of the primary tumour, taking care to avoid the eyes, optic nerves and brain stem; the final phase of the treatment is given with an anterior and two lateral wedged fields. The immediate lymphatic drainage in the upper half of the neck is treated electively with an anterior field to a dose of 5000 cGy in 5 weeks. In the case of an anaplastic carcinoma, it is necessary to give the primary only 6000 cGy in 6 weeks which can be done entirely with two lateral fields. The whole neck down to the clavicles should be treated at the same time with an anterior field to a dose of 5000 cGy in 5 weeks.

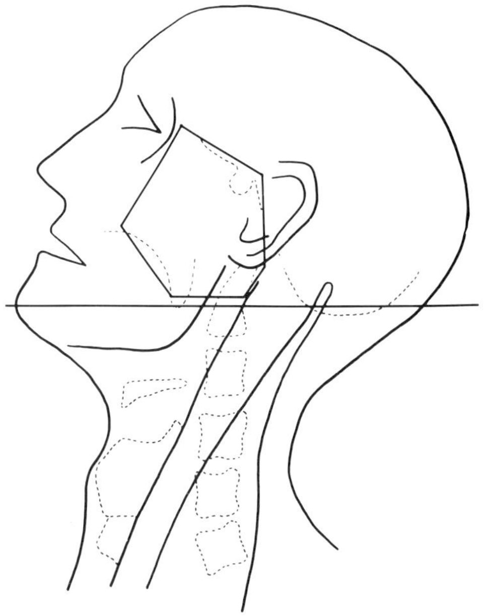

Figure 5.5 Radiotherapy fields for carcinoma of the nasopharynx

Adverse effects

During treatment, mucositis in the oropharynx causes dysphagia. Taste loss begins after the second week and usually lasts for several months after treatment is completed. The most unpleasant late effect is severe dryness of the mouth due to the lateral fields passing through both parotids, whose function is usually totally ablated. There is therefore, a great risk of caries, so good dental care is important. Occasional cases of damage to the spinal cord, brain stem or optic nerves have been described but should not occur with careful treatment planning. The pituitary gland is within the volume in most cases; there is often depression of pituitary function, detectable by chemical studies, but this hardly every results in clinical hypopituitarism.

Results

The outcome of treatment depends on clinical stage at presentation, and histological type. Survival rates are higher in anaplastic compared with squamous carcinoma. Mesic, Fletcher and Goepfert (1981) reported a 5-year survival of 65% for anaplastic carcinoma; the majority of the deaths were from distant metastases with only 2% of patients dying solely of local recurrence. By contrast, the 5-year survival with squamous carcinoma was 42% with about one-half of the deaths due to local disease. Survival figures correlate better with nodal staging than with T-staging, probably because of the difficulty in accurate assessment of extent of disease around the primary site. Survival rates correlate better with the level of nodal involvement in the neck than with size or fixity of nodes (Ho, 1982).

Juvenile angiofibroma

The juvenile angiofibroma of the nasopharynx, a rare lesion occurring in adolescent boys, is histologically benign but may run a clinically malignant cause. Severe haemorrhage or intracranial and orbital extension may be life threatening.

Accurate definition of the tumour extent by arteriography and CT scanning is an essential part of the management. Surgical resection is the treatment of choice wherever possible, but in many cases it may be very hazardous or impossible especially when there is infiltration beyond the nasopharynx. Radiotherapy is an alternative to surgery. A dose of 3000 cGy in 15 fractions in 3 weeks leads to resolution of the disease in nearly all cases although up to 2 years may elapse before disappearance of the lesion (Fitzpatrick, Briant and Berman, 1980). Radiotherapy is best reserved for inoperable cases because of the small but real risk of radiation-induced malignancy.

Carcinoma of the ear

From the point of view of treatment technique, carcinoma of the external auditory meatus and middle ear cavity can be considered together because of their similar clinical features, modes of spread and approach to treatment. Carcinoma at both these sites is exceedingly rare. Tumours of the external auditory canal are mainly squamous cell carcinomas but occasionally basal cell carcinomas occur; they are seen most frequently in women of middle age. Tumours of the middle ear are also mainly squamous cell carcinomas but adenocarcinoma of various types also occurs; most patients with squamous carcinoma of the middle ear have a long history of chronic otitis media and develop a carcinoma in later life.

Spread of the disease is initially in the soft tissues, tumours of the middle ear involving the external auditory meatus and vice versa. Invasion of the temporal bone occurs in the majority of cases with eventual involvement of the facial nerve and the adjacent brain. Lymphatic spread may occur to both preauricular and upper posterior deep cervical lymph nodes, especially in the case of tumours of the external auditory canal.

Diagnosis and staging

The diagnosis must be established by biopsy. At the same time a clinical assessment of the stage of the disease is essential. Clinical examination must include the ear, the cranial nerves, the surrounding soft tissues and the lymph nodes. Assessment of the degree of invasion of the temporal bone is difficult; plain X-rays of the petrous region and CT scanning are the most useful investigations for this purpose.

Treatment

Most cases are treated by resection and postoperative radiotherapy if the patient is fit enough and the tumour is not obviously inoperable. Contraindications to surgery include involvement of the carotid canal, intracranial extension, and fixed nodal metastases.

However, the value of surgery has not been clearly established; more radical operations introduced in recent years have failed to improve survival rates. Radical radiotherapy should be considered as an alternative to surgery, especially in the older or less fit patient. An advantage of surgery is the relief of pain which can be obtained even if the tumour is not completely removed.

Radiotherapy technique

The same technique is used for both radical and postoperative radiotherapy. Anterior and posterior oblique wedged fields are used to treat a target volume which includes the entire petrous bone, the parotid gland, and the preauricular and submastoid lymph nodes but just avoiding the brain stem and upper spinal cord (*Figure 5.6*). The treatment plane must be inclined so that the posterior field exits below the contralateral eye (*Figure 5.7*). A dose of around 6500 cGy in 6.5 weeks or equivalent is given.

Results

Most series report a 5-year survival of about 40% from surgery and postoperative radiotherapy, and 15% from radiotherapy alone (Hahn *et al.*, 1983). The more favourable cases are selected for surgery, so that overall the survival is about 20%.

In a small series reported by Holmes (1965) all patients were treated primarily by radical radiotherapy, with a 5-year survival of 54%.

Glomus jugulare tumour

This is a rare benign tumour belonging to the family of the non-chromaffin paragangliomas. It arises from chemoreceptor cells in the jugular bulb. It occurs more commonly in females than males with a peak incidence in the fourth and fifth decades. It may involve the middle ear causing deafness and tinnitus, and the lower six cranial nerves leading to a variety of neurological lesions. It is characteristically highly vascular. Its extent can be best delineated by digital angiography.

The most popular treatment now is surgical excision with prior embolization, but this is only feasible with relatively small lesions. Larger tumours are better treated by radiotherapy as surgery remains hazardous even with modern techniques. The same radiotherapy technique is used as for carcinoma of the middle ear. It is not necessary to give maximum tissue tolerance dosage: 5000 cGy in 25 fractions in 5 weeks is adequate.

Results of radiotherapy

Regression after radiotherapy is slow. Symptoms are gradually relieved over a period of weeks or several months. Clinical and radiological evidence of the tumour usually persists indefinitely but rarely causes further trouble (Maruyama, Gold and Kieffer, 1971). Long-term follow-up of many series treated by radiotherapy reveals that less than 20% of the tumours show evidence of regrowth within 20 years, and the mortality from the disease is less than 10%.

Carcinoma of the maxillary antrum

Carcinoma of the maxillary antrum characteristically presents at a late stage because it does not give rise to

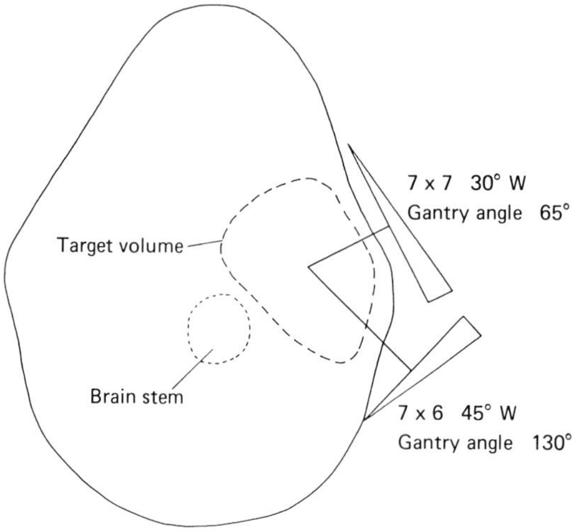

Figure 5.6 Field arrangement for treatment of carcinoma of the middle ear. 6 MeV, 100 cm f.s.d.

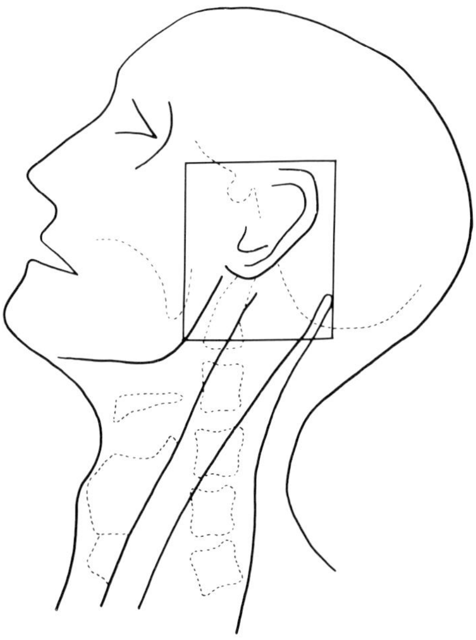

Figure 5.7 Lateral view of volume irradiated for carcinoma of the middle ear

symptoms until it penetrates through the bony walls of the antrum to involve other structures. Nevertheless, involvement of regional lymph nodes is uncommon. Spread occurs inferiorly through the floor of the antrum to involve the oral cavity, anteriorly into the cheek, laterally into the nasal cavity, superiorly into the orbit, and posteriorly into the pterygoid fossa.

Diagnosis and staging

The antrum should be explored and biopsy taken, preferably via a nasal antrostomy which will also provide drainage. The extent of spread of the disease must be established by clinical examination of the sinuses, mouth, orbit, cranial nerves and neck, together with X-rays and CT scanning.

There is no UICC staging system for carcinoma of the maxillary antrum. The AJC system recommends division of the antrum into two parts by means of Ohngren's line, a theoretical plane joining the medial canthus of the eye with the angle of mandible. Tumours arising anteroinferior to this line, i.e. in the 'infrastructure', have a better prognosis than those arising posterosuperior, in the 'suprastructure'. The AJC staging system for the primary tumour is as follows:

T1 tumour confined to antral mucosa of the infrastructure with no bone erosion or destruction
T2 tumour confined to the suprastructure mucosa without bone destruction or to infrastructure with destruction of the medial or inferior bony walls only
T3 more extensive tumour invading the skin of the cheek, orbit, anterior ethmoid sinuses, or pterygoid muscle
T4 massive tumour with invasion of cribriform plate, posterior ethmoids, sphenoid, nasopharynx, pterygoid plates, or base of the skull.

Treatment

Most unsuccessfully treated cases of carcinoma of the maxillary antrum die of persistent local disease. The problem is one of local control which is difficult because of the large bulk of the tumour present at diagnosis. Combined treatment with surgery and radiotherapy is preferable wherever possible. Unfortunately, a sizeable proportion of patients are unfit for surgery due to age, poor general condition or extent of disease. In these patients radiotherapy is the only radical treatment which can be attempted.

In patients who are considered potentially operable, preoperative radiotherapy is preferred. The principles of preoperative radiotherapy outlined above are not usually applied to antral carcinoma.

There is always the likelihood that when operation is undertaken it may not be possible to remove the entire tumour, so a full radical dose is advisable. Fortunately, the maxilla has a good blood supply so that the morbidity of surgery is not greatly increased by high dose radiotherapy preoperatively, unlike many other head and neck sites.

The maxillary antrum is the most favoured site in the head and neck for intra-arterial cytotoxic therapy in conjunction with radiotherapy. Most antral carcinomas derive their blood supply entirely from the maxillary and facial arteries and can therefore be perfused by the external carotid artery. Improved local control rates have been claimed from the use of fluorouracil (Sato *et al.*, 1970), and from methotrexate and bleomycin (Moseley *et al.*, 1981). However, mucositis and late normal tissue effects of radiation are also enhanced (Chan and Shukovsky, 1976). There is no clear evidence that the addition of chemotherapy either systemically or locally enhances the therapeutic ratio of radiotherapy.

Radiotherapy technique

Initial treatment is by external beam radiotherapy. The volume should include the entire maxilla, the pterygoid fossa, the whole of the ethmoid bone on both sides, the nasal fossa and the homolateral retropharyngeal lymph nodes. The cornea, lens, and lacrimal glands on the affected side can be shielded provided there is no involvement of the orbit. If the floor of the orbit is involved the whole orbital contents will need to be irradiated with inevitable loss of vision, but in any case the subsequent surgical procedure will include orbital exenteration — such surgery can be carried out 3–6 weeks after the finish of radiotherapy. Care must be taken to avoid any irradiation to the contralateral eye.

The usual technique is by anterior and lateral wedged fields using a 4 or 6 MeV linear accelerator (*Figures 5.8* and *5.9*). An alternative is to use a single anterior field with an electron beam of energy 25–35 MeV as described by Bataini and Ennuyer (1971). This is a simple method of giving a good uniform radiation distribution but compared with photon irradiation there is a greater skin reaction and more risk of scattered radiation to the eyes.

Intracavitary irradiation can be used after maxillectomy to treat areas of suspected residual disease or a frank recurrence on the surface of the cavity. Several different techniques can be used. Barley and Paine (1976) described a method of packing the cavity with radium ovoids. Alternatively, a mould can be constructed to fit the cavity, and loaded with ^{198}Au grains or ^{192}Ir wires. There is a rapid fall off of radiation dose below the surface so a tumoricidal effect can only be delivered to a depth of a few millimetres, therefore the technique has a very limited application.

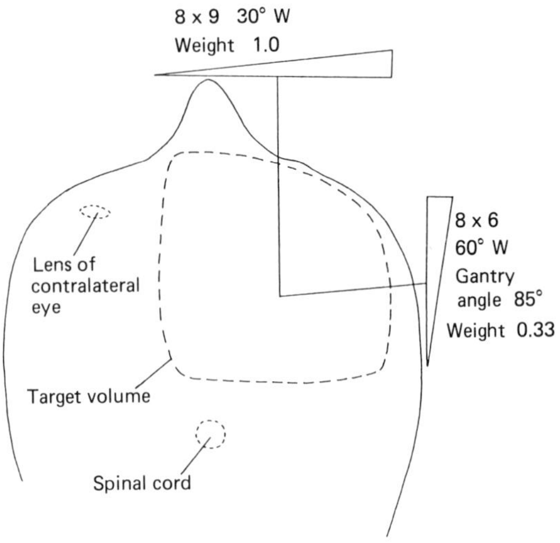

Figure 5.8 Field arrangement for treatment of carcinoma of the maxillary antrum. 6 MeV, 100 cm f.s.d.

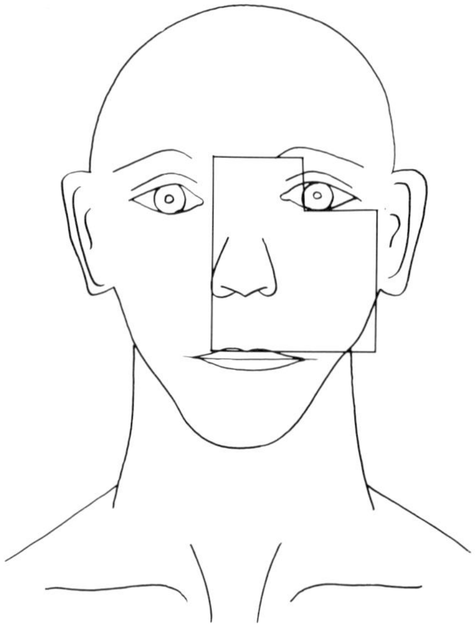

Figure 5.9 Anterior view of volume irradiated for carcinoma of the maxillary antrum

Results

The best survival figures obtained from combined treatment are between 30% and 40% at 5 years. On average the 5-year survival rates for patients treated by radical radiotherapy alone are around 15%, although a few series have reported over 30%, e.g. Amendola *et al.* (1981).

Tumours of the nasal fossa

Squamous carcinoma

Squamous carcinoma of the nasal fossa most often arises anteriorly in the nasal vestibule. It is slow-growing with a low incidence of node involvement.

It is often claimed that surgery is the treatment of choice for anterior nasal lesions on the grounds that cartilage necrosis is a likely sequel of radical radiotherapy. However, the control rates by radiotherapy are as good as those of surgery and the cosmetic results usually better. Cartilage necrosis is seen only occasionally; it is most frequent in the case of lesions which have invaded the cartilage of the nasal septum. The only common late effect of radiotherapy is atrophic rhinitis with crusting.

The ideal technique is to use a single anterior electron field of appropriate energy according to the depth of the lesion. If high energy electrons are not available an alternative is a pair of anterior oblique wedged fields from a cobalt unit or 4 MeV linear accelerator. Cure rates are in the region of 70%.

Other carcinomas

A variety of histological types of carcinoma arise from the respiratory epithelium of the nasal fossa posterior to the vestibule. All are uncommon, the least rare being adenocarcinoma and transitional cell carcinoma. Adenocarcinoma is especially associated with occupational exposure to carcinogens, e.g. in the furniture and boot industries.

The management of these tumours is similar to that of carcinoma of the maxillary antrum. Spread frequently occurs to the antrum and other paranasal sinuses; consequently the radiotherapy target volume should include the whole of the nasal fossa plus the paranasal sinuses on the same side as the tumour, and so is very similar to that described above for antral carcinoma.

Aesthesioneuroepithelioma (olfactory neuroblastoma)

This tumour arises from the olfactory epithelium. Although it resembles neuroblastoma microscopically it behaves in a very different manner from the neuroblastoma of childhood. It can occur at all ages being commonest in middle-aged adults; it grows slowly with a natural history of several years and metastases occur in only about 20% of cases. It is rare and so there is no general agreement on the best treatment policy. The best reported results have been obtained by radical surgical excision and high dose postoperative radiotherapy. Using this approach Bailey and Barton (1975) reported a 5-year recurrence-free survival rate of 67%.

Malignant granuloma

This is a destructive chronic inflammatory process beginning in the septum, causing necrosis of soft tissue, cartilage and bone, leading to gross mutilation of the face. There are two types generally recognized. Wegener's granulomatosis is a necrotizing giant cell vasculitis with lesions in the lungs and kidneys in addition to the nose. This is best treated by immunosuppressive drugs. Midline granuloma or Stewart's granuloma remains localized to the face; there is extensive necrosis but no vasculitis and no other organs become involved. Local tissue destruction is extensive.

Radiotherapy is probably the best treatment available for the Stewart's type of granuloma. High doses are necessary; Fauci, Johnson and Wolff (1976) reported 10 patients treated to a dose of 5000 cGy in 5 weeks, all of whom responded and only two recurred locally; on the other hand three patients receiving only 1000 cGy all developed recurrence.

Carcinoma of the larynx

Carcinoma of the larynx has a different behaviour according to the part of the organ in which it arises. Consequently, for the purposes of description and classification the larynx is divided into three regions.

Supraglottis — the part of the larynx above the vocal cords including the ventricular bands, the posterior surface of the epiglottis, the aryepiglottic folds and arytenoids.

Glottis — comprising the true vocal cords joined by the anterior and posterior commissures.

Subglottis — the region below the vocal cords which merges with the trachea at the level of the inferior border of the cricoid cartilage.

The vast majority of primary tumours of the larynx are squamous carcinomas which vary somewhat in behaviour according to their site of origin. However, there are certain general features common to the management of all laryngeal carcinomas.

Diagnosis and staging

Direct laryngoscopy and biopsy are essential to establish the diagnosis and to make an accurate assessment of the extent of the lesion. For T1 glottic carcinoma no further investigation is necessary. For all other sites and stages endoscopy alone may not reveal the full extent of the tumour, so radiological examination is advisable. This should include at least soft tissue X-rays of the neck and anteroposterior tomography. The place of contrast laryngography and CT scanning is less clear. CT scanning is useful to delineate extension into the pre-epiglottic and paralaryngeal tissues and mediastinum.

The UICC staging system for the primary tumour is as follows:

Supraglottis

T1 tumour confined to the region with normal mobility
T1a tumour confined to the laryngeal surface of the epiglottis, to an aryepiglottic fold, to a ventricular cavity or to a ventricular band
T1b tumour involving the epiglottis and extending to the ventricular cavities or bands
T2 tumour confined to the larynx with extension to adjacent site or sites or to the glottis without fixation
T3 tumour confined to the larynx with fixation and/or other evidence of deep infiltration
T4 tumour with direct extension beyond the larynx.

Glottis

T1 tumour confined to the region with normal mobility
T1a tumour confined to one cord
T1b tumour involving both cords
T2 tumour confined to the larynx with extension to either the supraglottis or the subglottis regions with normal or impaired mobility
T3 tumour confined to the larynx with fixation of one or both cords
T4 tumour with direct extension beyond the larynx

Subglottis

T1 tumour confined to the region
T1a tumour confined to one side of the region
T1b tumour with extension to both sides of the region
T2 tumour confined to the larynx with extension to one or both cords with normal or impaired mobility
T3 tumour confined to the larynx with fixation of one or both cords
T4 tumour with destruction of cartilage and/or with direct extension beyond the larynx.

Treatment

The management of laryngeal carcinoma depends on the site and stage of the disease. After successful radical radiotherapy the quality of the voice is better than after surgery, either partial or total laryngectomy. Consequently in most cases the preferred management is radical radiotherapy with close follow-up and salvage surgery for residual or recurrent tumour. Exceptions to the policy of radical radiotherapy occur in the following circumstances where in general elective laryngectomy is preferable.

(1) Extensive lesions where the chance of a radiotherapy cure is poor, especially where there is evidence of deep invasion of cartilage which often fails to heal after radiotherapy and leaves the patient with a chronically swollen and infected larynx.

(2) Airway obstruction, especially when it is due to deeply infiltrating tumour causing laryngeal oedema. In such a case radiotherapy cannot be given without a preliminary tracheostomy, which probably facilitates spread of the disease and worsens the prognosis.

(3) Mobile unilateral lymph node involvement where combined treatment with surgery and radiotherapy gives a better chance of local control than either method of treatment used singly.

(4) A patient with an advanced lesion who is unlikely to attend regularly for follow-up. In such a case, if radiotherapy fails the chance of successful salvage surgery may be missed.

Postoperative radiotherapy is advisable where there is histological evidence of lymph node involvement or spread beyond the larynx into the soft tissues of the neck.

Radiotherapy dosage

Most radiotherapists favour daily fractionation over 6 or more weeks. However, in the controlled trials mentioned above and in the BIR trial (Wiernik and Gunn, 1984) shorter treatments over 3 or 4 weeks and three fractions per week gave the same tumour control rates and late normal tissue effects as longer daily fractionation. Acute mucositis tends to be more severe but shorter lasting with the shorter treatment times. This is not a problem where small fields are used, and so for earlier disease using small fields the shorter treatment times are preferable on the grounds of economy and convenience. Where larger fields are used for more advanced disease it is advisable to minimize mucositis by using longer treatment times.

A number of studies show a steep dose–response relationship over the range of 6000–7000 cGy in 6 weeks for more advanced disease, especially T3 and

T4 supraglottic carcinoma. Doses near the upper end of this range give the highest tumour control rates but at the expense of greater morbidity. Local control of early disease has a shallower dose-response curve, so doses nearer the lower end of the range are preferable.

Glottic carcinoma

The vocal cord is the part of the larynx most commonly affected by carcinoma in the UK. Glottic carcinoma usually presents early, because a small tumour on a vocal cord will cause persistent hoarseness and lead the patient to seek medical advice. Spread occurs relatively slowly; the anterior commissure, the laryngeal ventricle and subglottic space may eventually be involved. Lymph node metastases are relatively uncommon.

Treatment

There is general agreement that early stage T1 and T2 disease should be treated primarily by radical radiotherapy.

The management of more advanced T3 and T4 glottic carcinoma remains controversial. Where there is extensive spread above and below the glottis with fixation of the vocal cord, the chance of tumour control by radiotherapy is much reduced. After radiotherapy the larynx often does not return completely to normal. There may be persistent oedema and limitation of movement but no obvious persistent tumour visible, so that it is difficult to be sure whether or not carcinoma is still present. Many laryngologists take the view that recurrence after radiotherapy may be diagnosed too late, and that salvage laryngectomy has a high rate of both morbidity and failure; accordingly they prefer a policy of immediate laryngectomy which they maintain gives a higher survival rate than radical radiotherapy and salvage surgery. Nevertheless, this view has not been tested by a controlled trial. A comparison of patients treated by radical radiotherapy or immediate laryngectomy in the same centre by Marshall, Mark and Bryce (1972) showed no difference in survival rates from the two policies, but over one-half of the survivors of radical radiotherapy retained the larynx. It is reasonable to adopt a policy of radical radiotherapy and salvage surgery for most patients with T3 glottic carconoma, with the exceptions of the circumstances mentioned above, i.e. cartilage invasion, airway obstruction, or nodal involvement.

Radiotherapy technique

There is no need to irradiate lymph nodes electively. In the case of early lesions, the target volume can be kept small (*Figure 5.10*) and treated by a pair of anterior oblique wedged fields. For advanced tumours and especially where there is subglottic spread a larger target volume must be treated (*Figure 5.11*) and either wedged oblique fields or lateral fields can be used.

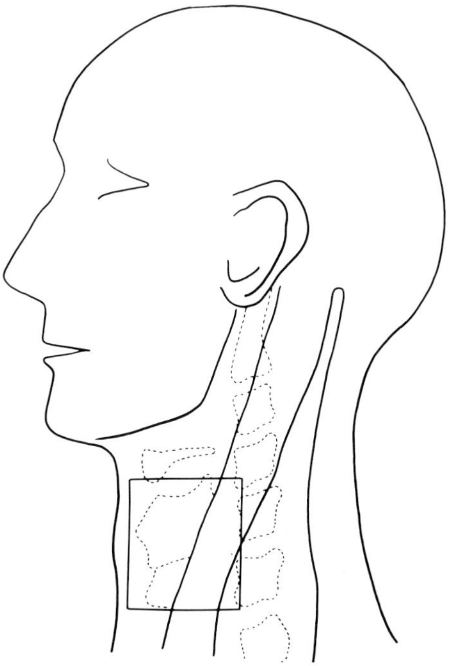

Figure 5.10 Lateral view of volume irradiated for early glottic carcinoma

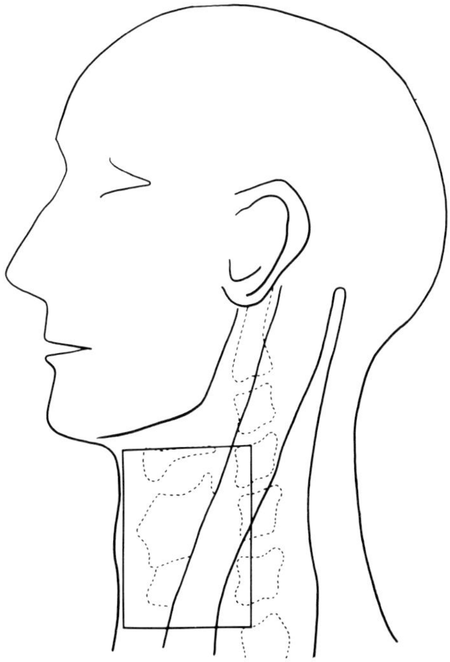

Figure 5.11 Lateral view of volume irradiated for advanced glottic carcinoma

Table 5.5 Typical results of a policy of radical radiotherapy for glottic carcinoma (from Harwood, 1982)

Stage		*Dying of cancer (%)*	*Local control by radiotherapy (%)*
T1a	N0	5	88
T1b	N0	12	81
T2	N0	16	68
T3	N0	26	50
T4	N0	36	56
TX	N+	47	30

Results

Typical results are shown in *Table 5.5*.

Supraglottic carcinoma

Supraglottic carcinoma does not usually give rise to symptoms until it is fairly extensive. It tends to grow rapidly and lymphatic spread occurs at an early stage, initially to the upper deep cervical and mid-cervical lymph nodes. About one-third of patients have involved lymph nodes palpable at presentation; microscopic involvement of nodes is found in about 70% of patients undergoing surgery.

For the rather uncommon early lesions the choice of treatment is between partial laryngeal surgery and radical radiotherapy. Small tumours of the epiglottis can be removed by horizontal partial laryngectomy, conserving the vocal cords, but restoration of swallowing after this operation is often difficult.

In general, a policy of radical radiotherapy is preferred. For the more commonly seen T3 and T4 tumours the choice lies between radical radiotherapy with salvage surgery, and total laryngectomy with block dissection. The indications for surgery in this group are as discussed above.

Radiotherapy technique

The whole larynx should be irradiated by parallel opposed lateral fields. Where no nodes are palpable the upper and mid deep cervical nodes should be included in the target volume (*Figure 5.12*). Where nodes are clinically involved it is advisable to include the entire lymph node chain on both sides of the neck.

Results

Typical results are shown in *Table 5.6*.

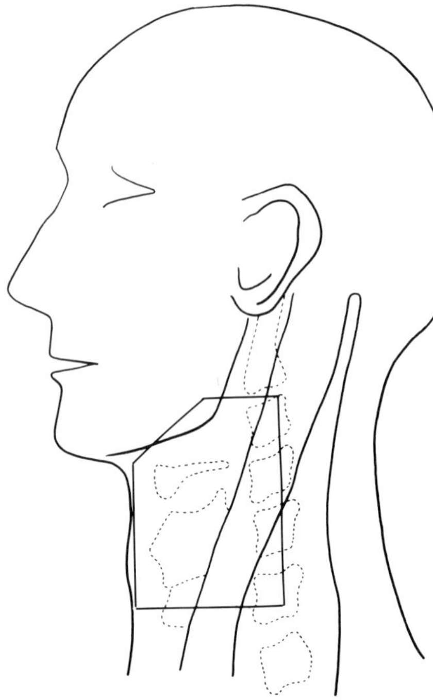

Figure 5.12 Lateral view of volume irradiated for supraglottic carcinoma

Table 5.6 Typical results of radical radiotherapy of supraglottic carcinoma (from Harwood, 1982)

Stage		*Dying of cancer (%)*	*Local control by radiotherapy (%)*
T1a	N0		78
T1b	N0	25	67
T2	N0		68
T3–4	N0	34	54
T3–4	N1	53	56
T3–4	N3	71	39

Subglottic carcinoma

Subglottic carcinoma is relatively rare. Lymphatic spread occurs readily to paratracheal and upper mediastinal lymph nodes. Accordingly, it is rarely possible to remove all the disease at operation. Where there is a reasonable airway, the best treatment is radical radiotherapy including the larynx and superior mediastinum. If there is airway obstruction necessitating tracheostomy immediate laryngectomy is preferable followed by postoperative radiotherapy to include the stoma and superior mediastinum.

Adverse effects

Mucositis occurs in most patients towards the end of the course of radiotherapy. Symptoms depend on field size; with large volumes the mucositis may be particularly troublesome causing pain, dysphagia, increasing hoarseness and excess production of sticky phlegm. The patient should be advised to avoid factors which irritate the ulcerated mucosa, especially smoking, spirits and spicy foods. Hydration and nutrition must be maintained; soft foods are advisable and liquid food supplements may be necessary. In some cases with very severe mucositis it is necessary to pass a fine bore feeding tube to maintain adequate fluid and calorie intake.

Acute laryngeal oedema occasionally occurs during the course of radiotherapy especially where more advanced tumours are being treated. If this becomes severe there is stridor and airway impairment. Treatment initally should be by conservative measures, i.e. bedrest, an antibiotic and a steroid, with the aim of avoiding tracheostomy if possible. However, if there is respiratory difficulty the blood gases should be monitored and tracheostomy performed as soon as there is evidence of respiratory insufficiency. Inhalation of an oxygen–helium mixture is useful to tide the patient over while preparation is being made for tracheostomy.

Care of patient after radical radiotherapy

In most cases, the visible tumour regresses and the mucosa heals over. Normally radiation oedema settles gradually over a period of 2 or 3 months and the larynx then returns to normal except for some persistent dryness. The patient should be followed up at monthly intervals for the first year and then if there is no recurrence the follow-up intervals can be gradually extended. In the event of difficulty in mirror examination of the larynx, regular direct examination under anaesthetic is advisable. Any suspicious areas should be biopsied and if there is evidence of recurrence salvage laryngectomy is performed.

In the occasional patient, most often where advanced disease has been treated, the larynx does not return completely to normal. A vocal cord may remain fixed or oedema may persist for many months. These signs do not in themselves necessarily indicate persistence of tumour. The results in a personal series of 43 patients with fixation of the vocal cord treated by radical radiotherapy are shown in *Table 5.7*. The outcome of patients with persisent post-radiotherapy oedema is shown in *Table 5.8*.

Late radiation damage to the normal tissues of the larynx is rare in the absence of persistent tumour, provided that the dose levels recommended above are not exceeded. The occasional patient develops radiation perichondritis. This is manifested by pain and tenderness in the laryngeal cartilages, persistent oedema, hoarseness, dysphagia and general ill health. It should be treated in the first instance with antibiotics and steroids. If it fails to improve with these conservative measures recurrence must be suspected and biopsy performed, although in these circumstances biopsy is often falsely negative and may worsen the symptoms.

In any patient with persistent oedema or symptoms of perichondritis which persist for several months and do not improve with conservative measures it is wisest to perform laryngectomy. Inevitably, a proportion of such larynges removed will prove on histological examination not to contain tumour, but the majority turns out to be positive. It is better to remove the occasional negative larynx than to miss the chance of successful salvage surgery of recurrence.

Table 5.7 Effect of radiotherapy on vocal cord fixation in glottic carcinoma. (From a series of 300 patients with carcinoma of the larynx treated in a regional radiotherapy centre between 1960 and 1970)

No. with fixation of vocal cord	43
Recurrence-free survivors at 5 years	23
Cord remained fixed	5
Cord became mobile	18

Table 5.8 Prognostic significance of persistent laryngeal oedema after radiotherapy for T3 and T4 carcinoma of the larynx. (From a series of 300 patients with carcinoma of the larynx treated in a regional radiotherapy centre between 1960 and 1970)

Gross oedema (necessitating tracheostomy)	6
Recurrence-free at 5 years	2
Recurred (2–45 months)	4 — all died
Moderate oedema	11
Recurrence-free at 5 years	5
Recurred (2–20 months)	6 — one salvaged surgically

Carcinoma of the hypopharynx

For the purpose of tumour classification the hypopharynx is divided into three parts, the pyriform fossa, the post-cricoid region and the posterior wall.

Diagnosis and staging

Endoscopy and biopsy are essential. It is often difficult to determine the lower limit of the tumour at endoscopy. A barium swallow and lateral soft tissue X-ray of the neck should be performed in all cases. Anteroposterior tomography of the larynx may demonstrate involvement of the subglottic region or trachea. CT scanning may reveal unsuspected mediastinal involvement.

The UICC staging system for the primary tumour is as follows:

T1 tumour confined to one site
T2 tumour with extension to adjacent site or region without fixation of hemilarynx
T3 tumour with extension to adjacent site or region with fixation of hemilarynx
T4 tumour with extension to bone, cartilage or soft tissues.

Carcinoma of the pyriform fossa

In its early stages carcinoma of the pyriform fossa gives rise to minimal symptoms; often it does not present until a late stage when there is invasion of the larynx or a mass in the neck. Lymph node involvement occurs commonly. Lymphatics pass to the upper end of the deep cervical chain so that there is a predilection for nodal metastases to become fixed to the base of skull. The behaviour of carcinoma of the pyriform fossa is similar to that of supraglottic carcinoma of the larynx and is in general treated according to similar principles.

Radical radiotherapy with salvage surgery is a suitable policy for an early tumour of the medial wall of the fossa which has not caused laryngeal fixation. A tumour on the lateral wall is likely to involve cartilage at an early stage, and so is better treated surgically. Surgery with postoperative radiotherapy is the treatment of choice for a patient with mobile unilateral lymph node involvement. However, the majority of patients who develop pyriform fossa carcinoma in the UK are unsuitable for surgical treatment. This is because the disease occurs mainly in elderly people, or in alcoholics, in poor general condition. In addition, many present at an inoperable stage with fixed lymph node metastases. In these patients, radiotherapy is the only possible potentially curative treatment.

Radiotherapy technique

Lateral fields are used similar to those for supraglottic carcinoma, but extended more inferiorly to cover the cricoid cartilage and at least 1 cm of the upper oesophagus. Where there is a large lymph node mass extending posteriorly to the lateral projection of the spinal cord, treatment to a radical tumour dose by parallel opposed lateral fields will result in a spinal cord dose above tolerance; in such a case the cord dose can be reduced by the use of two oblique wedged fields from the same side.

Results

In early disease without lymph node involvement 5-year survival rates of up to 50% have been reported from both radical radiotherapy and surgery. In the advanced and inoperable patients treated by radiotherapy the survival rate is less than 10% and, as the latter group constitute the majority, the overall 5-year survival rate is about 15%.

Post-cricoid carcinoma

Carcinoma of the post-cricoid region also often presents at a late stage. At least one-half of the patients who develop this tumour already have some swallowing difficulties because of the Paterson-Kelly syndrome or a post-cricoid web. The significance of worsening dysphagia is not always appreciated at first, so they often present with large annular tumours around the pharyngo-oesophageal junction with submucosal lymphatic spread into the oesophagus. They tend to be in poor condition and have lost a considerable amount of weight. Lymphatic spread occurs commonly and widely to lymph nodes high in the neck and in the mediastinum.

Treatment

Curative treatment is worth attempting only in a patient with no lymphatic spread and a potentially resectable primary. The chances of success are higher with surgery than with radical radiotherapy. It is necessary to remove the larynx, hypopharynx and oesophagus, and to restore the alimentary tract by a reconstructive procedure; the most satisfactory method is to pull the stomach up through the mediastinum and anastomose it to the pharynx. Postoperative radiotherapy is inadvisable after laryngopharyngectomy because there will be a portion of stomach within the high dose volume. The stomach cannot tolerate a high dose of irradiation so postoperative radiotherapy carries an appreciable risk of complications such as stricture and perforation. Accordingly, where combined treatment is considered advisable preoperative radiotherapy should be given. Radical radiotherapy is used for localized disease in a patient unsuitable for surgery. A patient with tumour infiltrating into the mediastinum, or with bilateral or fixed nodes in the neck, hardly ever survives more than 1 year however treated. Laryngopharyngectomy is sometimes suggested for palliation to restore swallowing, but on the whole it usually adds to the patient's misery and it is better to employ only minimal palliative measures.

Radiotherapy technique

A similar technique is used for both radical and preoperative radiotherapy. It is not possible to deliver a radical dose of radiotherapy to the primary tumour and all the regions of potential lymphatic spread, as the volume would include the entire neck up to the skull and the superior mediastinum. Hence only the primary site and the lower cervical nodes are irradiated.

In a patient with a long neck and a short lesion the simplest technique is to use lateral fields which can be angled down slightly to avoid the shoulders (*Figures 5.13* and *5.14*). With a longer lesion, or in a patient with a short neck, a more complex technique is required using two anterior oblique double wedged fields as described by Garrett (1971).

Results

Post-cricoid carcinoma has a very poor prognosis, the overall 5-year survival is less than 10%. In selected early cases 5-year survival rates of up to 35% have been reported from surgery. Pearson (1966) reported a 5-year survival rate of 25% from radical radiotherapy but most other series have failed to achieve such a high figure.

Carcinoma of the posterior pharyngeal wall

The posterior wall is the least common site for malignant tumours in the hypopharynx. There are no reported series large enough to compare the results of various methods of treatment. Radical radiotherapy using treatment techniques similar to those for post-cricoid carcinoma is the treatment of choice. Wang (1971) reported seven out of 15 patients treated radically by radiotherapy alive at 3 years.

Salivary gland tumours

Pleomorphic adenoma

The majority of pleomorphic adenomas of the parotid occur superficial to the facial nerve. Such tumours are best treated by superficial parotidectomy with preservation of the nerve. Postoperative radiotherapy should be reserved for those cases where the excision has been incomplete, this may occur with tumours of the deep lobe where complete removal would necessitate sacrifice of the facial nerve, or where the pseudo-capsule is breached at surgery. In

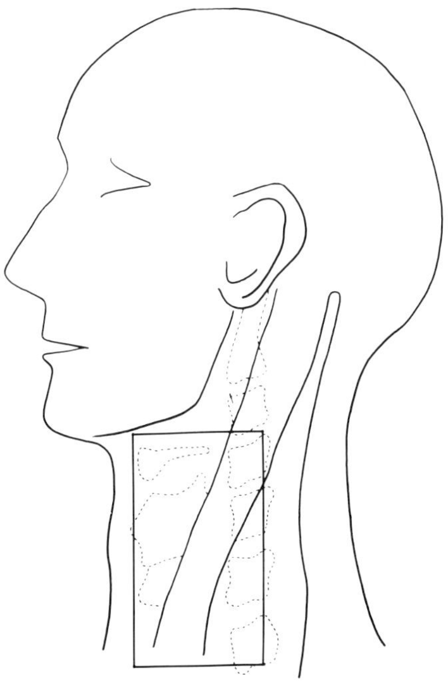

Figure 5.13 Lateral view of volume irradiated for post-cricoid carcinoma

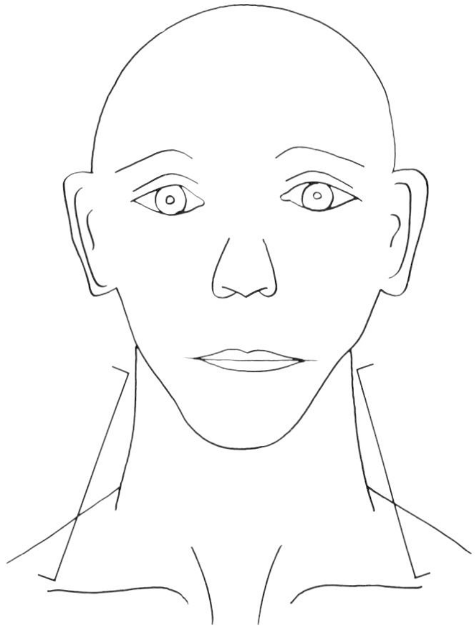

Figure 5.14 Technique of irradiation of post-cricoid carcinoma

these circumstances the use of postoperative radiotherapy reduces the risk of local recurrence from about 30% to 2% (Rafla, 1982), and it is important to avoid local recurrence because of the propensity of the pleomorphic adenoma to undergo malignant change if it persists or recurs over a number of years.

An alternative policy for the treatment of pleomorphic adenoma of the parotid frequently employed in the past but now less popular is enucleation and routine postoperative radiotherapy. The advocates of this policy (Armitstead, Smiddy and Frank, 1979) claim that it causes less deformity and less risk of facial nerve damage than superficial parotidectomy, and that the recurrence rate is only 2 or 3%. The routine use of radiotherapy for pleomorphic adenoma has been criticized mainly on the grounds that it may induce malignant change; there have been anecdotal reports of malignant change occurring in pleomorphic adenoma after radiotherapy (Patey, 1973), but there is no evidence that the incidence of malignant change or recurrence is greater in irradiated than non-irradiated patients, There is however, a slight risk of radiation-induced tumours in the adjacent normal tissue; Gleave, Whittaker and Nicholson (1979) reported one case of a fibrosarcoma occurring in the field of irradiation after a latent interval of 15 years, out of a series of 103 patients irradiated for recurrent pleomorphic adenoma. In general, a complete surgical excision is preferable to enucleation and radiotherapy but where complete removal is not achieved radiotherapy should not be withheld.

Carcinoma

Most salivary gland carcinomas present as an operable swelling; total removal is performed and a histological diagnosis made on the excised specimen. Postoperative radiotherapy is usually advisable except for tumours of low grade malignancy, such as the mucoepidermoid carcinoma and acinic-cell carcinoma, which have been completely excised. Some tumours are obviously malignant at presentation, as shown by fixation to the skin or deeper structures, involvement of the facial nerve, or rapid growth. Surgery should be the prior treatment wherever possible; preoperative radiotherapy without prior biopsy has been advocated (Corcoran, Cooke and Hobsley, 1983) to a dose of 4000 cGy in 4 weeks. There is no evidence that this approach gives better results than immediate surgery and postoperative radiotherapy, but it may have a place in the management of tumours of doubtful operability by rendering them easier to excise.

Inoperable tumours are treated by radiotherapy alone. Such treatment is often thought to be essentially palliative. However, in many cases the disease can be controlled for a considerable period and a small but appreciable cure rate obtained, so in general radical radiotherapy is usually worth attempting.

Radiotherapy technique

For parotid tumours the target volume must include the entire parotid bed and the operation scar (*Figure 5.15*). Any extension beyond the parotid bed must be covered. The upper margin of the target volume should be at least as high as the upper border of the zygomatic arch, and the lower border at least as low as the hyoid bone. A wider volume is required for malignant tumours, especially the adenoid cystic carcinoma with its propensity for perineural spread; the parapharyngeal space and adjacent base of skull should be included. For submandibular tumours the target volume should encompass the entire submandibular triangle from the midline to the posterior border of the sternomastoid muscle, and from the lower alveolus superiorly to below the hyoid bone inferiorly. No precise limits can be set for target volumes for minor salivary gland tumours, in view of their wide variety of position and spread; in general a wide margin around the known limits of the disease must be irradiated.

It is vital to include the lymphatic drainage on the same side of the neck, down to the level of the clavicle, for those tumour types where the incidence of lymph node metastases is high, especially squamous cell carcinoma and adenocarcinoma.

The technique most often employed for parotid tumours consists of anterior and posterior oblique wedged fields on a cobalt unit or linear accelerator making sure that the plane of the treatment is inclined so that the posterior field exits below the contralateral eye (*Figure 5.15*). Maximum tissue tolerance doses are required, i.e. of the order of 6500 cGy in 6.5 weeks or equivalent for postoperative or

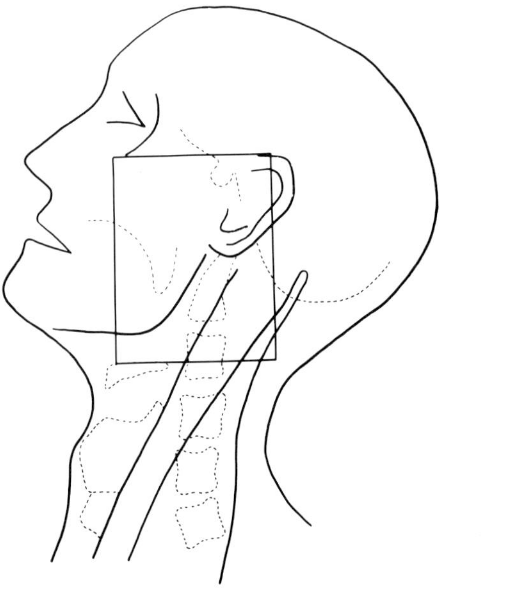

Figure 5.15 Lateral view of volume irradiated for a parotid tumour

radical treatment of malignant tumours. A slightly lower dose, e.g. 5500 cGy in 5.5 weeks or equivalent, is probably sufficient for pleomorphic adenoma.

Adverse effects

The side-effects of parotid irradiation are usually slight, there is often some discomfort in the ear on the irradiated side due in part to dryness and crusting in the external auditory meatus, and also to Eustachian tube obstruction especially where the parapharyngeal space is included in the target volume. There is often temporary loss of the sense of taste, and epilation around the occiput due to the exit dose from the anterior oblique field. An alternative technique is to use a single lateral field with 18 MeV electrons; this is only suitable for tumours not involving the deep lobe of the parotid because beyond a depth of 5 cm there is a fairly rapid fall off of dose. Electron therapy does however avoid epilation, and a smaller volume of normal tissue is irradiated compared to the wedged pair technique.

Results

The prognosis depends on the stage of the disease and its histology. Survival rates greater than 90% for low grade acinic-cell and mucoepidermoid tumours, and less than 20% for anaplastic and squamous carcinomas are usually quoted. The site also affects prognosis, tumours arising from the parotid having a better prognosis than those arising in minor salivary glands. Postoperative radiotherapy has not been tested by controlled trials but retrospective surveys strongly suggest a considerable reduction in local recurrence rates, e.g. MacNaney *et al.* (1983) reports a 13% local recurrence rate with radiotherapy, compared with 38% without. The influence of post-operative radiotherapy seems to be the same with all histological types. However, reported series must be interpreted with care, especially when only short-term results are quoted. Many salivary gland carcinomas have a long natural history. For example, in adenoid systic carcinoma of the minor salivary glands actuarial survival rates are about 60% at 5 years, but fall to 30% at 10 years and 13% at 20 years (Henk and Langdon, 1984).

In advanced inoperable tumours Rafla (1982) reported a series of 101 patients treated by radiotherapy alone, 50 of whom are alive at 5 years, 31 without evidence of disease. Response rates were much the same with all histological types. Slightly better results have been reported with fast neutron therapy; Catterall (1981) reported 19 out of 40 patients alive and recurrence-free at 5 years.

Orbital tumours

A large number of different types of both primary and secondary tumours occurs in the orbit, but all are relatively uncommon. *Table 5.9* shows these tumours and conditions in the orbit in which radiotherapy plays a part in management. Those which are most frequently seen by the radiotherapist are discussed below.

Table 5.9 Conditions arising in the orbit which may be treated by radiotherapy

Primary neoplasms
Lymphoma
Rhabdomyosarcoma
Other sarcomas, e.g. malignant fibrous histiocytoma
Lacrimal gland carcinoma
Melanoma
Secondary neoplasms
Local invasion from adjacent structures
paranasal sinus carcinoma
nasopharyngeal carcinoma
eyelid carcinoma
Blood-borne metastases
Leukaemic deposits
Non-malignant conditions
Pseudotumour
Malignant granuloma
Histiocytoma X
Endocrine exophthalmos

Lymphoma

Orbital lymphoma may occur in one of three different circumstances, as primary disease, as the presenting symptom of a generalized lymphoma, or as involvement at a later stage of the disease in a patient with a systemic lymphoma.

All histological types of lymphoma (*see* Chapter 8) may involve the orbit. Histological interpretation of orbital biopsy material is often difficult; it may not be possible to classify the type of lymphoma accurately, or even to say whether a lymphoid lesion is benign or malignant.

Where the histology report is of lymphocytes with evidence of lymphoid follicle formation the disease is probably benign, although may eventually turn out to be well-differentiated nodular lymphoma. In such a case the management will depend upon the symptoms and signs. If there is a large mass, or conjunctival nodules are causing irritation, treatment by radiotherapy to a dose of 2000 cGy in 2 weeks leads to complete resolution of the disease with no side-effects.

The most common histological report from a lymphoid lesion presenting in the orbit is that of mature lymphocytes with no clear features to suggest hyperplasia or malignancy. Most of such lesions are probably well-differentiated lymphocytic lymphomas. They should be treated by radiotherapy to a dose of 3000 cGy in 3 weeks if no evidence of systemic lymphoma can be found in the patient.

Unequivocal malignant lymphoma should be investigated as described in Chapter 8, and treated by radiotherapy only if localized to the orbit.

Radiotherapy technique

Where only subconjunctival disease is present the best technique is to use a single anterior field with orthovoltage irradiation, in the range 140–300 kV according to tumour thickness. A diaphragm system and field defining lamp is preferable to an applicator, as shielding of the cornea is easier. A small lead disc is suspended on fine cross wires and positioned in the beam so that its shadow just covers the cornea (*Figure 5.16*).

Where an orbital mass is present the whole orbit is treated by anterior and lateral wedged fields (*Figure 5.17*). The lateral field passes behind the lens of the eye on the affected side. The cornea and lens are shielded from the anterior field by a fine lead cylinder positioned along the line of the beam, this results in an area of low dosage immediately behind the globe, but as lymphoma rarely penetrates into the intraconal space this is of no consequence.

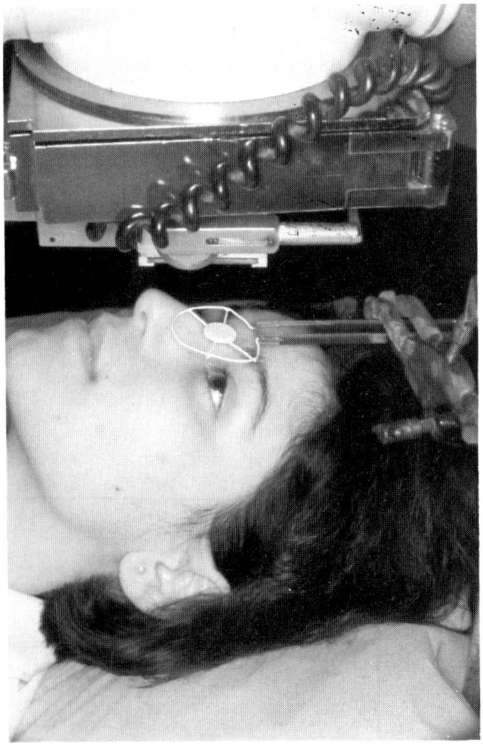

Figure 5.16 Method of corneal shielding for use with superficial X-irradiation of the conjunctival sac

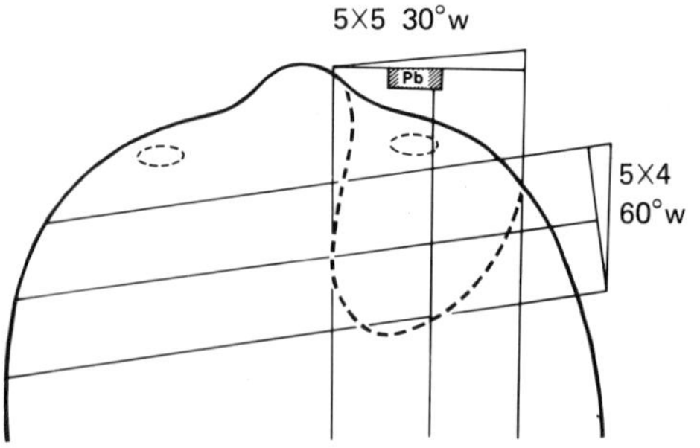

Figure 5.17 Field arrangement for treatment of orbital lymphoma. The cornea is shielded by a beam-shaped lead cylinder

In the treatment of primary lymphoma of the orbit the more malignant histological types should be given a tumour dose of 4000 cGy in 4 weeks, and the better differentiated types 3000 cGy in 3 weeks. For palliative irradiation of orbital deposits in a patient with known systemic lymphoma 2000 cGy in 2 weeks is adequate.

Results

Radiotherapy controls the local disease in all cases, local recurrence being virtually unknown (Kim, 1978, Henk, 1982). In the more malignant types the results of treatment and the prognosis are the same as those of lymphomas at other extra-nodal sites, (*see* Chapter 8). In the well-differentiated lymphocytic type and those where the histology is reported as an indeterminate lymphocytic lesion, about 25% eventually develop systemic disease, either disseminated lymphoma or chronic lymphatic leukaemia, which usually runs a protracted indolent course.

Rhabdomyosarcoma

The orbit is one of the more frequent sites of origin of rhabdomyosarcoma of childhood and one with a good prognosis. The cure rate with chemotherapy and radiotherapy is over 90% using the treatment regimes described in Chapter 10. When the orbit is irradiated in children under the age of 2 there is impairment of bone growth causing facial asymmetry and sometimes quite severe deformity. Consequently, the need for radiotherapy in this condition has been questioned, but it is not yet clear whether such high cure rates can be obtained by chemotherapy alone; clinical trials to answer this question are now in progress.

Radiotherapy technique

Most rhabdomyosarcomas arise anteriorly in the eyelids or at the canthi, and do not penetrate the intraconal space. They can therefore be treated by an anterior and lateral field as described for lymphoma.

About 10% arise in the intraconal space; these are best treated by lateral superior and inferior oblique fields passing behind the lens of the eye in the affected orbit, and exiting above and below the contralateral orbit.

Lacrimal gland tumours

The same histological types of tumour occur in the lacrimal gland as in the salivary glands. All are very rare; most masses presenting in the lacrimal fossa arise in some other tissue, for example, lymphoma, dermoid cyst or granuloma.

The commonest lacrimal gland neoplasm is the pleomorphic adenoma. This should be treated surgically; if the capsule is ruptured at operation local recurrence is likely, but postoperative radiotherapy is inadvisable because effective dosage to the whole area at risk is likely to lead to loss of vision.

The commonest malignant lacrimal gland tumour is the adenoid cystic carcinoma, which has a peak incidence in young adults. Other types of carcinoma are seen more often in later life. Radical surgery offers the best chance of cure of all types of lacrimal gland carcinoma, but involves orbital exenteration and excision of the bony roof and lateral wall of the orbit. Preoperative investigation of the extent of the disease by X-rays and CT scanning is essential. Unfortunately, many tumours prove inoperable due to involvement of the orbital apex or intracranial extension. An inoperable tumour without distant metastases should be treated by radiotherapy, using a technique similar to that described for lymphoma, to a dose of 6500 cGy in 32 fractions in 6.5 weeks. Vision will almost inevitably be lost, as this dose exceeds the tolerance of the optic nerve and retina; however the cornea should be shielded for at least part of the treatment so that it does not receive more than about 4000 cGy, thereby avoiding severe corneal reaction and its sequelae. Local control of the disease is achieved in about 20% of cases.

Pseudotumour

Pseudotumour is a term used to describe a non-neoplastic mass in the orbit of uncertain aetiology. This is a diagnosis made when all other causes of inflammatory masses have been excluded, for example sarcoidosis and Wegener's granuloma. It does however have certain characteristic clinical features. It is commonest between the ages of 40 and 60. The symptoms are proptosis, pain, diplopia, lid swelling and redness. CT scanning shows a diffuse infiltration of heterogeneous consistency. Histology shows a mixed picture with lymphocytes, plasma cells, eosinophils, macrophages and fibroblasts; any one of the cell types may predominate.

Pseudotumour is of interest to the radiotherapist as one of the few non-malignant conditions in which radiotherapy still plays a part in management (*see* Chapter 17). The initial tretment is to give a short course of steroids in high dosage, which in most cases leads to rapid resolution of the disease. However, in about one-half of the patients the condition recurs on withdrawal of the steroids, and in such cases radiotherapy giving a dose of 2500 cGy in 10 treatments is usually effective in eliminating the disease permanently and carries less risk than continued high dose steroid therapy. The patient who fails to respond to steroids usually also fails to respond to radiotherapy.

Adverse effects of radiotherapy of the orbit

Dryness

Doses in excess of 3000 cGy in 3 weeks cause significant dimunition of secretion of the lacrimal gland and the secretory glands of the conjunctiva. If the lacrimal gland and most of the conjunctival sac receive more than this dose some dryness of the eye results, with consequent corneal irritation. This may be relieved by regular instillation of hypromellose drops. Where dryness is severe there is a risk of corneal ulceration, in which case the cornea may be protected by a haptic contact lens.

Corneal damage

The cornea has a radiosensitivity similar to that of mucosal surfaces. With most orbital radiotherapy the cornea can be shielded, so that direct radiation injury is prevented. If the cornea cannot be shielded without under-dosing the tumour radiation changes occur. There is an acute reaction which is usually painful but can be relieved by steroid drops.

Permanent changes result from doses above 5000 cGy in 5 weeks. The acute reaction heals with scarring and there is often an associated iridocyclitis. Secondary glaucoma may supervene. The whole eye gradually atrophies over a period of several months after radiation.

Cataract

The lens is the most vulnerable structure in the eye to radiation. Death of cells in the periphery of the lens gradually leads to opacities at the posterior pole occurring at an interval of several years after radiation. Such opacities have been observed after only a few hundred cGy, but progressive cataract impairing visual acuity is not usually seen unless the dose to the lens exceeds 1000 cGy.

Where the dose has exceeded 2000 cGy cataract is almost inevitable. Radiation-induced cataract can be treated by lens extraction in the same way as other types of cataract.

Retinopathy

The retina and optic nerve have a similar radiation tolerance to other parts of the central nervous system. Acute effects are not seen and late changes are unusual unless the dose exceeds 5000 cGy in 5 weeks. Higher doses cause vascular damage leading to secondary changes in the retina, optic atrophy, and visual impairment.

Uveal melanoma

This is the commonest malignant tumour of the eye. It has a wide range of growth rate, often growing very slowly with a natural history spanning many years. Blood-borne metastases occur in about 50% of cases.

Biopsy of a choroidal lesion is not possible, so the diagnosis must be made on clinical grounds. The findings on fundoscopy, fluorescein angiography, and ultrasound help to distinguish melanoma from non-malignant lesions in the fundus.

Treatment

It is no longer accepted that enucleation of the eye should be performed as soon as the diagnosis is made. Some lesions will remain static for long periods of time and in most cases distant metastases, if they occur at all, do so late in the course of the disease. It is therefore reasonable to observe for evidence of growth before instituting any form of treatment (Gass, 1980). Zimmerman, McLean and Foster (1978) observed a higher metastatic rate in patients who had undergone enucleation than in patients treated conservatively with preservation of the eye; they suggested that enucleation may worsen the prognosis by disseminating malignant cells into the circulation. An alternative explanation for these findings, however, is that some conservatively treated lesions may be in fact non-malignant, and that more aggressive tumours with a higher metastatic potential are more likely to give rise to severe local symptoms and therefore be subjected to enucleation.

Enucleation is necessary only for large lesions where there is poor vision due to involvement of the macula or optic disc, and where there is pain from secondary glaucoma or extrascleral extension. Small lesions of less than 3 disc diameters which are increasing in size are treated by photocoagulation. Radiotherapy is best used for intermediate sized lesions too large for control by photocoagulation but not warranting enucleation.

Radiotherapy techniques

Local applicators

A radioactive applicator can be sutured to the posterior sclera immediately adjacent to the tumour and left in position until the required radiation dose has been delivered. Ideally a tumour suitable for this form of treatment should not exceed 5 mm in height over the scleral surface and 15 mm in diameter at the tumour base; it should not involve the ciliary body and its margin should be at least 1.5 disc diameters from the optic nerve head. Radioactive isotopes used for this purpose are cobalt–60 (Stallard, 1966) and ruthenium–106 (Lommatzsch, 1974). The latter, with its pure beta emission of average energy 3 MeV, gives a lower radiation dose to the lens and surrounding retina. With either isotope the aim should be to deliver a dose of at least 9000 cGy to the apex of the tumour in about 1 week.

Charged particles

The Bragg peak effect from a beam of heavy charged particles can be used as another method of highly localized irradiation. Particles are generated by high energy cyclotrons and so are available in only a very few specialized centres throughout the world. The largest experience is with 160 MeV protons (Gragoudas, Goiten and Koehler, 1977); helium ions have also been used. This method is an alternative to radioactive applicators, and can also be used for larger lesions unsuitable for applicators as an alternative to enucleation.

Postoperative radiotherapy

If extrascleral extension of tumour is found at enucleation there is a high risk of local recurrence in the orbit. Postoperative radiotherapy to the orbit is advisable in such cases using anterior and anterolateral oblique wedged fields. There is a possible advantage in using large dose fractions for melanoma, so 3500 cGy in seven fractions in 3 weeks is recommended.

Results of radiotherapy

Most series treated by radioactive applicators show a local tumour control rate of around 60%. Enucleation is required for progressive tumour in about 20%; a further 20% succumb from distant metastases.

Radiation effects on the retina are considerable, and only about one-quarter of successfully treated patients retain normal visual acuity in the treated eye.

It is too soon to assess the value of charged particle irradiation. Similar results to those of isotope applicators are being claimed but with more advanced tumours included.

References

ALCOCK, C.J., PAINE, C.H. and WEATHERBURN, (1984) Interstitial radiotherapy in treatment of supei.. cial tumours of the lower alveolar ridge. *Clinical Radiology*, **35**, 363–366

AMENDOLA, B.E., EISERT, D., HAZRA, T.A. and KING, E.R. (1981) Carcinoma of the maxillary antrum: surgery or radiation therapy. *International Journal of Radiation Oncology, Biology and Physics*, *7*, 743–746

AMERICAN JOINT COMMITTEE FOR CANCER STAGING AND END RESULTS (1977) Reporting Manual for Staging of Cancer. Chicago: American Joint Committee

ARMITSTEAD, P.R., SMIDDY, F.G. and FRANK, H.G. (1979) Simple enucleation and radiotherapy in the treatment of the pleomorphic salivary adenoma of the parotid gland. *British Journal of Surgery*, **66**, 716–717

BAILEY, B.J. and BARTON, S. (1975) Olfactory neuroblastoma: management and prognosis. *Archives of Otolaryngology*, **101**, 1–5

BARLEY, V.L. and PAINE, C.H. (1976) Carcinoma of the maxillary antrum. *Proceedings of the Royal Society of Medicine*, **69**, 697–700

BATAINI, J.P. and ENNUYER, A. (1971) Advanced carcinoma of the maxillary antrum treated by cobalt teletherapy and electron beam irradiation. *British Journal of Radiology*, **44**, 590–598

BEZWODA, W.R., DE MOOR, N.G. and DERMAN, D.P. (1979) Treatment of advanced head and neck cancer by means of radiation therapy plus chemotherapy — a randomised trial. *Medical and Paediatric Oncology*, **6**, 353–358

CATTERALL, M. (1981) The treatment of malignant salivary gland tumours with fast neutrons. *International Journal of Radiation Oncology, Biology and Physics*, **7**, 1737–1738

CATTERALL, M. and BEWLEY, D.K. (1979) *Fast Neutrons in the Treatment of Cancer*. London: Academic Press

CHAN, R.C. and SHUKOVSKY, L.J. (1976) Effects of irradiation on the eye. *Radiology*, **120**, 673–675

COFFIN, F. (1973) The control of radiation caries. *British Journal of Radiology*, **46**, 365–368

COHEN, L. (1982) Absence of a demonstrable gain factor for neutron beam therapy of epidermoid carcinoma of the head and neck. *International Journal of Radiation Oncology, Biology and Physics*, **8**, 2173–2176

CORCORAN, M.O., COOKE, H.P. and HOBSLEY, M. (1983) Radical surgery following radiotherapy for advanced parotid carcinoma. *British Journal of Surgery*, **70**, 261–263

DALY, T.E., DRANE, J.B. and MACCOMB, W.S. (1972) Management of problems of the teeth and jaws in patients undergoing irradiation. *American Journal of Surgery*, **124**, 539–542

DECROIX, Y. and GHOSSEIN, N.A. (1981) Experience of the Curie Institute in treatment of cancer of the mobile tongue. 1. Treatment policies and results. *Cancer*, *47*, 496–502

DUNCAN, W., ARNOTT, S.J., ORR, J.A. and KERR, G.R. (1982) The Edinburgh experience of fast neutron therapy. *International Journal of Radiation Oncology, Biology and Physics*, **8**, 2155–2157

DURRANT, K.R. and ELLIS, F. (1973) The treatment of squamous-cell carcinoma of the lower lip by rigid implants. *Clinical Radiology*, **24**, 502–505

FAUCI, A.S., JOHNSON, R.E. and WOLFF, S.M. (1976) Radiation therapy of mid-line granuloma. *Annals of Internal Medicine*, **84**, 140–147

FITZPATRICK, P.J., BRIANT, T.D.R. and BERMAN, J.M. (1980) The nasopharyngeal angiofibroma. *Archives of Otolaryngology*, **106**, 234–236

FLETCHER, G.H. (1972) Elective irradiation of sub-clinical disease in cancers of the head and neck. *Cancer*, **29**, 1450–1454

FLETCHER, G.H. (1973) *Textbook of Radiotherapy*. Philadelphia: Lea & Febiger

GARRETT, M.J. (1971) Megavoltage technique for the treatment of carcinoma of the post-cricoid region. *Clinical Radiology*, **22**, 136–138

GASS, J.D.M. (1980) Observation of suspected choroidal and ciliary body melanomas for evidence of growth prior to enucleation. *Ophthalmology*, **87**, 523–528

GLEAVE, E.N. (1980) Management of metastatic cervical nodes. *Proceedings of the Edinburgh Surgical Festival* 1980, 4–5

GLEAVE, E.N., WHITTAKER, J.S. and NICHOLSON, A. (1979) Salivary tumours — experience over thirty years. *Clinical Otolaryngology*, **4**, 247–257

GRAGOUDAS, E.S., GOITEN, M. and KOEHLER, A.M. (1977) Proton irradiation of small choroidal malignant melanomas. *American Journal of Ophthalmology*, **83**, 665–673

HAHN, S.S., KIM, J.A., GOODCHILD, N. and CONSTABLE, W.C. (1983) Carcinoma of the middle ear and external auditory canal. *International Journal of Radiation, Oncology, Biology and Physics*, **9**, 1003–1007

HARWOOD, A.R. (1982) Cancer of the larynx — the Toronto experience. *Journal of Otolaryngology*, Suppl 11, 3–21

HENK, J.M. (1975) Radiosensitivity of lymph node metastases. *Proceedings of the Royal Society of Medicine*, **68**, 85–86

HENK, J.M. (1978) Results of radiotherapy for carcinoma of the oropharynx. *Clinical Otolaryngology*, **3**, 137–143

HENK, J.M. (1982) Radiotherapy for orbital lymphoma and pseudo tumour. *Orbit*, **1**, 71–74

HENK, J.M. and JAMES, K.W. (1978) Comparative trial of large and small fractions in the radiotherapy of head and neck cancer. *Clinical Radiology*, **29**, 611–616

HENK, J.M. and LANGDON, J.D. (1984) *Malignant Tumours of the Oral Cavity*. London: Edward Arnold

HO, J.H.C. (1978) An epidemiological and clinical study of nasopharyngeal carcinoma. *International Journal of Radiation Oncology, Biology and Physics*, **4**, 181–198

HO, J.H.C. (1982) Nasopharynx. In *Treatment of Cancer*, edited by K.E. Halnan, pp. 249–268. London: Chapman and Hall

HOLMES, K.S. (1965) Carcinoma of the middle ear. *Clinical Radiology*, **16**, 400–404

JESSE, R.H. and FLETCHER, G.H. (1977) Treatment of the neck in patients with squamous cell carcinoma of the head and neck. *Cancer*, **39** (Suppl. 2), 868–872

JOHNSON, J.T., BARNES, E.L., MYERS, E.N., SCHRAMM, V.L., BOROCHOVITZ, D. and SIGLER, B.A. (1981) The extra capsular spread of tumours in cervical node metastases. *Archives of Otolaryngology*, **107**, 725–729

KIM, Y.H., FAYOS, J.V. and SCHNITZER, B. (1978) Extranodal head and neck lymphoma: results of radiation therapy. *International Journal of Radiation Oncology, Biology and Physics*, **4**, 789–794

LANGDON, J.D., HARVEY, P.W., RAPIDIS, A.D., PATEL, M.F., JOHNSON, N.W. and HOPPS, R.M. (1977) Oral cancer: the behaviour and response to treatment of 194 cases. *Journal of Maxillofacial Surgery*, **5**, 221–237

LOMMATZSCH, P.K. (1974) Treatment of choroidal melanomas with Ru-106/Rh-106 beta-ray applicators. *Survey of Ophthalmology*, **19**, 85-100

MARCUS, R.M., MILLION, R.R. and MITCHELL, T.P. (1980) A pre-loaded custom-designed implantation device for stage T1–T2 carcinoma of the floor of the mouth. *International Journal of Radiation Oncology, Biology and Physics*, **6**, 111–113

MARSHALL, H.F., MARK, A. and BRYCE, D.P. (1972) The management of advanced laryngeal cancer. *Journal of Laryngology and Otology*, *86*, 309–315

MARUYAMA, Y., GOLD, L.H.A. and KIEFFER, S.A. (1971) Radioactive cobalt treatment of glomus jugulare tumours. Clinical and angiographic investigation. *Acta Radiologica*, **10**, 239–247

McGUIRT, W.F. and McCABE, B.F. (1978) Significance of node biopsy before definitive treatment of cervical metastatic carcinoma. *Laryngoscope*, **88**, 594–597

McNANEY, D., McNEESE, M.D., GUILLAMONDEGUI, O.M., FLETCHER, G.H. and OSWALD, M.J. (1983) Postoperative irradiation in malignant epithelial tumours of the parotid. *International Journal of Radiation Oncology, Biology and Physics*, **9**, 1289–1295

MESIC, J.B., FLETCHER, G.H. and GOEPFERT, H. (1981) Megavoltage irradiation of epithelial tumours of the nasopharynx. *International Journal of Radiation Oncology, Biology and Physics*, **7**, 447–453

MOSELEY, H.S., THOMAS, L.R., EVERTS, E.C., STEVENS, K.R. and IRELAND, K.M. (1981) Advanced squamous cell carcinoma of the maxillary sinus. Results of combined regional infusion chemotherapy, radiation therapy and surgery. *American Journal of Surgery*, **141**, 522–525

MURTHY, A.K. and HENDRICKSON, F.R. (1980) Is contralateral neck treatment necessary in early carcinoma of the tonsils? *International Journal of Radiation Oncology, Biology and Physics*, **6**, 91–94

O'CONNOR, A.D., CLIFFORD, P., DALLEY, V.M., DURDEN-SMITH, D.J., EDWARDS, W. and HOLLIS, B.A. (1979) Advanced head and neck cancer treated by combined radiotherapy and VBM cytotoxic regimens: 4-year results. *Clinical Otolaryngology*, **4**, 329–337

PATEY, D. (1973) Radiotherapy and carcinoma of the parotid. *British Medical Journal*, **1**, 236

PEARSON, J. G. (1966) The radiotherapy of carcinoma of the oesophagus and post-cricoid region in south-east Scotland. *Clinical Radiology*, **17**, 242–257

PEREZ, C.A., PURDY, J.A., BREAUX, S.R., OGURA, J.H. and VON ESSEN, S. (1982) Carcinoma of the tonsillar fossa: a non-randomised comparison of preoperative radiation and surgery or irradiation alone: long-term results. *Cancer*, *50*, 2314–2322

PIERQUIN, B., CHASSAGNE, D., CASHIN, Y., BAILLET, F. and FOURNELLE LE BOIS, F. (1970) Carcinomes épidermoides de la langue mobile et du plancher buccal. *Acta Radiologica*, **9**, 465–480

PRICE, L.A. and HILL, B.T. (1982) Safe and effective induction chemotherapy without cisplatin of squamous cell carcinoma of the head and neck: impact of complete response rate and survival at 5 years following local therapy. *Medical and Paediatric Oncology*, **10**, 535–548

RAFLA, S. (1982) Salivary glands. In *Treatment of Cancer*, edited by K.E. Halnan, pp. 269–294 London: Chapman and Hall

SATO, Y., MORITA, M., TAKAHISHI, J., WOTANOBE, N. and KIRIKAE, I. (1970) Combined surgery, radiotherapy and regional chemotherapy in carcinoma of the paranasal sinuses. *Cancer*, **25**, 571–579

SCHNEIDER, J.J., FLETCHER, G.H. and BARKLEY, H.T. Jr (1975) Control by irradiation alone of non-fixed clinically positive lymph nodes from squamous cell carcinoma of the oral cavity, oropharynx, supraglottic, larynx and hypopharynx. *American Journal of Roentgenology*, **123**, 42–48

SHANTA, V. and KRISHNAMURTHI, S. (1977) Combined therapy of oral cancer: bleomycin and radiation. A clinical trial. *Clinical Radiology*, **28**, 427–429

STALLARD, H.B. (1966) Radiotherapy for malignant melanomas of the choroid. *British Journal of Ophthalmology*, **50**, 147–155

STELL, P.M., DALBY, J.E., STRICKLAND, P., FRASER, J.G., BRADLEY, P.J. and FLOOD, L.M. (1983) Sequential chemotherapy and radiotherapy in advanced head and neck cancers. *Clinical Radiology*, **34**, 463–467

STRONG, E.W. (1969) Pre-operative radiation and radical neck dissection. *Surgical Clinics of North America*, **49**, 271–276

SUIT, H.D., LINDBERG, R. and FLETCHER, G.H. (1965) Prognostic significance of extent of tumour regression at completion of radiation therapy. *Radiology*, **84**, 1100–1107

TERZ, J.M., KING, E.R. and LAWRENCE, W. (1981) Preoperative irradiation for head and neck cancer: results of a prospective study. *Surgery*, **89**, 449–453

UNION INTERNATIONALE CONTRE LE CANCER (1978) TNM classification of malignant tumours. 3rd edn. Geneva: UICC

VIKRAM, B., STRONG, E.W., SHAH, J.P. and SPIRO, R. (1984a) Failure in the neck following multimodality treatment for advanced head and neck cancer. *Head and*

Neck Surgery, **6**, 724–729
VIKRAM, B., STRONG, E.W., SHAH, J.P. and SPIRO, R. (1984b) Failure at the primary site following multimodality treatment in advanced head and neck cancer. *Head and Neck Surgery*, **6**, 720–723
WANG, C. C. (1971) Radiotherapeutic management of carcinoma of the posterior pharyngeal wall. *Cancer*, **27**, 894–896
WIERNIK, G. and GUNN, Y. (1984) The BIR fractionation trials of laryngopharyngeal radiotherapy. *British Journal of Radiology*, **57**, 277
ZIMMERMAN, L.E., McLEAN, I.W. and FOSTER, W.D. (1978) Does enucleation of the eye containing a malignant melanoma prevent or accelerate the dissemination of tumour cells? *British Journal of Ophthalmology*, **62**, 420–425

6

Soft tissue and bone sarcomas

S. J. Arnott

Soft tissue sarcoma

Soft tissue sarcomas are rare tumours accounting for less than 1% of all malignancies. The incidence is of the order of 0.5 to 0.8 per 100000 population per year: therefore in the UK there will be approximately 380 new cases diagnosed each year. These tumours assume a relatively greater importance under the age of 25 years when they account for 6% for all malignancies, the most common histological type being rhabdomyosarcoma (*see* Chapter 10).

Soft tissue tumours are of mesenchymal origin and are classified according to the cell type or tissue from which they are derived. The majority are most probably derived from intermediate mesenchymal cells (Enterline, 1981).

Histological subtypes

The classification of sarcomas usually employed is that prepared by the World Health Organization (Enzinger, Lattes and Torloni, 1969). The most common of these tumours and their relative incidence are shown in *Table 6.1* (Russell *et al.*, 1977). However, the rarity and variety frequently give rise to practical problems in classification. The differentiation of particular cell types is important as it may have an influence on therapeutic approaches, and add to knowledge concerning the relative frequency of various tumour subtypes and their natural history.

The classification of soft tissue sarcomas remains a matter os some controversy, and changes in nomenclature, and as a result relative prevalence, are still occurring. For example, true fibrosarcomas are now considered to be much less common than was originally believed. Malignant fibrous histiocytoma, on the other hand, is a tumour which has only recently been recognized following an appreciation that histiocytes could act as facultative fibroblasts and so give rise to a variety of tumours (Ozello, Stout and Murray, 1963). There remain a few sarcomas for which it is still impossible to assign a cell of origin. For these, descriptive terms are used, e.g. alveolar soft part sarcoma, clear cell sarcoma.

Table 6.1 Histopathological classification of sarcomas

Tumour type	*Incidence (%)*
Rhabdomyosarcoma	19.8
Fibrosarcoma	19.0
Liposarcoma	18.2
Malignant fibrous histiocytoma	10.5
Synovial sarcoma	10.0
Leiomyosarcoma	6.5
Neurogenic sarcoma	4.9
Angiosarcoma	2.7
Others	1.9

From the clinical and prognostic point of view, the exact histiological subtype is less important than the grade of an individual sarcoma and this is taken into consideration in the staging of these tumours (Werf-Messing and Unnik, 1965; Russell *et al.*, 1977). Grading of sarcomas is not based simply on the numbers of mitotic figures seen per high power field, but also takes into account other features such as degree of cellularity, pleomorphism and the production of extracellular substances such as collagen and mucin.

Age and sex incidence

If rhabdomyosarcoma is excluded, the majority of soft tissue sarcomas occur in middle and late life, the peak incidence occurring in the 40–70 age group (*Table 6.2*). The sex ratio is virtually equal, the male: female ratio being 1.12:1 (Russell *et al.*, 1977).

Table 6.2 Relationship of age and incidence of sarcomas

Age group	*Sarcoma type*
Late childhood	Rhabdomyosarcoma Fibrosarcoma
Early adult	Synovial sarcoma Alveolar soft part sarcoma Haemangiopericytoma
Middle age	Fibrosarcoma Liposarcoma Leiomyosarcoma Malignant fibrous histiocytoma Haemangiopericytoma Kaposi's sarcoma
Elderly	Liposarcoma Kaposi's sarcoma

Aetiology

The aetiology of these tumours is largely unknown although a variety of factors has been implicated. Trauma is now generally not considered to be of any aetiological significance (Morton, 1974). Genetic factors, on the other hand, are of importance in a small group of patients. For example, a higher frequency of sarcomas is seen in patients who have survived a previous retinoblastoma (Jensen and Miller, 1971), and desmoid tumours are seen more commonly in patients with familial polyposis (McAdam and Goligher, 1970). Malignant transformation may occur in a pre-existing benign tumour. For example, neurofibrosarcoma develops in approximately 10% of patients with multiple neurofibromatosis (Storm *et al.*, 1980). The development of sarcomas is a rare complication of radiotherapy, especially if this were given for the treatment of a benign condition, e.g. angioma.

Other postulated factors are less well documented. For example the causal relationship of sarcomas arising in scars or chronic granulation tissue, and the role of chemicals in human sarcoma development remains unclear. Exceptions are the associations of vinyl chloride and hepatic angiosarcomas and asbestos exposure and the development of pleural mesothelioma.

A matter of great interest at the present time is the possible aetiological role of viruses (Morton *et al.*, 1969; Harris and Sinkovics, 1976; Minson, 1984).

Site

One-half of all sarcomas will develop in an extremity, 40% occurring in the lower limbs. Of these, 80% will be found in the thigh. The remainder are distributed between the trunk and head and neck.

Spread

Sarcomas usually develop deeply within soft tissues and local growth is the predominant form of initial spread. Many are associated with profuse neovascularization which frequently leads to haemorrhage and necrosis. Of greater importance is the fact that tumour cells can readily enter these vessels, so leading to early metastasis.

True sarcomas are never encapsulated, although they may have a pseudo-capsule produced by compression of the periphery of the tumour and the surrounding tissues. This appearance may lead to inappropriate surgery such as enucleation which frequently accounts for the high rates of local recurrence seen with these tumours.

Growth also occurs along tissue spaces and along the line of nerves, blood vessels and bones which may, in turn, become invaded. However, Ligaments, tendons, fascial sheaths and intermuscular fibrous septa act as barriers for a considerable period of time. Spread through compartments may occur, but this usually happens only in association with tumours of large size. Skip lesions are seen with a number of sarcomas.

Whilst blood-borne metastases occur frequently, lymph node spread is relatively uncommon. It is seen, However, with greater frequency in association with certain histological subtypes, such as synovial sarcoma. Metastases principally occur in lungs, liver, bone and brain.

As a general rule, liposarcomas which have myxoid features, and most other well-differentiated tumours, frequently remain localized, whereas round cell and pleomorphic sarcomas have a greater tendency to metastasize.

Management

Clinical assessment

The initial clinical presentation of a peripherally situated sarcoma is of the recent development of an enlarging, painless swelling. However, some patients may indicate that a mass had been present for some considerable time, even up to 1 year, only slowly enlarging during this period. Other patients will present with features such as pain, indicating invasion or pressure on adjacent nerves, blood vessels or bone. Limb oedema may indicate extensive lymph node involvement in a few. Sarcomas may be associated with non-metastatic syndromes such as spontaneous hypoglycaemia, which may be a feature of large fibrosarcomas, and certain metabolic effects are seen with some malignant fibrous histiocytomas.

Lesions which may be confused with sarcomas are haematoma, abscess, muscular herniation, cysts, fat necrosis and benign neoplasms such as lipoma and neurofibroma. On occasions, a solitary subcutaneous metastasis from an unknown primary tumour may mimic a sarcoma. As a general rule, any new soft tissue swelling should be biopsied.

Tumours arising in other sites may be associated with a greater frequency of symptoms due to tumour invasion. This is particularly true of retroperitoneal sarcomas when ureteric or bowel obstruction may be presenting features. Alteration of bowel or urinary habit may be seen in pelvic tumours.

Investigations

Histological confirmation

An adequate biopsy of the tumour is essential. There is some controversy among surgeons concerning the best way to obtain a histological specimen. Most would agree that needle biopsy is inadequate. Some surgeons believe that excision biopsy may promote spread of tumour into surrounding muscle compartments (Markhede, Angervall and Stener, 1982) and most would advocate an incisional biopsy. Care must be taken regarding the site of the biopsy. It should be placed longitudinally in order not to compromise subsequent muscle group excisions and in such a situation to allow removal at definitive surgery or to be within possible radiotherapy fields.

Radiology

Radiological investigations are designed to evaluate not only the local extent of tumour, but also the site and number of metastases. Various radiological techniques may be employed ranging from conventional radiology, through ultrasonography to newer techniques of angiography, lymphangiography and computed tomography (CT). As a general rule, the simpler diagnostic techniques are used first. These may demonstrate widespread metastatic disease which obviates the need to use more sophisticated investigations.

Conventional radiography

Plain X-rays of the affected part together with a chest radiograph are required in all patients. The chest X-ray provides a good screening test for the presence of obvious and possibly widespread pulmonary metastases. X-rays of the primary tumour may delineate the local extent of an obvious soft tissue mass, although xero-radiography is usually better in this respect. Since the introduction of CT this latter investigation is now much less frequently employed. Conventional radiology of the primary tumour is of most help in determining the relationship of the soft tissue tumour to the bony skeleton and may demonstrate bone involvement or periosteal reaction.

Angiography

Prior to the availability of CT, angiography provided the most accurate information concerning the nature and extent of soft tissue tumours. Now, however, it is mainly used to solve problems unresolved by other techniques. Occasionally, it may be employed for palliative embolization. The features best demonstrated by angiography are the local extent of a tumour and its relationship to major vessels.

Computed tomography

This is the most useful radiological investigation in the assessment of both central and peripheral soft tissue sarcomas (de Santos *et al.*, 1978; Levine *et al.*, 1979). In the light of current knowledge it is difficult to justify patients not having CT performed. It provides accurate information concerning the exact local extent of a tumour, and its resectability. It is also extremely sensitive in the detection of recurrence after definitive treatment. CT will not, however, give accurate information concerning the histological nature of the tumour (Golding and Husband, 1982). There is now considerable evidence showing that CT is the most accurate technique for the detection of pulmonary metastases (Husband and Golding, 1982).

Other radiological investigations

A variety of other radiological investigations may be indicated in certain circumstances. Liver scintigraphy, for example, should be performed in patients with intra-abdominal tumours and in those with high grade sarcomas in other sites, as these are associated with an increased incidence of hepatic metastases. Ultrasonography is reserved for equivocal cases. The combination of these techniques is as accurate as Ct (Snow, Goldstein and Wallace, 1979; Lindell *et al.*, 1981).

Lymphangiography should be used when dealing with those tumours known to have a higher incidence of nodal involvement, e.g. synovial sarcoma. Bone scans are not usually necessary unless bone metastases are suspected.

Table 6.3 Staging system for soft tissue sarcomas. (After Russell *et al.*, 1981)

TNM classification	*Stage grouping*
Primary tumour (T)	*Stage I*
	IA G1 T1 N0 M0
T0 — no demonstrable tumour	B G1 T2 N0 M0
T1 — tumour < 5 cm in diameter	
T2 — tumour > 5 cm in diameter	*Stage II*
T3 — gross invasion of bone, vessel or nerve	
	IIA G2 T1 N0 M0
	B G2 T2 N0 M0
Nodes (N)	*Stage III*
N0 — no nodes verified	IIIA G3 T1 N0 M0
N1 — histologically involved regional nodes	B G3 T2 N0 M0
	C Any G, T1, 2 N1 M0
Metastases (M)	*Stage IV*
M0 — no known metastases	IVA Any G, T3 Any N M0
M1 — clinically detected metastases	B Any G Any T Any N M1
Grade (G)	
Histopathological grade G1 to G3	

Treatment policy

Staging

Staging is important as not only does it allow an assessment of prognosis to be made for the individual patient, but it also allows comparison to be made between different methods of treatment for those with equivalent disease. This is particularly important when dealing with rare tumours such as soft tissue sarcomas.

A summary of the modern TNM staging classification is given in *Table 6.3*. Kaposi's sarcoma, dermatofibrosarcoma and desmoid tumours are excluded from this staging system as are sarcomas arising in viscera and the brain.

General assessment

In all decisions regarding treatment, the age and general condition of the patient must be taken into consideration. What is appropriate treatment for the young may be totally inappropriate in the elderly. In this context, many clinics employ a scale of fitness such as the Karnofsky index or some modification of it (Karnofsky *et al.*, 1948).

Treatment choice

The choice of which treatment modalities are to be used will depend on such factors as the likely success of achieving local tumour control together with cosmetic and functional considerations.

Surgery

The site of the tumour has a great influence on the effectiveness of surgery, which is most successful in the management of sarcomas arising in an extremity. Lesions of the head and neck or retroperitoneal area are much less amenable to complete surgical removal and are frequently referred for primary radiotherapy.

There are three basic surgical approaches to a sarcoma arising in an extremity: simple enucleation or excision; wide monobloc resection; and amputation. As a general rule, the effectiveness of surgery is proportional to the functional loss and anatomical disfigurement produced by each procedure. For example, enucleation or simple excision will be associated with a high local recurrence rate of the order of 40–90% (Atkinson, Garvan and Newton, 1963; Markhede, Angervall and Stener, 1982), whereas amputations have a relatively low incidence (Shiu *et al.*, 1975; Simon and Enneking, 1976). The principle behind wide monobloc excision is resection of the affected part, including biopsy scars, without the surgeon visualizing the tumour at any time during the procedure. The plane of excision should be one fascial barrier around the palpable sarcoma. An example of such an operation is compartmentectomy. This procedure is not possible for very advanced tumours, nor is it appropriate in all anatomical sites. The problems associated with tumour recurrence following local excision, and those of the mutilation of amputation have led to the majority of surgeons employing wide excisional techniques whenever possible. In these procedures, the aim is to achieve as good a functional and cosmetic result as possible. The development of these techniques has been encouraged by the effectiveness of postoperative radiotherapy in improving local tumour control rates.

Radiotherapy

A great deal of pessimism still exists concerning the effectiveness of radiotherapy in the treatment of soft tissue sarcomas. This has arisen because the majority of cases referred for treatment have had large, inoperable or recurrent tumours, in which poor responses have been achieved. However, encouraging results have appeared which indicate that irradiation can make a significant contribution to both local tumour control and survival. One of the earliest reports describing the effectiveness of radiotherapy in patients with soft tissue sarcoma was by Cade (1951). He described the treatment by irradiation of a series of 22 patients with fibrosarcoma. In six there was long-standing complete tumour regression. Windeyer, Dische and Mansfield (1966) have presented similar effective treatment results.

More recently, the efficacy of combining surgery with postoperative radiotherapy has been described (Suit and Russell, 1977; Rosenberg and Glatstein, 1981). These reports suggest that local radical surgery combined with postoperative radiotherapy can achieve local tumour control rates and survival equivalent to those obtained by amputation. Certainly, the superior functional and cosmetic results of such a treatment policy are obvious. There are other advantages which make this approach preferable. For example, complete pathological examination of the specimen is possible. This provides the full details of tumour extent, degree of infiltration and histological grade which will influence any subsequent treatment given. In addition, definitive surgical treatment is not delayed and there is no contraindication to postoperative radiotherapy.

Patient assessment

Patients requiring radiotherapy will fall into three broad categories:

(1) Those in whom definitive surgery has been performed and no residual disease, or only microscopic tumour, is present
(2) Those in whom obvious tumour is present either because surgery has not been carried out, or because recurrence has developed following surgery
(3) Metastatic disease has been demonstrated. The primary tumour may still be *in situ* or the patient may be locally free from disease.

Treatment policy

A careful search must first be made to exclude metastatic disease.

In the absence of metastases, if gross local tumour is present, either definitive radical surgery or, if this is not possible, debulking of tumour should first be performed. This will enhance the effectiveness of radiotherapy and enable subsequent dose and field modifications to be made during treatment in order to achieve an optimal functional result.

Patient selection

Should an amputation have been performed, local radiotherapy is not indicated unless tumour is present at the resection margins and further surgery is impossible.

Similarly, postoperative radiotherapy is not required if a true monobloc excision has been performed for low grade tumours less than 5 cm in size, with minimal infiltration and in which wide excision margins have been achieved.

However, for all less well differentiated tumours and for larger tumours, even if low grade, postoperative radiotherapy is indicated. In these circumstances, grade has less influence on local recurrence. For example, a survey of 194 patients managed by wide excisional surgery alone, demonstrated that local recurrence occurred in 25% of low-grade tumours and 21% of moderate or high-grade lesions (Shiu and Hajdu, 1981).

If microsscopic residual disease is found on histological examination of the resected specimen, further surgery is unnecessary as the results of the combined treatment policy for this group of patients are as good as for those in whom excision appears complete (Schmitt, 1984).

Radiotherapy techniques

Peripheral tumours

A variety of radiotherapy techniques will be required in the irradiation of limb and superficial trunk lesions to achieve uniform dose distribution in the target volume. The size of the target volume will be influenced by the original size of the tumour, its site, histological grade and the extent of any surgical procedure. It is vital that knowledge of all these factors is obtained before treatment planning commences. This will involve discussions with the surgeon, pathologist and diagnostic radiologist. The insertion of liga clips is a gret help in delineating the surgical field and may be more useful than relying on the excision scar as a guide. CT is of great value. Generally speaking, poorly-differentiated sarcomas require a wider margin of treatment than do well-differentiated tumours.

Megavoltage radiotherapy is necessary because of its good depth dose characteristics, skin sparing and reduced absorption in bone. However, all scars must receive the maximum dose by using bolus to reduce the risk of scar recurrence (*Figure 6.1*).

As a general rule, single field treatments are inadequate. For lesions of the limbs, parallel opposed fields provide a good dose distribution. A margin of 5 cm proximal and distal to the site of the original tumour is usually adequate for low-grade tumours providing this includes the surgical scar. For poorly-differentiated lesions, a 10 cm margin is necessary. In this way, the whole of the tumour bed is irradiated with a sufficient margin to allow for longitudinal spread. Other treatment techniques are possible for limb tumours, but there is a risk that the depths of the tumour bed may be inadequately irradiated. When using parallel opposed fields, it is still possible, and indeed essential, to avoid treating the limb circumferentially to high doses. *Figure 6.2a* shows a cross section of the thigh and *Figure 6.2b* demonstrates the sparing of one part of the limb while at the same time fully irradiating the entire tumour area. Bearing in mind the positional problems of patients, *Figure 6.2c* illustrates the difficulties which may be encountered when using alternative treatment techniques. *Figure 6.3* demonstrates the reduced reaction obtained in the spared portion of the limb.

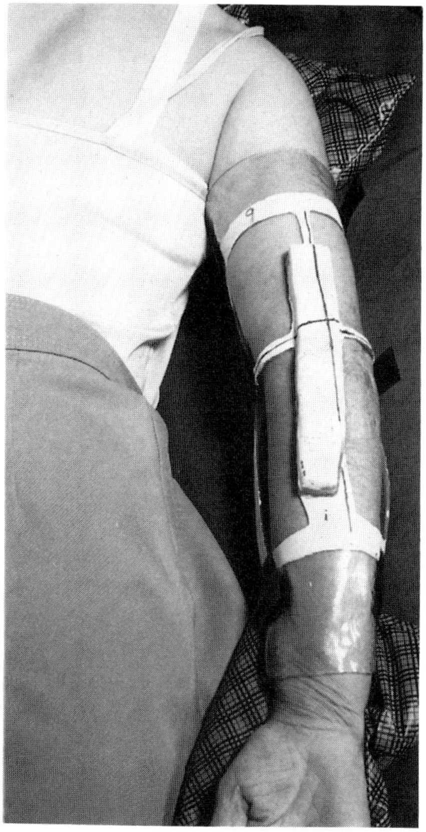

Figure 6.1 Arm in cast with bolus to scar

Reproducibility of treatment set-up is vital. Sometimes simple immobilization devices may be used together with skin marks or tattoos which, if possible, should be placed over skin which is relatively non-mobile (*Figure 6.4*). However, in more peripherally sited tumours, more sophisticated immobilization techniques are necessary (*Figure 6.5a and b*). Frequently joints need to be included. If at all possible, some shielding of the joint should be performed to spare at least one section of it from the full dose of radiotherapy.

In the region of the shoulder, tangential field arrangements are often necessary in order to spare the lungs. In the buttock also, more complex field arrangements are required to spare the bowel as much as possible (*Figure 6.6*).

However, in thigh tumours arising close to origins of muscles on the public rami, parallel opposed fields are required. Nevertheless, it is usually possible to shield off the bowel, at least in part, thus reducing morbidity.

Treatment planning and dose

Calculation of the target volume will dictate the field size to be used. There is some difference of opinion concerning whether this initial field size should continue to be used throughout treatment or whether a shrinking field technique is preferable.

The majority of centres will use shrinking field techniques at least in those situations where there is no residual disease or only microscopic tumour. Generally, treatment is given to the initial volume at a rate of 1000 cGy per week using five daily fractions up to a dose level of 4000 cGy in 20 fractions over 4 weeks. Thereafter, the field size is reduced to include the whole length of the scar with 1 cm of margin at either end. The width of the field is also reduced to avoid high dose circumferential irradiation. Treatment is continued for a further 2 weeks, giving an

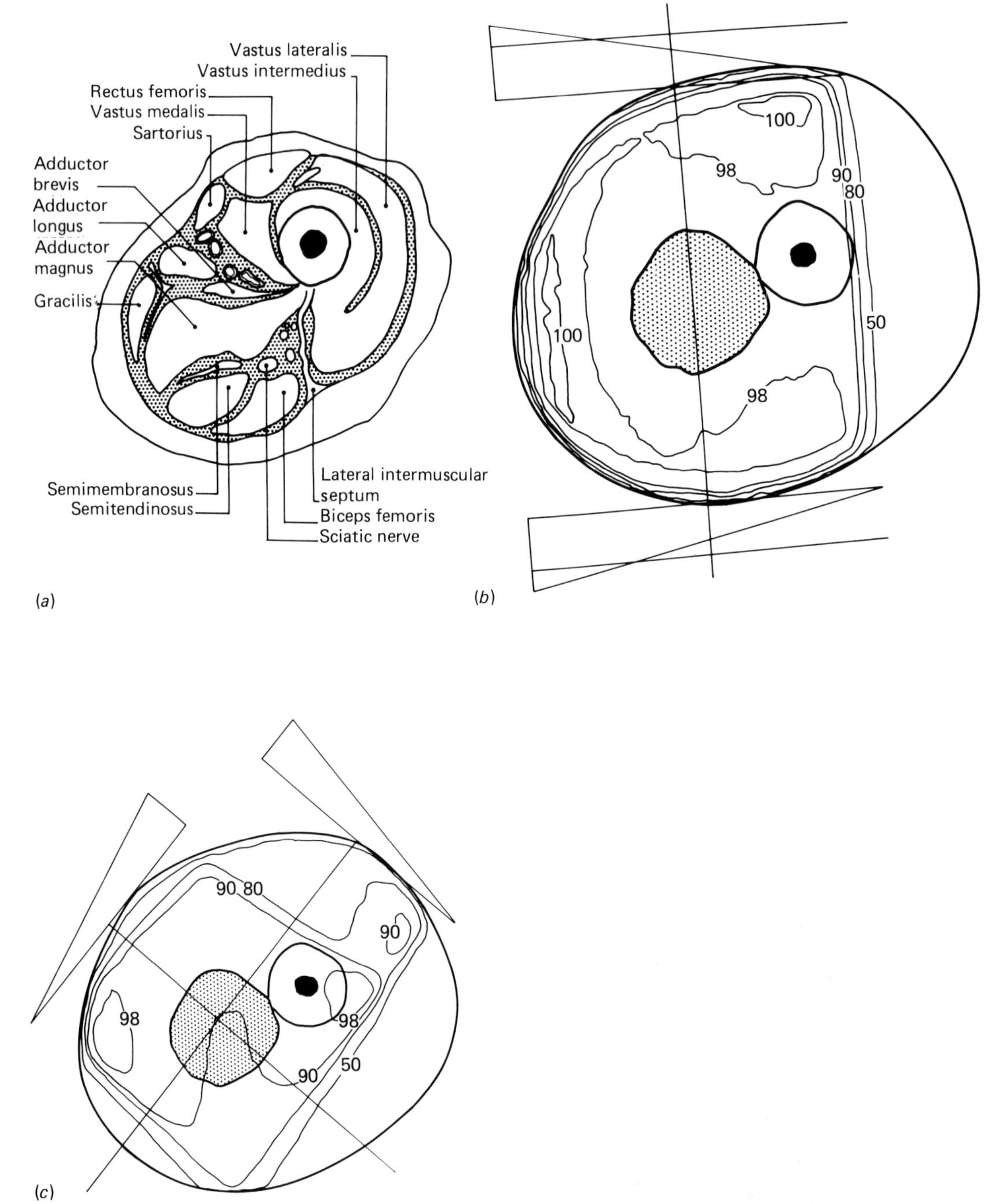

Figure 6.2 *(a)* Cross section of the thigh. *(b)* Good dose distribution using parallel opposed fields with adequate limb circumference sparing.
(c) Showing poorer distribution of dose which might occur when using wedged pair of fields

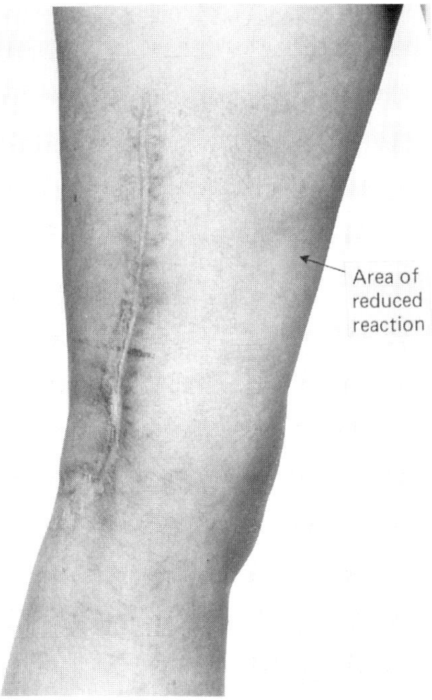

Figure 6.3 Avoidance of circumferential irradiation

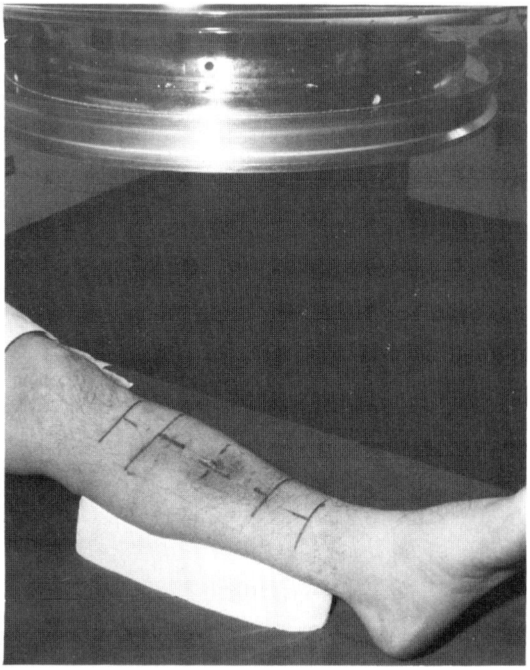

Figure 6.4 Simple immobilization device consisting of a posterior cast of plaster of Paris

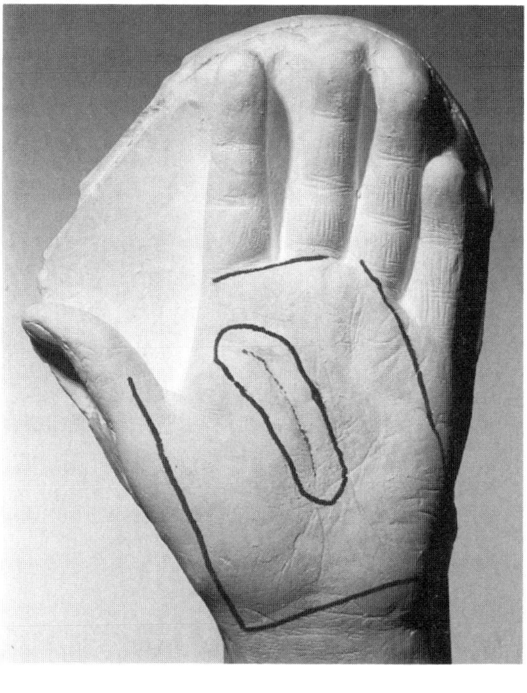

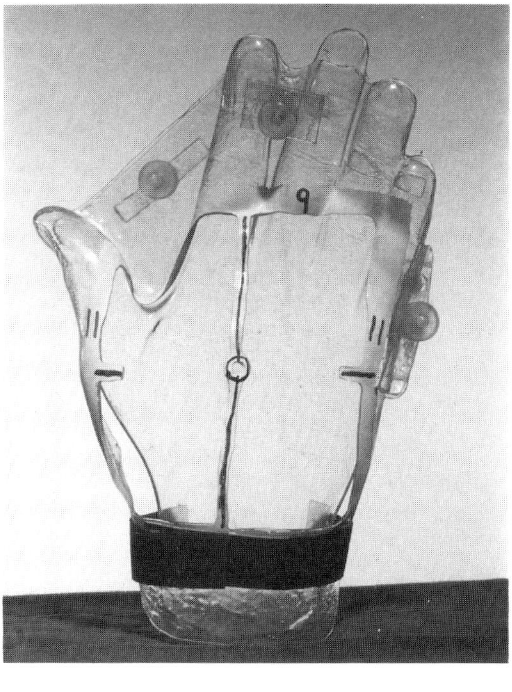

Figure 6.5 *(a)* Cast of hand showing site of excised tumour. *(b)* Bexoid shell for hand treatment

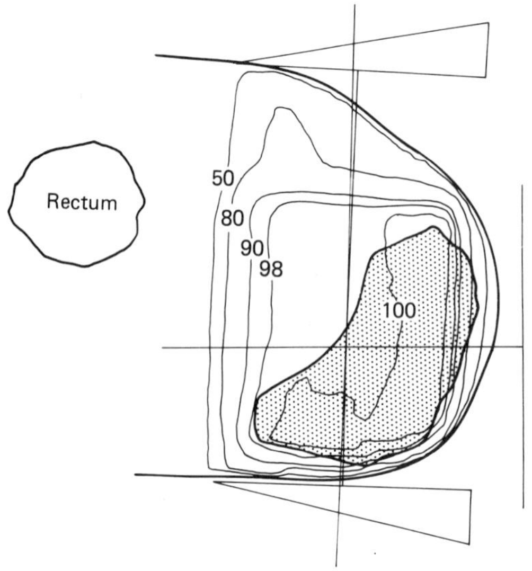

Figure 6.6 Tumour in buttock region: three field arrangement to spare rectum

additional 2000 cGy in 10 fractions during this period. Thus, the main tumour-bearing area will have received a dose of 6000 cGy in 30 fractions in an overall period of 6 weeks. In all patients, accurate simulation is necessary to delineate the target volume.

When macroscopic tumour is present, it is not possible to shrink the field to the same extent as margins of 5 cm around the tumour will still be required throughout treatment. Reduction of the total dose given may, therefore, be necessary depending on the treatment volume used so that a maximum of 5000 cGy is given in 30 fractions over the 6-week period.

The alternative approach is to give a dose equivalent to 5000 cGy in 4 weeks to the whole of the initial target volume. Where this is large, for example in excess of 150 cm^2, a dose reduction to 4500 cGy will be necessary. Whatever technique is used, all fields should be treated each day. Even when parallel opposed fields are employed, a computer planning progrmme is still helpful in order to obtain the optimum dose distribution.

When reduced doses are necessary because of volume considerations, boost doses of 1000 – 2000 cGy may be given with electrons or possibly by means of implants. These techniques are usually only applicable in selected cases of relatively superficial tumours. In the majority of instances, external beam therapy is the preferred treatment modality.

Apart from achieving reduced local tissue reactions, there is no evidence to suggest that protracted treatments using shrinking field techniques give better local tumour control rates than do shorter treatments with fixed field sizes.

Lesions in other sites

When sarcomas arise in the head and neck region, the techniques of treatment employed are similar to those normally used for squamous carcinomas in these sites. Usually the field sizes required will be smaller than in the treatment of limb tumours, and doses equivalent to 5500 cGy in 20 fractions over 4 weeks are necessary. The spinal cord and mid-brain must be avoided in treatment as must the eye if possible. *Figure 6.7* shows a typical treatment plan.

Superficial trunk lesions may require special techniques of immobilization together with tangential treatment fields in order to minimize dosage to underlying vital structures (*Figure 6.8*).

Retroperitoneal sarcomas

As a result of the insidious onset of retroperitoneal sarcomas, they are often of large size when diagnosed. This limits the surgery which can be performed and, for many patients, all that is possible is biopsy. Even in aggressive surgical hands, the resection rate is low and operative mortality high (Fortner *et al.*, 1981). The survival rates of each patients reflect these problems, and while some enthusiastic reports have suggested that 5-year survival rates of the order of 30% may be achieved (Kinne *et al.*, 1973), most centres have few, if any, long-term survivors. Thus, the basic approach to these patients is one of palliation, treatment being required for relief of symptoms. If possible, relatively high doses should be given as these will produce better long-term local tumour control. Usually only parallel opposed field arrangements are suitable and doses of the order of 4500 cGy in 20 fractions over 4 weeks are the maximum possible. Protection of the kidneys may be necessary depending on the site of the tumour irradiated. However, part or all of one kidney may be included in treatment if this would otherwise involve shielding of tumour.

Treatment reactions

Acute

In the treatment of limb and superficial trunk tumours, the skin reaction is the only problem likely to be encountered. This is usually mild, rarely exceeding erythema and dry desquamation over the majority of the field area. However, more severe

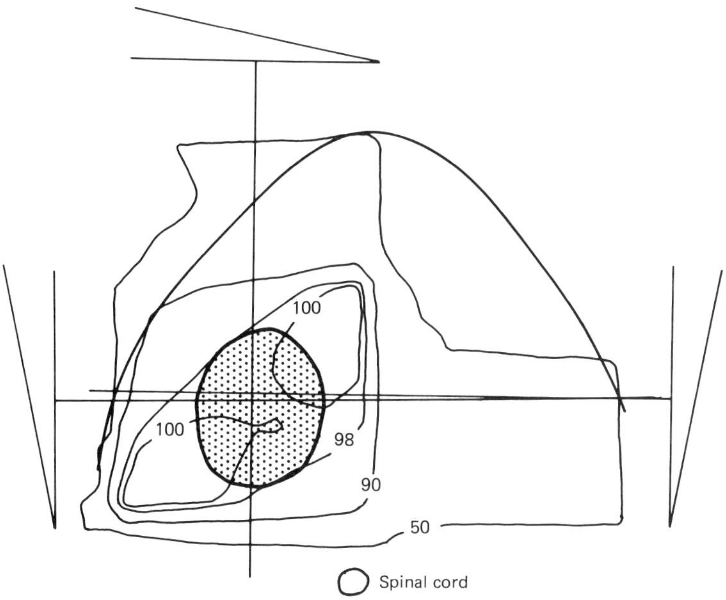

Figure 6.7 Typical dose distribution for sarcoma arising on soft palate

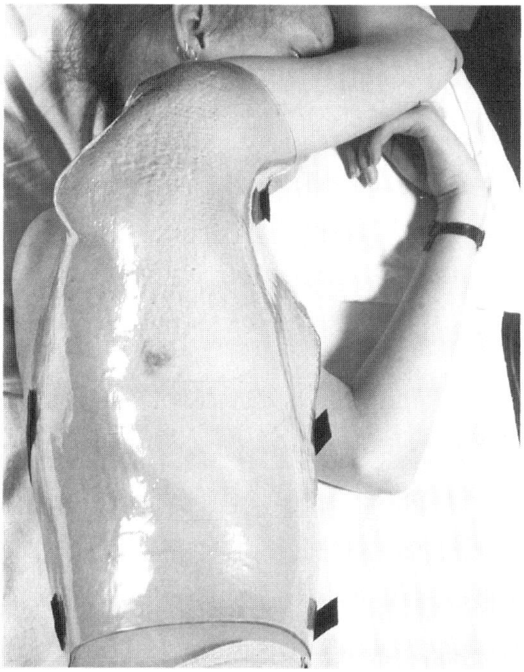

Figure 6.8 Body shell to immobilize patient during treatment of chest wall tumour

reactions will be seen when irradiating the groins, perineum and axilla, and patchy, moist desquamation may be seen at any skin crease.

Simple measures are usually all that are necessary for treatment. The skin should be kept as cool and as dry as possible during radiotherapy. Thereafter, oilatum cream will help in the management of dry desquamative reactions. When moist desquamation occurs, graneodin or similar ointment will help promote healing.

Late

The late reactions following courses of radiotherapy for sarcomas limit the doses which may be given. Late skin reactions are seldom a problem, except when the lower third of the leg has been treated, or on the rare occasions when tumours arising in the hand and foot have been irradiated. Trauma is often a precipitating factor whenever skin breakdown occurs.

While no direct effects on muscle are recognizable during the acute reaction phase, the patient may complain of muscle fatigue. However, late changes similar to those of atrophy of the skin and subcutaneous fibrous tissue, also occur in muscle. This may be manifest as loss of muscle bulk and woody induration. Fibrosis of the intermuscular septa may also interfere with muscle function, leading to stiffness. This may also be due to effects on joints. However, stiffness is not usually due to direct effects on the joint surfaces, but more commonly as a result of fibrotic changes in the joint capsule.

The radiopathological basis of late muscle changes is related to radiation effects on blood vessels and connective tissues (Rubin and Casarett, 1968). These vascular and connective tissue reactions lead to delayed secondary degeneration causing atrophy and fibrosis of the irradiated muscles. In the vast majority of patients, carefully applied treatment produces few late problems. Stiffness, which may develop, is largely preventable by early and continued physiotherapy.

In most situations, long segments of bone will inevitably be included in treatment. Acute reactions are usually not demonstrable in adult irradiated bone, but late changes may occur as a result of injury to the cellular and vascular components. For example, high dose treatment may cause periosteal damage which in turn leads to death of underlying bone. In addition, there may be damage of the cellular components, osteoclasts being more resistant than osteoblasts. This can result in osteoporosis, progressing to osteonecrosis. This complication occurs with greater frequency if the bone is directly invaded by tumour. In most other instances, it arises from the use of very high doses of radiation, poorly fractionated treatments, or re-treatments. The significance of osteonecrosis depends on the site affected. Rib fractures may be painful, but often have little other significance. However, necrosis of a weight-bearing bone such as the femur is serious, but with good, modern, beam-directed, megavoltage techniques this should be a problem of the past.

A rare late complication of bone irradiation is the induction of a new primary sarcoma. It is difficult to quantify the risk, but it has been suggested that it may be of the order of 0.2% in patients irradiated for breast carcinoma (Hatfield and Schulz, 1970).

Irradiation of retroperitoneal sarcomas may produce those late changes which are seen following abdominal radiotherapy for other malignancies (*see* Chapter 10).

Palliation

Palliative radiotherapy is required in a variety of circumstances. It may be necessary to relieve symptoms from an uncontrolled primary tumour, for example in the presence of widespread metastatic disease, or where the age and general condition of the patient preclude radical treatment. Alternatively, it may be necessary for the control of symptoms due to metastases in various sites.

Primary tumour

When palliative treatment is being given, only simple treatment arrangements are necessary. These may take the form of single applied fields, or parallel opposed fields. Electrons of suitable energy may be used as an alternative.

The margin of irradiation may be reduced to cover the tumour with a minimum of margin. This is to permit moderately high doses of treatment to be given, as low doses are less likely to be of benefit. The dose of radiotherapy required is of the order of 3500–3750 cGy in 10 fractions over a period of 2 weeks, treating all fields each day.

A useful alternative approach is employed in some centres, in which radiotherapy is given at weekly intervals, judging the total dose given according to the reaction produced. This is the so-called 'growth restraint approach'. Dose fractions of the order of 300–350 cGy are given at weekly intervals, sometimes over long periods of time, and may offer good palliative benefit.

Lung metastases

Radiotherapy to lung metastases may be of great benefit, especially when used at a stage when the disease is of small bulk. In spite of the fact that only low doses may be used, clearance of metastases is the rule. This regression may last from 3 to 6 months (*Figure 6.9a and b*).

Parallel opposed fields are used to cover both lung fields. Care must be taken to ensure that the lung apices and bases are fully included. A useful measure is to take a simulator film with the patient holding a breath in deep inspiration as the lung markings are often difficult to visualize under screening conditions. Care must be taken if a straight X-ray rather than a simulator film is used, as this may introduce errors of parallax. Using a correction factor for lung, a central dose of 2500 cGy in 20 fractions over a period of 4 weeks is given. Both fields are treated each day. When large lung deposits are causing symptoms, small field treatments may be helpful, enclosing only the metastases in question. Treatment, in these circumstances, is given in a much shorter period of time. A useful regimen is to give a central dose of 2000 cGy in five fractions over 1 week, using a parallel opposed pair of fields.

Reports which have suggested a benefit from prophylactic lung irradiation in osteosarcoma (Breur *et al.*, 1977; Newton and Barrett, 1978) have stimulated consideration of a similar approach in patients with soft tissue sarcoma (Coe, Madden and Mould, 1981). However, there is now real doubt about any such benefit, and in these circumstances the routine use of this form of treatment cannot be justified.

Bone metastases

Painful metastatic deposits in bone can be alleviated

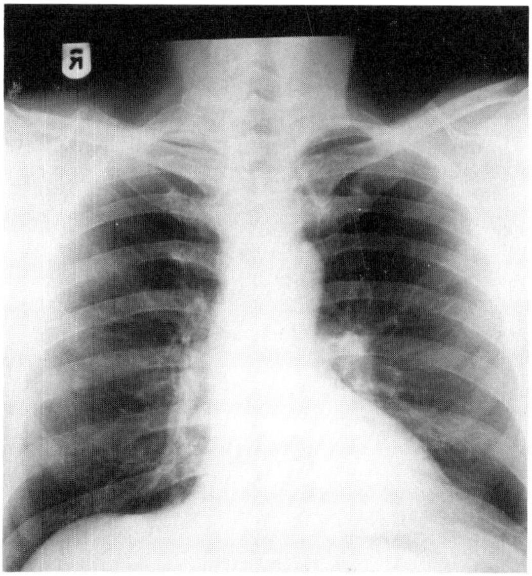

Figure 6.9 *(a)* Bilateral pulmonary metastases in a patient with synovial sarcoma.

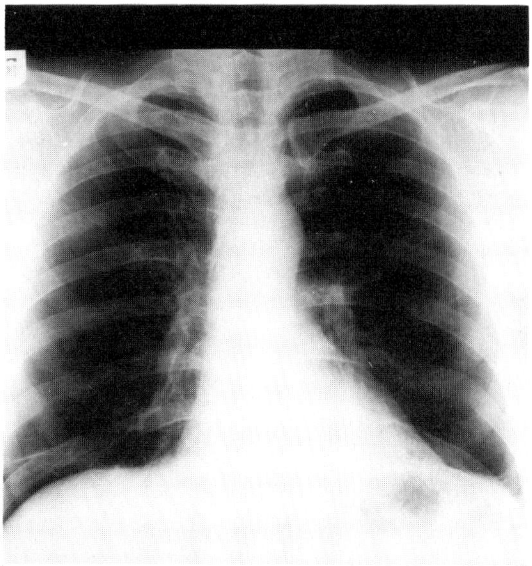

Figure 6.9 *(b)* X-ray taken after whole lung irradiation showing complete clearance of metastases

by palliative radiotherapy in the majority of patients. For a limb bone a parallel opposed pair of fields is required, whereas for deposits in the spine, a single applied field is usually adequate. Again, short treatment times are preferable. While some centres advocate the use of single treatments, these are usually associated with a greater degree of systemic upset than fractionated radiotherapy. A week's course of treatment is a good compromise, giving either a central or maximum dose of 2000 cGy in five fractions, depending on the site to be treated.

Metastases in other sites

While it is not usually appropriate to treat metastases in sites such as the liver and brain, radiotherapy for these may be considered in certain circumstances — for example in patients in good general condition with significant symptoms due to the deposits. A long interval between the initial presentation and the development of the metastasis is a useful additional criterion. Poorly-differentiated tumours are likely to demonstrate a more worthwhile response.

When irradiating the liver, treatment should be given only to that area grossly involved by tumour using either a single applied field or a parallel opposed pair of fields, depending on the site. A central or maximum dose of 3000 cGy in 10 fractions over 2 weeks is effective. A slightly longer overall time is used in order to reduce systemic effects.

The treatment of cerebral metastases necessitates the use of whole brain irradiation using a parallel opposed pair of fields, giving a central dose of 2000 cGy in five fractions over 1 week. Dexamethasone therapy will be required in addition, modifying the dose after radiotherapy, according to symptoms (*see* Chapter 15).

Other techniques of radiotherapy

Various alternative techniques of radiotherapy have been employed in the management of patients with soft tissue sarcomas in an attempt to improve local tumour control rates. These have included combined treatment regimens and also the use of newer forms of radiotherapy.

Radiotherapy under hypoxic conditions

Attempts to improve the results of postoperative combined treatment have included giving radiotherapy after conditions of tourniquet-induced hypoxia (Suit and Russell, 1977). The rationale for this treatment method is that a proportion of local treatment failures is due to the presence of viable, hypoxic tumour cells during the period of radiotherapy which are relatively radioresistant. The use of the tourniquet induces hypoxia in the surrounding normal tissues and thus reduces the differential radiosensitivity between normal and tumour cells and hopefully, therefore, improves the therapeutic ratio.

Unfortunately, a preliminary study of this form of radiotherapy performed at the M.D. Anderson Hospital in Houston, Texas demonstrated severe late normal tissue effects which led to amputation being necessary in no fewer than seven out of a total of 21 patients treated (Suit and Russell, 1977). This was, at least in part, due to large treatment fields being used which resulted in large volumes of normal tissues being irradiated to unacceptably high dose levels. Further analysis showed that in terms of local tumour control and survival, tourniquet radiotherapy was no more effective than conventional postoperative radiotherapy.

Preoperative radiotherapy

There has been some enthusiasm in the USA for the use of preoperative radiotherapy, in some cases also employing a postoperative supplementary treatment boost. However, the numbers of patients so treated have been small (Atkinson, Garvan and Newton, 1963; Martini, Lindberg and Russell, 1977; Suit, Proppe and Bramwell, 1982).

It is difficult to justify this approach as routine treatment. For example, a number of tumours will not require, or indeed benefit from, adjuvant radiotherapy. Many of the criteria concerning which tumours would best be given radiotherapy can only be determined by full histological examination of the resected specimen. There is no evidence to suggest that postoperative treatment is in any way inferior to preoperative radiotherapy and more information is available to enable accurate treatment to be given.

Initial radiotherapy, however, may be given to some tumours believed to be inoperable, which then regress to such an extent that resection can be performed. At the present time this sequential form of treatment is the only form of preoperative radiotherapy recommended in the treatment of soft tissue sarcoma.

Fast neutron therapy

The rationale for the use of fast neutrons in the treatment of soft tissue sarcomas is based on experimental evidence that neutron irradiation is more effective, by a factor of about three, in the destruction of hypoxic tumour cells (*see* Chapters 1 and 2). Areas of necrosis are a prominent feature of soft tissue sarcomas and cells surrounding these areas may be hypoxic yet viable, and relatively radioresistant. These cells may be a cause of local treatment failure. In addition, tumours such as sarcomas, with long volume doubling times, have a great ability to recover from sublethal radiation damage. However, this property is reduced following neutron therapy and therefore, theoretically, better responses should be seen. Encouraging results have been reported from Hammersmith Hospital where local tumour control rates of 75% have been reported for inoperable tumours (Catterall and Bewley, 1979). However, work in other centres has suggested that local normal tissue complications following neutron treatments are high (Schmitt *et al.*, 1983). This has certainly been the experience in Edinburgh where a small series of only 20 patients has been treated by fast neutrons. In these patients, overall local tumour control rates of 44% have been achieved, results which are similar to those obtained using conventional X-ray therapy (Gilbert, Kagan and Winkley, 1974). Unfortunately, significant normal tissue complications occurred in 40% of the neutron treated patients and these were particularly marked when limbs were irradiated. This is, at least in part, due to the increased absorption of neutrons in subcutaneous fatty tissues leading to excessive fibrosis and soft tissue contracture. At present there is no evidence to suggest that fast neutrons are in any way superior to excisional surgery and postoperative X-ray treatment in the management of soft tissue sarcomas.

Chemotherapy

Considerable controversy exists concerning the place of chemotherapy in the management of patients with adult soft tissue sarcoma. This is in complete contradistinction to the situation in rhabdomyosarcoma of childhood, where chemotherapy has an undoubted place and has contributed significantly to improved survival rates (*see* Chapter 10).

The wide variety of histological types of tumours in adults and their rarity has made the assessment of the effectiveness of chemotherapy difficult. In addition, differences in patterns of referral to individual centres pose problems in the analysis of reported series. A number of drugs have been shown to have effectiveness when used as single agents in metastatic disease. The most important of these are: hydroxydaunorubicin, cyclophosphamide, DTIC, vincristine, methotrexate and cisplatin. More recent drugs such as mitozantrone and ifosphamide, which are related to hydroxydaunorubicin and cyclophosphamide respectively, are currently undergoing investigation. These newer drugs have the advantage of reduced toxicity. Chemotherapy may be considered for the treatment of established metastases and also as an adjuvant treatment.

Treatment of metastatic disease

The results of treating metastases by single agent chemotherapy have been disappointing. Response rates, mainly partial regression rates, at the order of 20% have been quoted (Gottlieb *et al.*, 1975). Many combinations of drugs have also been used, the most effective being those which include hydroxydaunorubicin (Benjamin, Wiernick and Bachur, 1974; Suit, Proppe and Bramwell, 1982). However, the toxicity of these combined regimens is substantially greater. Possibly the most effective regimen available is that employing hydroxydaunorubicin, cyclophosphamide and methotrexate (Rosenberg *et al.*, 1983). However, chemotherapy for metastatic disease is only suitable for relatively young, fit patients, able to tolerate the toxicity of treatment. It should be remembered that, for a number of patients, the progress of the disease might well be slow and long periods of good quality life are possible without treatment of any kind. There is no evidence, for example, that chemotherapy prolongs survival in patients with metastases.

Adjuvant chemotherapy

The use of adjuvant chemotherapy in patients with soft tissue sarcoma remains an unsolved issue. Various conflicting reports have appeared over the years, the most enthusiastic of which have appeared from the USA. One of the major problems in assessing results has been that frequently the periods of follow-up have been short, and the patient numbers small. For example, a recent enthusiastic report from the National Cancer Institute (NCI) in America described the use of adjuvant chemotherapy in a group of 65 patients in whom initial assessment was carried out only 3 months after the trial closed. Much of the claimed survival improvement was, therefore, projected (Rosenberg *et al.*, 1983). A different investigation carried out at the M.D. Anderson Hospital in Texas, on the other hand, did not show such an advantage, although apparently identical patients were investigated and the drugs used were similar (Lindberg *et al.*, 1977).

Much further investigation is necessary to evaluate the use of adjuvant chemotherapy in soft tissue sarcoma. Meaningful results are only likely to come from prospective, randomized, multicentre trials.

Results of treatment

Care is necessary in the evaluation of results of individual reported series as patient selection will have a considerable influence. For example, analysis of large series shows that up to 5% of patients will have metastatic disease at the time of presentation and that about one-third will have locally advanced tumours invading bone, vessel or nerve (T3).

Excisional surgery and postoperative radiotherapy will give survival rates of the order of 50 – 60% at 5 years. Survival will be influenced by stage, being 70 – 75% for patients with T1 tumours, 60 – 65% for those with T2 tumours and only 30 – 35% for T3 lesions. When all gross tumour is removed at the time of surgery or where only microscopic tumour remains, the overall survival rate will be around 65%. If gross tumour is present after surgery, survival will fall to 30%. The grade of tumour is also important. The survival of patients with well-differentiated tumours lies between 55% and 60%, whereas that of patients with poorly-differentiated lesions is only 25 – 30%. If allowances are made for differences in patient selection, these results are similar to those quoted for radical ablative surgery.

As a general rule, and independent of the therapeutic approach, patients under the age of 30 have a poorer survival, as do those in the older age group, the best prognosis being seen in patients between 30 and 40. Site is an important factor in determining prognosis in that lesions in the buttock have a poorer outlook.

There is a close correlation between local recurrence, the development of metastases and survival. It is difficult to assess whether there is a casual relationship between local recurrence and metastatic disease. It may be argued, for example, that local recurrence will act as a focus for subsequent metastases. However, it is likely in most instances, that both local recurrence and metastases are indicators of the degree of agression of a tumour, rather than being casually related to each other. However, purely from the point of view of quality of life, the importance of achieving local tumour control cannot be overstressed.

Bone sarcomas

Primary malignant bone tumours are, like soft tissue sarcomas, rare tumours which account for only just over 1% of all malignancies. Conversely, the skeleton is one of the most frequent sites of metastatic disease. The most common primary malignant tumour of bone is osteosarcoma, followed by chondrosarcoma, Ewing's sarcoma and giant cell tumour (Dahlin, 1957). All the others are extremely rare. Ewing's sarcoma is discussed in detail in Chapter 10.

Osteosarcoma

The classical definition of this tumour is that of a primary malignant tumour of bone whose cells produce osteoid, even if in only small foci (Dahlin and Coventry, 1967). Sometimes the tumour will be found to have predominantly chondroblastic or fibroblastic elements and the majority are poorly differentiated.

Age and sex incidence

Osteosarcoma occurs slightly more frequently in

males, the male:female ratio being 3:2, and its greatest incidence is in the 10 – 25 age group. Thereafter, the incidence falls to lower levels, which persist until later life when there is a further rise due to tumours arising in association with Paget's disease in patients over the age of 60.

Site

While any bone may be involved by osteosarcoma, the vast majority (80%) arise around the knee (Lichtenstein, 1977). About 90% will arise in long bones, the most common site being the lower end of the femur, followed by the upper ends of the tibia and the humerus. However, occasionally a sarcoma will arise in a vertebra, the iliac bone or jaw. In a long bone, the metaphysis is usually affected, but infrequently the tumour may arise more in the mid-shaft region. On rare occasions, the tumour may be multicentric. A further variant is the parosteal sarcoma arising in the periosteal tissues of the bone. These tumours have a much better prognosis.

Aetiology

This is unknown in the majority of patients, but because of the age and site at which these tumours principally arise, it has been postulated that disturbances of growth and maturation are causative factors.

Trauma has been implicated, but probably simply draws attention to the presence of the tumour. Rarely, osteosarcoma arises in association with pre-existing bone abnormalities such as osteitis deformans and osteochondroma, and occasionally may follow irradiation. In the older age group there is a clear association with Paget's disease of bone.

Clinical picture

Pain and swelling of the affected part are the most common presenting features and may be associated with reduced mobility of the adjacent joint. Pathological fracture may occur, as may systemic symptoms such as fever or those due to anaemia.

Investigations

Radiological investigations are those which are most important. Bone destruction in association with bone formation may be seen. Frequently there is cortical bone destruction and soft tissue extension. Sometimes so-called sun-ray spicules may be seen in the subperiosteal tumour cuff, and there may be lifting of the periosteum at the growing edge of the tumour, forming a Codman's triangle. The detailed extent of the tumour within the bone is best determined using tomography or CT.

Careful assessment of metastatic disease is mandatory and involves chest X-ray, bone scan and CT of the chest. If this latter investigation is not available, whole lung tomography should be performed. There is now considerable evidence, as seen in soft tissue sarcomas, to show that CT scanning is a more sensitive investigation than whole lung tomography which, in turn, is significantly more sensitive than conventional chest radiography (Husband and Golding, 1982).

Spread

Spread occurs into the medulla of the bone and there is also local destruction of cancellous and cortical bone. The principal problem with this tumour, however, is the early spread to lungs, although metastases do occur to other bones and, less commonly, lymph nodes.

Developments in management

Cade Technique

There have been many changes in the management of patients with osteosarcomna during the past 30 years. However, it is not yet clear which is the optimum approach and there are still many unanswered questions.

The traditional management in the UK, until relatively recently, was that of the 'Cade' approach (Cade, 1955). Basically, this consisted of giving patients radical radiotherapy to the primary tumour and then observing them at frequent intervals thereafter, searching during this period for the development of pulmonary metastases. Should the patient remain metastasis-free after an interval of 6 – 9 months, amputation was carried out, the basic philosophy being that the vast majority would inevitably develop pulmonary metastases, usually within 9 months of diagnosis, and that it was, therefore, inhumane to carry out what would be an unnecessary amputation in most patients.

A subsequent review of British patients referred to major oncological centres in the UK seemed to confirm that delayed amputation preceded by radical radiotherapy was at least as effective as immediate amputation. (Sweetnam, Knowelden and Seddon, 1971). This analysis showed that in 192 patients evaluated, the 5-year survival was 28% in the combined management group, compared with 23% in those undergoing immediate amputation. However, this review also indicated that subsequent amputation might be required, even in the presence of metastases, for painful local tumour recurrence and pathological fracture. The problem of the uncontrolled primary tumour following radiotherapy was emphasized by Jenkin, Allt and Fitzpatrick (1972). A further difficulty of this approach was the problem of persuading patients who were making apparently good progress, to have an amputation.

Chemotherapy

Not surprisingly, in the early 1970's when enthusiastic reports of the value of chemotherapy began to appear, the 'Cade' technique was abandoned. One of the first reports indicating the effectiveness of chemotherapy was by Jaffe (1972) which described worthwhile responses of metastatic disease in a group of 10 patients given high dose methotrexate. Subsequently, the same drug regimen was used in an adjuvant fashion in a further group of 23 patients (Jaffe *et al.*, 1974). High doses of methotrexate were advocated, as it was implied that low doses were ineffective. Primary amputation was performed in all patients as it was alleged that any tumour poorly controlled by radiotherapy might act as a focus for the development of drug-resistant cells. An argument which is difficult to substantiate. Encouraging preliminary results were reported, 19 of the 23 patients being alive and free from disease. However, assessment was made at only very short periods of time following treatment. In addition, four of the successfully treated patients in this study had parosteal sarcomas and a further three osteochondrosarcomas, both of which carry a better prognosis.

Further reports began to appear about the same time, demonstrating the effectiveness of other drugs such as hydroxydaunorubicin (Cortes *et al.*, 1974) and that combinations of drugs such as the Conpadri-l regimen, consisting of cyclophosphamide, vincristine, melphalan and hydroxydaunorubicin, might have increased effectiveness (Sutow, Sullivan and Fernbach, 1975). However, in all these studies, comparisons were made with historical controls, which makes their evaluation difficult. The same was true for a prospective randomized, multicentre investigation, started in 1975 and organized by the Medical Research Council in the UK. In this trial, lower doses of methotrexate were employed. However, as yet, there have not been any published results.

Evaluation of results

The validity of using historical controls in order to assess the effectiveness of modern chemotherapy regimens is questionable. This has been highlighted by reports from the Mayo Clinic in America and also from Sweden which have suggested that for a variety of reasons, survival rates in patients managed by primary surgery alone have improved over the years without the use of adjuvant chemotherapy, and are now of the order of 50% at 3 years (Taylor *et al.*, 1978; Brostrom *et al.*, 1980). Several reasons may be considered to account for this improvement. One explanation might be that the natural history of the disease is changing, although there is little evidence of this. Alternatively, variations in patient selection could influence the results reported by specialist centres. Further, the introduction of sophisticated screening techniques for metastases would now exclude some patients who would have been included in historical studies. In addition, more aggressive salvage treatment for metastases, including multiple thoracotomies, is now being widely adopted. Certainly, there can be no doubt that, largely due to increased public awareness, patients are now referred at an earlier stage and, on the whole, do have tumours which are less locally advanced and which, as a result, may be associated with a lower frequency of metastases (Brostrom *et al.*, 1980).

The problems of assessing the claims of published results are emphasized by the fact that more recent updated reports of earlier chemotherapy studies now indicate that the long-term survival rates following the use of adjuvant chemotherapy have fallen to around 50%, and therefore are not significantly different from those quoted from surgical series (Cortes, Holland and Glidewell, 1978; Ettinger *et al.*, 1981). This stresses the importance of not relying on historical controls in any comparison. Sadly, there is only one report in the literature of a prospective, randomized, controlled trial comparing patients receiving adjuvant chemotherapy with a similar group managed by surgery alone (Edmonson *et al.*, 1980). This study, which was also carried out at the Mayo Clinic, has failed to demonstrate any survival advantage from the use of adjuvant chemotherapy. However, only 37 patients have so far been included in the trial and their follow-up period has been short.

Limb sparing techniques

Limb preservation techniques were pioneered at the Memorial Hospital in New York in conjunction with the development of their chemotherapy schedules (Rosen *et al.*, 1976). Patients were initially treated with aggressive chemotherapy consisting of high dose methotrexate, hydroxydaunorubicin and cyclophosphamide. During this period, a specific endoprosthesis was fashioned ready to be inserted at the completion of initial chemotherapy. Resection of only the tumour-bearing area of bone was performed, together with an adequate margin.

The first reports describing this technique were enthusiastic, indicating that survival rates in excess of 80% were possible. However, later analysis has shown that long-term survival has fallen to around 50% (Rosen *et al.*, 1979). Disappointment with these survival figures has led to a series of modifications of the chemotherapy regimen, first by the addition of bleomycin and actinomycin D, and then more recently by introducing changes in the regimen used postoperatively according to the response seen in the resected specimen following initial chemotherapy (Rosen *et al.*, 1982). Once more, survival rates of around 90% are being quoted at short follow-up periods after the initial treatment of small numbers of patients. Although other centres are using a similar approach, no-one has yet been able to match these results (Lange and Levine, 1982), which is a matter of concern. Whatever the validity of the survival figures quoted from the Memorial Hospital, their approach has stimulated world-wide interest in the possibilities of limb conservation. In the UK, for example, the surgical aspects of this approach are now being investigated intensively. It is important to remember, however, that not every patient will be suitable for limb conservation. Local excision and reconstruction are only possible when the tumour is of small size, confined to bone or with only a small extra-osseous soft tissue extension. Involvement of nerves or blood vessels usually precludes preservation of the limb. It is not yet clear whether survival rates following conservative surgery are as good as those following amputation, although there are undoubted psychological advantages to limb conservation. Further unanswered questions concern the efficacy of any adjuvant chemotherapy which might be used and the length of time for which it should be given.

Several studies, throughout the world, have now been established in order to evaluate the efficacy of the regimen proposed by Rosen *et al.* (1982). In Europe, a large multicentre investigation has started, the purpose of which is to assess the efficacy or need for high dose methotrexate in patients with non-metastatic osteosarcoma, together with an evaluation of the effectiveness of chemotherapy given over much shorter periods of time than traditionally employed (European Osteosarcoma Intergroup, 1983). It will be some time before the results of these investigations are available, meanwhile the controversy persists. In these circumstances, all patients with osteosarcoma should be managed only in specialist centres.

Pulmonary metastases

Recognition of the fact that the lungs are the principal sites of metastases in osteosarcoma has led to attempts to prevent their development and also the evaluation of methods of management of established disease. The use of prophylactic treatment, other than chemotherapy, has added to the controversy surrounding the management of patients with osteosarcoma.

Whole lung irradiation

Although osteosarcoma has generally been regarded as a tumour which is relatively radioresistant, regression of disease has been observed following treatment of the primary tumour (Cade, 1955). Following from this, it was argued that if the tumour to be irradiated was of only small bulk, improved responses might be observed. In the absence of any data suggesting the efficacy of chemotherapy, evaluation of the use of prophylactic whole lung irradiation was carried out in the late 1960s and early 1970s (Newton, 1972). These initial reports were encouraging. In 1970 the European Organization for Research on the Treatment of Cancer (EORTC) Radiotherapy Cooperative Group initiated a prospective, randomized trial designed to evaluate the place of prophylactic lung irradiation in patients deemed to be metastasis free. Publication of the results was delayed in order to allow an adequate follow-up period to have elapsed in the majority of patients. Unfortunately, the enthusiastic reporting of the use of adjuvant chemotherapy led to the EORTC trial being abandoned in 1975 with the inclusion of only 86 patients. In spite of this, an improvement in survival was seen in those receiving prophylactic radiotherapy, although this only achieved statistical significance in patients below the age of 17 (Breur *et al.*, 1978). A worrying feature, however, was that this benefit was not seen in every participating centre. In view of this, it was decided to launch a new trial comparing the use of adjuvant lung irradiation to adjuvant chemotherapy. This trial closed in 1983, but results are not yet available. However, other recently reported studies have been less optimistic about the value of this form of treatment (Newton and Barrett, 1978).

Undoubtedly, however, whole lung irradiation is of benefit in patients with established disease, and responses similar to those described in patients with soft tissue sarcomas may be observed. The technique and dosage employed are identical. Greater care may need to be exercised in patients with osteosarcoma because of the increased risk of radiation pneumonitis in patients who may have received chemotherapy, especially if bleomycin had been incorporated. This would necessitate a reduction in dosage from 2500 to 1750 cGy in 20 fractions over 4 weeks.

Resection of lung metastases

The surgical resection of solitary metastases has been established practice for many years. More recently, however, reports have appeared indicating that multiple thoracotomies may lead to long-term survival in selected patients (Martini *et al.*, 1971). While this is a technical possibility, the advisability of this approach must seriously be questioned.

Following the widespread introduction of chemotherapy in osteosarcoma, results of a combined approach utilizing drug treatment followed by resection, have been presented (Beattie, Martini and Rosen, 1975). However, it is generally acknowledged that most patients developing pulmonary metastases will eventually die from recurrent pulmonary disease or other distant metastases. As with reports of the use of adjuvant systemic chemotherapy, the numbers of patients treated in this way are small and therefore careful patient selection is required before embarking on surgical removal of pulmonary metastases.

Radiotherapy in osteosarcoma

As a result of the many developments which have occurred in the management of osteosarcoma, the place of radiotherapy remains unclear except in certain well-defined situations. There can be no doubt that irradiation of the primary tumour is of value in the presence of metastatic disease (Tefft, Chabora and Rosen, 1977). This may be combined with systemic chemotherapy. For limb bones, parallel opposed fields are required and a central dose of the order of 3500 cGy in 10 fractions in 2 weeks will give good palliation. This dose does not compromise the use of chemotherapy.

In certain anatomical sites, surgery for the primary tumour may not be a feasible proposition. For example, when tumours arise in vertebrae, the sacrum, or in the ilium. In these circumstances, a radical dose of radiotherapy should be given. For vertebral lesions it is necessary to include the vertebrae above and below the level affected. Except below the level of L2, spinal cord tolerance will limit the dose which may be given. It is necessary to employ a wedged pair or three field technique to achieve a good dose distribution (*Figure 6.10*) and doses equivalent to 4750 cGy in 25 fractions over 5 weeks are required. While this may produce control of the tumour for a period of time, even for as long as 4 or 5 years, regrowth usually occurs. Care must be taken when considering the use of adjuvant chemotherapy as this may increase the risk of radiation damage to the spinal cord.

Similar doses are necessary for the treatment of iliac lesions. Often the tolerance of bowel and the size of the fields required for therapy limit the maximum doses which may be employed. The technique of treatment used will vary. In some cases only parallel opposed field arrangements are possible. On occasions, the distribution of dose will be improved by adding a lateral field to such an arrangement as with the irradiation of pelvic soft tissue sarcomas.

Other bone tumours

Chondrosarcoma

These are tumours of cartilagenous histogenesis arising principally between the ages of 30 and 60. Their treatment is surgical, although this may not be possible for certain centrally placed tumours or may be inadvisable in the presence of metastases. It has been suggested that razoxane may improve the response to radiotherapy (Rhomberg, 1978), but the

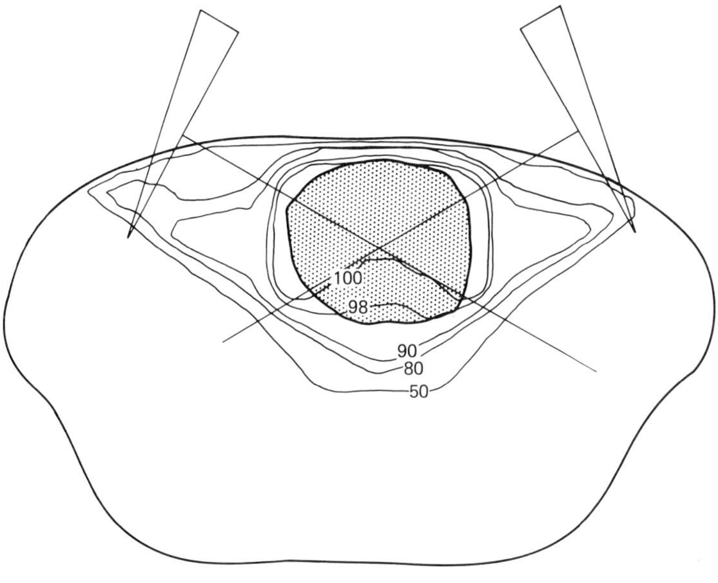

Figure 6.10 Wedged pair treatment for a vertebral sarcoma

evidence for this is scanty. Occasional good responses have been reported (Ryall *et al.*, 1979).

For palliation, a useful approach is that of the 'growth restraint' technique as used for soft tissue sarcomas. Careful patient assessment is necessary before offering any form of radiotherapy for these tumours as the majority will show little, if any, response. There are, however, cases where the site of the tumour, the general condition of the patient, or the refusal of radical surgery leave radiotherapy as the only possible form of treatment. This is most commonly the situation with pelvic tumours. In these circumstances, the treatment volumes must be kept as small as possible, the tumour being irradiated without taking a very wide margin. Parallel opposed fields may be used, but bowel tolerance is often a problem with this technique. A three field arrangement using anterior and posterior fields combined with a lateral field, such as described in the treatment of soft tissue sarcomas of the pelvis (*see Figure 6.6*) gives a preferable dose distribution and is usually better tolerated. Even though the aim of treatment is palliation, doses of the order of 5000 cGy in 20 fractions over 4 weeks are necessary to produce worthwhile growth restraint.

Giant cell tumours

Giant cell tumours are usually benign. A few are undoubtedly malignant *de novo*, and a number undergo malignant transformation. For the majority, surgical excision or curettage followed by packing with bone chips is the treatment of choice. Occasionally, for centrally placed tumours such as those arising in vertebrae, or those in such a situation that amputation might be required, radiotherapy may be used as an alternative. When vertebral tumours are to be irradiated a technique such as that described for the irradiation of osteosarcoma of the spine is necessary (*Figure 6.10*). However, for giant cell tumours such a wide margin is not usually necessary and only one-third to one-half of the vertebrae above and below the affected bone need be included within the treatment volume.

For peripheral lesions where radiotherapy is being given in an attempt to avoid amputation, a parallel opposed pair technique is generally satisfactory.

Doses in the range of 3500 cGy in 15 fractions over 3 weeks are usually adequate to control the majority of these tumours. However, there is some controversy over the influence of radiotherapy in causing malignant transformation.

For malignant lesions, wide surgical excision is advocated. Where surgery is inappropriate, radiotherapy may be employed. In these circumstances, higher doses of the order of 5000 cGy in 20–25 fractions in 4 – 5 weeks are necessary, depending on the site to be irradiated. There is little evidence suggesting that chemotherapy is effective.

Lymphoma of bone

Lymphomatous infiltration of bone may take place as a manifestation of generalized lymphoma (*see* Chapter 8). Rarely primary lymphoma of bone may occur. Careful investigation of the patient must be performed to exclude lymphoma in other sites.

For localized lymphoma, radiotherapy is effective in controlling the primary tumour in the majority of patients. The whole bone must be irradiated and doses of the order of 4500 cGy in 20 fractions in 4 weeks are required.

Conclusions

The place of radiotherapy in the management of patients with bone tumours has changed dramatically in recent years. It is of central importance in the management of Ewing's sarcoma (*see* Chapter 10). In other tumours it is now largely used for the treatment of inoperable lesions and metastases. Its prophylactic use in an attempt to prevent the development of pulmonary metastases in osteosarcoma remains controversial.

References

ATKINSON, L., GARVAN, J.M. and NEWTON, N.C.(1963) Behaviour and management of soft tissue sarcomas. *Cancer*, **16**, 1552–1562

BEATTIE, E.J., MARTINI, N. and ROSEN, G. (1975) The management of pulmonary metastases in children with osteogenic sarcoma with surgical resection combined with chemotherapy. *Cancer*, **35**, 618–621

BENJAMIN, R.S., WIERNICK, P.H. and BACHUR, N.R. (1974) Adriamycin chemotherapy—efficacy, safety and pharmacological basis of an intermittent single high-dosage schedule. *Cancer*, **33**, 19–27

BROSTROM, L.A., APARISI, T., INGEMARSSON, S. *et al.* (1980) Can historical controls be used in current clinical trials in osteosarcoma? Analysis of prognostic factors. *International Journal of Radiation Oncology, Biology and Physics*, **6**, 1711–1715

BREUR, K., COHEN, O., SCHWEISGUTH, O. and HART, A.M.M. (1977) Irradiation of the lungs as an adjuvant therapy in the treatment of osteosarcoma of the limbs: an EORTC randomized study. *European Journal of Cancer*, **14**, 461–471

CADE, S. (1951) Soft tissue tumours: their natural history and treatment. *Proceedings of the Royal Society of Medicine*, **44**, 19–36

CADE, S. (1955) Osteogenic sarcoma; a study based on 133 patients. *Journal of the Royal College of Surgeons of Edinburgh*, **1**, 79–111

CATTERALL, M. and BEWLEY, D.K. (1979) *Fast neutrons in the treatment of cancer*. London: Academic Press

COE, M.A., MADDEN, F.J. and MOULD, R.F. (1981) The role of radiotherapy in the treatment of soft tissue sarcoma: a retrospective study, 1958–1973. *Clinical Radiology*, **32**, 47–51

CORTES, E.P., HOLLAND, J.F. and GLIDEWELL, O. (1978) Amputation and adriamycin in primary osteosarcoma: a five-year report. *Cancer Treatment Reports*, **62**, 271–298

CORTES, E.P., HOLLAND, J.F., WANG, J.J. *et al.* (1974) Amputation and adriamycin in primary osteosarcoma. *New England Journal of Medicine*, **291**, 998–1000

DAHLIN, D.C. (1957) Bone Tumours. Springfield, Illinois: Thomas

DAHLIN, D.C. and COVENTRY, M.B. (1967) Osteogenic sarcoma. A study of six hundred cases. *Journal of Bone and Joint Surgery*, **49**, 101–110

DE SANTOS, L.A., GOLDSTEIN, H.M., MURRAY, J.A. and WALLACE, S. (1978) Computed tomography in the evaluation of musculoskeletal neoplasms. *Radiology*, **128**, 89–94

EDMONSON, J.H., GREEN, S.J., IVINS, J.C. *et al.* (1980) Methotrexate as adjuvant treatment for primary osteosarcoma. *New England Journal of Medicine*, **303**, 642–643

ENTERLINE, H.T. (1981) Histopathology of sarcomas. *Seminars in Oncology*, **8**, 133–155

ENZINGER, F.M., LATTES, R. and TORLONI, H. (1969) *Histological typing of soft tissue tumours*. Geneva: World Health Organisation

ETTINGER, L.J., DOUGLASS, H.O., HIGBY, D.J. *et al.* (1981) Adjuvant adriamycin and cis-diammine dichloroplatinum (Cis-platinum) in primary osteosarcoma. **Cancer**, **47**, 248–254

EUROPEAN OSTEOSARCOMA INTERGROUP PROTOCOL 80831 (1983) Randomized pilot study to asses the tolerability and efficacy of two drug combinations in patients with osteosarcoma. Brussels

FORTNER, J.G., MARTIN, S., HAJDU, S.I. and TURNBULL, A. (1981) Primary sarcoma of the retroperitoneum. *Seminars in Oncology*, **8**, 180–184

GILBERT, H.A., KAGAN, A.R. and WINKLEY, J. (1974) Management of soft tissue sarcomas of the extremities. *Surgery, Gynaecology and Obstetrics*, **139**, 914–918

GOLDING, S.J. and HUSBAND, J.E. (1982) The role of computed tomography in the management of soft tissue sarcomas. *British Journal of Radiology*, **55**, 740–747

GOTTLIEB, J.A., BAKER, L.H., O'BRYAN, R.M. *et al.* (1975) Adriamycin used alone and in combination for soft tissue and bone sarcomas. *Cancer Chemotherapy Reports*, **6**, 271–282

HARRIS, J.E. and SINKOVICS, J.G. (1976) Immunology and immunotherapy of human tumors. In *The Immunology of Malignant Disease*, pp. 411–429. St. Louis, Missouri: C.V. Mosby

HATFIELD, P.M. and SCHULZ, M.D. (1970) Post-irradiation sarcoma: including five cases after X-ray therapy for breast carcinoma. *Radiology*, **96**, 593–602

HUSBAND, J.E. and GOLDING, S.J. (1982) Computed tomography of the body: when should it be used? *British Medical Journal*, **284**, 4–8

JAFFE, N. (1972) Recent advances in the chemotherapy of metastatic osteosarcoma. *Cancer*, **30**, 1627–1638

JAFFE, N., FREI, E., TRAGGIS, D. *et al.* (1974) Adjuvant methotrexate and citrovorum factor treatment of osteogenic sarcoma. *New England Journal of Medicine*, **291**, 994–997

JENKIN, R.D.T., ALLT, W.E.C. and FITZPATRICK, P.J. (1972) Osteosarcoma: an assessment of management with particular reference to primary irradiation and selective delayed amputation. *Cancer*, **30**, 393–400

JENSEN, R.D. and MILLER, R.W. (1971) Retinoblastoma: epidemiologic characteristics. *New England Journal of Medicine*, **285**, 307

KARNOFSKY, D.A., ABELMAN, W.H., CRAVER, L.F. and BURCHENALL. J.H. (1948) The use of the nitrogen mustards in the palliative treatment of cancer: with particular reference to bronchogenic cancer. *Cancer*, **1**, 634–656

KINNE, D.W., CHU, F.C.H., HUVOS, A.G. *et al.* (1973) Treatment of primary and recurrent retroperitoneal liposarcoma. Twenty-five year experience at Memorial Hospital. *Cancer*, **31**, 53–64

LANGE, B. and LEVINE, A.S. (1982) Is it ethical not to conduct a prospectively controlled trial of adjuvant chemotherapy in osteosarcoma? *Cancer Treatment Reports*, **66**, 1699–1704

LEVINE, E., LEE, K.R., NEFF, J.R. *et al.* (1979) Comparison of computed tomography and other imaging modalities in the evaluation of musculoskeletal tumours. *Radiology*, **131**, 431–437

LICHTENSTEIN, L. (1977) *Bone Tumours*. St. Louis, Missouri: C.V. Mosby Co

LINDBERG, R.D., MURPHY, W.K., BENJAMIN, R.S. *et al.* (1977) Adjuvant chemotherapy in the treatment of soft tissue sarcomas. A preliminary report. In *Management of Primary Bone and Soft Tissue Tumours*, compiled by L.W. Dybala, S.B. Freitag and D.C. Culhane pp. 343–352. Chicago: Year Book Medical Publishers Inc

LINDELL, M.M., WALLACE, S., DE SANTOS, L.A. and BERNADINO, M.E. (1981) Diagnostic technique for the evaluation of the soft tissue sarcoma. *Seminars in Oncology*, **8**, 160–171

McADAM, W.A.F. and GOLIGHER, J.C. (1970) The occurrence of desmoids in patients with familial polyposis coli. *British Journal of Surgery*, **57**, 618–631

MARKHEDE, G., ANGERVALL, L. and STENER, B. (1982) A multivariate analysis of the prognosis after surgical treatment of malignant soft tissue tumours. *Cancer*, **49**, 1721–1733

MARTINI, N., HUVOS, A.G., MIKE, V. *et al.* (1971) Multiple pulmonary resections in the treatment of osteogenic sarcoma. *Annals of Thoracic Surgery*, **12**, 271–280

MARTINI, R.G., LINDBERG, R.D. and RUSSELL, W.O. (1977) Preoperative radiotherapy and surgery in the management of soft tissue sarcoma. In *Management of Primary Bone and Soft Tissue Tumours*, compiled by L.W. Dybala, S.B. Freitag and D.C. Culhane pp. 299–307. Chicago: Year Book Medical Publishers Inc

MINSON, A.C. (1984) Cell transformation and oncogenesis by herpes simplex virus and human cytomegalovirus. In *Cancer Surveys 3*, edited by J. Wyke and R. Weiss, pp. 91–112

MORTON, D.L. (1974) Soft tissue sarcomas. In *Cancer Medicine*, edited by J. Holland and E. Frei, pp. 1854–1861. Philadelphia: Lea and Febiger

MORTON, D.L., MALMGREN, R.A., HALL, W.T. *et al.* (1969) Immunologic and virus studies with human sarcomas. *Surgery*, **66**, 152-161

NEWTON, K.A. (1972) Prophylactic irradiation of the lung in bone sarcoma. In *Bone — Certain Aspects of Neoplasia*, edited by C.H.G. Price and F.G.M. Ross. London: Butterworths

NEWTON, K.A. and BARRETT, A. (1978) Prophylactic lung irradiation in the treatment of osteogenic sarcoma. *Clinical Radiology*, **29**, 493–496

OZELLO, L., STOUT, A.P. and MURRAY, M.R. (1963) Cultural characteristics of malignant histiocytomas and fibrous xanthomas. *Cancer*, **16**, 331–344

RHOMBERG, W.U. (1978) Radiotherapy combined with ICRF 159 (NSC 129943). *International Journal of Radiation Oncology, Biology and Physics*, **4**, 121–126

ROSEN, G., CAPARROS, B., HUVOS, A.C. *et al.* (1982) Preoperative chemotherapy for osteogenic sarcoma: a selection of post-operative adjuvant chemotherapy based upon the response of the primary tumour to preoperative chemotherapy. *Cancer*, **49**, 1221–1230

ROSEN, G., MARCOVE, R.C., CAPARROS, B. *et al.* (1979) Primary osteogenic sarcoma. The rationale for preoperative chemotherapy and delayed surgery. *Cancer*, **43**, 2163–2177

ROSEN, G., MURPHY, M.L., HUVOS, A.G. *et al.* (1976) Chemotherapy, en bloc resection and prosthetic bone replacement in the treatment of osteogenic sarcoma. *Cancer*, **37**, 1–11

ROSENBERG, S.A. and GLATSTEIN, E.J. (1981) Perspectives on the role of surgery and radiation therapy in the treatment of soft tissue sarcomas of the extremities. *Seminars in Oncology*, **8**, 190–200

ROSENBERG, S.A., TEPPER, J., GLATSTEIN, E. *et al.* (1983) Prospective randomized evaluation of adjuvant chemotherapy in adults with soft tissue sarcomas of the extremities. *Cancer*, **52**, 424–434

RUBIN, P. and CASARETT, G.W. (1968) *Clinical Radiation Pathology*. Philadelphia: W.B. Saunders Co

RUSSELL, W.O., COHEN, J., ENZINGER, F. *et al.* (1977) A clinical and pathological staging system for soft tissue sarcomas. *Cancer*, **40**, 1562–1570

RYALL, R.D.H., BATES, T., NEWTON, K.A. and HELLMAN, K. (1979) Combination of radiotherapy and razoxane (ICRF 159) for chondrosarcoma. *Cancer*, **44**, 891–895

SCHMITT, G. (1985) Fast neutron therapy of soft tissue sarcomas. In *EORTC Monograph on Management of Bone and Soft Tissue Sarcomas*, The Hague

SCHMITT, G., SCHNABEL, K., SAUERWEIN, W. and SCHERER, E. (1983) Neutron and neutron-boost irradiation of soft tissue sarcomas: a four and a half year analysis of 139 patients. *Radiotherapy and Oncology*, **1**, 23–29

SHIU, M.H., CASTRO, E.B., HAJDU, S.I. *et al.* (1975) Surgical treatment of 297 soft tissue sarcomas of the lower extremity. *Annals of Surgery*, **182**, 597–602

SHIU, M.H. and HAJDU, S.I. (1981) Management of soft tissue sarcoma of the extremity. *Seminars in Oncology*, **8**, 172–179

SIMON, M.A. and ENNEKING, W.F. (1976) The management of soft tissue sarcomas of the extremities. *Journal of Bone and Joint Surgery*, **58A**, 317–327

SNOW, J.H. JR., GOLDSTEIN. H.M. and WALLACE, S. (1979) Comparison of scintigraphy, sonography and computed tomography in the evaluation of hepatic neoplasms. *American Journal of Roentgenology, Radium Therapy and Nuclear Medicine*, **132**, 915–918

STORM, F.K., EILBER, F.R., MIRRA, J. *et al.* (1980) Neurofibrosarcoma. *Cancer*, **45**, 126–129

SUIT, H.D., PROPPE, K.H. and BRAMWELL, V.H.C. (1982) In *Treatment of Cancer*, edited by K.E. Halman, pp. 607–622. London: Chapman and Hall

SUIT, H.D. and RUSSELL, W.O. (1977) Soft part tumours. *Cancer*, **39**, 830–836

SUTOW, W.W., SULLIVAN, M.P. and FERNBACH, D.J. (1975) Adjuvant chemotherapy in primary treatment of osteogenic sarcoma: a south-west oncology group study. *Cancer*, **36**, 1598–1602

SWEETNAM, R., KNOWELDEN, J. and SEDDON, H. (1971) Bone sarcoma: treatment by irradiation, amputation and combination of the two. *British Medical Journal*, **2**, 363–366

TAYLOR, W.F., IVINS, J.C., DAHLIN, D.C. *et al.* (1978) Trends and variability in survival from osteosarcoma. *Mayo Clinic Proceedings*, **53**, 695–700

TEFFT, M., CHABORA, B.McC. and ROSEN, G. (1977) Radiation in bone sarcomas: a re-evaluation in the era of intensive systemic chemotherapy. *Cancer*, **39**, 806–816

WERF-MESSING, B. VAN DER and UNNIK, J.A.M. VAN (1965) Fibrosarcoma of the soft tissues — a clinicopathological study. *Cancer*, **18**, 1113–1123

WINDEYER, B., DISCHE, S. and MANSFIELD, C.M. (1966) The place of radiotherapy in the management of fibrosarcoma of the soft tissues. *British Journal of Cancer*, **24**, 696–704

7

Intrathoracic tumours

B. S. Mantell

Bronchial carcinoma

Bronchial carcinoma remains one of the major causes of death in the Western world. Its incidence is still rising in women, although no longer in men. It is also steadily gaining a hold in the Third World as the tobacco habit spreads. Most patients present with advanced disease; the primary tumour is massive with involvement of mediastinal structures, and distant metastasis is already established even if not readily detectable. Perhaps one patient in five is suitable for an attempt at curative treatment by surgery or radiotherapy, but the rest can be offered only palliation of their symptoms, and a life expectancy of perhaps a few months. Nevertheless, much can be done by the radiotherapist to help these people, and in many cases to enable them to enjoy a reasonable standard of health, even if only for a limited time. For this reason patients with bronchial carcinoma form a very large part of the work load of any radiotherapy department, and a number of simple but effective techniques have been developed to deal with the various manifestations of this disease.

Selection of patients for treatment

Treatment for lung cancer may be radical, aimed at cure, or palliative, intended only for relief of symptoms. In deciding upon treatment it is necessary to make a diagnosis that includes not only proof that lung cancer is present, but also an assessment of the extent of the tumour both locally and systemically, and its histological type. For practical purposes affecting the treatment selected, the following histological classification is suitable.

Squamous cell carcinoma
Adenocarcinoma
Large-cell anaplastic carcinoma
Small-cell anaplastic (oat-cell) carcinoma
Alveolar-cell carcinoma

Some patients present with evidence of metastasis such as enlarged supraclavicular nodes, bone pain, or neurological disorder. Proof of the diagnosis will often be obtainable by cytological examination of sputum, or by a small biopsy taken from a skin nodule or a lymph node. It may be felt necessary to carry out a bronchoscopy; but if a patient with *metastatic* disease has a chest X-ray appearance typical of lung cancer but no histological or cytological proof is obtainable, one may well feel justified in avoiding this more invasive procedure.

In the absence of clinically recognizable metastases, bronchoscopy is mandatory except for the more peripheral tumours. With the introduction of the fibreoptic bronchoscope this has become a much simpler procedure than with the rigid bronchoscope. It is readily performed, even on outpatients, using local anaesthesia and sedation rather than a general anaesthetic. The vocal cords are examined for paralysis, and the trachea is inspected for compression or tumour invasion. Widening of the carina due to subcarinal lymph nodes is looked for, and the main bronchi and the lobar and segmental orifices are examined in turn. Any suspicious area of mucosa is biopsied, and if necessary cytological material may be sought by collecting a trap specimen of bronchial secretions or washings. Being flexible, the fibreoptic bronchoscope may be used to visualize air passages out of reach of the rigid instrument. Some lesions which are not visible by the bronchoscope may still be biopsied by a transbronchial needle passed down the flexible bronchoscope and thrust through the bronchial wall.

More peripheral lesions may be biopsied by a drill or needle passed through the chest wall under radiological control.

Curative treatment for bronchial carcinoma

Perhaps 20% of all patients diagnosed as having lung cancer are found to be suitable for an attempt at curative treatment, which in most cases is surgical. There must be no evidence of distant metastasis clinically, radiologically, nor on isotope bone scan. Liver metastases must be excluded by biochemical, ultrasound and isotope scan investigation. There must be no phrenic or recurrent laryngeal palsy to indicate locally advanced disease, nor any significant pleural effusion. Computerized axial tomography (CAT) is a recent introduction which is helpful in assessing the size and attachments of a tumour and the presence or otherwise of mediastinal invasion. There must be sufficient healthy mucosa between the tumour and the carina to permit resection with an adequate margin, and the patient's general health and respiratory reserve must be such as to allow lobectomy or pneumonectomy. These are major procedures with operative mortalities of about 3% for lobectomy and 6% for pneumonectomy, the risk being greater with increasing age above 60 years (Ginsberg *et al.*, 1983). About 30% of those who survive surgery live for 5 years. There remains therefore a group of patients with small localized tumours who are rejected for surgery for technical or medical reasons or because of age, or who may refuse surgery. Radical radiotherapy can be considered as an alternative for this group.

Radical radiotherapy for lung cancer

If radiotherapy is to be curative no metastases can be present, and the same investigations as those carried out before radical surgery are required. Then, the tumour must be small enough to be raised to a radical dose, in the region of 1800 to 1900 ret: that is 5500 cGy in 20 daily fractions or the biological equivalent. The tumour, with a margin of perhaps 2 cm of normal tissue all around, must be enclosed in a volume which will tolerate a dose of this size. Such a volume may be up to 500 or at most 1000 ml; a larger volume will result in an unacceptable level of disturbance during treatment and of fibrosis afterwards. The patient's respiratory reserve must be assessed, but with modern equipment and careful and accurate planning it is possible to keep the amount of lung tissue destroyed by fibrosis to a minimum. A patient whose respiratory reserve is too poor to permit pneumonectomy or even lobectomy may still be suitable for an attempt at radical radiotherapy.

Even a tumour as small as an egg is likely to contain a substantial proportion of anoxic cells, the radioresistance of which militates against cure. Assessment of the size and precise location of a growth has improved immensely with the introduction of CAT. The demonstration of enlarged mediastinal nodes, not revealed by chest X-ray or ordinary tomography, can save a patient a useless thoracotomy as well as a futile attempt at radical radiotherapy. Unfortunately, even with the aid of CAT, the thoracic surgeon still finds the case which all criteria had suggested was operable but where thoracotomy reveals extensive mediastinal disease. This patient, if treated by radiotherapy, would undergo meticulous planning and a month's course of high-dose irradiation in the vain hope of cure. Therefore, it is difficult to compare the results of surgery and radiotherapy for lung cancer unless the surgical figures include all patients operated upon, and not just those in whom resection was achieved. Furthermore, the operative mortality associated with surgery is not suffered by those patients treated with radiotherapy.

Most patients treated by radical radiotherapy are likely to have squamous cell carcinomas. The less differentiated growths are usually too advanced at presentation for consideration of any radical treatment, either surgical or radiotherapeutic. Adenocarcinomas have a reputation for radioresistance for which it is hard to find any objective supporting evidence. It is perhaps arguable that a tumour which appears in the chest where early symptoms are often negligible, yet which is found at the time of treatment to be relatively small, is probably one which does not behave in a particularly aggressive manner, and which may be compatible with prolonged survival irrespective of treatment of any kind (Geddes, 1979). It is therefore not surprising that, in some series at least, radical radiotherapy has produced results broadly comparable with those of surgery. As long ago as 1956 Smart and Hilton reported a group of 33 patients among whom of 12 who could have survived 5 years, four did so. In a later report on a total of 40 patients, Smart (1966) had nine (22.5%) 5-year survivors.

A prospective trial of surgery versus radiotherapy in operable lung cancer (Morrison, Deeley and Cleland, 1963) produced results strongly in favour of surgery with 23% of survivors at 4 years compared with only 7% for radiotherapy. However, the radiation dose employed — 4500 cGy in 4 weeks — would not be regarded by the present author as adequate to sterilize a carcinoma with any degree of reliability. Another prospective trial, by the Medical Research Council, was confined to oat-cell carcinoma (Fox and Scadding, 1973). Of the 73 patients drawn for radiotherapy 62 were treated radically, but of the 71 allotted to surgery only 32 actually had a resection. No patient treated surgically lived for 5 years; three of those who had radical radiotherapy survived 5 years and all of these three continued to 10 years. These abysmal results are entirely in keeping with the aggressive nature of oat-cell carcinoma. It is of interest to note in passing, however, that Lennox *et al.* (1968) claimed 29% 2-year survivors in 41 peripherally situated oat-cell carcinomas treated surgically, and Bates *et al.* (1974) carried out pneumonectomies in 24 cases of lung carcinoma who had each received a preoperative dose of 1750 cGy to the mediastinum in seven treatments over 8 days. Eighteen were confirmed as oat-cell carcinomas on the surgical specimens, and five of these survived at least 4 years.

Technique of radical radiotherapy

The first step is to localize the tumour accurately. The chest film, tomograms and bronchoscopy findings are all utilized here. In recent years CAT has added a new dimension to localization and delimiting of tumours, and in the subsequent planning of accurate beam-directed radiotherapy. An increasing number of radiotherapy centres have access to CAT with a radiotherapy planning facility.

For a planning scan the patient lies on a special flat insert to the usually curved-section scanner table, in order to simulate the flat-surfaced radiotherapy treatment couch. Marks placed on the patient's skin are indicated by radiopaque markers thin enough not to produce artefacts on the scan; plastic capillary tubing filled with barium suspension is suitable. The patient lies in the position to be adopted during radiotherapy; most commonly this is supine, with the head resting on a foam block about 5 cm thick. The hands are placed on top of the head so that the arms are kept well clear of the treatment beams which will be used later. Scans to cover the proposed treatment volume are made with the patient breathing normally, as the tissues will move with respiration during treatment. The upper and lower limits of the tumour are identified on the images produced. A representative cut through the centre of the volume is transferred by means of a floppy disc to the combined viewing and planning equipment. This produces upon the same cathode ray screen both the scan and isodose curves of the required beams (*Figure 7.1*). As with all computerized planning systems this takes into account variables such as curvature of the skin surface and differential absorption of radiation in lung and other tissue. A suitable plan to irradiate the tumour while limiting the dose to lung and avoiding the spinal cord may thus be produced (*Figure 7.2*).

Not every department has access to such sophisticated planning equipment, but most have a radiotherapy simulator. This is used with the patient in the treatment position as described above. Anteroposterior and lateral films are taken centred on a mark on the patient's skin placed according to the findings on X-ray and bronchoscopy. The field-wires of the simulator are set to represent fields of, for example, 8 × 8 cm (*Figures 7.3 and 7.4*). High kV diagnostic X-rays are used to produce well penetrated views which will enable the bronchial tree to be seen clearly

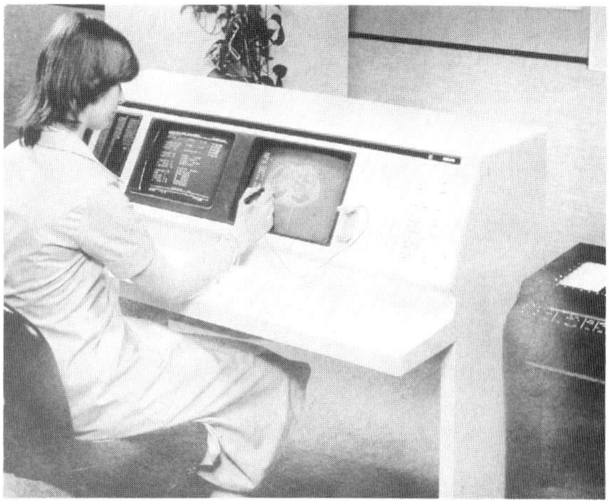

Figure 7.1 Planning radical radiotherapy using a computerized tomography system. (Courtesy of Philips Medical Systems)

in the anteroposterior view. This permits the information derived from bronchoscopy to be used to mark the position of the tumour on the film. It is essential to take the lateral film with the patient's hands on his head, otherwise the arms obscure detail, and later obstruct the therapy beams. It is usually possible to visualize the tumour on the anteroposterior film, and it may also be possible on the lateral. Important landmarks on the lateral film are the trachea, and the posterior line of the vertebral bodies which enables the position of the spinal cord to be marked. A transverse contour section of the patient's body is obtained through the chosen treatment centre, and knowing the magnifications of the films obtained from the simulator, the treatment volume containing the tumour and a margin of about 2 cm all around is marked onto the contour (*Figure 7.5a*). The position of the spinal cord can be similarly marked. The amount and disposition of the lung tissue in the plane of treatment is of very great importance for accuracy and dosimetry, as the radiation dose after transmission through lung is increased by a factor of about 3% per cm compared with soft tissue (Meredith and Massey, 1972). Unfortunately, in the absence of CAT this important factor relies on educated guesswork as to the shape of the lung-sections. A method of improving this position employs a CAT facility which does not provide for direct radiotherapy planning. The simulator localization technique is carried out as described and a CAT scan is obtained through the centre of the treatment volume with the patient in the treatment position. The resulting scan (*Figure 7.6*) is enlarged photographically to the same size as the drawn contour which is then superimposed upon it on a light-box. This serves first to verify the position of the treatment volume and the spinal cord obtained from the

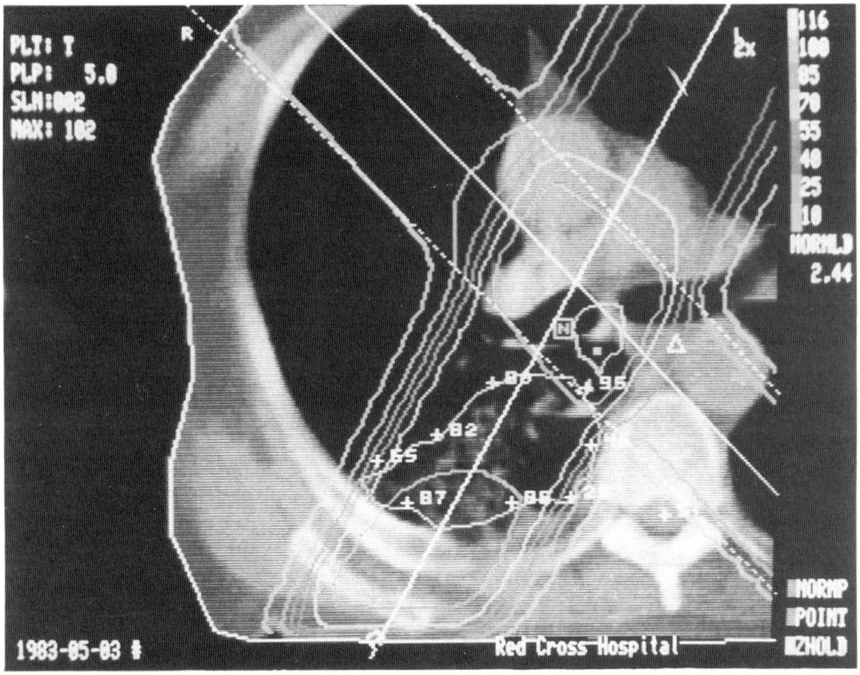

Figure 7.2 A plan produced by the Philips computerized tomography system. A colour-television type screen is used, and different isodose levels are represented by a colour code. (Courtesy of Philips Medical Systems)

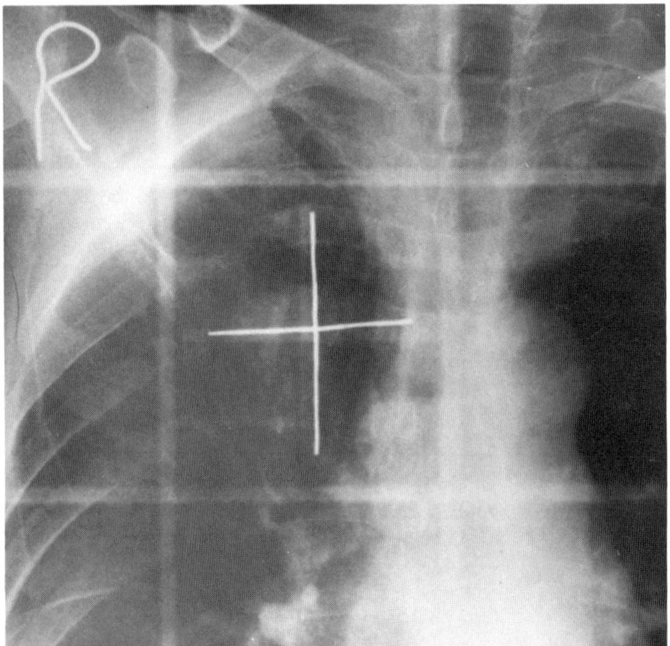

Figure 7.3 Radical radiotherapy for lung cancer: the anteroposterior simulator film

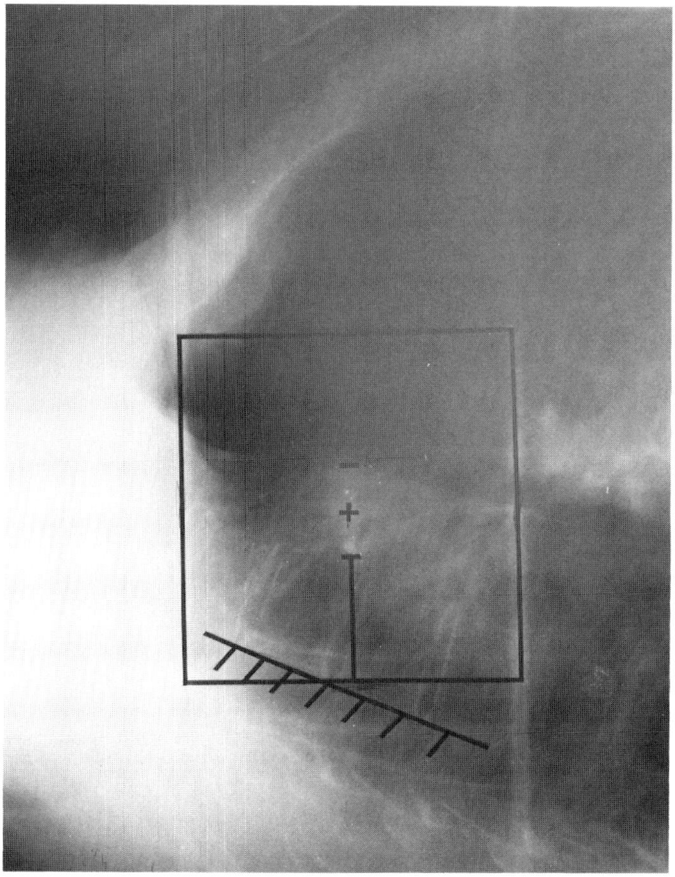

Figure 7.4 The lateral simulator film. The position of the spinal cord and the limits of the treatment volume have been marked

simulator films, and second, by tracing, the lungs the tumour and the mediastinal structures can be drawn onto the contour.

Localization having been completed, planning then proceeds using a planning computer for preference, but alternatively, manually. Three fields are commonly used, arranged to limit the dose to the spinal cord as far as possible; it should not be necessary to give more than 3500 cGy to any part of the spinal cord for a tumour dose of 5500 cGy. The amount of lung tissue irradiated to more than 2500 cGy should also be kept to the minimum. It must be remembered, however, that pulmonary function will only be impaired by the amount of lung damage within the treated section of the thorax, while injury even to a very short section of the spinal cord may have disastrous consequences.

Treatment is best given using a linear accelerator, but an isocentric cobalt unit is an alternative except in the largest patients. It is the present author's practice to treat all fields daily, as to do otherwise may result in later subcutaneous fibrosis.

Care of the patient during radical radiotherapy

The course of 20 treatments, five times a week, may be tedious but is normally well tolerated as an outpatient. Very little specific medical care is required apart from correction of any anaemia and control of intercurrent infection. Nausea is unlikely, and there should be no skin reaction using megavoltage radiation. Dysphagia due to radiation oesophagitis may arise after about 2 weeks of treatment, and usually responds to a local anaesthetic-containing preparation such as Mucaine.

Radiotherapy as an adjuvant to surgery

This has proved of little value in bronchial carcinoma.

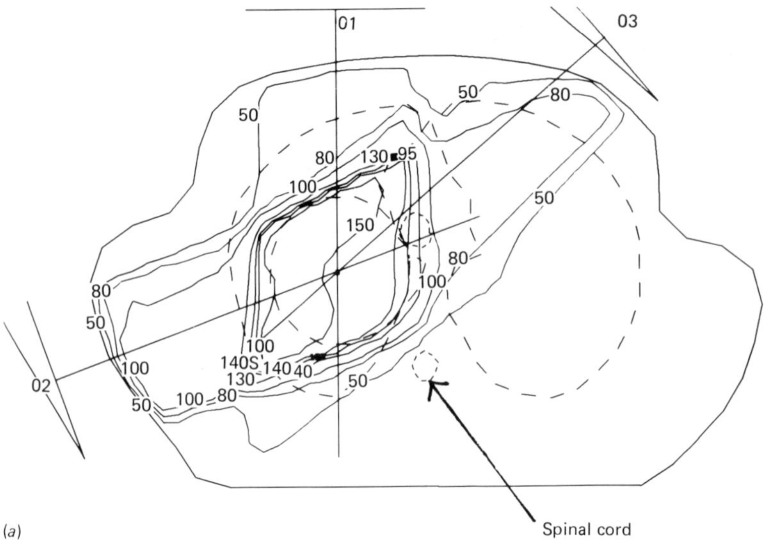

(a)

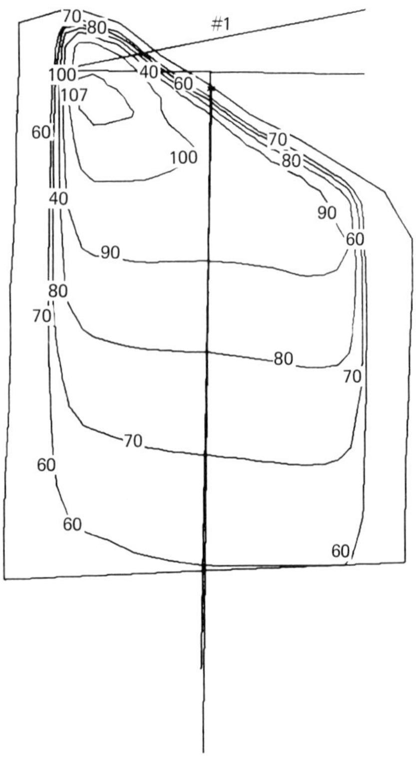

(b)

Figure 7.5 (a) A plan for radical radiotherapy of lung cancer produced by a RAD-8 planning computer. The plan is constructed on a transverse contour of the patient, on which the treatment volume, the lungs and the spinal cord have been marked. (b) Use of a wedge filter in the anterior beam to compensate for the slope of the sternum

The small series of oat-cell carcinomas reported by Bates *et al.* (1974) and discussed above, is one of the few accounts supporting the use of preoperative irradiation. Paulson (1975) gave doses of the order of 3000 cGy in 10 daily treatments, followed 3–6 weeks later by radical surgery, in selected cases of superior sulcus carcinoma. Sixteen out of 46 patients survived for 5 years. A small pilot study by Kazem *et al.* (1984) in which preoperative telecobalt irradiation of 2000 cGy in five daily treatments was given to the mediastinum in cases of operable non-small-cell carcinoma, produced a crude 5-year survival of 58% compared with 43% of cases not irradiated preoperatively. On the other hand, Shields *et al.* (1970), in a randomized prospective trial, had worse survival figures after preoperative radiotherapy. Paterson and Russell (1962) reported a randomized prospective trial of mediastinal irradiation after pneumonectomy but were unable to show any gain. Radiotherapy may sometimes be considered when gross tumour has been left behind at surgery or where histological examination of the resected specimen shows transection of tumour. Radiotherapy in these circumstances carries a substantial risk of bronchopleural fistula, and a delay of perhaps 6 weeks is advised if it is to be used at all. Guttman (1965) found the results of radiotherapy, when used after incomplete resection, were even worse in terms of survival than the 7.4% 5-year survivors she obtained in those cases who were regarded as inoperable at thoracotomy and in whom no resection had been attempted.

Palliative radiotherapy for lung cancer

About 80% of patients attending hospital with lung cancer have disease which is too advanced for any

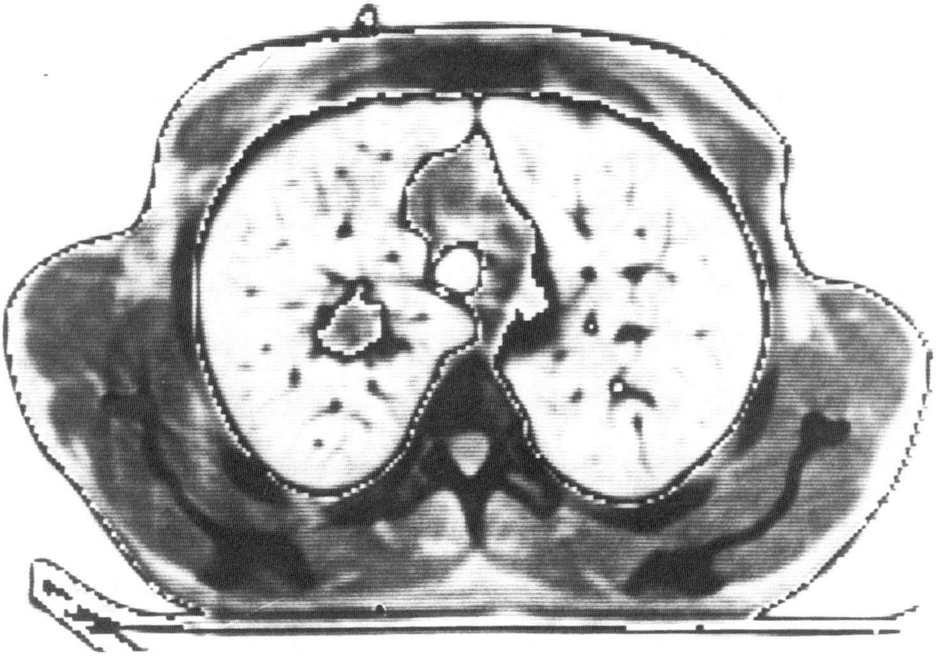

Figure 7.6 Radical radiotherapy for lung cancer: a CT scan through the centre of the treatment volume, enlarged photographically to fit the contour taken around the patient. The skin mark is represented by a capillary tube filled with radiographic barium, and is seen vertically above the tumour

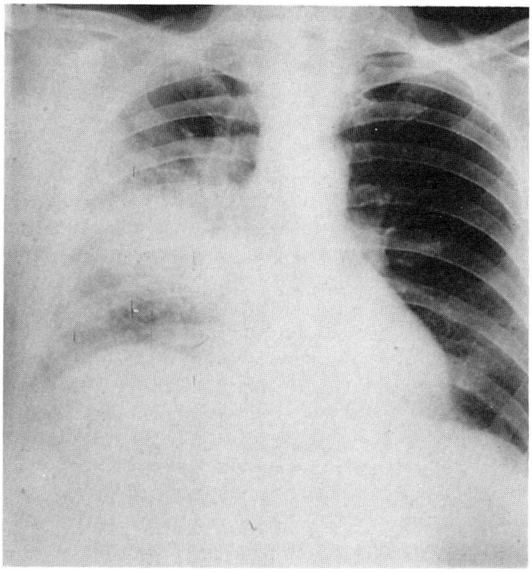

Figure 7.7 Locally advanced lung cancer

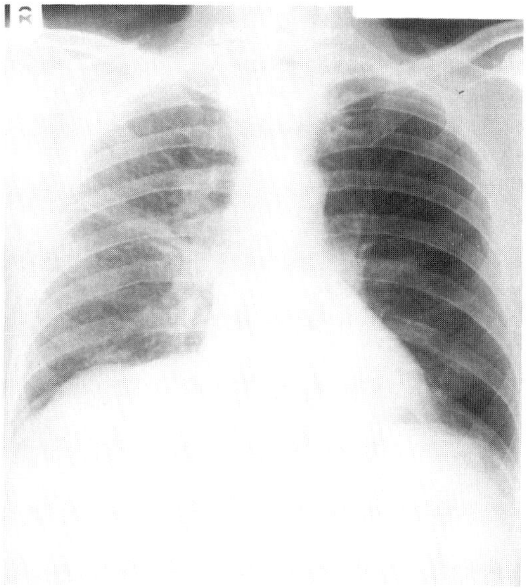

Figure 7.8 Locally advanced lung cancer after palliative radiotherapy

attempt at curative treatment by surgery or radiotherapy (*Figures 7.7 and 7.8*). These patients are likely to survive less than 1 year from diagnosis. Apart from those cases where an immediately life-threatening complication such as respiratory obstruction can be relieved, or in those patients with oat-cell carcinoma who respond to chemotherapy and who may possibly enjoy a longer survival, there is no evidence that treatment of any sort prolongs life. Durrant *et al.* (1971) reported an investigation in which four groups of patients were compared. The first had no treatment until required for the relief of symptoms; the second had palliative radiotherapy; the third received nitrogen mustard; and the fourth both nitrogen mustard and palliative radiotherapy. All four groups had a mean survival of about 8.5 months, and the degree of symptom relief seemed to be about the same. There seems therefore no reason to advise any treatment for most patients with lung cancer unless for the relief of symptoms. On the other hand, a patient who has been discovered on routine chest X-ray to have an abnormality shown to be an inoperable lung cancer will almost certainly expect something to be done about it if he learns the diagnosis, and it will then be extremely difficult to refuse to treat him. Furthermore, every radiotherapist has had the occasional patient whose advanced disease was apparently held in check for many years after palliative radiotherapy, although it must be admitted that there are also those patients who survive for years with their lung cancers in the absence of treatment!

In this context it is interesting to speculate that some of these patients may in fact have no metastases. Saunders *et al.* (1984) reported a study of the use of misonidazole as a radiosensitizer in lung cancer. The patients had non-small-cell carcinoma apparently confined to the primary site and immediate lymphatic drainage, distant metastases being excluded as far as possible. Survival was comparable to that of similar cases in other series and was not affected by misonidazole. However, of 42 patients who underwent necropsy, 14 showed no evidence of metastasis. It seems possible, therefore, that within the mass of patients usually irradiated palliatively there may be some who indeed have no metastases. Perhaps some of these might be cured by vigorous local irradiation, in spite of the poor outlook for the group as a whole.

Technique of palliative radiotherapy

The aim is to relieve symptoms in patients who probably have but a few months to live. It follows therefore that the treatment should not produce any new symptoms of its own, and that it should occupy as little of the patient's remaining life as possible. The radiation dose used should be the minimum to give sustained symptomatic relief. Deeley (1966) carried out a trial in which two groups, each of 51 patients all with anaplastic histology, were compared. One group received 3000 cGy and had a mean survival of 9.3 months, while the other treated with 4000 cGy had a mean survival of only 6 months. The only other difference noted was that there was a greater degree of radiation fibrosis in the higher dose group; the frequency of residual disease within the chest and of distant metastasis was the same in the two groups. Johnson *et al.* (1973) treated 100 patients in three approximately equal groups. Two groups were treated using telecobalt to a dose of either 4800 cGy in 20 fractions over 4 weeks, or 2800 cGy in four fractions over 10 days. The third group also received the second regimen, but using 35 MeV electrons. In all three groups 30% survived for 1 year and 6% for 5 years, while the degree of palliation seemed to be the same.

It is the present author's policy to use a dose of 2800 cGy in seven treatments given three times a week in most cases. An alternative dose of 3000 cGy in 10 daily fractions is used for fields larger than about 300 cm^2, as the individual fractions are smaller and therefore more easily tolerated on larger volumes. This second regimen is also prescribed if the patient is to remain in hospital for radiotherapy, as the overall treatment time is then shorter. It is also used for re-treatment if required, after an interval of 3 months, and may even be used for a third course. Most patients are treated on an outpatient basis. Although orthovoltage radiation has been used successfully in the past, megavoltage equipment — either linear accelerator or telecobalt — should now be chosen whenever possible. Megavoltage enables the required dose to be delivered with little or no skin reaction, the greatest speed, and the least disturbance to the patient. If for any reason one is obliged to use orthovoltage X-rays it is important to calculate the radiation actually received on the skin. This consists of the applied dose together with the transmitted dose from the opposing field. It should not be allowed to exceed 3250 cGy in 10 daily fractions if the skin reaction is not to proceed beyond a dry desquamation and so add to the patient's discomfort. It will be necessary to accept a midplane dose of 2000 – 2500 cGy or so with orthovoltage if the recommended maximum skin dose is not to be exceeded.

Technique and dosage are the same irrespective of the histological type of carcinoma. In general, the less well differentiated a tumour the more rapid its growth rate and the more quickly it will respond to radiotherapy. Palliation may thus be obtained gratifyingly rapidly in an anaplastic carcinoma, although local recurrence and distant metastasis are correspondingly quick to manifest themselves.

Common symptoms requiring palliation are cough, haemoptysis, dyspnoea and chest pain. Some special situations will be considered separately.

The planning of palliative radiotherapy

Most cases can be dealt with by a pair of parallel opposed megavoltage fields with the patient supine. The occasional patient who is unable to lie down may

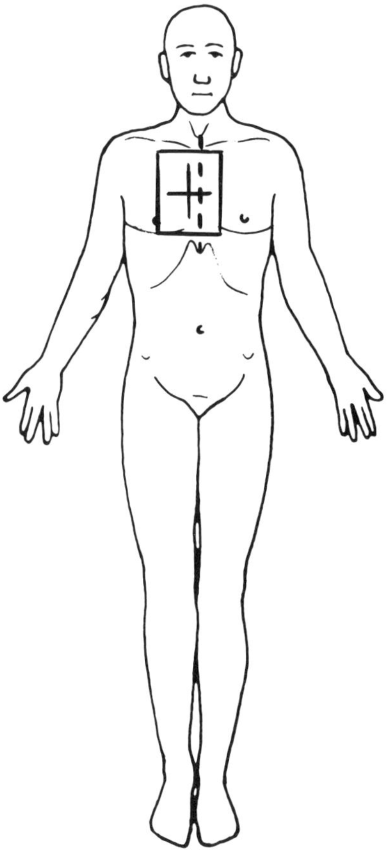

Figure 7.9 Typical field for palliative radiotherapy of carcinoma of the right lung, showing relationship to midline

be treated sitting using a back-pointer, or even semi-recumbent with one anterior field and as high an energy as is available. A good quality chest X-ray, and preferably a highly penetrated film which will show the bronchial tree, are needed. A report of the bronchoscopy findings is invaluable, and a CAT scan if available may also be helpful, although less so than in planning radical radiotherapy. If the patient's underlying respiratory function is poor due to chronic bronchitis or emphysema this will need to be taken into account in deciding upon the size of the fields, as the dose of radiation to be given is sufficient to cause pneumonitis which might further embarrass the patient's breathing. Chest infection should be brought under control before starting radiotherapy, and severe degrees of anaemia, i.e. below 1.4 mmol/ℓ (9 g/dl) should be corrected.

A useful preliminary step is to mark the patient's midline from the suprasternal notch to the xiphisternum (*Figure 7.9*). In most cases it is then possible to mark the anterior treatment field onto the patient's skin using the ordinary posteroanterior chest X-ray. This is true even though the film has been taken with the patient standing with the scapulae rotated laterally, while for planning the patient is supine with the arms by the sides. The limits of the tumour superiorly and inferiorly are noted in relation to the anterior endsof the ribs as seen on the chest film, and are transferred to the patient's skin by counting down the ribs. The medial and lateral limits are measured from the midline of the film and similarly transferred to the patient's skin using the midline already marked. Bronchoscopy findings are helpful here in ensuring that the tumour is adequately covered. A typical field thus marked might measure 16 cm superoinferiorly and 12 cm transversely, with its centre 2 cm to the side of the midline on which the tumour is situated, and

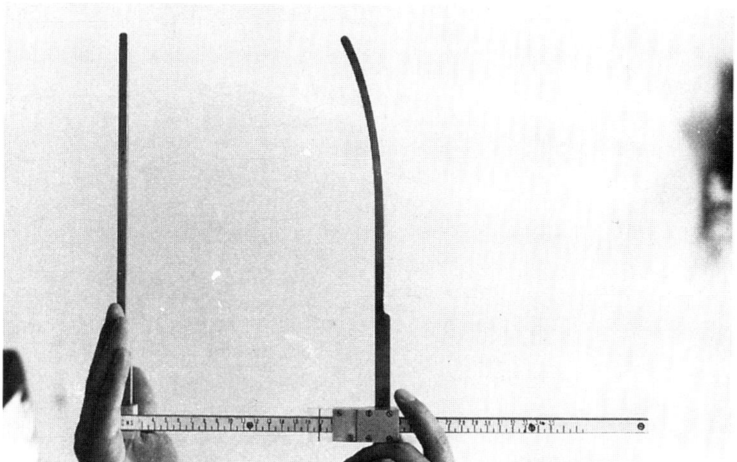

Figure 7.10 Calipers for measuring separation of fields

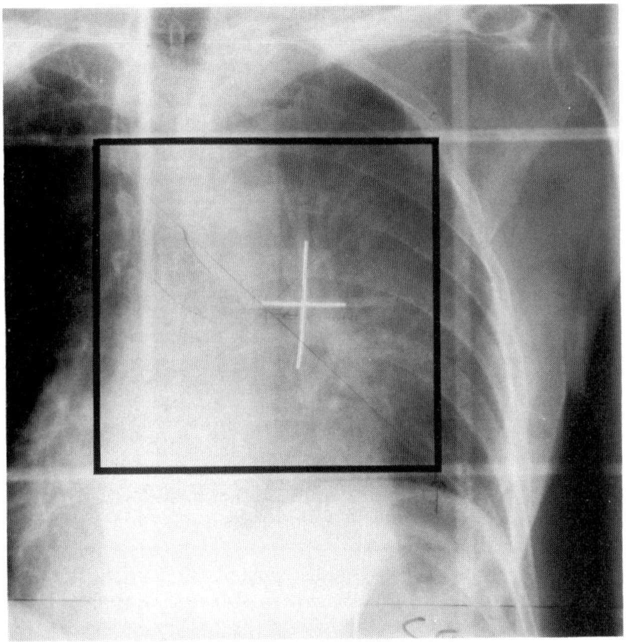

Figure 7.11 Palliative radiotherapy for lung cancer: a simulator check-film. The field borders have been amended, and are marked together with the new centre

Figure 7.12 A marker film of the corrected field, taken on an 8 MeV linear accelerator. A double exposure has been used, the wider field showing the relationship of the therapy field to the rest of the chest

extending from the upper margin of the manubrium down to the fifth rib. As far as possible the field should not be allowed to extend into the suprasternal notch as this may result in particularly severe dysphagia from radiation oesophagitis. The antero-posterior separation of the patient is measured using suitable calipers (*Figure 7.10*) through the midpoint of the field and the size and position of the field is then checked radiographically (*Figure 7.11*). A radiotherapy simulator is the best equipment for this purpose but, alternatively, a marker film (*Figure 7.12*) may be obtained using the therapy machine itself with appropriate industrial quality film and lead foil intensifying screens. If necessary the fields are corrected by moving the patient's skin marks, or by adjusting the field size, and the separation is finally checked. The author normally uses only the midpoint separation for calculating the dose to be given to each field, but in some centres maximum and minimum separations are measured and a mean taken for the calculation. Treatment is delivered using an isocentric technique.

If metastatic lymph nodes are present in one or both supraclavicular fossae one may wish to extend the fields upward to include them, remembering to shield the suprasternal area by lead blocks if at all possible. It is often simpler to treat these nodes with a separate single anterior field from a vertical beam, allowing a gap of about 1 cm between the lower edge of this field and the upper edge of the opposed fields.

Care of the patient during palliative radiotherapy

Palliative radiotherapy as described is well tolerated and nausea or vomiting rarely occur. With megavoltage beams there should be no skin reaction. The most frequent side-effect is radiation oesophagitis which produces burning dysphagia after a week of treatment. This is short lived and is usually controlled by a local anaesthetic preparation such as Mucaine, or even soluble aspirin. However, it can be distressing, and every effort should be made to prevent it by avoiding the suprasternal notch where the narrow separation results in a larger midpoint dose than at the central axis of the beams. Should the patient develop a chest infection during radiotherapy it is best to stop treatment until the infection has been brought under control by antibiotics.

Patients whose general condition is poor may be improved sufficiently to enable them to benefit from palliative radiotherapy by the use of prednisolone 30 mg/day. This improves appetite and sense of well-being, but carries the usual risks of steroid therapy. It may diminish the oesophageal reaction to some extent but, on the other hand, may encourage the growth of monilia in the mouth and oesophagus, causing particularly unpleasant soreness and dysphagia and requiring treatment by fungicidal drugs such as amphotericin.

There are some special situations requiring palliative radiotherapy which merit individual consideration. These are superior vena caval obstruction, respiratory obstruction, dysphagia, and the Pancoast syndrome.

Superior vena caval obstruction

This distressing condition may justifiably be regarded as a radiotherapeutic emergency. It is due to a mass in the right upper mediastinum occluding the superior vena cava. Most often caused by lung cancer, it may also occur with lymphomas, thymomas, and very rarely in non-malignant conditions (Chajek and Fainaru, 1973). There is venous congestion and oedema of the head, neck and arms, with local cyanosis and characteristic collateral veins on the chest wall (*Figure 7.13*). The X-ray picture is classical (*Figure 7.14*). There may be orthopnoea, so that some patients are unable to lie supine for treatment and may have to be irradiated in a sitting position. The condition usually responds very rapidly to palliative radiotherapy (*Figure 7.15*), but Szur and Bromley (1956) noted that it may recur in about 20% of cases. These patients may respond to irradiation a second time, after an interval of at least 3 months. Some of these recurrences, and some cases who fail to respond in the first instance, are due to thrombosis of the superior vena caval system. Hope-Stone and Key (1961) used venography to identify these patients, some of whom may improve with anticoagulant therapy.

In planning radiotherapy for superior vena caval obstruction it is important to ensure that the fields come high enough to include the entire obstruction. This usually means extending the irradiation above the right clavicle. It may not be possible to avoid including the suprasternal notch in these fields.

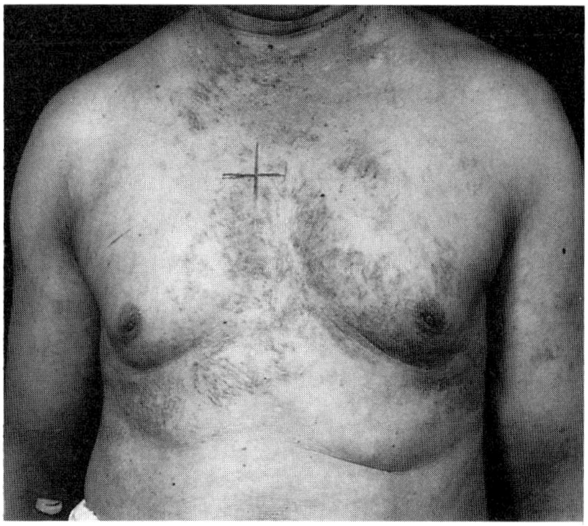

Figure 7.13 Patient with superior vena caval obstruction

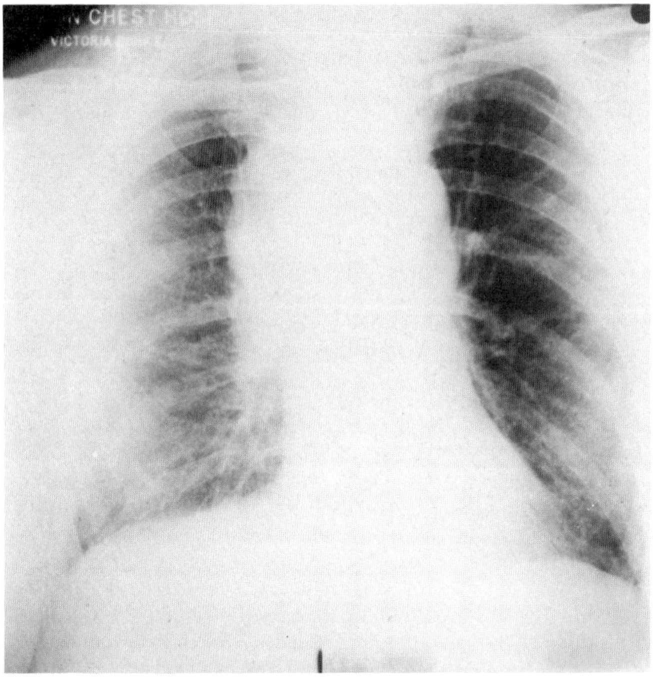

Figure 7.14 The chest X-ray showing right upper mediastinal mass

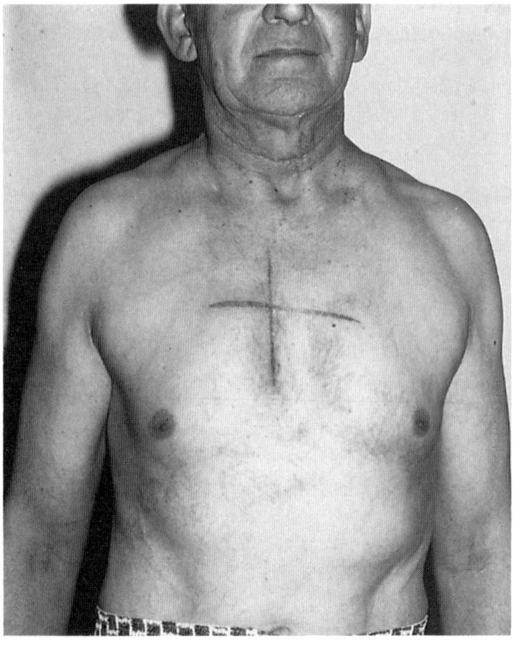

Figure 7.15 Patient after palliative radiotherapy

Respiratory obstruction

The lumen of a main or lobar bronchus may be narrowed by extrinsic compression by tumour mass, or by intrinsic growth. When occlusion eventually occurs the corresponding lung or lobe collapses. This collapse may often be reversed by palliative radiotherapy (*Figures 7.16 and 7.17*). Re-aeration sometimes appears so quickly that it is the present author's practice to repeat the simulator marker film half-way through the course of treatment so that the fields may be moved if necessary to take account of any shift of the mediastinum back towards the normal as the collapse resolves. Sometimes there is no improvement, probably because after the collapse has been established for a certain period fibrosis develops and prevents re-aeration.

When the trachea or both main bronchi are obstructed the situation is life-threatening, and must be regarded as an acute emergency. The obstruction may often be relieved by immediate radiotherapy, but sometimes the patient's condition deteriorates further shortly after the start of treatment. This is usually ascribed to increase of oedema; Cameron *et al.* (1969) demonstrated a worsening of airways obstruction as measured by the FEV_1, persisting for 4 days from the beginning of radiotherapy. Later Cameron *et al.* (1972) reported abolition of this deterioration by prednisolone or mustine before

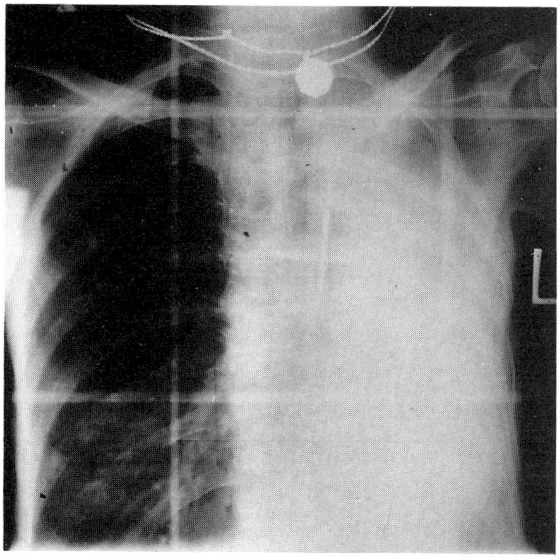

Figure 7.16 Simulator film: collapse of left lung due to a carcinoma occluding left main bronchus

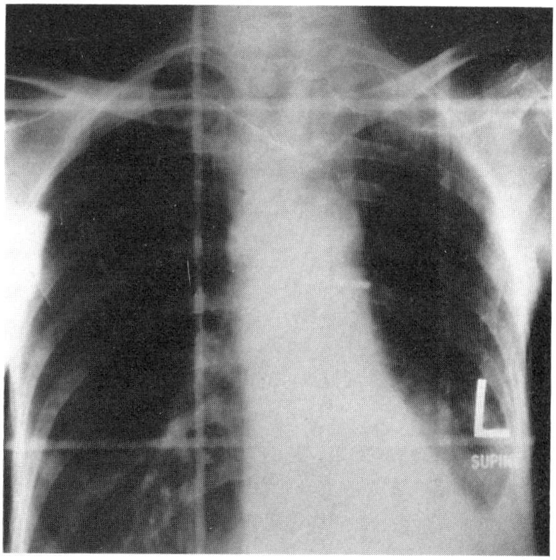

Figure 7.17 Check simulator film, half way through a palliative course of irradiation

irradiation. They found that prednisolone started at a dose of 20 mg/day, 24 hours before radiotherapy, was particularly effective, as well as being simpler to use and less toxic than mustine. It is the present author's policy to start all such patients on dexamethasone 4 mg 6-hourly immediately and then begin palliative radiotherapy within hours. The situation is so perilous that dexamethasone is used in all cases irrespective of the risk of peptic ulceration or diabetes mellitus, appropriate action being taken with cimetidine or insulin if necessary in these respective circumstances.

An interesting alternative technique for the relief of bronchial obstruction is the use of the fibreoptic bronchoscope to carry a laser beam to visible parts of the tumour, with instant evaporation of tissue (Hetzel *et al.*, 1981). A further refinement is to give a light-sensitive material (haematoporphyrin D) intravenously, which appears to be concentrated in the tumour and so permits a more selective response. Unfortunately, the patient may also develop light sensitivity of the skin for weeks afterwards.

These methods are still being evaluated, and may well prove useful for immediate unblocking of an air passage, but can only work on the intrabronchial portion of the tumour, so that palliative radiotherapy may still be required to reduce the bulk of the growth.

Dysphagia

This is commonly due to compression of the oesophagus by a mass of tumour in the mediastinum (*Figures 7.18 and 7.19*); it progresses from difficulty with hard solids to soft solids, then liquids, and may ultimately become complete. This complication can usually be improved or completely relieved by palliative radiotherapy; as long ago as 1955 Blanshard reported relief in three out of four patients. These cases are usually admitted to hospital for treatment if the dysphagia is at all severe. If the patient is unable to maintain a positive fluid balance of at least 1500 ml/24 hours, consideration should be given to the use of a nasogastric tube or, if necessary, intravenous fluids, until swallowing is adequate.

A particular situation obtains when the oesophagus is directly invaded by tumour; this is particularly likely to occur with carcinomas of the left main bronchus, which comes into close proximity with the oesophagus. Regression of the tumour with irradiation may hasten development of a fistula, which may also of course occur spontaneously (*Figure 7.20*). This produces a characteristic form of dysphagia in which any attempt to take food or drink is followed almost immediately by a violent explosive coughing out of the ingested material. This complication is lethal, but may be controlled for a while by the introduction of a suitable prosthetic tube such as that described by Atkinson, Ferguson and Ogilvie (1979).

In the assessment of a patient with dysphagia associated with lung cancer the author advises a barium swallow to ascertain the site and nature of the obstruction. If the mucosa appears irregular suggesting invasion by carcinoma, especially if the left main bronchus is known to be involved, then endoscopy should be carried out. If frank tumour is present in the oesophagus, radiotherapy is probably best avoided and a prosthetic tube inserted at the same procedure.

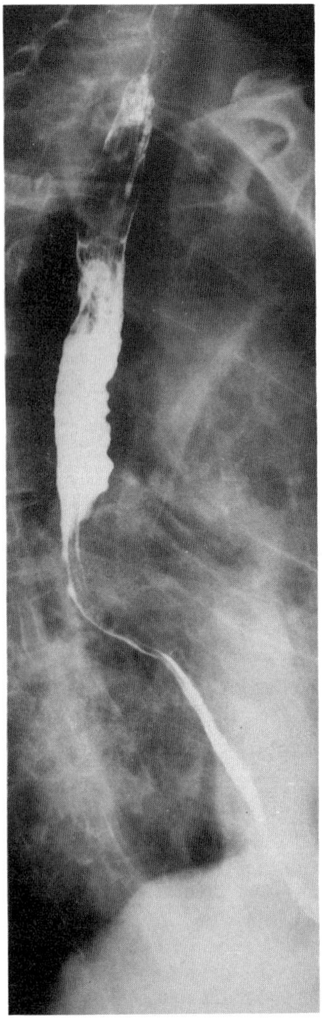

Figure 7.18 Compression of oesophagus in bronchial carcinoma

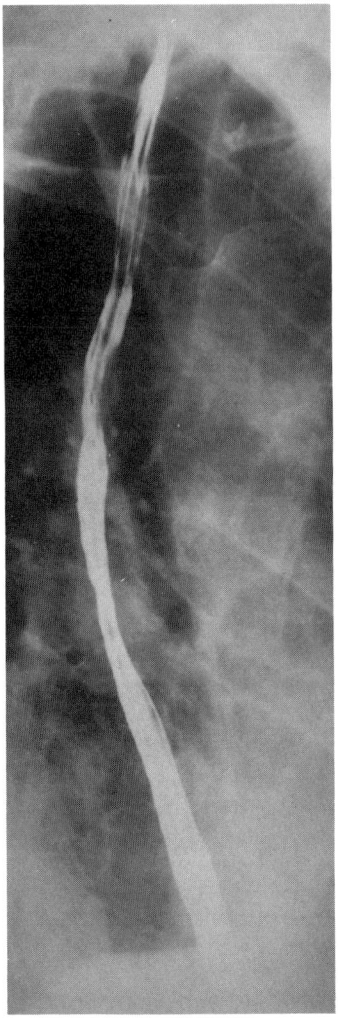

Figure 7.19 Bronchial carcinoma shown in *Figure 7.18* after palliative radiotherapy; dysphagia has been relieved

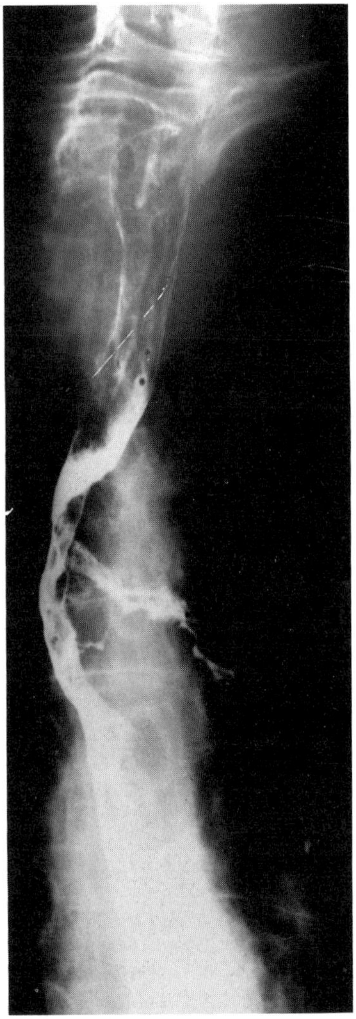

Figure 7.20 Fistula between oesophagus and left main bronchus in bronchial carcinoma. Radiotherapy has not been given, and is contraindicated

When dysphagia appears several months after a radical course of radiotherapy, or after a second course of palliative treatment, the possibility of narrowing of the oesophagus by fibrosis should be considered. This may be confirmed at endoscopy, and if present treated by bouginage.

Sometimes a form of dysphagia occurs with recurrent laryngeal palsy. This is almost always left-sided due to involvement of the nerve as it passes around the aortic arch; the right nerve is only affected when there is growth high in the region of the right supraclavicular region. In addition to a hoarse voice and characteristic bovine cough the patient often complains of difficulty in swallowing, particularly of fluids. These seem to 'go down the wrong way'. Radiotherapy very rarely relieves recurrent laryngeal palsy, but most patients seem to learn to cope with it and quickly develop a knack of swallowing without inhalation of fluid.

The Pancoast syndrome

This syndrome, in which a carcinoma of the lung apex produces both pain down the arm and Horner's syndrome, was described by the American radiologist Henry Pancoast in 1932. It is due to involvement of the brachial plexus and the cervical sympathetic system by the tumour. Almost a century before Pancoast, Hare (1838) wrote a meticulous clinical and post-mortem account of a patient with this syndrome. He described the ptosis and miosis of what is now known as Horner's syndrome, in this patient, when Horner himself was only seven. Hare described the involvement of the last cervical and first dorsal nerve roots and the invasion of the tumour into the intervertebral foramina and up to the dura. His patient developed paraplegia as may still be seen occasionally in this condition.

The Pancoast syndrome has a reputation for being intractable to radiotherapy (Rowlandson, 1968). The present author has found radiotherapyin moderate doses to be highly effective in relieving the pain (Mantell, 1973) and is sometimes followed by long survival. The key to success seems to be inclusion of the vertebral canal in the radiation fields (*Figure 7.21*) in accordance with Hare's 1838 description of the penetration of the vertebral canal by the tumour. Morris and Abadir (1979) agreed that radiotherapy is effective but reported that a dose of 6000 cGy in 20 fractions was needed for all patients to obtain pain relief, smaller doses controlling pain in only half. The present author, using doses of 3000 cGy in 10 fractions to 4000 cGy in 15 fractions, obtained complete pain relief in seven out of 10 patients, and partial relief in two more (Mantell, 1973).

Improved survival rates have been claimed for preoperative radiotherapy followed by radical surgery (Paulson, 1975). Paulson was able to resect 61 of 92 cases with two operative deaths, 3 – 6 weeks after irradiation to 3000 cGy in 10 daily treatments, with an actuarial 5-year survival of 34% in those patients who completed treatment. However, Morris and Abadir (1979) quoted the experience of the Memorial Hospital New York, that only 9% of Pancoast tumours were found to be resectable.

In the present author's experience some patients are certainly cured by radiotherapy alone (*Figure 7.22*), which is understandable as this must be regarded as a peripheral lung tumour and might be expected to carry a somewhat better prognosis than a centrally sited growth.

Technique of radiotherapy for the Pancoast syndrome

The patient lies supine; it is often advantageous to have the ipsilateral arm abducted at the shoulder with the hand on the hip to keep the upper arm out of the beam. Anterior and posterior parallel opposed fields are used, sufficiently large to encompass the tumour, as seen on X-ray, with an adequate margin. The superior border must extend well above the clavicle

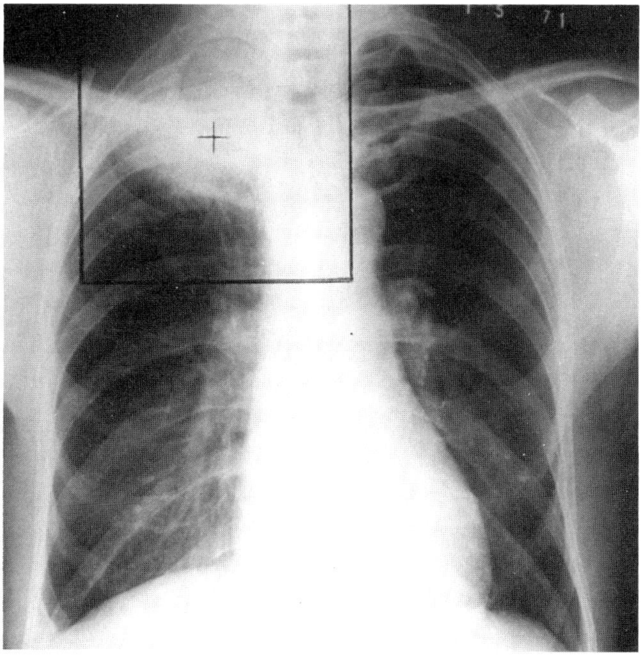

Figure 7.21 Pancoast syndrome: the radiation field. Note inclusion of the vertebral canal. The third right rib is eroded. The diagnosis was proved by needle biopsy

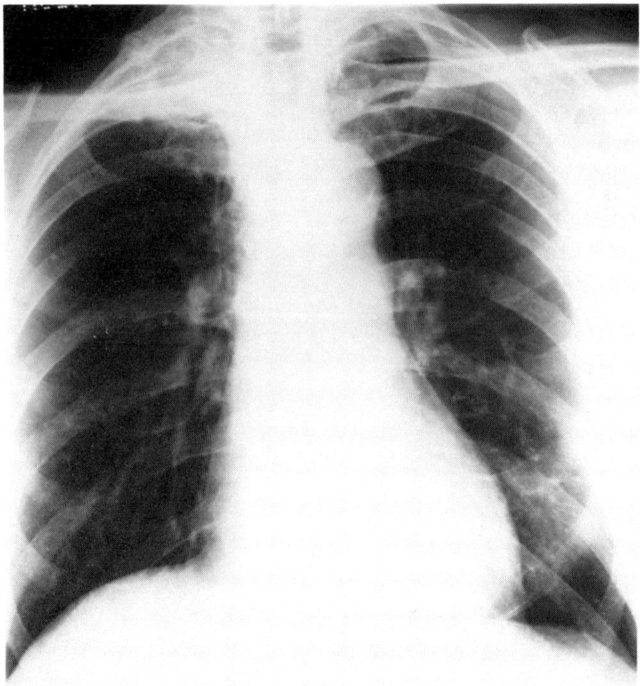

Figure 7.22 Radiograph of the patient in *Figure 7.21*, 13 years later

into the root of the neck, and the inferior border will probably be at or below the third rib anteriorly. The medial border comes across the midline at least to the contralateral vertebral pedicles so as to include the spinal canal. The lateral border may well be at or near the coracoid (*see Figure 7.21*). Megavoltage radiation is needed; the present author gives a central axis dose of 3000 – 4000 cGy in 10 – 15 daily treatments without the use of compensation to allow for the rapidly changing contour in this region of the chest. Inclusion of the spinal cord in the treated volume requires limitation of the dose to the levels suggested.

Chest wall invasion

Advanced lung cancers may invade the chest wall, usually with rib destruction and often with the production of a palpable and tender mass (*Figure 7.23*). The severe pain associated with this complication may be difficult to relieve by radiotherapy. It is probably better to use a pair of opposed megavoltage fields than a single field, as the tumour mass is usually bulky and a single field may not deliver an adequate dose throughout. Localization is achieved radiographically using a simulator as described above; if a mass is palpable the treatment volume may be indicated by this. A dose of the order of 3000 cGy in 10 daily fractions should be given; if pain is not relieved after this dose the present author is prepared to continue to a total of 3900 cGy in three more exposures. If pain remains uncontrolled after this, and very large doses of analgesics are required, cordotomy may justifiably be considered.

Pleural effusion

While a small exudate in a costo-phrenic angle is not necessarily indicative of advanced disease, a large effusion means that a great deal of tumour is present with nodules of growth scattered over the pleurae. The patient complains of dyspnoea which is relieved by aspiration of the fluid. Unfortunately this recurs, often within days. Control of recurrence depends upon the creation of a pleurodesis, for which a variety of agents including mustine, bleomycin, mepacrine, tetracycline and *Corynebacterium parvum* have been used. In all of these, the key to success is to aspirate the effusion to dryness by syringe or by an intercostal catheter with underwater seal drainage before introducing the irritant material. In some cases thoracoscopy is required for talc to be blown over the pleural surfaces before the lung is re-expanded. This procedure needs general anaesthesia but is a highly effective method of pleurodesis. Occasionally, irradiation of a hemithorax (*see* Pleural mesothelioma) is justified as an attempt to control an effusion, especially if it is associated with pain due to invasion of the chest wall.

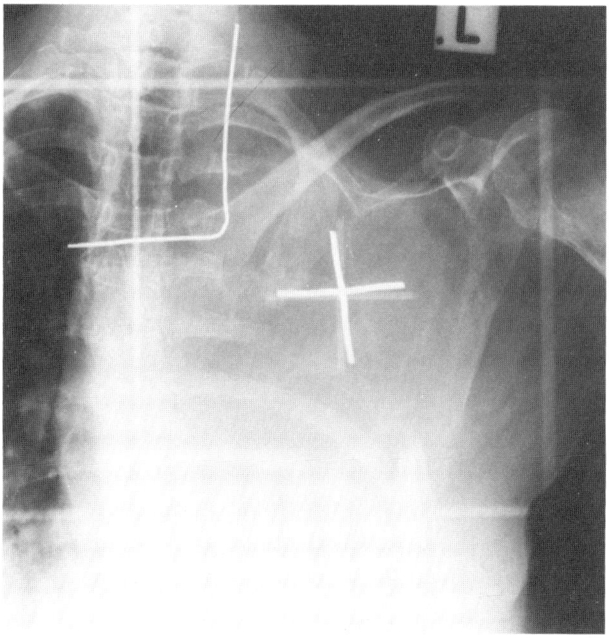

Figure 7.23 Destruction of the chest wall by direct invasion by a bronchial carcinoma

Treatment of metastases

Unlike breast carcinoma, in which patients with metastatic disease may survive in relatively good health for many years, metastases from lung cancer usually herald the terminal stages of the disease. Treatment offered must take into account the fact that the patient probably has only a few weeks to live, with steadily deteriorating health. Metastases in bone, brain and liver often co-exist, and hypercalcaemia may be present causing malaise, nausea and thirst. Any radiotherapy used must be given in as short a time as is reasonably possible, bearing in mind the patient's short prognosis.

Strong analgesics must be used freely, the dose being increased boldly and the drugs given sufficiently frequently to prevent the onset of pain as far as possible. Prednisolone 30 mg/day in the first instance, is extremely valuable for increasing the patient's sense of well-being and improving appetite. This dosage combined with a liberal fluid intake may also be sufficient to control hypercalcaemia. Even in patients with a history of peptic ulceration prednisolone may sometimes be justifiably employed under cover of a protective drug such as cimetidine.

In spite of this grim outlook radiotherapy still has a place in the care of the patient with metastatic lung cancer.

Bone metastases

Deposits in the limb bones may be treated with single exposures of megavoltage radiation. The linear accelerator enables a dose of 1500 cGy to be delivered from a single field to a depth of 2 or 3 cm in about 4 minutes. The site of the metastasis can be marked at the point of maximal tenderness, aided by the X-ray appearance. A generous field can be used. It is advisable to confirm the position of the field by the light-beam of the machine immediately before exposure, and to stop the treatment half-way to ensure that the patient has not moved.

There is often a transient increase of pain after a large single dose of radiation, but this is usually prevented by prednisolone in a dose of about 30 mg/day. Pain is usually eased considerably by the third day.

Spinal metastases may be localized and treated similarly. A large single dose from a megavoltage beam on the lower dorsal or the lumbar spine can cause transient but severe nausea and vomiting, and should always be covered by an antiemetic such as metoclopramide. If a length of 15 or 20 cm of the spine is to be treated the preferred treatment is orthovoltage X-rays giving an incident dose of 2800 cGy in seven fractions, three times a week. For pelvic bone metastases, a hemipelvis may be treated by this same schedule given at the midplane using a megavoltage unit isocentrically. When there are widespread bony metastases throughout the pelvis, palliation of pain can be achieved simply and rapidly by irradiating the whole of the bony pelvis, including if necessary the lower lumbar spine and the upper parts of the femora in a pair of large opposed lateral megavoltage fields and delivering a mid-plane dose of 1000 cGy in five daily treatments. Because of the large coronal separation the dose in the hip bones is greater than that in the midline where the bowel lies. Anti-emetics are always prescribed for this technique.

Metastases in the cervical spine are best treated in a sitting position by a posterior orthovoltage field, as megavoltage delivered from the back of the neck causes severe dysphagia due to a radiation reaction in the pharynx. The width of the orthovoltage field should be limited to about 6 cm, which is adequate to treat the cervical spine without also irradiating the parotid glands which would cause a dry mouth. A supporting collar should be provided. Localized rib metastases are also best treated by orthovoltage as deep penetration is undesirable. If short (10 cm) focus-skin distance applicators are available these will further reduce the excessive depth dose while adequately irradiating the lesion. In some centres half-body irradiation to a single dose of 800 cGy has been used effectively for the treatment of widespread metastases (Fitzpatrick and Rider, 1976). This technique is also discussed in Chapter 3.

Skin metastases

These occur particularly in the more anaplastic cancers. They are occasionally painful, and may distress the patient merely by their presence. They may break down causing unpleasant ulcers. They are readily treated using superficial (140 kV) X-rays, or if very thick by orthovoltage (250–300 kV) or electron beam, giving a single exposure of 1500 cGy (*Figures 7.24 and 7.25*).

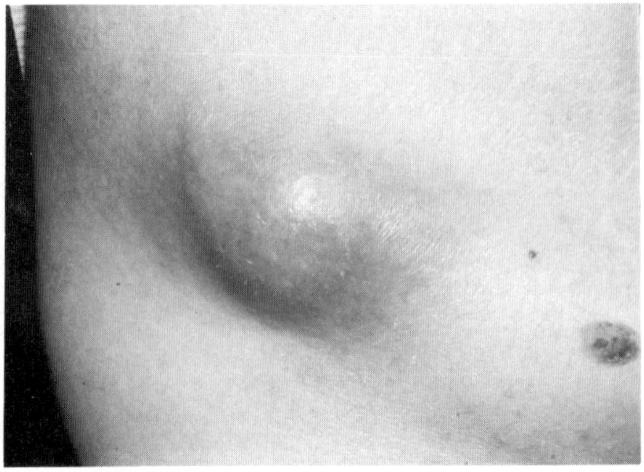

Figure 7.24 A large skin metastasis from a poorly differentiated bronchial carcinoma

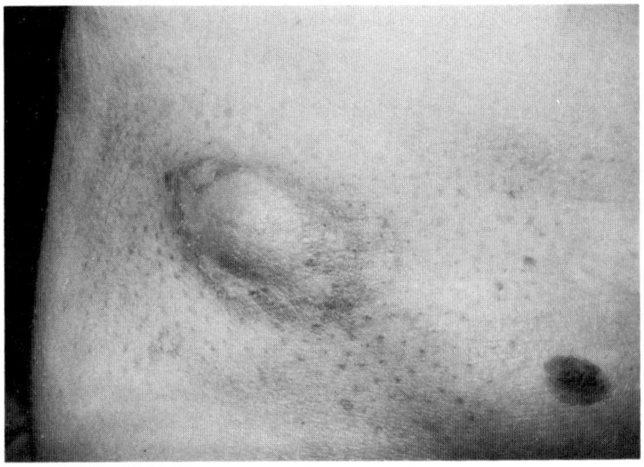

Figure 7.25 The skin metastasis shown in *Figure 7.24* after a single exposure of 1500 cGy. Because of the thickness of the deposit, 10 MeV electrons were used instead of superficial X-rays

Liver metastasis

This is common in the terminal stages of lung cancer, causing malaise, anorexia and jaundice. Radiotherapy has nothing to offer, but prednisolone 30–40 mg/day may make the patient feel less ill.

Sometimes jaundice occurs in the absence of any evidence of significant liver enlargement. Biliary obstruction due to a mass of nodes in the porta hepatis may then be suspected. Ultrasound examination may demonstrate not only the nodes but also dilatation of the biliary passages. If the tumour is poorly differentiated it may respond sufficiently rapidly to radiation to justify an attempt at relieving the jaundice by palliative radiotherapy. Anterior and posterior parallel opposed megavoltage fields are used, centred on the right costal margin about 4 cm to the right of the midline, and measuring about 15 × 15 cm. A dose of 3000 cGy in 10 daily fractions is given using an antiemetic such as metoclopramide.

The central nervous system

As well as non-metastatic effects upon the central nervous system, intracranial deposits are common in lung cancer. The spinal cord is frequently involved when vertebral metastases cause collapse of bone and pressure upon it. Sometime meningeal plaques of metastatic tumour involve spinal or cranial nerves in the absence of any detectable bone damage. Spinal cord deposits have also been described in small-cell lung cancer (Holoye *et al.*, 1984)

Brain secondaries may be single or multiple. They usually occur in the presence of widespread disease, but Deeley and Rice Edwards (1968) found no extra-cranial metastases in 15 of 63 autopsies of patients with brain secondaries from bronchial carcinoma. There may be raised intracranial pressure especially with posterior fossa deposits. Mental deterioration, speech disorders, motor and sensory defects and visual field losses are all common, as are Jacksonian fits and generalized seizures. In recent years the diagnosis has been greatly facilitated by the advent of CAT.

Intracranial secondaries are particularly devastating, and most patients spend the greater part of their remaining life in hospital. Of 88 patients treated by Deeley and Rice Edwards (1968) with whole brain irradiation, only 29 were able to return home for at least 1 month and of these most were dead within 3 months. Twenty-seven patients died during treatment and 32 others gained no benefit. There is however, the occasional long survivor; Deeley and Rice Edwards had two patients who survived more than 3 years.

Dramatic improvement in the clinical manifestations may be produced by dexamethasone 4 mg every 6 hours. An aphasic hemiplegic patient may recover both speech and power within a few hours of starting this drug. This probably means that the neurological defects are due predominantly to intracranial oedema rather than destruction of nervous tissue by tumour. Under these circumstances, the present author is prepared to irradiate the whole brain (*see* Chapter 15) to a dose of 3000 cGy in 10 daily fractions in the hope of being able to reduce or even withdraw dexamethasone, which in this large dose soon produces marked features of Cushing's syndrome. If there has been no improvement with dexamethasone it is doubtful if cranial irradiation is justified except perhaps for the relief of intractable headache.

Involvement of the vertebrae by metastases is common. Collapse of a vertebra may cause spinal cord compression; in the cervical region this is potentially lethal. Paraplegia resulting from collapse of a dorsal vertebra, and cauda equina involvement from the upper lumbar vertebrae, are both extremely distressing to the patient and add to the nursing difficulties. Irradiation of spinal metastases is therefore amply justified in the hope of preventing these complications.

Once spinal cord involvement has developed urgent decompression is needed; this should be effected within 24 hours if any recovery of function is to be obtained. In tumours such as breast carcinoma, where the prognosis may be several years, emergency laminectomy is mandatory. In lung cancer, however, the expectation of survival is of the order of weeks; even if decompression is successful the patient may not leave hospital. For this reason a laminectomy would be contraindicated. Nevertheless, an attempt at treatment using dexamethasone and radiotherapy should be instituted. A loading dose of dexamethasone 8 mg is given parenterally, and the steroid is continued orally in a dose of 4 mg every 6 hours. The standard nursing procedure for paraplegia is carried out; this requires an indwelling catheter and protection of pressure points. Palliative radiotherapy to the affected area of the spine is begun immediately, giving a dose of 3000 cGy in 10 daily treatments as an incident dose if orthovoltage is used, or at the 100% dose level with megavoltage. Dexamethasone dosage is reduced after 1 week and is gradually tailed off. If there is no improvement in the paraplegia within 1 day of beginning treatment the chance of obtaining a response becomes increasingly unlikely. Nevertheless, radiotherapy should be continued as it will at least help to control local pain.

Occasionally evidence of spinal cord compression occurs in the absence of obvious vertebral disease. A meningeal plaque of tumour may be demonstrated by myelography and treated as above with dexamethasone and radiation. Such plaques may be very extensive and require very long radiotherapy fields to cover them (*see* Chapter 15).

The systemic treatment of lung cancer

In lung cancer, where most patients die of metastatic disease, and where widespread malignancy is often evident when the patients first present, it is natural that means for systemic treatment should be sought. For many years chemotherapy with nitrogen mustard and later cyclophosphamide was used to obtain transient shrinkage of masses of tumour, occasionally with some benefit to the patient in the relief of superior vena caval or bronchial obstruction. Small-cell cancer was always the most frequent responder to these simple techniques, and to date remains the only histological type in which there is any convincing evidence of useful palliation or prolongation of life.

Muggia, Blum and Foreman (1984) have reviewed the developments to date in the use of cytotoxic therapy for non-small-cell cancers, including both advanced disease and, in combination with surgery or radiotherapy, the earlier stages. They consider that regimens containing cisplatin compounds may be particularly advantageous. Reported results concentrate upon response rates which vary from 24 to 68%. The likelihood of any real benefit to patients seems remote at present.

Small-cell lung cancer behaves in so aggressive a fashion that in general it is best regarded as generalized from the outset. Apart from the substantial number of long-term survivors from purely localized treatment claimed by Lennox *et al.* (1968) and Bates *et al.* (1974), most workers agree that it is essentially a systemic disease and that some form of systemic treatment is necessary for any long-term control. Many studies are in progress at the moment. These include the use of repeated courses of multiple drug chemotherapy, massive single doses of cyclophosphamide with protection of the urothelium by mesna (2-mercaptoethane-sulphonate) followed by autologous bone marrow replacement, and whole body irradiation. Many regimens involve the addition of local irradiation to sites of bulk disease in the mediastinum and supraclavicular fossae. Souhami *et al.* (1984) were unable to show any advantage in either survival or local recurrence rate when such radiotherapy to a dose of 4000 cGy followed chemotherapy with hydroxydaunorubicin, vincristine, cyclophosphamide and methotrexate.

Clinical evidence of central nervous system metastases occurs in as many as 49% of patients with small-cell lung cancer (Nugent *et al.*, 1979). The incidence seems to be reducible by prophylactic whole brain irradiation (Jackson *et al.*, 1977), but life expectancy is not improved because of the development of metastatic disease elsewhere. However, the effect of intracranial metastases is so devastating, and produces so much requirement for hospital care, that its routine use for those patients whose disease responds to systemic therapy may well be justified. A dose of 2000 cGy in five daily treatments is suggested (*see* Chapter 15).

Since small-cell lung cancer is a particularly radio-responsive tumour whole body irradiation has been tried as a form of systemic treatment. Urtasun *et al.* (1982) reported a randomized trial to compare a three drug chemotherapy regimen with irradiation of the upper half of the body to a midplane single dose of 800 cGy repeated to the lower half of the body 6 weeks later. All patients had irradiation to the mediastinum. The median survival was similar in the two groups; with 'early' disease, 42 weeks in the chemotherapy group and 43 weeks in the radiation group. However, in those patients with clinically advanced disease the median survival, 44 and 15 weeks respectively, favoured chemotherapy. Urtasun *et al.* (1983) suggest that this technique of radiotherapy may be useful as a means of consolidation and maintenance after chemotherapy, and are proceeding with a study of this.

Pleural mesothelioma

This distressing tumour causes severe and progressive chest pain and increasing dyspnoea. There is no curative treatment and the disease runs a course of steady deterioration to death in about 2 years. Many patients have a history of exposure to asbestos at work, and if so may qualify for financial compensation. It is also frequent in populations living near asbestos factories and mines.

Mesothelioma develops as waxy, white or yellow masses on both visceral and parietal pleura. Calcified asbestos plaques may be present, but there is no evidence that the tumour actually arises in these (Parkes, 1973). The growth erodes the ribs and may produce painful swellings on the chest wall. There may be compression and obstruction of the mediastinal contents, and effusion is common. Distant metastases are unusual, but local lymph nodes may be involved. Histologically, there may be papillary and tubular formation as well as anaplastic and spindle cells. There may be difficulty in deciding whether a tumour is indeed a true mesothelioma or an adenocarcinoma involving the pleura, which may produce a very similar clinical and macroscopic picture. Biopsies are obtained by needle, by thoracoscopy or by open surgery; incisions into the chest wall, however, carry a risk of fungation of tumour.

Surgery has a limited place in the treatment of mesothelioma. Considerable amounts of tumour may be removed by pleurectomy, and involved portions of the diaphragm can be excised if involved by the growth. Temporary pain relief may result from such surgery, but the tumour soon regrows and the pain recurs, with nodules of mesothelioma appearing in the thoracotomy scar.

Radiotherapy also has little to offer, but palliation of pain can sometimes be obtained by irradiation of a large volume, usually a full hemithorax. This may also slow down the formation of effusion. Any residual lung function on the treated side will be destroyed, so the patient must have sufficient reserve to tolerate this loss; in most cases there is probably little useful respiratory function in the affected hemithorax.

Megavoltage radiation is used with large parallel opposed anterior and posterior fields (*Figure 7.26*).

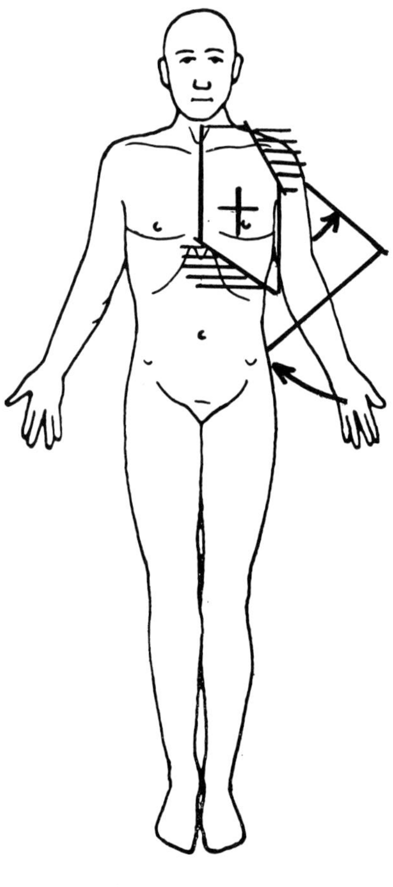

Figure 7.26 Field for irradiation of the left hemithorax. The patient's hand is placed on the hip

The patient lies supine with the hands on the hips, and by means of an isocentric technique both fields are treated without moving the patient. An antero-posterior film is taken on a radiotherapy simulator centred on an arbitrary point in the region of the nipple. The field to be treated is marked on the film and the centre moved accordingly. It is the present author's practice to place the medial edge of the field on the midline. The lateral edge lies 2 or 3 cm lateral to the chest wall. The apex is included and inferiorly the field extends down to the tenth rib. Lead blocks are used to shield the shoulder joint and the abdominal contents lying below the line of the tenth rib (*Figures 7.27 and 7.28*). This shielding is marked on the film and a template is prepared for position of the blocks on the treatment machine. A maximum dose of 3000 – 3500 cGy in 15 daily fractions is given; antiemetics are prescribed routinely.

Hilaris *et al.* (1984) reported 41 patients with pleural mesothelioma treated by a combination of surgery, radiotherapy and, in some cases, chemotherapy. Debulking of the tumour by as complete a parietal pleurectomy as possible was first carried out. Residual disease was treated by interstitial radiotherapy in 15 patients, using iodine-125 at the time of surgery, or iridium-192, 3–5 days later giving a dose

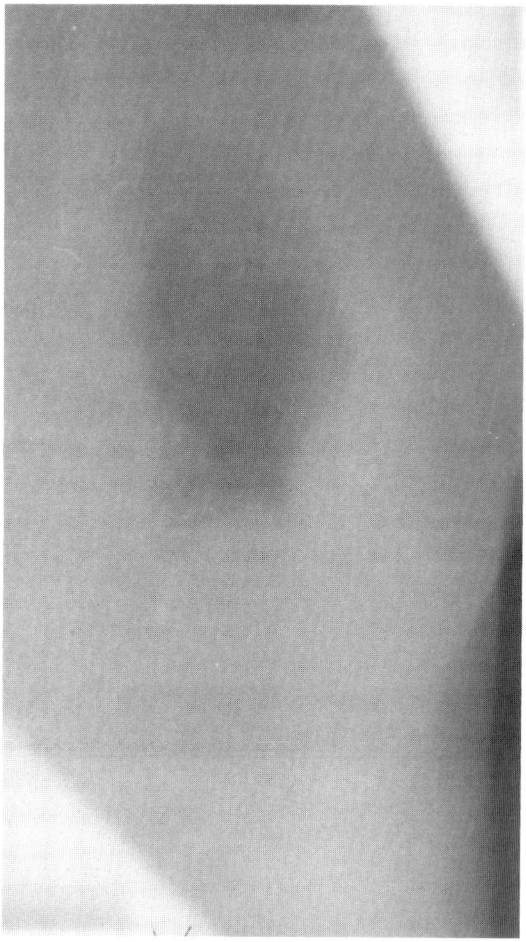

Figure 7.28 Hemithorax irradiation: marker film produced on the therapy unit, with shielding blocks in position

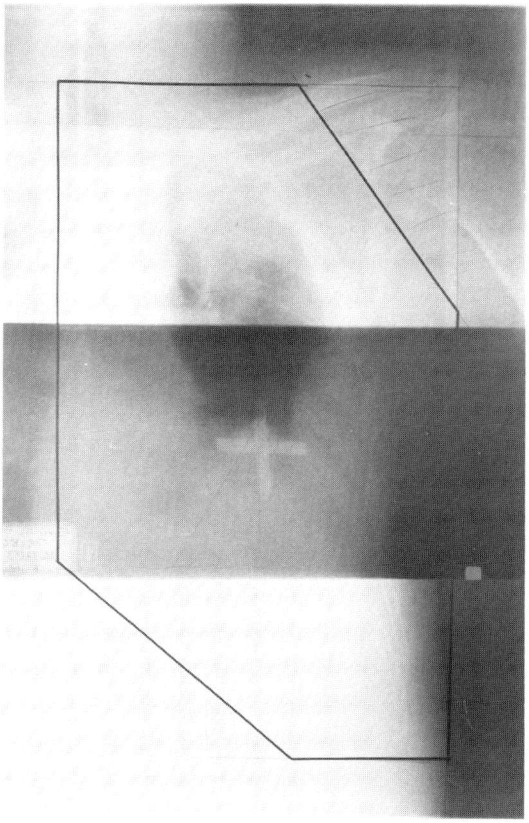

Figure 7.27 Simulator film for hemithorax irradiation. Two exposures have been made using the same centre because of the length of the field. The field limits have been marked ready for preparation of the template for the shielding blocks

of 3000 cGy at 1 cm. The whole hemithorax was irradiated 4–6 weeks postoperatively using a combination of photon and electron megavoltage radiation designed to minimize the lung dose, so that the pleura received a maximum of 4500 cGy in 4.5 weeks, while most of the lung was kept below 2000 cGy. Some patients also received chemotherapy with cyclophosphamide, hydroxydaunorubicin or cisplatin, or intrapleural phosphorus-32.

The 2-year survival was 40%, and only one-third of these patients were disease-free. The median survival was 25 months; but even these meagre results were better than those from a previous group treated by the same authors with surgery and external radiotherapy, where the median survival was only 6 months.

Carcinoma of the oesophagus

The main symptom of carcinoma of the oesophagus is dysphagia. This progresses from trouble with solids and then liquids to complete aphagia. The relief of dysphagia is the most pressing aim of treatment; permanent cure, although possible, is difficult to achieve.

Most oesophageal cancers are squamous celled, but there are true oesophageal adenocarcinomas as well as the more common infiltration of the lower end by gastric carcinoma. A rare oat-cell carcinoma has also been described (Doherty, McIntyre and Arnott, 1984).

Surgical treatment is commonly attempted. This involves excision of a sufficient length of the oesophagus to clear the extensive submucosal spread which is characteristic of this tumour. It follows that the longer the area of involvement by gross tumour, the less likely it is that resection will be possible. Earlam and Cunha-Melo (1980), reviewing the literature, consider that only 39% of squamous cell carcinomas are resectable, with an operative mortality of 33% and a 5-year survival of about 10%. They point out that radiotherapy can produce a similar final result, without the operative mortality, in spite of having much less well selected patients than surgery.

Surgery is least difficult for growths in the lower third of the oesophagus. Radiotherapy, on the other hand, is more readily applicable to the upper and middle thirds; the marked anterior and leftward curvature of the oesophagus in the lower third makes the production of a plan adequate for high dose radiation particularly difficult, but a small palliative dose can be delivered using simple parallel opposed fields.

Oesophageal cancer can be cured by radiotherapy. Pearson (1966) claimed an actuarial 5-year survival of 23% for middle-third tumours and 17% for the lower third. The present author would suggest that radiotherapy should be regarded as the treatment of choice for all but the lower-third tumours. Modern techniques of palliative intubation, while they may provide immediate relief of dysphagia, may also fail because of the insufficient length of the tube to clear the tumour or because of displacement of the tube itself. Atkinson, Ferguson and Ogilvie (1979) reported a mortality of 11% from endoscopic intubation. Intubation is best reserved for those cases who have failed to benefit from radiotherapy, or whose dysphagia has returned due to recurrent tumour. Recurrent dysphagia due to radiation fibrosis involving the oesophagus can usually be managed by careful endoscopic dilatation without the introduction of a prosthetic tube with its increased risk of perforation.

Preparation of the patient for treatment

Patients with carcinoma of the oesophagus may be dehydrated and emaciated, and correction of fluid and vitamin depletion and anaemia are of immediate importance. The diagnosis is suggested by barium swallow and confirmed by oesophagoscopy and biopsy. Patients with complete aphagia may have a nasogastric tube passed at the time of endoscopy; if this is not possible parenteral feeding may be required. If metastatic lymph nodes are detected by palpation in the supraclavicular fossa, or by CAT in the mediastinum or coeliac axis region, radiotherapy is limited to palliation using anterior and posterior opposed fields, and a dose of 3000 cGy in 10 daily fractions.

Technique of radical radiotherapy

A simulator with an image intensifier screening facility is invaluable in planning radiotherapy. The patient lies supine with the hands above the head so that the humeri do not obstruct the lateral view of the oesophagus. The patient is asked to swallow a mouthful of barium; if this cannot be done the mediastinum is irradiated with a pair of anterior and posterior parallel opposed fields and the attempt repeated after a limited dose of radiation has been given. It is the present author's practice to make this attempt after four treatments each of 275 cGy.

On screening it may be possible to visualize some or much of the oesophagus, because of the barium already swallowed. Usually it is necessary for the patient to swallow further mouthfuls of barium during screening. The course of the oesophagus may be marked by a line of ink dots on the skin of the front of the chest. The upper and lower limits of the stricture can be indicated by marks (*Figure 7.29*). The line of dots passes from the midline in the region of the manubrium inclining to the left as it descends until it bends fairly sharply to the left as it approaches the stomach. The axis of the treatment volume can then

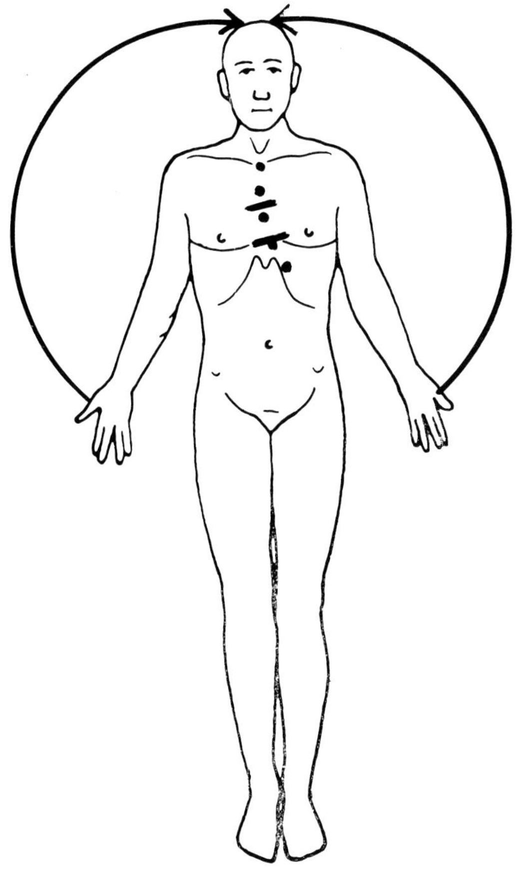

Figure 7.29 Line of oesophagus with the upper and lower radiographic limits of the tumour marked on the skin. The patient's hands are on the head

be marked onto the skin of the chest as a straight line inclining to the left from above downward, with its centre in the middle of the stricture and the upper and lower limits at least 5 cm beyond the ends of the stricture to allow for submucosal spread. An anteroposterior film is then taken on the simulator with barium in the oesophagus; the magnification of this film is obtainable from the focus-skin and focus film distances and the anteroposterior thickness of the patient's chest (*Figure 7.30*).

The X-ray tube is then rotated through 90° to point horizontally at the patient. The simulator couch is turned so that the line of the treatment volume as marked on the front of the patient's chest lies at right angles to the central axis of the X-ray beam, and therefore is parallel to the film carrier which has rotated with the X-ray tube (*Figure 7.31*). Thus, when a second and lateral film is taken with barium in the oesophagus there is no foreshortening of the image of the treatment volume, now projected in the lateral view. To obtain the magnification of this film

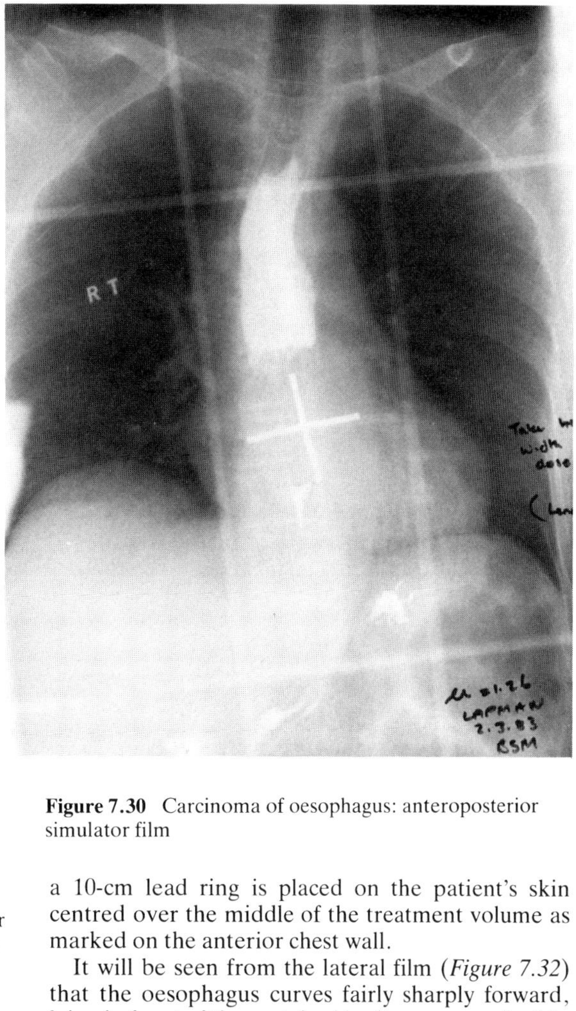

Figure 7.30 Carcinoma of oesophagus: anteroposterior simulator film

a 10-cm lead ring is placed on the patient's skin centred over the middle of the treatment volume as marked on the anterior chest wall.

It will be seen from the lateral film (*Figure 7.32*) that the oesophagus curves fairly sharply forward, lying in front of the vertebral bodies over much of its course, and then moving even further forward to join the stomach. The position of the spinal cord can also be seen, lying immediately posterior to the vertebral bodies. This is carefully marked onto the film as it must be kept out of the high dose volume which is to be planned. The centre of the stricture can be identified lying vertically below the centre that has been marked on the anterior chest wall, and a line parallel to the edge of the film passes through the anterior centre and the middle of the stricture.

A piece of semi-transparent graph paper is then taken and a rectangle is marked onto it to represent the treatment volume as seen in the lateral film, magnified to the same degree as the film (*Figure 7.33*). Several such rectangles may be prepared to represent different diameters of treatment volume, e.g. 6, 7 and 8 cm. The graph paper is fixed to an X-ray viewing screen, or preferably a light-table, and the lateral film superimposed upon it, with the line passing through the anterior centre and the middle of the stricture also passing through the centre of the rectangle marked on the graph paper. The film is then moved until the rectangle includes the stricture and the required margin of oesophagus while avoiding any part of the spinal cord. The oesophagus should lie as close to the central axis of the rectangle as possible, and the smallest rectangle to fulfil these requirements is chosen. The centre and edges of the chosen rectangle are then traced onto the film (*Figure 7.34*). Finally, the marking of the treatment volume onto the anteroposterior film may be completed, by choosing a suitable width allowing for the known magnification of this film; this is usually but not necessarily the same as the width represented on the lateral film. Thus we are left with two orthogonal films on which the treatment volume is marked. The lateral film should carry an accurate representation of the volume, but it will probably be slightly foreshortened on the anterior film because of the anterior curvature of the oesophagus.

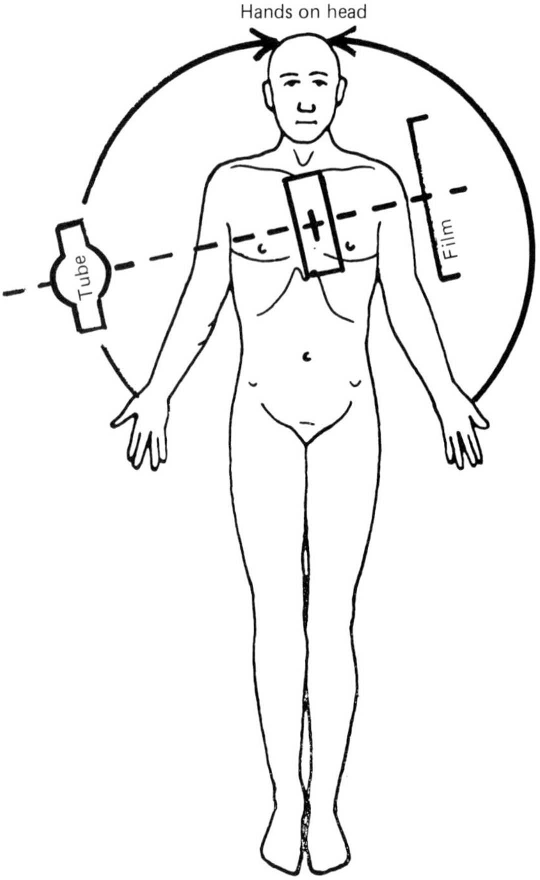

Figure 7.31 Barium swallow localization: disposition of patient in relation to diagnostic X-ray beam

Figure 7.32 Carcinoma of oesophagus: lateral simulator film. Spinal cord and the treatment volume have been marked

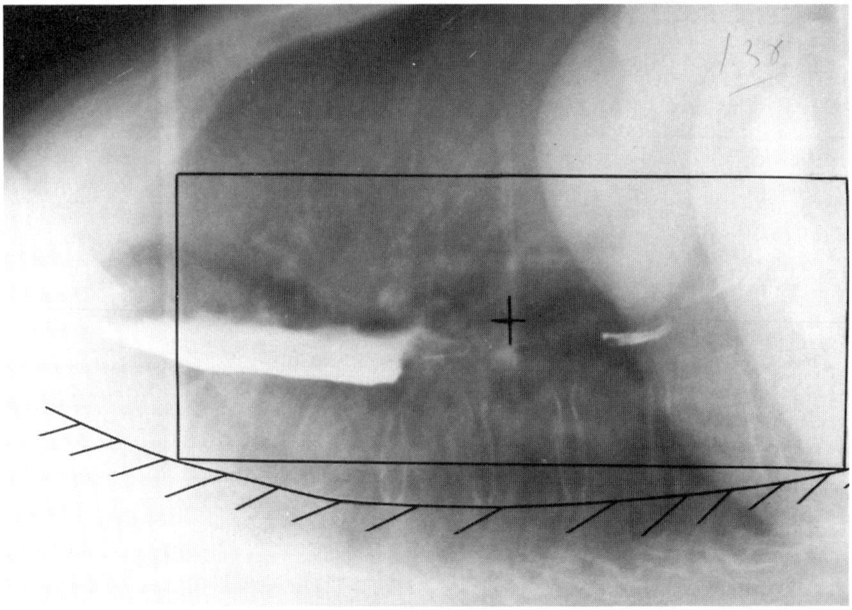

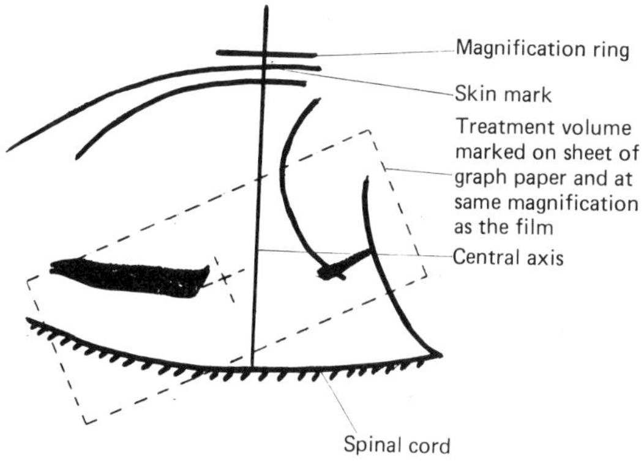

Figure 7.33 Selecting the treatment volume on the lateral film

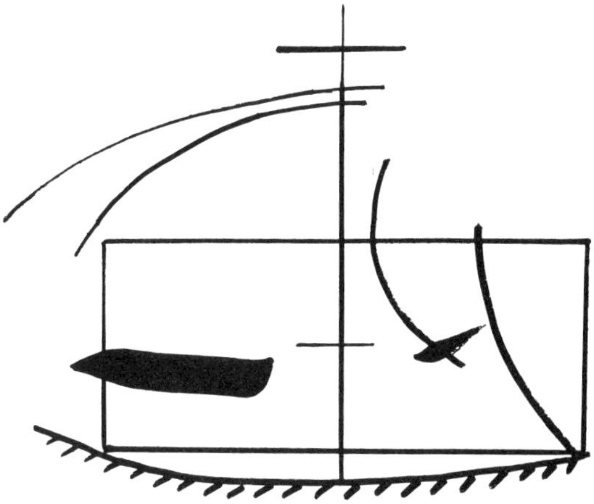

Figure 7.34 The treatment volume selected

Contours are taken around the patient's body at the upper, middle and lower points of the treatment volume thus determined. On each of these contours the treatment volume is marked together with the position of the spinal cord. It is also necessary to mark onto these contours the lung tissue, as this will greatly influence the size and distribution of the radiation dose within the treatment volume; CT is useful for this purpose. Sections are taken corresponding to each of the three contours, with the patient lying in the treatment position upon a flat couch-top. The couch and the scanner gantry are rotated so that the sections are taken in the planes of the three contours. These sections are enlarged photographically and used to trace the lung outlines onto the contours; the positions of the spinal cord are also verified by this means (*Figure 7.35*). Modern planning equipment now becoming more widely available enables this manoeuvre to be carried out on the screen of the viewing unit in the course of computerized planning without the need to take contours or the intervention of photography. The treatment plan is produced by means of a radiotherapy planning computer if available, or manually. It aims at creating a cylinder of high

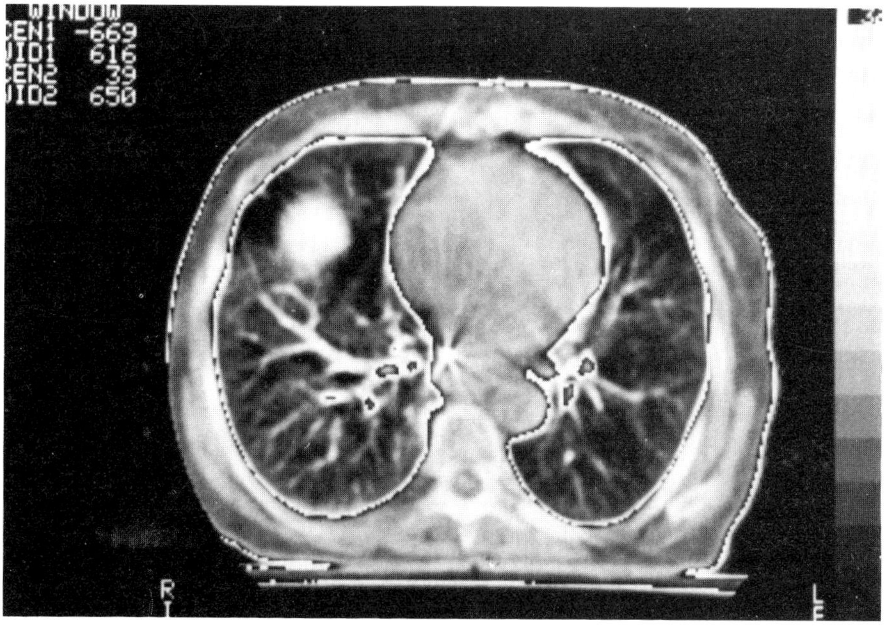

Figure 7.35 Carcinoma of oesophagus: planning CT scan taken at right angles to the long axis of the treatment volume

radiation dose which includes the tumour with an adequate margin of oesophagus, while avoiding the spinal cord and reducing to a minimum the volume of lung which receives sufficient radiation to cause pneumonitis. Three fields at 120°, one anterior and two posterior-lateral, are usually chosen (*Figure 7.36a and b*). The line of the isocentre is almost always found to be tilted out of the horizontal, because of the direction of the oesophagus. Fleming and Orchard (1974) describe the special calculations required to determine the correct angles of the treatment head, gantry and couch to ensure that the fields encompass the treatment volume along its entire length.

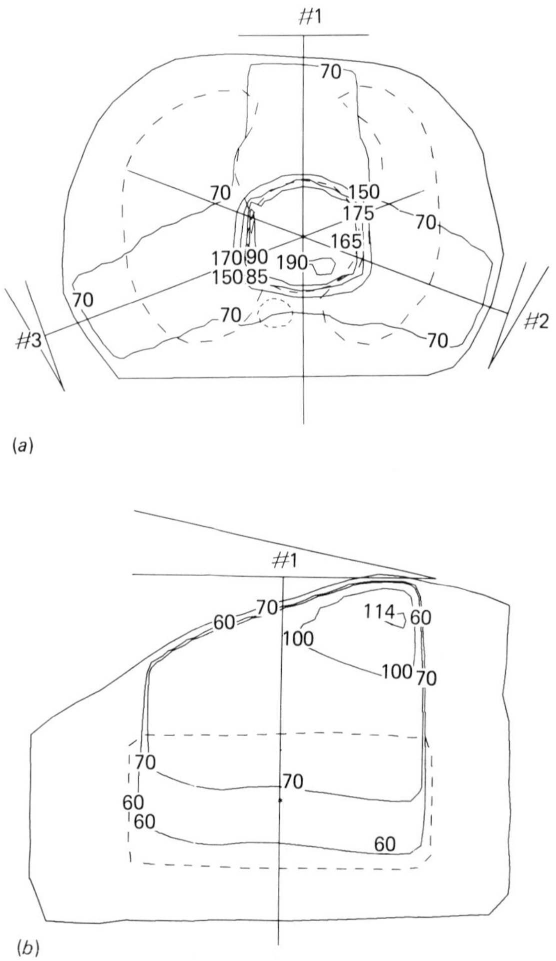

Figure 7.36 (*a*) Plan for radical irradiation of oesophageal carcinoma prepared by a RAD-8 computer for 8 MeV X-rays. On the patient's contour the spinal cord, the lungs and the treatment volume are represented by dotted lines. (*b*) Use of a wedge filter in the anterior beam to compensate for the slope of the sternum

In the future a tracking technique may well prove to be particularly valuable for treating oesophageal carcinoma (Brace *et al.*, 1981).

Care of the patient during radiotherapy

Swallowing may improve during the course of treatment and it is usually possible to maintain an adequate intake of fluid calories and vitamins by mouth. Help should be sought from a dietician in designing a suitable diet; a liquidizer is invaluable for those patients who can swallow fluids only. Some patients require a nasogastric tube until swallowing improves; endoscopic intubation with a suitable prosthesis is also sometimes used, but it must be remembered that this procedure is itself potentially risky, and may carry a mortality as high as 11% (Atkinson, Ferguson and Ogilvie, 1979).

There may be transient deterioration in swallowing due to a painful radiation oesophagitis after 2 or 3 weeks of treatment. This is usually controllable by a local analgesic preparation such as Mucaine. There is no skin reaction when a linear accelerator is used and rarely any clinical evidence of radiation pneumonitis. In general, radiotherapy is well tolerated, and should carry little morbidity and no mortality.

Carcinoma involving the lowermost part of the oesophagus

This area does not lend itself readily to radical radiotherapy because of the sharp curvature of the oesophagus anteriorly and to the left and the close proximity of the gastric mucosa which may ulcerate after doses in excess of 4500 cGy (Brick, 1955). On the other hand, it is fairly easily accessible to the surgeon and attempts at curative treatment should probably be surgical. However, palliation can often be achieved by a limited dose of radiation given through simple anterior and posterior parallel opposed fields (*Figure 7.37*). Adenocarcinoma of the stomach is frequently but erroneously regarded as radioresistant. It responds well and frequently enough to megavoltage radiotherapy in a dose of only 3000 cGy in 10 daily treatments to allow such irradiation to be a simple, safe and well-tolerated means of palliation when the gastric cardia and the lowermost part of the oesophagus are involved by carcinoma causing dysphagia (Mantell, 1982).

Thymic tumours

These are rare; a busy radiotherapy department may rarely see more than one case a year (Penn and Hope-Stone, 1972). Patients may present with neck, chest or arm pain, hoarseness, swelling of the chest wall, or less specific symptoms such as tiredness or anorexia.

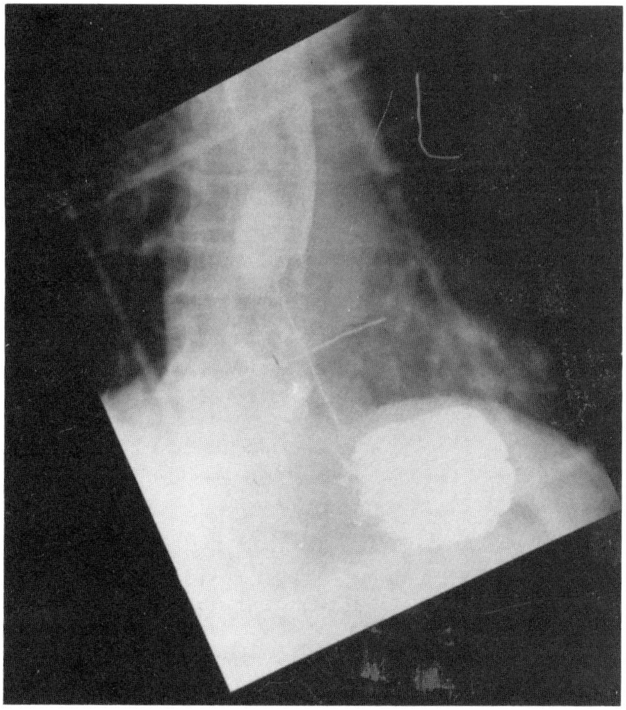

Figure 7.37 Simulator film for palliative radiotherapy of carcinoma of the cardia and lower oesophagus

About one-half of the cases are discovered by incidental chest radiography in asymptomatic patients. Myasthenia gravis may be present in perhaps one-third of the patients; conversely, rather less than one-third of cases of myasthenia gravis are associated with a thymic tumour. Blood dyscrasias may occur, e.g. red cell aplasia (Havard and Scott, 1960).

Distant metastases from thymic tumours are particularly rare; Rachmaninoff and Fentress (1964) in reporting a case, found only nine more in the literature. The degree of aggressiveness of a thymoma may be difficult to assess from its histological appearance.

Classification of thymomas

Thomson and Thackray (1957) divided thymomas into epithelial, lymphocytic and teratomatous groups. The first group included the lymphoepitheliomas, some of which may be associated with myasthenia gravis, and also a wide range of epidermoid, oval- and spindle-celled and undifferentiated growths. Granulomatous thymomas, histologically indistinguishable from Hodgkin's disease, were also included in this group. The lymphocytic group included lymphosarcomas as well as tumours composed of masses of apparently benign lymphocytes. The teratomas included both benign and malignant forms. Germ cell tumours arising in the anterior mediastinum and resembling seminomas, dysgerminomas and testicular teratomas are also encountered, but are not true thymic tumours (*see below*).

Diagnosis of thymic tumours

An anterior mediastinal mass is demonstrated by chest X-ray with a lateral film (*Figures 7.38a, b and 7.39*). Further imaging to show the site, size and extent of the tumour is nowadays usually provided by CAT, which is also valuable in planning radiotherapy. Thoracotomy is necessary; it may be possible to remove the tumour completely, but usually there is extensive infiltration of mediastinal structures and lung rendering the thymoma inoperable; in this case a large biopsy should be taken.

Radiotherapy for thymic tumours

If the tumour has been completely excised it may be justifiable to withhold radiotherapy. However, if the growth is shown to be invasive on histological examination it is probably wise to give postoperative irradiation even if excision seems to be complete (Penn and Hope-Stone, 1972). Radiotherapy should always be given for inoperable and incompletely excised

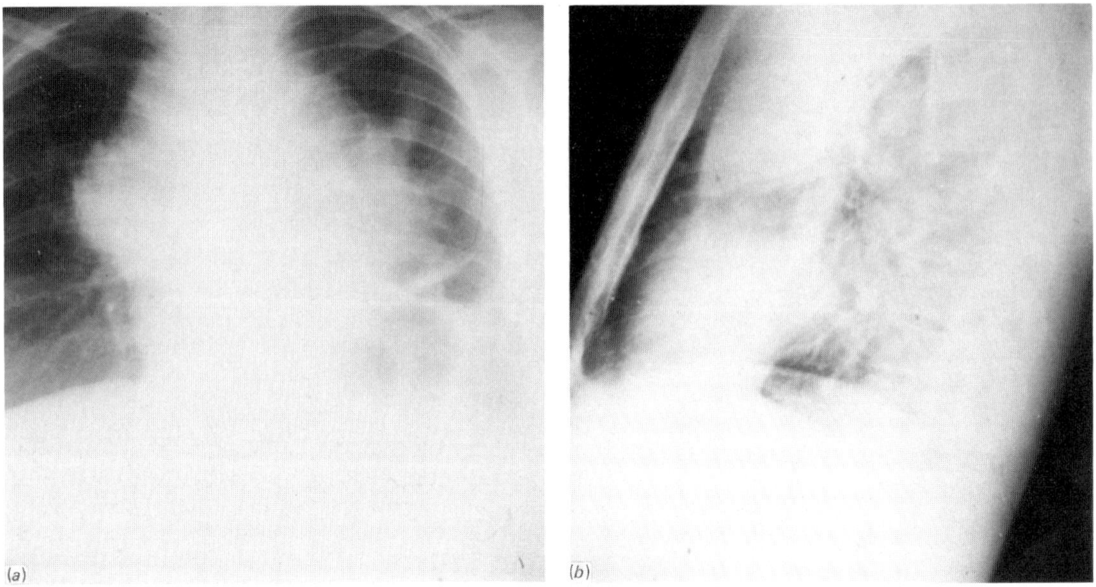

Figure 7.38 (*a*) Thymoma: anteroposterior view. (*b*) Lateral view of thymoma

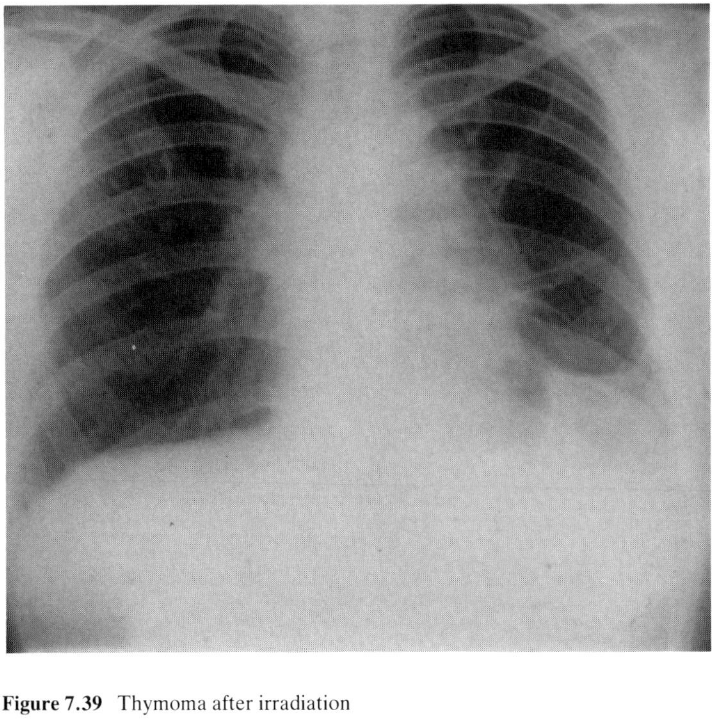

Figure 7.39 Thymoma after irradiation

tumours. Myasthenia gravis, if present, must be controlled during radiotherapy so that the patient can cooperate in his treatment (Skeggs, 1968).

The patient is treated supine. Considering the large volume of tissue which must be irradiated in most cases, a dose of 4500 cGy in 20 daily fractions over 4 weeks is likely to be the maximum that can be given. The tumour is localized initially by anterior and lateral films taken on a radiotherapy simulator, as described for lung cancer; the fields must include any palpable supraclavicular nodes. Tissues at risk from radiation damage include the lungs and the spinal cord; Skeggs (1968) described mediastinitis and pericarditis, but after much higher doses than above. CAT not only enables the limits of the tumour to be mapped out but also shows the disposition of lung tissue and the spinal cord in relation to the thymoma. A dedicated radiotherapy planning system linked to a CAT installation is preferable; failing this a photographic method may be used as described for bronchial and oesophageal carcinoma. A plan is produced to give the dose suggested while keeping the spinal cord below about 3000 cGy, and limiting the amount of lung tissue that receives more than 2000 cGy to the smallest volume possible (*Figure 7.40*).

In many cases a pair of anterior oblique wedged megavoltage fields will give the distribution required. Some very bulky tumours may need irradiation by a pair of parallel opposed anterior and posterior fields to an initial dose of 2500 cGy in 10 daily treatments to reduce the size sufficiently for more accurate planning as above. The dose already received by lung and spinal cord must be taken into account in planning the second part of the course, when the tumour dose is raised to a total of 4500 cGy.

In so rare a tumour, the results of radiotherapy are difficult to assess. In Penn and Hope-Stone's series (1972), only seven of 18 patients were treated to a 'radical' dose which was regarded as 4000 cGy. All seven survived 3 years and three are known to have lived 10 years. It seems justifiable to use radiotherapy for invasive thymomas as described.

Mediastinal germ-cell tumours

These rare tumours histologically resemble seminomas, dysgerminomas and testicular teratomas. Like their genital counterparts they may metastasize widely, and some are rapidly responsive to small doses of radiation. They also respond like testicular tumours to the newer regimens of chemotherapy using cisplatin combinations, which may be curative even in the metastatic case, and this is probably the treatment of choice.

Cox (1975) reviewed the literature and reported a study of 24 cases. Ages ranged from 18 to 50 years, and 22 were males. Presenting symptoms included chest pain, cough, haemoptysis, dyspnoea and superior venal caval obstruction. Six asymptomatic patients were referred after an anterior mediastinal mass was noted on chest X-ray. Treatment was by radiotherapy in 19 cases, resection in one, and chemotherapy in four. The drugs used included alkylating agents, vincristine and actinomycin D, but not cisplatin. Five patients were alive at the time of

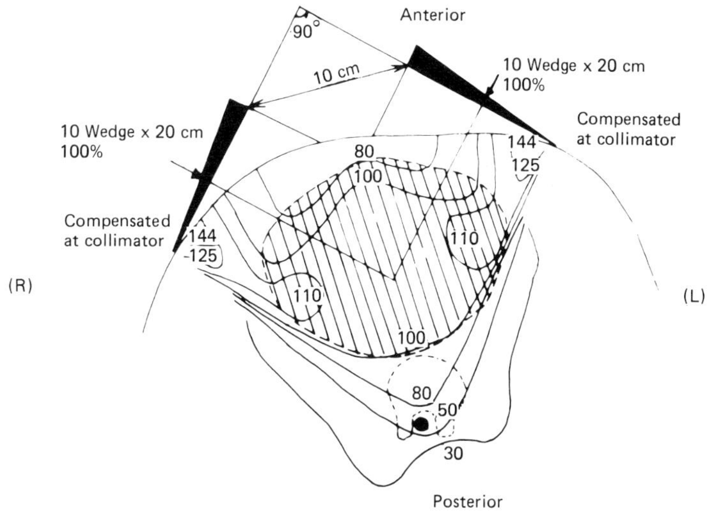

Figure 7.40 Thymoma: diagram of a typical radiotherapy plan

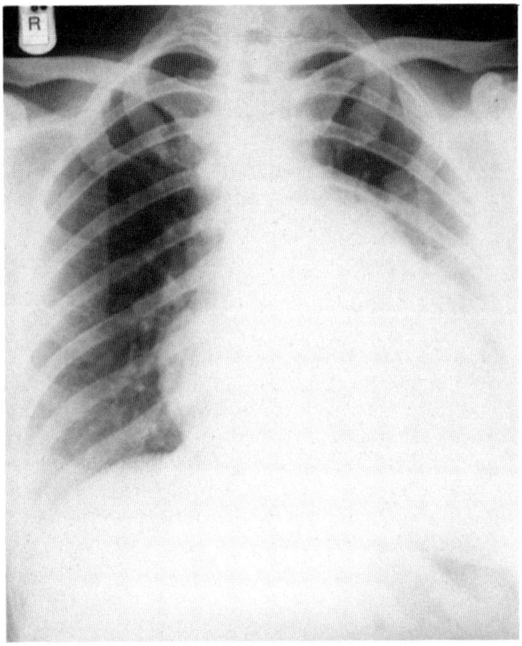

Figure 7.41 Mediastinal germ-cell tumour

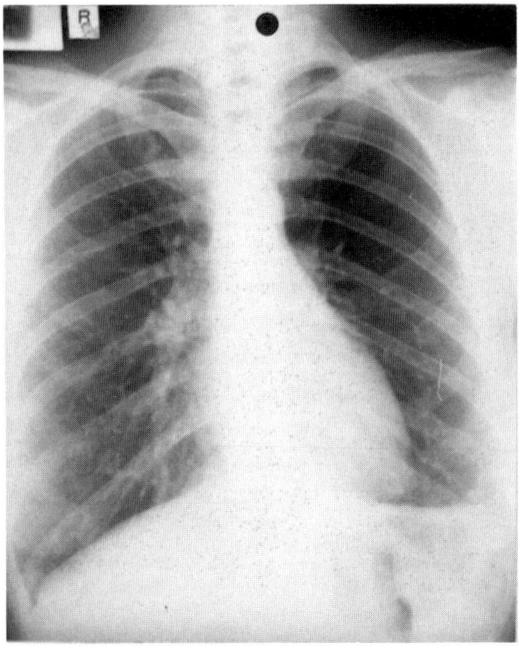

Figure 7.42 Mediastinal germ-cell tumour shown in *Figure 7.41* after treatment with a cisplatin chemotherapy regimen. (Courtesy Dr R. T. D. Oliver)

the report having survived for periods of between 2 and 18 years, and another had died of a cardiac infarct with no evidence of tumour after 7 years. All of these patients had histological seminomas, or mixed tumours containing seminoma, and all had been treated by radiotherapy. Nowadays they should be treated in the same way as metastasizing testicular tumours (*Figures 7.41 and 7.42*) (*see* Chapter 3).

References

ATKINSON, M., FERGUSON, R. and OGILVIE, A.L. (1979) Management of malignant dysphagia by intubation at endoscopy. *Journal of the Royal Society of Medicine*, **72**, 894–897

BATES, M., HURT, R.L., LEVISON, V.B. and SUTTON, M. (1974) Treatment of oat-cell carcinoma of bronchus by preoperative radiotherapy and surgery. *Lancet*, **1**, 1134–1135

BLANSHARD, G. (1955) The palliation of bronchial carcinoma by radiotherapy. *Lancet*, **2**, 897–901

BRACE, J.A., DAVY, T.J., SKEGGS, D.B.L. and WILLIAMS, H.S. (1981) Conformation therapy at the Royal Free Hospital. A progress report on the tracking cobalt project. *British Journal of Radiology*, **54**, 1068–1074

BRICK, I.B. (1955) Effect of million volt irradiation on the gastrointestinal tract. *Archives of Internal Medicine*, **96**, 26–31

CAMERON, S.J., GRANT, I.W.B., LUTZ, W. and PEARSON, J.G. (1969) The early effect of irradiation on ventilatory function in bronchial carcinoma. *Clinical Radiology*, **20**, 12–18

CAMERON, S.J., GRANT, I.W.B., PEARSON, J.G. and MARQUES, C. (1972) Prednisolone and mustine in prevention of tumour swelling during pulmonary irradiation. *British Medical Journal*, **1**, 535–537

CHAJEK, T. and FAINARU, M. (1973) Behcet's disease with decreased fibrinolysis and superior vena caval occlusion. *British Medical Journal*, **1**, 782–783

COX, J.D. (1975) Primary malignant germinal tumors of the mediastinum. A study of 24 cases. *Cancer*, **36**, 1162–1168

DEELEY, T.J. (1966) A clinical trial to compare two different tumour dose levels in the treatment of advanced carcinoma of the bronchus. *Clinical Radiology*, **17**, 199–301

DEELEY, T.J. and RICE EDWARDS, J.M. (1968) Radiotherapy in the management of cerebral secondaries from bronchial carcinoma. *Lancet*, **1**, 1209–1212

DOHERTY, M.A., McINTYRE, M. and ARNOTT, S.J. (1984) Oat-cell carcinoma of esophagus: a report of six British patients with a review of the literature. *International Journal of Radiation Oncology, Biology and Physics*, **10**, 147–152

DURRANT, K.R., BERRY, R.S., ELLIS, F., RIDEHALGH, F.R., BLACK, J.M. and HAMILTON, W.S. (1971) Comparison of treatment policies in inoperable bronchial carcinoma. *Lancet*, **1**, 715–719

EARLAM, R.J. and CUNHA-MELO, J.R. (1980) Oesophageal squamous-cell carcinoma. 1. A critical review of surgery, and 2. a critical review of radiotherapy. *British Journal of Surgery*, **67**, 318–390 and 457–461

FITZPATRICK, P.J. and RIDER, W.D. (1976) Half body radiotherapy. *International Journal of Radiation Oncology, Biology and Physics*, **1**, 197–207

FLEMING, J.S. and ORCHARD, P.G. (1974) Isocentric radiotherapy treatment planning where the treatment axis is not horizontal. *British Journal of Radiology*, **47**, 34–36

FOX, W. and SCADDING, J.G. (1973) Medical Research Council comparative trial of surgery and radiotherapy for primary treatment of small-celled or oat-celled carcinoma of bronchus. Ten-year follow-up. *Lancet*, **2**, 63–65

GEDDES, D.M. (1979) The natural history of lung cancer. A review based on rates of tumour growth. *British Journal of Diseases of the Chest*, **73**, 1–17

GINSBERG, R.J., HILL, L.D., EAGAN R.T. *et al.* (1983) Modern 30-day operative mortality for surgical resections in lung cancer. *Journal of Thoracic and Cardiovascular Surgery*, **86**, 654–658

GUTTMAN, R.J. (1965) Results of radiation therapy in patients with inoperable carcinoma of the lung whose status was established at exploratory thoracotomy. *American Journal of Roentgenology, Radium Therapy and Nuclear Medicine*, **93**, 99–103

HARE, E.S. (1838) Tumor involving certain nerves. *London Medical Gazette*, **23**, 16–18

HAVARD, C.W.H. and SCOTT, R.B. (1960) Thymic tumour and erythroblastic aplasia. Report of three cases and a review of the syndrome. *British Journal of Haematology*, **6**, 178–190

HETZEL, M.R., MILLARD, F.J.C., AYESH, R. *et al.* (1983) Laser treatment for carcinoma of the bronchus. *British Medical Journal*, **286**, 12–16

HILARIS, B.S., NORI, D., KWONG, E., KUTCHER, G.J. and MARTIN, N. (1984) Pleurectomy and intraoperative brachytherapy and postoperative radiation in the treatment of malignant pleural mesothelioma. *International Journal of Radiation Oncology, Biology and Physics*, **10**, 325–331

HOLOYE, P., LIBNOCH, J., COX, J. **et al.** (1984). Spinal cord metastasis in small-cell carcinoma of the lung. *International Journal of Radiation Oncology, Biology and Physics*, **10**, 349–356

HOPE-STONE, H.F. and KEY, J.J. (1961) Anticoagulant therapy in superior mediastinal obstruction. *British Medical Journal*, **2**, 1126–1128

JACKSON, D.V., RICHARDS, F., COOPER, M.R. *et al.* (1977) Prophylactic cranial irradiation in small-cell carcinoma of the lung. *Journal of the American Medical Association*, **237**, 2730–2733

JOHNSON, R.J.R., WALTON, R.J., LIM, M.L., ZYLAK, C.J. and PAINCHAUD, L.A. (1973) A randomized study on survival of bronchogenic carcinoma treated with conventional or short fractionation radiation. *Clinical Radiology*, **24**, 494–497

KAZEM, I., JONGERIUS, C.M., LAQUET, L.K., KRAMER, G. and HUYGEN, P.L.M. (1984) Evaluation of short course preoperative irradiation in the treatment of resectable bronchus carcinoma: long-term analysis of a randomized pilot-study. *International Journal of Radiation Oncology, Biology and Physics*, **10**, 981–985

LENNOX, S.C., FLAVELL, S.G., POLLOCK, D.J., THOMPSON, V.C. and WILKINS, J.L. (1968) Results of resection for oat-cell carcinoma of the lung. *Lancet*, **2**, 925–927

MANTELL, B.S. (1973) Superior sulcus (Pancoast) tumours: results of radiotherapy. *British Journal of Diseases of the Chest*, **67**, 315–318

MANTELL, B.S. (1982) Radiotherapy for dysphagia due to gastric carcinoma. *British Journal of Surgery*, **69**, 69–70

MEREDITH, W.J. and MASSEY, J.B. (1972) Patient dosage. In *Fundamental Physics of Radiology*, p.417. Bristol: John Wright and Sons Ltd

MORRIS, R.W. and ABADIR, R. (1979) Pancoast tumor: the value of high dose radiation therapy. *Radiology*, **132**, 717–719

MORRISON, R., DEELEY, T.J. and CLELAND, W.P. (1963) The treatment of carcinoma of the bronchus. A clinical trial to compare surgery and supervoltage radiotherapy. *Lancet*, **1**, 683–684

MUGGIA, F.M., BLUM, R.H. and FOREMAN, J.D. (1984) Role of chemotherapy in the treatment of lung cancer: evolving strategies for non-small cell histologies. *International Journal of Radiation Oncology, Biology and Physics*, **10**, 137–145

NUGENT, J.L., BUNN, P.A.Jr., MATTHEWS, M.J. *et al.* (1979) CNS metastases in small-cell bronchogenic carcinoma: increasing frequency and changing pattern with lengthening survival. *Cancer*, **44**, 1885–1893

PANCOAST, H.K. (1932) Superior pulmonary sulcus tumor characterised by pain, Horner's syndrome, destruction of bone and atrophy of hand muscles. *Journal of the American Medical Association*, **99**, 1391–1396

PARKES, W.R. (1973) Asbestos-related disorders. *British Journal of Diseases of the Chest*, **67**, 261–300

PATERSON, R. and RUSSELL, M.H. (1962) Clinical trials in malignant disease. Part IV — Lung cancer. Value of post-operative radiotherapy. *Clinical Radiology*, **13**, 141–144

PAULSON, D.L. (1975) Carcinomas in the superior pulmonary sulcus. *Journal of Thoracic and Cardiovascular Surgery*, **70**, 1095–1104

PEARSON, J.G. (1966) Radiotherapy of carcinoma of the oesophagus and post-cricoid region in South-east Scotland. *Clinical Radiology*, **17**, 242–257

PENN, C.R.H. and HOPE-STONE, H.F. (1972) The role of radiotherapy in the management of malignant thymoma. *British Journal of Surgery*, **59**, 533–539

RACHMANINOFF, N. and FENTRESS, V. (1964) Thymoma with metastasis to the brain. *American Journal of Clinical Pathology*, **41**, 618–625

ROWLANDSON, R. (1968) Results of treatment of pain down the arm associated with lung tumours. *British Journal of Diseases of the Chest*, **62**, 135–138

SAUNDERS, M.I., BENNETT, M.H., DISCHE, S. and ANDERSON, P.J. (1984) Primary tumor control after radiotherapy for carcinoma of the bronchus. *International Journal of Radiation Oncology, Biology and Physics*, **10**, 499–501

SHIELDS, T.W., HIGGINS, G.A., LAWTON R., HEILBRUNN, A. and KAHN, R.J. (1970) Preoperative X-ray therapy as an adjuvant in the treatment of bronchogenic carcinoma. *Journal of Thoracic and Cardiovascular Surgery*, **59**, 49–61

SKEGGS, D.B.L. (1968) Radiotherapy of thymic tumours in myasthenia gravis. *Proceedings of the Royal Society of Medicine*, **61**, 760–762

SMART, J. (1966) Can lung cancer be cured by irradiation alone? *Journal of the American Medical Association*, **195**, 1034–1035

SMART, J. and HILTON, G. (1956) Radiotherapy of cancer of the lung. Results in a selected group of cases. *Lancet*, **1**, 880–881

SOUHAMI, R.L., GEDDES, D.M., SPIRO, S.G. *et al.* (1984) Radiotherapy in small-cell cancer of the lung treated with combination chemotherapy: a controlled trial.

British Medical Journal, **288**, 1643–1646

SZUR, L. and BROMLEY, L.L. (1956) Obstruction of the superior vena cava in carcinoma of bronchus. *British Medical Journal*, **2**, 1273–1276

THOMSON, A.D. and THACKRAY, A.C. (1957) The histology of tumours of the thymus. *British Journal of Cancer*, **11**, 348

URTASUN, R.C., BELCH, A.R. and BODNAR, D. (1983) Hemibody radiation, an active therapeutic modality for the management of patients with small cell lung cancer. *International Journal of Radiation Oncology, Biology and Physics*, **9**, 1575–1578

URTASUN, R.C., BELCH, A.R., McKINNON, S., HIGGINS, E., SAUNDERS, W. and FELDSTEIN, M. (1982) Small-cell lung cancer: initial treatment with sequential hemibody irradiation vs. 3-drug systemic chemotherapy. *British Journal of Cancer*, **46**, 228–235

8

Hodgkin's disease and non-Hodgkin's lymphomas

A. M. Jelliffe

The lymphomas are tumours arising primarily from lymphatic tissue, most commonly lymph nodes, but also elsewhere in the body, particularly in those organs well endowed with lymphatic tissue, such as the alimentary canal. There is tremendous variation in their behaviour, prognosis and response to treatment. In general, the lymphomas are highly sensitive to ionizing irradiation, and many can be regarded as locally radiocurable.

Hodgkin's disease (HD) is often localized in extent and therefore is more often cured by irradiation, as was recognized in the publication of Gilbert (1939). Reports by Peters (1950), Nice and Stenstrom (1954), Jelliffe and Thomson (1955), Kaplan (1962), Easson and Russell (1963), Craver (1964), Jelliffe (1965) and others confirmed that up to about 40% of patients with clinically localized disease could survive for 10 or more years after irradiation. The cases included in these reports were investigated inadequately by modern standards, and it is now known that a large number of the failures were due to undetected widespread disease which received no irradiation.

As it became increasingly accepted that HD could be radiocurable, efforts were intensified to investigate the extent of the disease, culminating in the introduction of diagnostic laparotomy by Kaplan (Glatstein *et al.*, 1969). This obsession with the determination of the exact extent of the disease almost excluded interest in other factors which affect the natural history and thus the treatment of HD. An early concession to the importance of some of those other factors was made by Peters, who recognized that generalized symptoms impaired the prognosis. At Rye (Rosenberg, 1966) and Ann Arbor (Carbone *et al.*, 1971) symptoms worsening the prognosis were officially recognized by the inclusion of the symbol 'B' in the formal staging. More recently, attempts have been made to relate the treatment requirements not only to the anatomic extent of disease, but also to all the other many factors which are now recognized as being closely related to the activity of the disease, to the patient's reaction to it or to both (*see below*).

With non-Hodgkin's lymphoma (NHL), four out of five patients have widespread involvement of both lymph nodes and extranodal tissue when first seen, and for this reason radiotherapy alone is often assumed to be an ineffective method of treatment. With the accumulation of information it has become increasingly obvious that although most patients with NHL have generalized disease, many of those with localized disease can be controlled indefinitely with irradiation alone, and the patient regarded as cured. The recognition of this type of case has become increasingly important.

Radiotherapy in the treatment of lymphomas cannot be considered in isolation. In the following pages reference will also be made to those highly effective cytotoxic agents which may be used either in preference to, or in combination with irradiation, and to their place — as well as that of radiotherapy and surgery — in the management of this group of diseases.

Hodgkin's disease

General features

Hodgkin's disease is a malignant tumour of 'lymphoid' tissue, possibly arising from the histiocytic – monocytic cell population, but which is more often accepted today as originating from the T-type lymphocyte. Some of the features of the natural history of the different histological types of HD suggest that the term 'Hodgkin's disease' may embrace at least two totally different tumours which are dissimilar in their response to treatment and prognosis.

Many patients with HD have disease limited at its onset to lymph nodes. Extranodal involvement is uncommon in early cases but is frequent in generalized or relapsing disease. Painless lymph node enlargement occurs most commonly in the upper half of the body, particularly in the neck. This enlargement is usually described in standard text books of medicine as progressive, which is frequently inaccurate. One typical feature of HD is that in at least one-quarter of patients the disease waxes and wanes, producing intermittent systemic manifestations. This fluctuation varies from a small but measurable change to the complete disappearance of all disease, sometimes for up to several months. Such gross variation in size encourages the medical adviser to believe that the process is inflammatory, confirmed by its 'response' to the inevitable course of antibiotics. Presumably this variation in size is part of the 'intermittent syndrome' which includes periodic attacks of pyrexia, sweating, malaise, weight loss and anaemia, first referred to in 1887 by Pel and by Ebstein. Although HD presents most commonly in the neck, lymph node enlargement may be found anywhere in the body. The spleen and the liver may be palpable. Involvement of almost any structure in the body may occur with generalized or relapsing disease, but it is unusual for HD to appear to arise in *and* be localized to extranodal structures. The only organ which is almost never directly involved in the course of progressive HD is the central nervous system proper. It is common for extradural deposits to produce pressure on the spinal cord and infiltration of the cranial nerves at the base of the skull, but the disease is almost never found in the actual substance of the brain and spinal column.

Investigations frequently demonstrate HD in the mediastinum, which may enlarge to produce a huge mass, occupying one-half or more of the internal width of the thorax. It is always remarkable to see such a huge mass in a patient who is sometimes free from respiratory symptoms, but this can be explained on anatomical grounds. The largest mediastinal masses are anterior; in the past many of these cases were described as 'granulomatous thymomas'. In this position the mass will exert relatively little pressure on the main respiratory tract. Compression of the superior vena cava is rarely a presenting feature in HD.

Pulmonary involvement is seen most commonly as a streaky linear extension outwards from hilar lymph nodes, but discrete intrapulmonary opacities are not uncommon, varying in size and number from a fine miliary mottling, simulating tuberculosis, up to one or a few rounded masses which if single are almost always misdiagnosed as a primary lung cancer.

Liver involvement is usually patchy. Sometimes there are large discrete nodules. It is rarely of the generalized fine diffuse pattern seen commonly in grade 1 NHL. Jaundice may be produced by intrahepatic disease or by hilar node masses. It is very rare for jaundice to be caused by haemolysis unless there is associated hepatic dysfunction.

Bone involvement is uncommon in early cases. It has certain interesting features. Unlike most other cancers, bony deposits in HD are classically sclerotic, simulating those seen in prostatic cancer. Occasionally they are purely lytic, and sometimes they are mixed. Biopsy of these deposits may demonstrate the classical appearance of Hodgkin's disease, or more non-specific infiltration of lymphomatous small round cells. The present author has three patients presenting with biopsy proven 'small round cell' tumours of bone, all of whom were simultaneously or subsequently shown to have histologically confirmed HD. Contrary to generalized belief, bone involvement in HD is not necessarily associated with a bad prognosis. Long-term survival and sometimes cure may be achieved with suitable treatment.

Bone marrow infiltration is rarely demonstrated except in advanced cases, but anaemia is common in association with hypersplenism, haemolysis, thrombocytopenia, haemodilution or the cachexia associated with any advanced malignant disease. The presentation haemoglobin level can be related directly to the prognosis (MacLennan *et al.*, 1983), and is an important factor in the determination of the prognosis (*see below*).

The clinical picture may be complicated by metabolic abnormalities, of which the most common are hypercalcaemia and inappropriate antidiuretic hormone secretion. The nephrotic syndrome may be produced by tubular dysfunction associated with severe fluid retention. The process is reversible with control of the HD. Two little understood abnormalities which may be considered here are pruritus — which usually occurs in association with classical B symptoms — and alcohol pain, which can occur with localized disease, and is associated with nodular sclerotic HD.

The association of HD with systemic manifestations, referred to above, has been recognized since 1887. The precise relationship of these manifestations to the prognosis and treatment of HD was at first difficult to specify. Jelliffe and Thomson (1955) suggested that the presence of two or more 'systemic manifestations' placed patients in a poor prognosis group. Most of the 'systemic manifestations' referred to at that time were difficult to define and impossible to measure; some had a marked subjective element. For example, 'malaise' in Hodgkin's disease could quite reasonably be related to a patient's appreciation of his 'inevitably fatal' condition. The International (Ann Arbor) Classification (Carbone *et al.*, 1971) defined three B symptoms which are generally regarded as worsening the prognosis: pyrexia, night sweats and weight loss.

Histology

Hodgkin's disease characteristically shows complete replacement of involved lymph nodes with a pleiomorphic tissue. The characteristic Reed-Sternberg cells are multinucleate, but may be mononucleate. Variable numbers of other cells include neutrophils, plasma cells, lymphocytes, eosinophils, histocytes, fibroblasts and mature fibrous tissue. Since 1966 the morphological classification published by Lukes and Butler has been widely accepted.

Lymphocyte predominance (LP) is characterized by an infiltrate composed almost entirely of small lymphocytes with scanty Reed-Sternberg cells.

Nodular sclerosis (NS) shows well marked fibrosis, the node being subdivided by bands of fibrous tissue which may be so thick that they are clearly visible on naked eye examination of stained sections.

Mixed cellularity (MC) shows the typical features of 'average' HD: a uniform pleomorphic appearance without bands of fibrous tissue or an excess, or absence, of any of the characteristic cell types. This group is defined largely by exclusion. If a section shows no characteristic features of LP, NS or LD disease, then it will be classified as MC.

Lymphocyte depletion (LD), as originally described by Lukes and Butler, is rare. Its characteristic features include reticulum cell proliferation with a fine diffuse fibrosis, a large number of Reed-Sternberg cells, many of which show mitosis, and scanty lymphocytes.

The introduction of this new classification in 1966 was welcomed enthusiastically, as it appeared to provide a reliable new guide to prognosis. Certainly, when accurately defined as described originally by Lukes and Butler, LD HD carries an extremely bad prognosis. About 20% of patients with this form of HD survive 5 years. Fortunately, from the patient's viewpoint, this is a rare form of HD.

Unfortunately, from the scientific viewpoint, this small group is the only one in which the histological appearances could be related unequivocally to the prognosis. By far the commonest form of HD in Europe and North America is NS, in some reports up to 75% of cases, and many groups of workers have found very little difference between the long-term results of LP, NS and MC HD. The early experiences of the British National Lymphoma Investigation (BNLI) indicated that the prognosis of these three subgroups was similar (*Figure 8.1*). It began to appear that histology had little or no value in the management of HD, so much so that many centres questioned the need for anything more than a simple diagnosis of HD. At that time Bennett and colleagues reviewed all the sections from patients entered into the BNLI up to 1980. This required detailed re-examination of sections from 1500 patients, adhering strictly to the original criteria of the Lukes and Butler classification and, in addition, examining and classifying the nodal cellularity of NS cases according to their content of LP, MC and LD — a total of 1156 BNLI cases with NS HD. From this work, Bennett and colleagues have produced an easily reproducible method for subdividing patients with HD into those with low grade or with high grade malignancy, with a highly significant difference in prognosis (Bennett, Tu and Vaughan Hudson, 1981; Bennett *et al.*, 1983, 1985; MacLennan *et al.*, 1985). The histological appearance of HD is now of very great importance in its management and will be referred to again later (*Figure 8.2*).

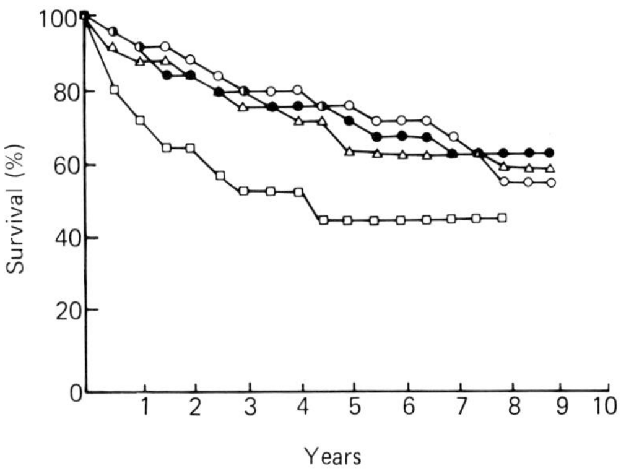

Figure 8.1 Survival of BNLI patients with Hodgkin's disease divided into four histological types, LP, NS, MC and LD (1979). There is no difference in survival between LP, NS or MC HD. ●LP (97) 8%; ○NS (841) 71%; △ MC (208) 17%; □ LD (43) 4%

Investigation

After a detailed clinical history and thorough clinical examination, the most important investigative procedure is the biopsy.

Biopsy

The importance of the initial biopsy in the management of all the lymphomas cannot be over-emphasized. Correct treatment is possible only if adequate biopsy is performed, preferably removing a whole node, or at least a large piece of a node. At this stage a needle biopsy is useless, and may be positively harmful. The interpretation of sections from a lymph node may be straightforward, but it can be extremely difficult, and the pattern of the node is an important feature. It is crucial to be sure of the initial diagnosis. The modern management of many lymphomas involves exceedingly powerful and potentially dangerous therapeutic regimens which must not be embarked on without absolute proof of the nature of the disease.

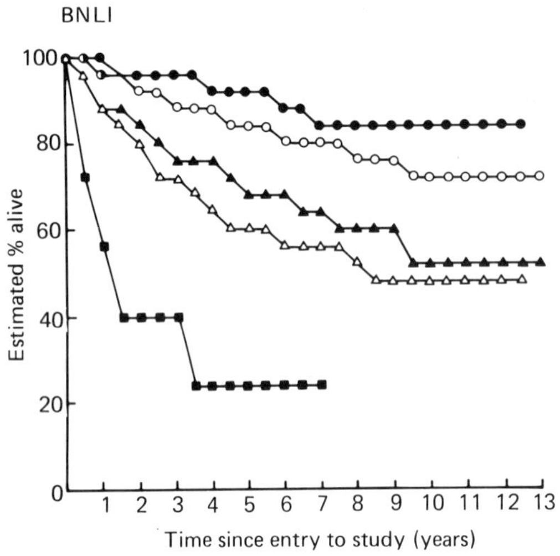

Figure 8.2 NS HD subdivided into grade 1 and grade 2. Survivals plotted with survival of LP, MC and LD HD. Patients with HD can now be divided into two major clear-cut categories. ●LP (71) 5%; ○NSI (829) 55% ▲ MC (249) 16.5%; △ NSII (329) 22%; ■ LD (22) 1.5%

Close cooperation between colleagues is essential. The best results are obtained when an adequate biopsy is despatched immediately by the surgeon to an experienced pathologist. Fresh unfixed specimens received in this way may be stained for surface markers which may help in establishing the final diagnosis. Spontaneous variation in the size of lymph nodes in HD has been referred to previously. When nodes wax and wane, an attempted biopsy at the wrong time may be useless. Occasionally nodes have shrunk so much that they cannot be found at operation. Sometimes previously enlarged nodes which are shrinking may be suitable for biopsy, but histological examination shows almost complete replacement by necrotic tissue surrounded by a thin rind of lymphoma cells which cannot be identified precisely. In such cases the most opportune moment for a node biopsy is when the nodes are enlarging, and a biopsy should then be embarked on as an emergency procedure.

Haematological investigations

A full blood count is essential in order to ensure safe treatment. In addition, the initial haemoglobin, total lymphocyte count and erythrocyte sedimentation rate (ESR) are important factors indicating the prognosis and probable treatment. Bone marrow examination after both aspirate and trephine rarely shows any infiltration with HD with clinically early disease, but should be carried out routinely because of the potential myelotoxicity of all effective treatment. Blood biochemical studies should include standard liver, kidney and bone investigations. In addition, there may be special abnormalities affecting calcium and salt and water metabolism.

Organ imaging

Posteroanterior and lateral chest X-ray

The value of this investigation has been recognized since the turn of the century. Its limitations have become more apparent with the introduction of the CT scan.

Lymphography

Until the early 1960s subdiaphragmatic extension of HD could be demonstrated reliably only by palpation. By modern standards, intra-abdominal HD could be diagnosed therefore only when massive disease was present. Before modern methods of organ imaging were available, the discovery of intra-abdominal HD was synonymous with a sentence of death, as was recognized in the staging classification used by some early workers (Jelliffe and Thomson, 1955).

The lymphogram was the first reliable, sensitive and humane method of demonstrating subdiaphragmatic disease while it was still limited in extent (Hreshehyshin, Sheehan and Holland, 1961). Its value in HD is because lymph node involvement is so often limited to the main central axis groups. Bipedal lymphography will fill only the iliac and para-aortic nodes up to the second lumbar vertebra, but fortunately other intra-abdominal lymph node groups, including the mesenteric, are not commonly involved in early HD. The most important limitation of the lymphogram was that it failed to visualize nodes between the body of L2 and the diaphragm. Many clinicians still regard the lymphogram as highly as the CT scan in the diagnosis of early retroperitoneal HD (Shiels *et al.*, 1984). The CT scan shows only the shape and size of the lymph node. The lymphogram shows shape, size and filling pattern.

Radioactive isotope scanning

Radioactive isotope scanning has not proven generally acceptable as a method of demonstrating lymph node involvement. Liver and spleen enlargement can be visualized, but involvement will be demonstrated only if relatively massive patchy HD is present. Radioactive isotope scanning of the skeleton is without any doubt the most sensitive method of detecting bony involvement at an early stage.

Ultrasound scanning

This is a relatively inexpensive method of detecting

abdominal lymph node involvement and measuring its response to treatment. However, this technique is highly dependent upon the expertise of the operator and is therefore likely to become of decreasing value as it is used more and more widely by diagnosticians whose work is not limited to ultrasound. Ultrasound is particularly useful in the examination of the liver. Bulky, localized HD infiltrating the liver can be detected by almost any modern organ imaging technique, but a fine diffuse lymphomatous infiltration may be demonstrable only by ultrasound.

CT scanning

CT scanning has greatly improved the accurate determination of the extent of HD in a way that is particularly satisfying to clinicians because of the anatomical nature of the demonstration. It is especially valuable in examining the anterior mediastinum and the retroperitoneal region. Responses to treatment are followed with greater confidence when accompanied by measurable improvement in lymph node masses.

Closed biopsy

Closed biopsy of many areas of the body, including the retroperitoneal region, has become a reliable confirmatory diagnostic procedure, usually under direct vision in combination with one of the newer imaging techniques described above. Reference has been made above to the limitations of needle biopsy as an initial diagnostic step. However, as an investigation of the extent of, or a recurrence of already histologically confirmed disease, it is becoming increasingly accepted.

Diagnostic laparotomy

Introduced by Kaplan in 1968 (Glatstein *et al.*, 1969), this procedure rapidly established itself as the only investigation which provided a 'true' picture of the extent of HD. It was accepted with tremendous enthusiasm because, at the time of its introduction, it appeared that long-term cure was only obtainable by radiotherapy, and for this to be effective treatment has to be given to all known sites of the disease. At the time of its introduction it was a bold and imaginative stride forward. Much new useful information was obtained on the natural history of HD and also on the accuracy of various tests including lymphography. Initially it appeared that because otherwise undiagnosable foci of disease were being demonstrated, the long-term results of treatment must be bettered. However, with the passage of time, it appears that in special cases a diagnostic laparotomy may offer immediate benefits which are related to more accurate determination of the extent of the disease, but that these are counterbalanced by operative morbidity and mortality and by future complications associated with removal of the spleen.

Long-term follow-up of laparotomized BNLI patients has shown an overall serious complication rate of about 8% of which at least one-half proves to be fatal. More recently, increasing interest has been focused on other factors influencing the prognosis in HD and of the interplay between these factors which are referred to later. By combining them in a Cox-type multifactorial analysis it is possible to prepare prognostic indices. The first groups of patients to be analysed in this way by the BNLI include all those presenting between 1970 and 1980 with clinical stage I, IIA (upper half) HD, whether or not they were subjected to laparotomy and the staging altered or left undisturbed (Haybittle *et al.*, 1975). Those patients found to have more extensive disease were treated with either total nodal irradiation or combination chemotherapy, and all others received relatively localized irradiation. All patients, none of whom had B symptoms, were analysed according to the age, sex, extent of disease (stage I or II), mediastinal involvement (of any type; non-bulky as well as bulky), histological grading, ESR, absolute lymphocyte count and laparotomy (*see below*).

This analysis showed that the factors which had a statistically significant effect on the prognosis included age, sex, ESR, mediastinal involvement and histological grading. Using these factors it was possible to prepare a prognostic index which related to survival. With this index it is possible to divide stage I, IIA patients into three groups. In the first group with low grade disease, subdiaphragmatic spread is unlikely, but in the event of it occurring it will develop slowly and will respond well to chemotherapy. A diagnostic laparotomy is unnecessary. In the third group with most active disease, occult subdiaphragmatic spread is likely to be present initially or will occur later, and is likely to be aggresive. In addition, many grade 2 NS HD relapse at the irradiation site and chemotherapy becomes necessary. Primary treatment should probably be with the chemotherapy, and a laparotomy is meddlesome medicine.

There remains a middle group in which a laparotomy may sometimes be helpful. For example, a young person in this group with asymptomatic limited upper half HD may be found to have an equivocal lymphogram for which the radiologist recommends a repeat in 6 months. The patient prefers to avoid cytotoxic drugs with the risk of reproductive organ damage. A laparotomy may provide more concrete evidence of the extent of the disease, allowing a more balanced therapeutic approach. It goes without saying that this procedure must be carried out in a centre of excellence by an experienced surgeon with the support of an excellent pathology team, so that risks can be reduced to a minimum and misinterpretation avoided.

An additional possible advantage of a staging laparotomy is that it allows an oophoropexy (Trueblood *et al.*, 1970). At operation, the ovaries can be transposed either to the midline or laterally over the ilium where they can be marked with metal clips and shielded with lead blocks from any subsequent irradiation. However, more recently it has been reported that even after oophoropexy ovarian function can be damaged by pelvic irradiation, and the procedure appears to be of limited value (Glees *et al.*, 1982).

Staging laparotomy has little or no place in patients with more advanced disease or with B symptoms. B symptoms are most rapidly relieved by cytotoxic drugs and stage IV cases cannot be managed by radiotherapy. There may be a place for total nodal irradiation in patients shown to have stage IIIA disease with a negative spleen, but the results of treatment with cytotoxic drugs are equally good, and in general it seems unreasonable to advise laparotomy in clinical stage III cases in order to determine whether or not the spleen is involved. More than three out of five cases with stage IIIA HD do have splenic infiltration and will need cytotoxic drugs.

Staging laparotomy will probably continue for a while, especially at centres of great expertise, but the indications for its use have become increasingly restricted. In the future it is likely to disappear completely as a diagnostic procedure, except in special circumstances such as those indicated above (Jelliffe and Vaughan Hudson, 1985). If prognostic indices can predict the natural history of cases of HD reliably, staging laparotomy will eventually disappear. However, at present prognostic indices are of unproven value in forecasting the future. The BNLI is currently carrying out a prospective study of stage I, IIA HD with the aim of evaluating the BNLI prognostic index.

Factors influencing the prognosis

Staging

The staging of most forms of cancer has been in vogue for many years, and continues to enjoy scientific support in spite of some of its serious limitations. When applied to widespread tumours which are to be treated with cytotoxic drugs, staging can be misleading, because it may provide no real idea of the total tumour burden which is present. For example, with HD the present author recalls two patients who, after laparotomy, had stage IIIA disease; both were males in their twenties and were entirely similar regarding all other factors known to affect the prognosis. One died less than 3 years after diagnosis, and the other is in rude health, married with three children, coping with an important job in industry 14 years since he was first seen. The second patient had disease apparently arising in one epitrochlear node with involvement of one ipsilateral axillary node. Two minute nodules were discovered in the spleen after painstaking examination. The first patient had palpable nodes in every region of the body. X-ray examination showed gross involvement of the mediastinum and para-aortic regions, and the spleen was almost replaced by HD.

The currently accepted Ann Arbor classification is as follows:

Stage I

Involvement of a single lymph node region or of a single extralymphatic site (IE), above or below the diaphragm.

Stage II

Involvement of two or more lymph node regions above or below the diaphragm. Localized involvement of one extralymphatic site may be included as one of the two (or more) regions (IIE).

Stage III

Involvement of lymph node regions above and below the diaphragm. Localized involvement of one extralymphatic site may be included as one of the regions (IIIE).

Stage IV

Diffuse or disseminated involvement of one or more extralymphatic sites, usually associated with obvious nodal involvement.

For the purpose of this classification, both the spleen and Waldeyer's ring are included as lymph node regions. Patients with any of the significant symptoms of pyrexia, night sweats and weight loss of 10% or more are indicated by the symbol B, and those without symptoms by the symbol A.

After the introduction of the staging laparotomy (Glatstein *et al.*, 1969), it became apparent that the presumed diagnosis of freedom from involvement, or involvement of, some regions and organs by HD as established clinically or by organ imaging could not always be confirmed histologically. It was therefore impossible to make direct comparison between non-laparotomized and laparotomized patients. Because of this a comparable pathological staging evolved, which included symbols in all cases referring to the involvement or not of organs examined histologically after the laparotomy. Thus, before a diagnostic laparotomy a patient might be staged as CSIIAE with HD apparently limited to the neck and mediastinum with extension into the immediately adjacent lung parenchyma. After laparotomy, the staging might be altered to PS IV AE N+S+H+M− because of histological evidence of involvement of the spleen and liver but not the bone marrow.

There is no doubt that staging provides important information relating to the prognosis and treatment. When radiotherapy was the only hope of cure, patients with widespread disease almost inevitably died, although this event could be postponed for years if the disease was indolent. Apparently localized HD could be cured in up to one-half of cases given adequate irradiation. The introduction of highly effective chemotherapy with its potential of curing generalized HD has changed our entire approach to this illness, and the picture has been complicated further by the realization of the potential dangers of modern high-dose irradiation and of combination chemotherapy, particularly when used sequentially, which are becoming increasingly obvious with time. There are now many other well recognized factors which are at least as important as staging in the prognosis and treatment of HD, which provide accurate indications of the activity and intensity of the disease and of the response and defences of the patient.

Factors influencing prognosis other than staging

Sex

The effect of sex on survival has been known for many years (Peters, 1950; Jelliffe and Thomson, 1955; Kaplan, 1972). More recently an analysis of more than 1500 BNLI cases has confirmed that there is a small overall difference in survival in favour of females over a 10-year period.

Age

Age has an important influence on survival. Up to the age of 50 there is a slow but perceptible reduction in prognosis. After 50 survival falls rapidly, and this fall is much greater than can be attributed to normal ageing. Age is a major factor influencing the prognosis (Vaughan Hudson *et al.*, 1983).

Histology

The importance of the histological picture was briefly referred to earlier. Until recently, the morphology of the node was considered by many to be almost unrelated to the prognosis. Since 1980 the work of Bennett and colleagues has completely changed this situation (Bennett *et al.*, 1985), so much so that any publication related to almost any aspect of the treatment of HD is virtually valueless unless due consideration is given to the exact morphological type of the HD under discussion. The most important point made by Bennett and colleagues is the recognition of nodular sclerotic grade 2 HD. In spite of the feeling that the 'classical' classification of HD is of little value as a prognostic indicator, it is still generally considered that the prognosis of nodular sclerotic HD ought to be good. Unexpected failure to control such a curable disease therefore has to be explained in a rational way. Perhaps the radiotherapy plan (carried out by a very good but rather junior registrar) was suspect? Could the failure be attributed to 'bulk disease'? Was the physicist in error? Perhaps the machine required recalibration? A witch hunt can be avoided, and a rational explanation discovered for many radiation failures by a careful re-examination of the nodal cellularity of NS cases.

The special clinical characteristics of NS grade 2 were recently described at a meeting of the Radiology Section of the Royal Society of Medicine (Jelliffe, 1983). During an analysis of 412 BNLI cases with stage I, IIA (upper half) disease, the disease extent having been confirmed by laparotomy, patients were divided into four main morphological groups, LP, NS1,NS2 and MC.There was a marked difference between the groups in their initial response to radiotherapy and in the possibility of later relapse at the irradiation site. The following summarized the characteristic features of the four subgroups in their local response to radiotherapy:

LP	Complete response:all cases	Local relapse: 3%
NS1	Complete response:almost all cases	Local relapse: 8%
NS2	Complete response:87%	Local relapse:18%
MC	Complete response:almost all cases	Local relapse: 5%

All cases have been followed-up since this report. The latest total figure of radiotherapy failure (failure to achieve complete response and relapse at radiotherapy site) with NS2 is 25%.

B symptoms and the ESR

The three B symptoms which the Ann Arbor meeting accepted as being indicative of a poor prognosis were otherwise unexplained pyrexia, night sweats and 10% weight loss. These symptoms have been accepted for many years as harbingers of evil. Many clinicians in the past accepted that it was infinitely better to have stage IIIA HD than stage IIB disease. Effective chemotherapy has improved both symptomatic relief and the possibility of cure. There is an association of B symptoms with NS2 HD which can be remorseless in its progress.

B symptoms are, of course, entirely non-specific. Identical symptoms can be produced by a multitude of disease processes. The ESR is a similar totally non-specific manifestation of illness, and a raised ESR can best be considered in the context of HD as a measurable B symptom, to which it has a similar significance. In the presence of other B symptoms it is of no prognostic value, but in the absence of other systemic manifestations it is by itself of serious import (*Figure 8.3*).

Total lymphocyte count

It has been recognized that patients with HD may present with a blood lymphocytopenia (Bunting, 1914; Aisenburg, 1965; Brown *et al.*, 1967) and reports including small numbers of patients have been published relating a poor prognosis to lym-

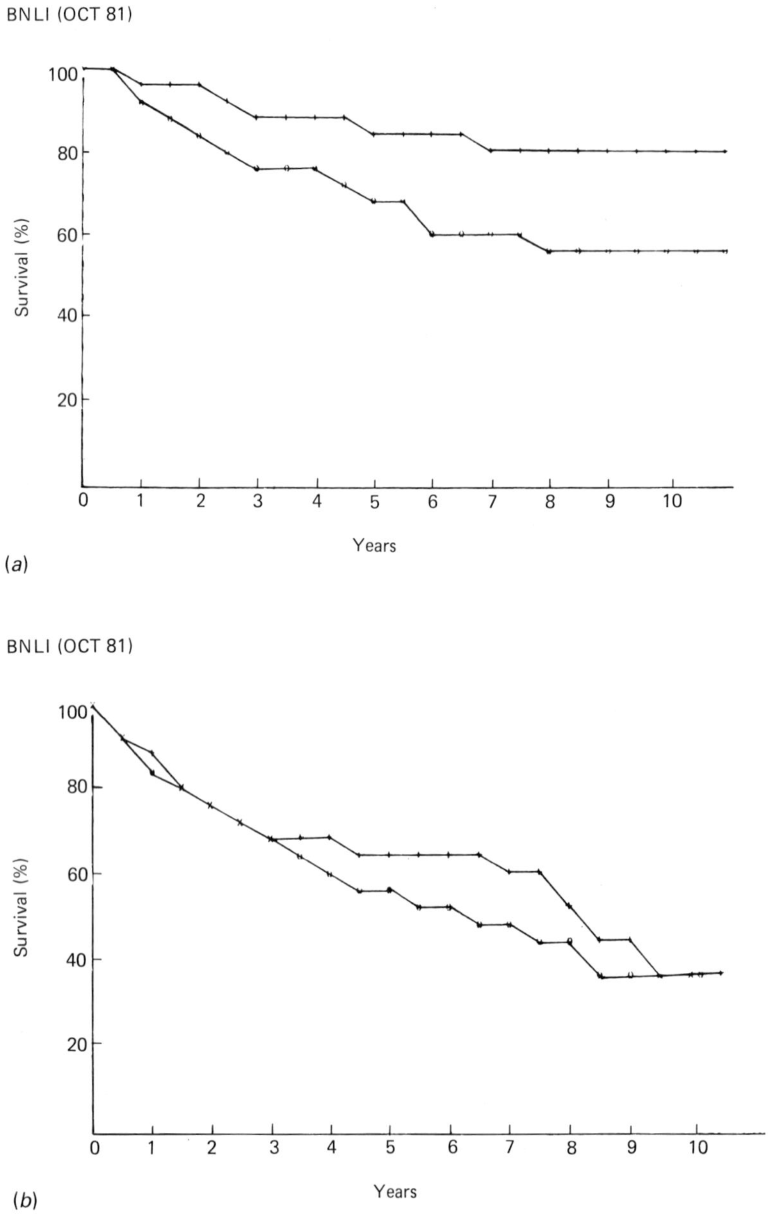

Figure 8.3 (*a*) The importance of the ESR in 'A' patients. +++ ESR under 40 (605); ooo ESR over 40 (192). (*b*) With 'B' symptoms the ESR is of no significance. +++ ESR under 40 (129); ooo ESR over 40 (273)

phocytopenia. The BNLI published a report on 1100 patients followed for up to 10 years, relating the presence of B symptoms and the prognosis to the initial total lymphocyte count. This report shows that there is an inverse relationship between the total lymphocyte count and the occurrence of systemic symptoms. An abnormal lymphocyte count affects the prognosis adversely (MacLennan *et al.*, 1981). This factor is a particularly useful indicator in widespread disease, in all morphological subgroups except NS.

Haemoglobin level

It has been suggested for many years that patients with HD who present with an anaemia have a poor prognosis (Jelliffe and Thomson, 1965; Westling, 1965; Tubiana *et al.*, 1971; Lee and Sprat, 1974). Until recently there have been no reports relating presenting anaemia to the prognosis in each anatomical stage. A report on 1103 patients in the BNLI was recently analysed and the presentation haemoglobin related to the anatomical stage, morphological subtype and the presence of B symptoms (MacLennan *et al.*, 1983). This analysis shows that a low haemoglobin is related to more advanced disease, aggressive histological subtypes and B symptoms, and a markedly decreased survival rate.

Treatment

Radiotherapy

Since the turn of the century it had been hinted that HD might be a radiocurable condition (Pusey, 1902), but the first really convincing publication was that of Gilbert (1939). His results were disregarded by the medical profession as a whole, who continued to regard HD as a death sentence until the 1970s, in spite of optimistic reports by Peters (1950), Jelliffe and Thomson (1955), Kaplan (1962), Easson and Russell (1963) and others. The outcome of the management of a pessimistic patient by a despondent doctor requires little imagination.

Retrospectively, it is now quite clear that by the 1950s at the latest there was incontrovertible proof that many patients with HD could be cured by radioerapy. Once it is accepted that HD is curable by irradiation, two questions require an answer: what is the optimum dose? and what is the optimum extent of treatment?

Treatment dose

It must be remembered that the roentgen was only accepted generally as a reliable unit of measurement in therapy by the early 1930s, so many early reports are not quantitively acceptable. Early publications (Jelliffe and Thomson, 1955; Jelliffe 1965) indicated that the best prospects for the local cure of HD followed a dose of 3500–4000 cGy (rads) in 3–4 weeks usually with daily fractions. A smaller dose could control HD completely, but did so less frequently. Kaplan (1966) reviewed his own cases and those in the literature, and prepared an elegant graph which is accepted as the ultimate statement on the subject. Today it is recognized that there are other important factors apart from dose which affect the radiocurability of HD, especially the histological subtype NS2. However, the general principles that this graph demonstrates remain valid. It shows that the prospect of local control of HD improves in a linear fashion. Irradiation achieves a 95% local cure rate with 4000 cGy and 100% with 4400 cGy. It is worth noting that this second dose is just above the tolerance of some normal tissues. Using this dose to the mediastinum there is a small but definite risk of late spinal cord damage, and many radiotherapists prefer to limit the dose to the cord to 3000 cGy. It is also worth noting that failure to reach the 4000 cGy level is not synonymous with treatment failure; it is simply that the probability of cure is reduced. Rarely, irradiation produces disastrous symptoms. In these circumstances, the total dose can be reduced or the overall treatment prolonged. A fit patient achieving 3500 cGy is preferable to a desperately sick person 'successfully' treated to the full textbook dose. The present author's experience includes several patients who received treatment to a less than optimum dose due to extreme intolerance, and who have survived disease free for many years and are presumably cured. Fortunately, HD is often remarkably radiosensitive.

Extent of treatment

The curative effects of irradiation are due to the direct action on tissues involved by HD. If irradiation is the accepted treatment, the fields used must encompass all the tumour-bearing volume. As it became accepted that HD responded well to irradiation, attempts were made to give prophylactic, extended field or — as it is known nowadays — adjuvant irradiation (Gilbert, 1939, Kaplan, 1962). The logical reason for this before the 1950s was the appreciation that it was not then possible to demonstrate occult disease, especially below the diaphragm. If prophylactic irradiation was given to areas of probable lymph node involvement before they became clinically apparent, many more patients might be cured. The publications of Peters (Peters, 1950; Peters and Middlemiss, 1958) which reported excellent results, attributed much of this improvement to the use of prophylactic irradiation to all the main node groups of the body. Peters' results were the best in the world at that time, but with hindsight it is unlikely that the small doses used for prophylaxis provided much benefit. Her excellent results were almost certainly due to energetic and meticulous irradiation delivered to and around the demonstrated tumour sites.

The first workers really to investigate the value of high dose adjuvant irradiation were Kaplan and his colleagues (1962) who commenced a series of studies comparing local with wider field irradiation. His early work was carried out after the introduction of the lymphogram and, in 1968, the Stanford School commenced investigating the staging laparotomy as the ultimate method of demonstrating the extent of the disease process. By the early 1970s it had become accepted that the only logical approach to the management of HD lay in full investigation of all possible areas of disease, followed by irradiation to all involved areas. Chemotherapy was also coming to be accepted as an effective treatment method. In certain cases where the prognosis was regarded as bad, for example with extensive disease in the spleen, combination chemotherapy was added to the irradiation, and by the 1970s no patient was considered for local irradiation alone. The minimal treatment recommended by the Stanford team was total nodal irradiation, even when the disease was shown by full investigation — including a staging laparotomy — to involve only one region.

The BNLI was not convinced that there was a need for such wide field treatment when the disease could be demonstrated to be limited in extent. Early workers had reported up to 40% survival 5–10 years after localized irradiation in clinically localized disease (Jelliffe, 1965; Hope-Stone, 1969; Hope-Stone, 1981). The demonstration by modern investigations of occult disease below the diaphragm, especially in the spleen, in about 40% of patients with clinically 'early' disease provided an explanation for the failure of local treatment to control the disease in many patients. In 1970 the BNLI commenced a prospective randomized study of stage I, IIA cases comparing the irradiation of locally involved regions only with local and prophylactic (extended field) irradiation. In the upper half the body, prophylactic irradiation usually involved the use of a full mantle field. Regions with known disease were given 4000 cGy in 4 weeks and adjacent, prophylactically irradiated regions received 3500 cGy over the same time period.

The 10-year results of this study were reported in 1981 by Hope-Stone. At that time it included 356 patients with stage I, IIA (upper half) HD who had had a diagnostic laparotomy and 215 who had not. In the laparotomized group, 90% of patients achieved a 10-year survival, and there was no difference in survival between patients treated initially with either local or prophylactic irradiation. In the non-laparotomized group, the 10-year survival rate was 75%, once again with no difference between the two subgroups. At that time it was believed that this suggested that laparotomy might improve the prognosis. It is now clear that the apparent improvement associated with laparotomy was due largely to case selection, the non-laparotomized group containing a larger number of patients with bad prognostic indicators. This study indicated that the long-term survival was not improved by prophylactic as opposed to local irradiation. It is interesting to note that Kaplan's early series comparing local with total nodal irradiation also showed no long-term difference in survival between the two groups (Rosenberg and Kaplan, 1970; Glatstein, 1977). Although survival is the same after local or prophylactic irradiation, patients treated locally have a 10% initial relapse rate in an adjacent area which would have been included if mantle type irradiation had been used. However, this type of relapse is almost always curable, often with further local irradiation.

Relapse may need combination chemotherapy. The risk of leukaemogenesis after combination chemotherapy, especially after wide field irradiation, is well documented (Papa *et al.*, 1984). BNLI protocols have avoided wide field irradiation as far as possible. This may be one of the reasons why the BNLI has records of only 11 patients in a total of about 1000 at risk who have developed leukaemia or a second lymphoma.

Mantle field irradiation has been well established for many years (Kaplan, 1972; Peckham, McElwain and Barrett, 1982). The mantle field advocated by the BNLI is shown in *Figure 8.4*. Local field irradiation includes the whole of the affected region, and may extend either 5 cm or one-third into neighbouring regions to cover any undetected spread along anatomical lines.

HD is rarely localized to the lower half of the body. During the same 10-year period (1970–1980) while 571 patients with upper half stage I, IIA were entered into studies, the BNLI recorded 53 patients with lower half I, IIA HD. This number is too small for statistical analysis. The overall 10-year survival rate of the 53 cases was 86%. Splenic involvement was found in five of the 31 laparotomized patients, a frequency less than in upper half disease.

With stage IIIA disease there is every reason to consider total nodal irradiation as advocated originally by Kaplan for HD involving lymph nodes in the upper and lower halves of the body (*Figure 8.5*). This technique is safe, and was originally considered by the BNLI to be generally more effective than chemotherapy. In a report in 1976 (BNLI Report no. 3) of a randomized comparison of total nodal irradiation with MOPP (mustine, vincristine, procarbazine and prednisone) in stage IIIA laparotomized patients, there was a 90% 4-year survival rate in both arms of the study. Relapse in either group was salvaged efficiently by either radiotherapy or chemotherapy as indicated. However, the BNLI recommended total nodal irradiation as the initial treatment of choice because it had a complete remission rate of 95% as opposed to one of 75% with MOPP.

When this study was first reported the total number of patients included was only 81. Forty-two were treated by total nodal irradiation after a laparotomy, and at that time the number was too small to indicate whether or not splenic involvement affected the prognosis. Up to August 1979 the BNLI accrued a total of 108 cases of stage IIIA HD treated with total nodal irradiation after laparotomy. Examination of this larger number showed that the 9-year survival rate was 75% whether or not the spleen was involved. But the relapse-free survival rate was very different. With the 27 patients without splenic

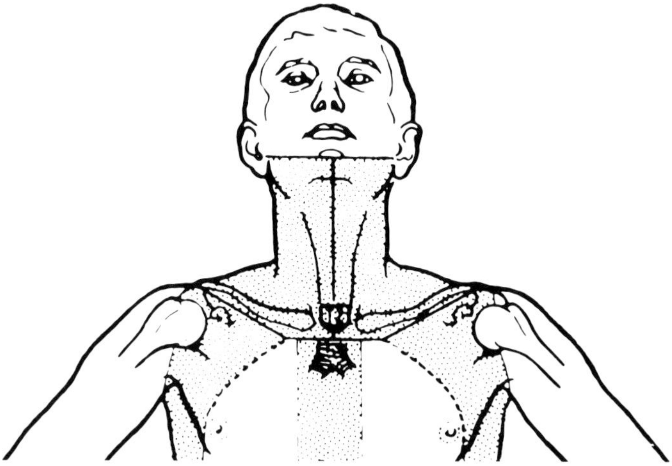

Figure 8.4 Distribution of irradiation in typical mantle field. Mediastinal field is taken down to D10 and the width is at least 8 cm

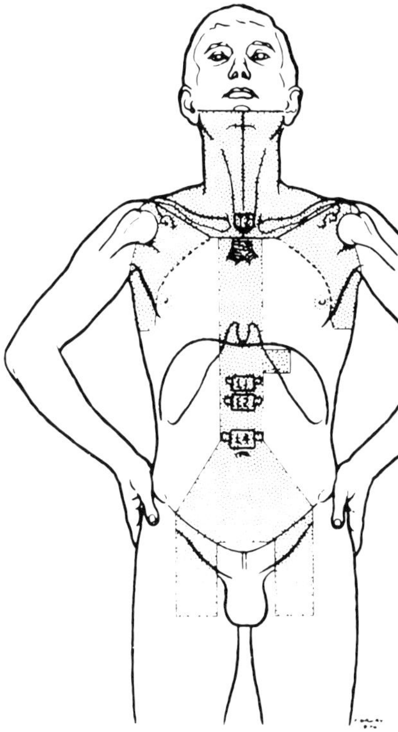

Figure 8.5 Distribution of irradiation total nodal irradiation. The spleen has been removed in this figure but irradiation is given to the splenic ligament. Normally the area is divided at about the level of the diaphragm or at L2 and the upper half is usually irradiated first. The second half is irradiated after an interval of about 4 weeks

involvement only 5% required salvage therapy with MOPP. With the 81 patients with splenic involvement relapse requiring MOPP occurred in 40% (Worthy, 1981). Patients receiving total nodal irradiation and combination chemotherapy, as opposed to more localized radiotherapy, are well known to be potential candidates for leukaemia. The BNLI now believes that total nodal irradiation should not be used as initial treatment for stage IIIA HD unless it is known that the spleen is free of disease. Because the spleen is so frequently involved it is a moot point as to whether or not laparotomy and splenectomy are justified to determine if total nodal irradiation can be given with a reasonable chance of long-term relapse-free survival.

Radiation techniques

From the technical point of view, the irradiation of localized HD has been simplified by the introduction of megavoltage units which have a relatively sharply defined beam edge and allow the treatment of mediastinal, neck and axillary nodes *en bloc*. Unfortunately, the shape of the thorax makes it extremely difficult to achieve uniform irradiation of main lymph nodes in the upper half of the body. The aim is a dose of 4000 cGy (according to Kaplan, 4400 cGy) throughout all the known tumour bearing sites and 3500 cGy to non-involved adjacent sites. This is usually effected by using two opposing fields shaped with lead blocks to protect the lungs creating the well known mantle field (Kaplan, 1972; Peckham, McElwain and Barrett, 1982). Unfortunately, it may be unsafe to expose the whole length of the cervical and thoracic cord to this dose of irradiation. The most common practice is to protect the spinal cord with a posterior lead strip commencing halfway through the course at the 2000 cGy level. On completion of the full course the spinal cord will have received a total maximum dose of 3000 cGy in 4 weeks which is well below the level of tolerance. Unfortunately, this shielding will also protect the centre of the mediastinum which is commonly involved by HD. A possible compromise is to treat mainly from the anterior field adding a posterior field with spinal cord shielding only when spinal cord tolerance has been recorded. This is a logical approach in patients with disease localized mainly to the anterior half of the thorax. Obviously this will lead to a higher dose to the myocardium and pericardium (Stewart *et al.*, 1967). The relative dangers of underdosing the tumour or overdosing the spinal cord or pericardium have to be considered in each individual. When the patient is slim and the disease is entirely limited to the front half of the chest, irradiation mainly from the front may offer advantages. With a more thick-set patient and more centrally placed disease it would be more logical to treat with two equally weighted opposed fields, and this latter technique is the one more commonly used. As well as protecting the lungs and spinal cord, allowance has to be made for variation in the source-skin distance in the different parts of the thorax. The axillary nodes will receive 10-15% more and the cervical nodes 15-20% more than the mediastinum, because of the relative thinness of the neck and axilla. Correction for this difference can be made either by using a compensating filter mounted on the treatment head or by reducing the field size on one occasion each week so that the axillae and neck receive the same total dose as the mediastinum.

Mantle

Treatment is normally given with the patient supine and prone. The hands are placed on the hips and the scapulae are rotated laterally to bring the lymph nodes along the lateral borders well into the axillary treatment fields. The neck is fully extended so that the upper edge of the field can pass from the tip of the extended chin backwards to the occiput. Assuming that there is no evidence of parenchymal infiltration, the lungs are protected by blocks which are shaped so that any central node mass is totally encompassed by the irradiation field. If there is no visible node mass a mediastinal field 8 cm wide is adequate. The upper border of the protecting lead blocks runs opposite the lower border of the fourth rib posteriorly and the lateral chest wall below the lower end of the scapula is shielded. The lower edge of the mediastinal field will extend down to the tenth to eleventh intervertebral disc, unless extensive mediastinal disease makes it necessary to extend this field further downwards.

Planning is best carried out on a simulator using the same focal skin distance as will be used for treatment. When the treatment field and areas to be leaded off have been decided, prone and supine simulator radiographs are taken. The field that is to be shielded is drawn on these films and an equivalent shape is cut in an expanded polystyrene block using a hot wire fixed at an equivalent point as the focal spot of the treatment machine. The gaps in the polystyrene block are then filled with a suitable molten alloy and the correctness of their position verified by further check films, taken on the megavoltage machine itself.

Inverted Y

Patients with limited disease below the diaphragm may be treated with this technique which involves similar steps to those taken with upper half disease. Normally, the upper border of this field corresponds to the lower border of the mantle field and the irradiation field is shaped similarly by lead blocks to cover the para-aortic, iliac and inguinal nodes. For obvious reasons, cord protection below L2 can be ignored. The position of the kidneys must be established and shielded, and if an oophoropexy has been carried out previously the ovaries must be protected with appropriate lead blocks. The dose received by the para-aortic and iliac nodes is reasonably uniform, but the inguinal nodes receive about 15% more.

Total nodal irradiation

A combination of mantle and inverted-Y fields offers an excellent method of irradiating all the main axis lymph nodes, for example in patients with stage IIIA disease without splenic involvement. The main technique is exactly as described for each half separately with the additional complication of avoiding a dangerously high dose overlap on the spinal cord at the junction of the upper and lower half field, while attempting to avoid underdosing any lymph nodes at this point. The gap between the two fields must be calculated in each case in such a way that the physical edges of the diverging fields do not overlap, producing a higher than acceptable spinal cord dose. In some centres the possibility of overlap on the spinal cord is avoided by taking the lower edge of the mantle down to the second lumbar vertebrae. This has the disadvantage of making the mantle much larger than the inverted Y, but eliminates any risk of late spinal cord damage.

Prophylactic (extended field) versus local (involved field) irradiation

Randomized trials comparing these two techniques in stage I, IIA HD have been carried out since the 1960s (Kaplan and Rosenburg, 1966; Collaborative Study, 1976; Hope-Stone, 1981). All these reported studies indicate that the relapse rate is higher in those patients treated locally, but that the long-term survival rate is the same in both groups. The approach that is chosen by the clinician is therefore a matter of personal opinion. However, the use of the BNLI prognostic index may make this choice more scientific. There seems to be no doubt that stage IA patients with a good prognostic index can be cured with local irradiation, without a previous laparotomy. The present BNLI studies prospectively evaluating this prognostic index may demonstrate that patients with more extensive disease and a poor prognostic index are better off with prophylactic irradiation of the mantle type.

Irradiation of Hodgkin's disease at special sites

Although Hodgkin's disease usually presents with enlarged lymph nodes, occasionally it appears to originate in an extranodal organ, when it is diagnosed usually only after histological examination of biopsied material. The infrequency of this occurrence is in sharp contradistinction with NHL. The management of HD presenting extranodally is dependent upon its extent and upon the presence of various factors influencing the prognosis. More commonly, extranodal involvement is usually discovered to be one part of widespread disease.

When the disease is apparently limited to one particular site, radical treatment should be given, in an attempt to cure the patient. The relative radiosensitivity of HD makes this worthwhile even when the local disease is extensive. The treatment aim should be 4000 cGy in 4 weeks shielding off any specially sensitive organs such as the kidneys. Obviously shielding of a relatively radiosensitive organ such as the kidney implies that the patient will probably survive for long enough to develop postradiation complications.

Head and neck

Hodgkin's disease rarely presents in Waldeyer's ring. When the disease is apparently limited in extent it is customary to irradiate either using a full mantle or with more local fields encompassing only the neck. With either technique, the treatment must be taken up to include, if necessary, the whole of the pharynx to the skull base and the highest cervical nodes. It is extremely debilitating, and the patient may suffer for many months from anorexia, dysphagia associated with dry mucous membranes and loss of taste.

Stomach and large bowel

Hodgkin's disease rarely presents in the alimentary canal, but involvement may occur as a late manifestation, often associated with recurrent disease in the para-aortic nodes. Unless precluded by previous heavy irradiation to the same site, the most effective local treatment is provided by local radiotherapy. Bleeding and abdominal pain can be rapidly controlled. Obviously the long-term value of such treatment depends upon the extent of the disease elsewhere.

Central nervous system

Hodgkin's disease almost never develops inside the central nervous system proper. It is a good working rule automatically to look elsewhere for a primary site when a patient with known HD develops clinical manifestations suggesting multiple intracranial deposits.

However, central nervous system symptoms are common, due to invasion of the meninges, most often with extradural deposits which may produce spinal cord compression. The symptomatology of extranodal spinal cord compression varies considerably according to the speed with which pressure builds up and whether or not this pressure occludes a penetrating branch of the spinal artery. These vessels are end arteries and their occlusion is followed by cord infarction. Weakness is usually, but not always, preceded by pain radiating round from the affected segment of the cord which is most commonly lower dorsal or upper lumbar.

Paralysis progressing rapidly, reaching total paraplegia over a few hours, is always due to spinal artery compression, and changes of this type will not be improved by treatment. The slow development of weakness of both legs, with or without anaesthesia below the level of the lesion and associated bladder symptoms is highly suggestive of an extradural deposit of HD which is eminently treatable. The radiosensitivity of HD is such that irradition alone is capable of reversing the process, but immediate surgical decompression has certain advantages. First, the pressure on the cord is relieved immediately. Second, the procedure allows histological confirmation of the diagnosis. It is important to exclude other primary tumours for which different treatments may be preferable (*see* Chapter 15).

When managing such a patient presenting with weakness of the legs, the diagnosis must be confirmed by myelography. This also provides exact localization of the deposit. The next step is urgent surgical decompression. It is unusual for all the tumour to be removed at operation, and postoperative irradiation will be necessary. This treatment is normally commenced immediately after the removal of stitches. A single field, extending about 5 cm above and below the level of the extradural deposit, provides adequate irradiation. The usual dose is 3000–3500 cGy over 4 weeks, treating 5 days each week.

Although this is usually one manifestation of generalized disease, occasionally it is impossible to demonstrate HD elsewhere, and treatment may then be followed by cure. Presumably the HD originated in adjacent high retroperitoneal lymph nodes and then spread directly backwards into the extradural region. Primary lymphoma of the brain, 'microgliomatosis', is discussed in Chapter 15.

Chemotherapy

Investigation of the use of combination chemotherapy in the management of Hodgkin's disease commenced at the NCI in 1963. The combination of nitrogen mustard, vincristine, procarbazine and prednisone, known as MOPP, was introduced in 1964, and by 1970 it had become established as an effective form of treatment by De Vita, Serpick and Carbone (1970) whose results have never been bettered (Jelliffe, 1979). After various studies using radiotherapy, the BNLI has accepted that combination chemotherapy is in general the initial treatment of choice in all stage IV and stage IIIA (spleen involved) cases and all patients presenting with B symptoms. It is also possible that some patients with stage I, IIA HD who have a poor prognostic index may be better treated initially with a large mediastinal mass, microscopically NS2 HD, a low lymphocyte count and haemoglobin, and a high ESR; the words 'may be' are chosen deliberately. It is true that initial irradiation of such a lymphoma produces a poor result, but there is so far no evidence that initial chemotherapy is followed by a better result. The fact is that this type of HD is aggressive and exceedingly difficult to control, and possibly many cases of this type are incurable using any combination of the currently available treatment methods. There is need for a study comparing initial chemotherapy with initial irradiation in stage I, IIA cases with a bad prognosis index, and this has been commenced by the BNLI.

There is a growing tendency throughout the world to recommend combination chemotherapy rather than radiotherapy for cases of stage I, IIA HD, including those without any indications of a possibly bad prognosis. Unless evidence is produced from a carefully conducted clinical trial that initial combination chemotherapy cures more patients than initial localized irradiation, it is unethical to consider treating such cases with currently available chemotherapeutic regimens rather than irradiation. Most cases which fail irradiation have one or more positive factors indicating a poor prognosis. In a paper from the BNLI presented at the Royal Society of Medicine (Jelliffe, 1983), all deaths in a group of 412 stage I,IIA HD were analysed. Of 18 patients dying of unequivocally active HD, 12 had grade 2 histology, six had an ESR of 40 or more, six had a low lymphocyte count and three had gross mediastinal disease. With few factors indicating a poor prognosis, at least 90% of patients with stage I, IIA (upper half) HD will survive for 10 years after irradiation, and if all factors are favourable the 10-year survival rate will be almost 100%. To provide statistical proof that initial combination chemotherapy produces a significantly better 10-year survival than at least 90% and possibly nearly 100% will require an enormous number of patients. Many of the hundreds of patients in this study will run the risk of sterilization and developing other manifestations of sexual dysfunction and, much later, leukaemogenesis. Those patients cured with localized irradiation will run none of these risks. It is difficult to imagine the satisfactory organization of such a study if all local ethical committees insist on fully informed consent.

In correctly chosen cases, combination chemotherapy may be dramatic in its effects. Using MOPP, or the effective equivalent but much less toxic LOPP (*see below*), complete response rates of from 60–80% or more have been reported, the exact figure depending on case selection and on the local definition of the term. Whatever the complete response rate reported, up to 40% of all treated patients can hope for cure. Regretfully, there has been no overall improvement in the cure rate of chemotherapy since the introduction of MOPP. Because it is known that steroids used as single agents produce little objective benefit in HD, the BNLI decided to omit prednisone from the combination and carry out a prospective comparison of MOPP with MOP. By 1974 analysis of the accumulated data showed that MOPP gave better results than MOP (Goldman, 1981), especially in the old and in cases with poor prognostic signs. The BNLI then tried to improve the results of MOPP by adding bleomycin. A study comparing MOPP with B-MOPP was completed in 1979, with no advantage to the patients in either arm (Goldman, 1981).

CHLVPP had been reported by McElwain *et al.* (1977) as an effective MOPP substitute, replacing mustine with oral chlorambucil and thus avoiding the periodic vomiting so typical of mustine. In 1979 the BNLI decided to compare MOPP with LOPP (*Table 8.1*). LOPP is identical with CHLVPP except for the substitution of vinblastine by vincristine (Oncovin), and the production of a more euphonious four letter word. This study commenced in 1980 and was completed in 1983, by which time it was clear that there was no difference in survival rates. A preliminary report on this trial was presented on behalf of the BNLI at Amsterdam (Jelliffe, 1983) and a full BNLI report with adequate follow-up is awaiting publication (Hancock, 1985). We conclude that at present LOPP is preferable to MOPP in the management of HD.

A possible improvement in the control of generalized HD has been reported from Milan, where recent work from Bonadonna and colleagues (1978) suggested that alternating MOPP with another combination, ABVD (Adriamycin (hydroxydaunorubicin), bleomycin, vinblastine, DTIC), can improve the long-term survival rate. This approach offers possible hope for the future. Collaborators in the BNLI have not been impressed in the past with ABVD. It is very toxic, it contains some agents which

Table 8.1 LOPP

Leukeran (chlorambucil)	10	mg daily	Orally	Days 1–10
Oncovin (vincristine)	1.4	mg/m^2 (max 2 mg)	i.v.	Days 1 + 8
Procarbazine	100	mg/m^2 (max 200 mg)	Orally	Days 1–10
Prednisone/prednisolone	25	mg/m^2 (max 60 mg)	Orally	Days 1–14

Duration LOPP will normally be continued for six courses, when initial complete remission is recorded after the third course. If initial complete remission is not recorded until later, a further three courses will be given after initial complete remission is recorded.

are not very effective against HD when used as single agents, and their experience with ABVD in relapsing disease is that it is often ineffective. Hydroxydaunorubicin is certainly an effective single agent, as is VP16 (Etoposide). The BNLI decided to investigate the principle of alternating treatment using a new combination of VP16, vinblastine, hydroxydaunorubicin and prednisone (EVAP). The current study is comparing LOPP (CHLVPP) with LOPP alternating with EVAP. As yet it is too early to report on this.

Effective cancer chemotherapy drug combinations are usually serendipitous, although there is usually no lack of scientific explanation when a new system succeeds. We have no exact knowledge as to how long chemotherapy should be continued in order to provide the best possible chance of cure with the least possible complication rate in an individual. When MOPP became widely used some clinicians decided that 12 was the correct number of courses — others six. Scientific logic is lacking from these choices, although of course they are both multiples of the divinely effective number three. When the BNLI commenced its comparison of MOPP with MOP it was decided to choose a minimum of six, but a compromise with the conscience was reached by deciding to include a randomized maintenance course for 6 months using either MOPP or MOP. This study showed neither value nor disadvantage to the maintenance arm. Later the BNLI commenced the MOPP vs B-MOPP study, and this included a randomized study of CVB (CCNU, vinblastine, bleomycin) as maintenance treatment. The BNLI has found no evidence from the literature or from its own work that maintenance therapy improves the prognosis, and the escalating evidence that prolonged chemotherapy increases the risk of leukaemogenesis has encouraged the abandonment of all further studies of this type.

Surgery

Surgery has little part to play in the cure of HD, other than in its vital role in establishing the initial diagnosis by biopsy. This aspect of the management of lymphomas is discussed in the next section on NHL, where surgery has a more definite although still limited place.

Conclusions

(1) Choice of treatment depends upon more than disease distribution. Equally important are disease activity and patient response. Staging laparotomy may be helpful in a very small number of patients, but better guidance will probably be provided by careful investigation and the use of more suitable prognostic indices.

(2) Radiotherapy provides the most effective and the safest method of curing relatively localized HD, for which there is no substitute at present.

(3) Chemotherapy is the initial treatment of choice in stage IV, stage III (spleen positive) and 'B' HD. Patients with stage I, IIA HD with a poor prognostic index may also be better treated initially with chemotherapy.

(4) Assuming that there are no dramatic developments in the management of HD, improvements will follow persistent efforts to reduce early and late complications of routine treatment. In the management of localized, good prognosis HD, relatively localized radiotherapy is preferable to wide field irradiation such as total nodal irradiation. There is no evidence that routine use of adjuvant chemotherapy improves the results of treatment. Chemotherapy may be the initial treatment of choice in localized HD, for example if the prognostic index is bad, or if there are technical reasons as with bulky mediastinal disease.

(5) With generalized or polysymptomatic HD, chemotherapy is indicated initially. There is no evidence that additional maintenance treatment after an adequate number of courses of combination chemotherapy provides any benefit. The BNLI advise a minimum of six courses of LOPP and at least three courses after a complete response has been recorded.

(6) The results of treatment with combination chemotherapy may be improved by alternating different combinations of drugs. This attractive idea is currently under study.

Non-Hodgkin's lymphomas

The non-Hodgkin's lymphomas are a confusing group of tumours. They show morphological heterogeneity, a wide spectrum of disease complexes and often unpredictable responses to treatment. Clinically, they vary from fulminant conditions which may kill within a few weeks, to chronic indolent processes with symptoms which are far less disturbing than the treatment recommended by their medical advisers.

The management of NHL cannot be equated with that of HD. There are many striking differences between NHL and HD. NHL occurs most commonly in the second half of life, it often appears to arise in extranodal structures, it has generalized in four out of five patients when first seen and cure is less likely with irradiation or cytotoxic drugs. There is no typical 'neoplastic cell' similar to the Reed-Sternberg cell providing a common thread for all the NHL.

It was suggested earlier that HD may include at least two disease processes. Many clinicians working with NHL believe that this portmanteau name is a retrograde step, packing together a number of diseases which are totally different in their management.

Histology

The NHL have been classified morphologically by many different authors. The first 'new' classification was by Robb-Smith (1938, 1964). This system was not accepted by clinicians who preferred to continue with a simple grouping of 'lymphosarcomas' — (giant) follicular lymphoma, (lymphocytic) lymphosarcoma, lymphoblastic lymphosarcoma and reticulum-cell sarcoma. At that time this simple classification was adequate for clinicians who prefer to reject complicated nomenclatures which are of no practical value. In the 1940s 'lymphosarcoma' was considered to be untreatable. The only question in the clinician's mind was whether the patient was likely to die in the near future or after a period of years to which the old simple classification provided an adequate answer. In 1956 a new classification, introduced by Rappaport, was accepted with enthusiasm throughout North America.

The first new 'modern' classification was that of Lukes and Collins (1975) which divided lymphomas into groups according to their cell of origin: B, T or U lymphocytes, true histiocytes or unclassifiable. The most common NHL is of B-cell origin and is of follicular appearance. This classification was exciting and innovative, but unfortunately it required special immunological investigations which are not generally available. Even when they are available, they are not always reliable and are not comparable between centres because of many variables (Taylor, 1977).

For the next few years morphological classification will remain a routine method of assessing NHL with a view to their clinical management. A good morphological classification must be understandable to clinicians and useful in the treatment of patients. It should take into account new ideas and allow ongoing studies which may lead to improvements in management in the future. The BNLI has developed such a classification based on morphological appearances, but making use of more modern concepts. It is understandable to clinicians as it has no confusing neologisms and it can be used by the routine histopathologist with a light microscope (*Table 8.2*). Presented initially by Bennett and colleagues at an international pathological workshop at the University of Chicago (Bennett, Farrer-Brown, and Henry, 1973) and reported briefly in 1974 (Bennett *et al.*, 1974), the BNLI classification was published in detail in 1977 and 1978 (Carr *et al.*, 1977; Henry, Bennett and Farrer-Brown, 1978). It is interesting to note that this classification closely resembles the Working Formulation for Clinical Usage agreed by an NCI-sponsored International Study of Classifications of NHL (National Cancer Institute, 1982). The BNLI classification has continued in use for 12 years, confirming its practical value and reproducibility. The major division of the BNLI classification into grade 1 and grade 2 is of practical value to the clinician because of the clear cut difference between the prognosis and management of the two grades.

BNLI classification of NHL

Grade 1 NHL

Follicular lymphoma (FL)

This entity is characterized by the persistence of the follicular pattern. Some follicles may be greatly enlarged. The cells within the follicles may be predominantly small, mixed small and large, or predominantly large. When the cells are predominantly large, the prognosis is marginally worse and more aggressive treatment may be necessary. Follicular lymphomas are, in general, slowly progressive. Many show the spontaneous waxing and waning described earlier as characteristic of many cases of HD.

Diffuse lymphomas (DL)

These vary enormously in appearance and prognosis. Two are included with FL as grade 1 lymphomas.

Diffuse lymphocytic well differentiated (DLWD, small round cell)

The normal lymph node is completely replaced with small round cells with dark nuclei and minimal cytoplasm. These are identical with the circulating cells in

Table 8.2 BNLI classification of non-Hodgkin's lymphomas. The final differentiation into grade 1 and grade 2 facilitates the clinicians's treatment choice

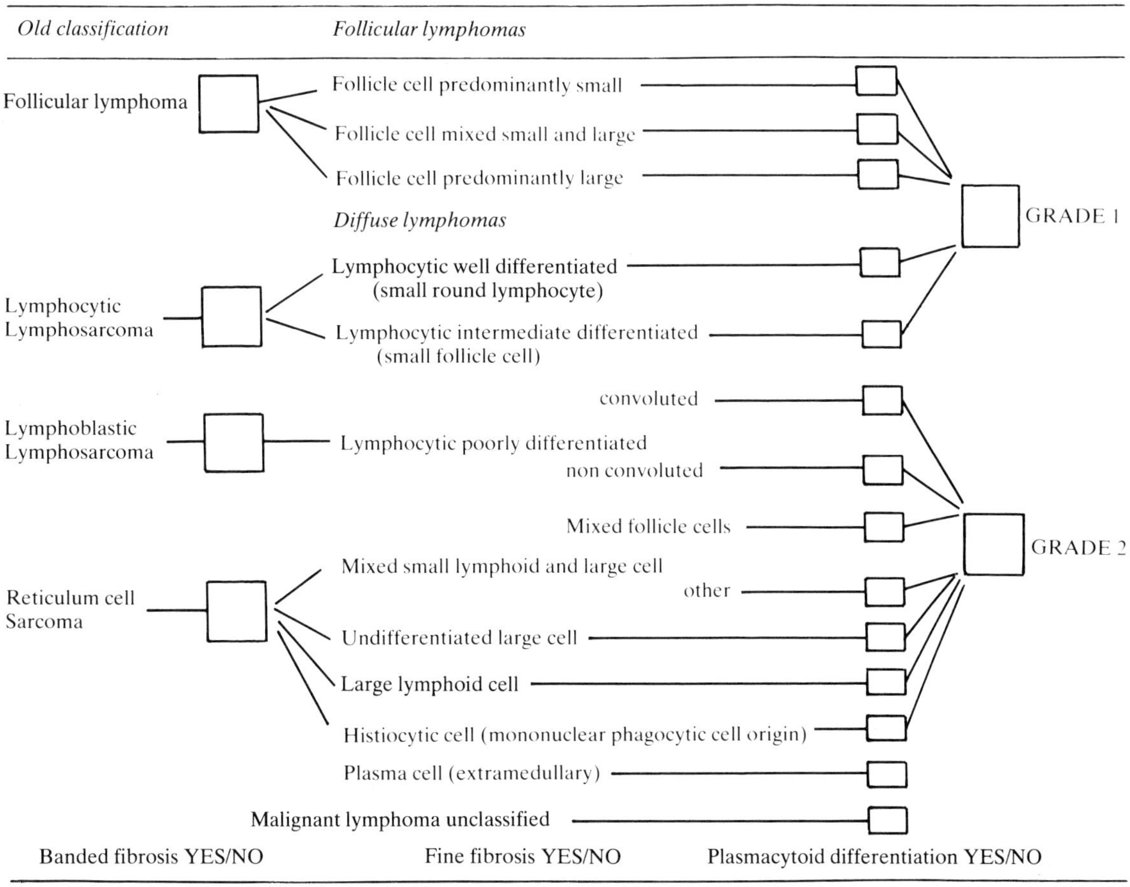

chronic lymphatic leukaemia, with which DLWD overlaps. There may be plasmacytoid differentiation with a gammopathy.

Diffuse lymphocytic intermediate differentiated (DLID, small cleaved cell, small follicle cell)

In DLID the diffuse infiltration is with small cleaved cells and this lymphoma may be regarded as the diffuse counterpart of the predominantly small cell FL.

The term 'differentiated' is not related to the function of these cells. The term was used in this classification as it was felt that it would be acceptable to clinicians as an indication of disease tempo.

Grade 2 NHL

All the remaining diffuse lymphomas are classified as grade 2. Although they cover a wide spectrum of disease they are in general more aggressive tumours than those in grade 1 and are controllable only with more vigorous treatment.

Diffuse lymphocytic poorly differentiated (DLPD)

This group of lymphomas includes three subdivisions. Burkitt's tumour typically shows the classical starry sky appearance. This is not seen in the second non-Burkitt type of DLPD. The third group of DLPD NHL presents typically in young people as a huge anterior mediastinal tumour: the convoluted appearance of the nucleus of the cell led to is description by Lukes and Collins as 'chicken-claw'. There is a close association with acute lymphatic leukaemia. This last type of lymphoma is probably of T-cell origin whereas most lymphocytic NHL arises in B cells.

Diffuse lymphocytic mixed (DLMX, mixed follicle cell)

The basic cells in this group of lymphomas are large lymphoid cells which are the transformed lymphocytes of Lukes and Collins. Sometimes there are bizarre giant cells present, and fibrosis. These lymphomas are sometimes diagnosed as lymphocyte depleted HD.

Histiocytic cell (mononuclear phagocytic cell)

Although these tumours of true histiocytic origin were originally diagnosed by the electron microscope, they are now recognizable by routine morphological methods. Some are composed of cells closely resembling normal histiocytes. Others show sheets of large poorly differentiated cells with characteristic histological features (Henry, 1975).

Plasma cell tumours

Extramedullary plasmacytomas have been considered to be uncommon until recently. It is now recognized that primary lymphomas of the gastrointestinal tract include many plasma cell tumours showing the typical features of plasma cells elsewhere in the body (MacLennan *et al.*, 1981).

Investigation

The investigation of NHL is generally similar to that of HD, but there are certain differences.

Biopsy

An excellent biopsy is as important as with HD, but surface markers and cytochemical studies may be especially helpful, and these can be performed only on fresh, unfixed specimens. Because NHL are frequently extranodal in origin, the possibility should always be in the surgeon's mind when a tumour arises in a site commonly involved by NHL, such as the tonsil or stomach. If the possibility is considered, the pathologist can be forewarned, and arrangements made for any special investigations.

Clinical findings

Whereas HD occurs most commonly between the ages of 15 and 45, NHL are found commonly in the fifth to seventh decades, and treatment becomes more difficult because of associated degenerative conditions. It is important to have an expert ENT examination because of the frequency of involvement of Waldeyers ring, including the nasopharynx.

Organ imaging

The generalized nature of the lymph node involvement reduces the value of the lymphogram. Involvement of nodes other than those in the central axis makes CT or ultrasound scanning more suitable.

It is not uncommon to find NHL in the head and neck, and abdomen, skipping the mediastinum. This is in sharp contradistinction to HD, where mediastinal disease is common. Because of the diffuse pattern of involvement, isotope scanning of the liver and spleen often shows no abnormality apart from organ enlargement. Diffuse hepatic infiltration can be demonstrated more reliably by ultrasound. Isotope scanning of the skeleton is potentially valuable, because bone involvement is common in NHL.

Percutaneous needle biopsy

Percutaneous needle biopsy of the liver is more likely to reveal positive results than in HD because of the diffuse nature of the disease.

Marrow examination

Aspiration and biopsy are both of greater value in NHL than HD. Diffuse invasion of the marrow is said by some workers to be demonstrable in up to four out of every five patients with grade 1 NHL, especially if multiple marrow biopsies are taken. Large biopsies with a Striker saw increase the chance of a positive result.

Diagnostic (staging) laparotomy

With NHL this procedure never achieved the popularity that it did with Hodgkin's disease for three reasons:

(1) The peak incidence of NHL occurs in the second half of life, and a diagnostic laparotomy becomes increasingly hazardous from the fifth to the eighth decade.
(2) As NHL generalizes it often produces a diffuse infiltration of organs such as the marrow and liver. Simple needle biopsies are frequently positive,
removing the need for a hazardous major procedure.
(3) There is no indication that a diagnostic laparotomy has made treatment simpler or more effective.

A few reports on the subject were published in the mid 1970s (Chabner *et al.*, 1975; Jelliffe, 1975; Bonadonna *et al.*, 1978) following which the procedure lost favour.

Primary extranodal non-Hodgkin's lymphoma

Although extranodal NHL may originate in any organ of the body, it is found most frequently in the head and neck and in the alimentary canal.

Head and neck (excluding CNS and eye)

A large rounded proliferative vascular tumour should always suggest the possibility of NHL, especially if the tumour is bilateral. The commonest site is in Waldeyer's ring. Involvement of salivary glands may present with diffuse enlargement of one or more glands, or the lymphoma may be discovered unexpectedly after removal of a salivary gland for a lump considered to be a pleomorphic adenoma. NHL originating in a paranasal sinus presents as a carcinoma and can be diagnosed only after histological examination. It may also occur in the orbit and primarily in the thyroid gland (*see* Chapter 13).

As with primary nodal NHL, extranodal grade 1 lymphomas respond well to a lower dose of 3500–4000 cGy over 4 weeks. Some grade 2 lymphomas respond to a dose of this order but many require a dose of up to 5500–6000 cGy in 6 weeks. With a lymphoma arising in Waldeyer's ring it is customary to irradiate the entire cervical chain of lymph nodes on both sides of the neck, whether or not they are clinically involved.

Irradiation of the entire neck and pharynx produces severe symptoms which may persist as permanent disabilities if too high a dose is given. It is impossible to avoid a confluent mucositis and dysphagia with a dose of 3500–4000 cGy over 4–5 weeks. The acute reaction will settle over 3–4 weeks but, inevitably, the patient will be left with a dry mucosa from which recovery is slow, taking place sometimes over many months. Early recovery is associated with the production of sticky, viscid saliva which becomes increasingly liquid with the passage of time. The patient's discomfort is accentuated by distortion and loss of taste, which is often associated with loss of appetite. Referral to a dental oral hygienist and the use of artificial saliva may help to alleviate the symptoms (*see* Chapter 18). Recovery from these extremely distressing symptoms is eventually complete, provided that a higher dose is not given to the whole block of tissue.

This group of lymphomas is best managed by irradiating *en bloc* the lymph nodes of the whole neck and the primary site to a dose of 3500 cGy in 4 weeks, using two opposing fields, followed by a further 1500 cGy using small fields to the primary site (e.g. nasopharynx) or to any residual (grade 2) lymph node mass which has not responded to the smaller dose (*see below*). In this way it is possible to deliver a maximum curative tumour dose while minimizing the distressing side-effects.

It is important to recognize these tumours for two reasons. First they are more radiosensitive than a primary carcinoma, and second, the patient must be investigated generally. Widespread disease may be discovered which may be controlled with suitable chemotherapy. When the disease is found to be strictly localized, radical irradiation offers a good chance of cure. Occasionally it may be considered that the local grade 2 NHL has been eradicated by surgery, as is sometimes seen following superficial radical parotidectomy, and postoperative irradiation is then not essential.

Gastrointestinal tract

NHL commonly arises in the stomach, small intestine and large bowel, in this order of frequency. NHL orginating in the stomach most commonly presents with epigastric pain, often radiating into the small of the back and waking the patient in the small hours of the morning. Haemorrhage or perforation are less common. Clinical examination may reveal an epigastric mass. The characteristic feature on radiological examination of the stomach is an enormous thickening of the rugae. If the surgeon is alerted by this finding, he will be able to undertake the different management at laparotomy which NHL entails. Primary NHL of the small intestine should always be considered if a patient is found to have a neoplasm in this site, because NHL is the most common small bowel malignancy. Because it is so rare, primary colonic NHL is almost always misdiagnosed as a bowel cancer. NHL arising in the intestine presents with haemorrhage, perforation or obstructive symptoms.

The diagnosis of NHL presenting in the gut may be made especially difficult because of associated circumstances. An extremely ill patient may be admitted in the small hours of the morning, and an emergency laparotomy performed by an inexperienced surgical registrar. When an advanced growth is discovered, little time is spent determining its nature or exact extent, and an emergency biopsy or resection is carried out as rapidly as possible. Sometimes no attempt is made to obtain material for histological examination. Retrospectively, it is difficult to recall the exact tumour extent and accurate 'staging' is impossible.

Crowther and Blackledge (1978) proposed a staging classification of gastrointestinal lymphoma which they related to clinical management. Wide local excision alone provides ample treatment for stage I and IIA tumours with limited local disease or with no more than immediately adjacent node involvement.

If the disease is more advanced, surgical removal must be followed by combination chemotherapy. In general, radiotherapy has little part to play in the management of this type of disease. This is largely because of the technical difficulties of irradiating the whole abdomen. Treatment is slow, spreading over many weeks. Many of these lymphomas are aggressive grade 2 tumours which may disseminate widely during this time. Initial combination chemotherapy will provide adequate local as well as generalized treatment and is preferable because of its flexibility.

Bone

Primary lymphoma of bone can be considered as an entity. For practical purposes it presents as one of a group of small round cell tumours of bone. The differential diagnosis includes Ewing's sarcoma, neuroblastoma, atypical myeloma and metastasis from a poorly differentiated carcinoma. The microscopical characteristics of these tumours may allow differentiation. Typically, primary bone lymphoma shows no fibrous septa, a diffuse reticulum pattern, and no perivascular cuffing or rosette formation (Arthur *et al.*, 1970).

Full investigation is always necessary in order to exclude generalized disease. If the lymphoma is limited to the original bone, radical radiotherapy is preferable to surgical ablation. The whole bone is irradiated to a tumour dose of 4000 cGy in 4–5 weeks using two opposed fields with daily fractionation. If possible, the fields are then reduced to protect major joints and a further 1500 cGy may be given in 2 weeks to the original main tumour volume. Efforts are made to protect a longitudinal strip of normal tissue in order to prevent the later development of totally encircling fibrous tissue which will interfere with the peripheral blood supply of the limb (*see* Chapter 6).

Testicle

Primary testicular lymphoma is uncommon. One of the largest published reviews is that of Gowing (1976) who reported 140 cases among a total of 2106 referred to the Testicular Tumour Panel and Registry. Of these, 120 were acceptable as having a localized primary testicular lymphoma. In 20% the disease was bilateral at presentation or became so later. The peak age incidence was between 60 and 80 years.

Histologically almost all testicular lymphomas are grade 2 and the prognosis is very poor. The primary is usually removed and it is customary to irradiate the retroperitoneal lymph node to 3000–3500 cGy in 4–5 weeks. The technique used to irradiate retroperitoneal lymph nodes is almost identical with that used in the control of seminoma (*see* Chapter 3). The kidneys are localized with an intravenous pyelogram and the position and degree of involvement of the retroperitoneal lymph nodes draining the testicle are determined by lymphography. The lymph nodes of the retroperitoneal iliac and inguinal regions are covered with two opposing fields and, because in at least one out of five cases the lymphoma is bilateral at presentation or will become so in the future, no attempt is made to shield the apparently unaffected testicle. Treatment may have to be prolonged because of radiation sickness or depression of the white blood cell count and platelets. The poor long-term results have stimulated interest in adjuvant combination chemotherapy, even when the disease is apparently limited to the testicle, but experience in the BNLI is that this makes no difference to the prognosis.

Treatment of primary nodal non-Hodgkin's lymphoma

Radiotherapy

The extreme radiosensitivity of some NHL has been appreciated for many years. For example, FL was known to respond for many years to relatively small doses of irradiation to local gland masses troubling the patient (Levitt, 1952). However, spontaneous variations in the size of lymph nodes and the absence of a detailed classification and of adequate organ imaging made the evaluation of treatment difficult and all types of NHL were generally regarded as incurable. Nowadays, with modern pathological classifications and organ imaging methods it is possible to manage patients with NHL in a logical fashion, and it is now clear that the disease is radiocurable in some patients.

In general, irradiation is only effective when it can encompass the whole tumour undergoing treatment. Permanent control is therefore likely only when a lymphoma is localized. However, because some NHL are exquisitely radiosensitive, attempts have been made to treat NHL with large volume irradiation up to total body irradiation.

Localized irradiation

With modern investigations, many patients with apparently localized NHL can be shown to have generalized disease, and only about one-quarter are finally considered to have localized disease after full study. These patients have potentially radiocurable disease.

During the last decade there have been many reports of long-term survivors after irradiation for localized NHL (Werf-Messing, 1968; Millett *et al.*; 1969, Prosnitz *et al.*, 1969; Robinson, Fischer and Vera, 1971; Lipton and Lee, 1971; Hellman *et al.*, 1977). It is not possible to compare most of these reports exactly because they use different histological classifications and because they refer to patients treated before the introduction of modern investigations, but even with these reservations certain themes can be detected. Localized grade 1 lymphomas (e.g. FL) may be controlled for many years. A 5-year disease-free survival rate of 80–100% has been reported in some small series. With long-term follow-up many, but not all, patients with localized grade 1 lymphomas eventually relapse. Localized grade 2 NHL is less commonly controlled for long by local irradiation, but patients surviving for 5 years or longer without relapse are probably cured. The BNLI has had the opportunity to follow a large number of patients with apparently localized NHL, treated with local irradiation. All cases have been routinely investigated according to modern standards with particular emphasis on the function of the marrow and liver. Examination of these cases reveals some interesting facts.

Localized grade 1 NHL

Between 1974 and the end of 1980, the BNLI carried out a randomized comparison of local irradiation alone with local irradiation followed by adjuvant chlorambucil (Phillips, 1981). Ninety patients who received irradiation only have been reported recently (Spry *et al.*, 1986). The overall 10-year survival rate was 70% and the relapse-free survival rate 35%. Three-quarters of relapses occurred elsewhere, confirming the long-held view that many patients with apparently limited lymphomas already have widespread disease that cannot be detected by current methods. The plateau suggests that a number of these patients can be cured at no cost to themselves. Localized radiotherapy has no serious complications, and, if relapse occurs, treatment with cytotoxic drugs has not been compromised. Factors influencing the survival in this group of patients include the extent of the disease, production of complete response and the administered dose. The original protocol specified 3500 cGy in 4 weeks, treating five times weekly, or its radiobiological equivalent. When resolution is slow, additional irradiation should be given provided that normal tissues are not compromised. There is a close relationship between the dose and complete response. At 4000 cGy or more the complete response rate is 97%; from 3500–3999 cGy, 93%; from 3000–3499 cGy, 86%; and below 3000 cGy, only 56%. It is therefore important to give a minimum of 3500 cGy in 3–4 weeks.

Localized grade 2 NHL

An earlier BNLI study compared local radiotherapy alone with localized radiotherapy followed by combination chemotherapy (Phillips, 1981). A recent report from the BNLI analysed 85 patients with grade 2 NHL treated by radiotherapy alone (Lamb *et al.*, 1984). Most relapses were distant from the irradiation site, suggesting that local cure was possible. Various factors affected the local response to irradiation and the survival. Failure to induce complete response was followed by a 15% 5-year survival compared with a 75% 5-year survival after complete response. The disease-free survival at 5 years with stage I cases was 65%, compared with 27% for stage II cases. The radiotherapy dose was extremely important. The BNLI recommended dose was 4000 cGy in 4 weeks, and when resolution was slow this could be increased to 6000 cGy in 6 weeks, provided normal tissues were not compromised. When the dose exceeded 4500 cGy complete response was obtained in almost 100% of cases. Below 4000 cGy the complete response rate fell rapidly to 65% or less, emphasizing, as in grade 1 NHL, the importance of adequate irradiation. As with localized grade 1 NHL, both survival and the disease-free survival curves flatten out, suggesting that localized grade 2 NHL can be cured with adequate local radiotherapy in about 40% of patients.

Total nodal irradiation

Hodgkin's disease can often be treated successfully using a combination of mantle and inverted-Y fields, because it is usually limited to the central axis lymph nodes. It is known that NHL frequently involves mesenteric nodes and the alimentary canal, and total nodal irradiation should therefore include the whole abdomen. The Stanford group have developed a safe and apparently effective method of total abdominal irradiation using shrinking fields (Goffinet *et al.*, 1976; Glatstein *et al.*, 1976). This technique has been devised to adminster a dose of 4400 cGy to the para-aortic and mesenteric lymph nodes while restricting the dose to the kidneys and right side of the liver to less than 2000 cGy. In the first phase of treatment the whole abdomen and the pelvic lymph nodes are treated with opposing anterior and posterior fields to a midline dose of 1500 cGy while shielding off the right lobe of the liver. The upper abdominal contents are then irradiated with two opposing lateral fields. Finally, during the third phase, opposing anterior and posterior fields, with shielding of the kidneys and the right half of the liver, take the final dose to 4000 cGy while sparing the kidneys and liver. This excellent treatment method has not been adopted generally, presumably because modern cytotoxic drugs are as effective and less complicated.

Total body irradiation

This technique was first used by Heublein (1932) and later by Medinger and Craver (1942) in the management of generalized lymphomas. By the 1950s effective chemotherapy had become available and was replacing the X-ray bath (Levitt, 1952).

Total body irradiation recently enjoyed a resurgence following its popularization by Johnson (1975). Johnson's many publications on the subject described techniques which were well tolerated by patients. A common complication was a fall in the platelet count about 2 weeks after completion of treatment. With grade 1 tumours this reversible change was of little significance. Johnson reported a 5-year survival rate of 80%. Since then total body irradiation has disappeared from routine treatment. In 1974 the BNLI decided to compare total body irradiation with modified CHOP (*see Table 8.3*) in the management of generalized grade 2 NHL. The response to total body irradiation was reasonable but not as good as to CHOP. Moreover, the low platelet count after completion of treatment provided an obstruction to further therapy, and total body irradiation was abandoned in 1978. (For technique *see* Chapter 11.)

Chemotherapy

In the early days of cytotoxic drug therapy, effective responses of various NHL were reported using single agents such as chlorambucil. Relapse was common, and it became generally accepted that cytotoxic drugs were of temporary palliative benefit. Following the early success of aggressive combination chemotherapy in the management of leukaemia and HD, similar regimens were introduced into the management of NHL. Many of the earlier reports were favourable, suggesting that combination chemotherapy gave much better results than single agent therapy (Hoogstraten *et al.*, 1969). These early reports were misleading, largely because of current confusion in the histological interpretation of these lymphomas. It has now been established that a completely different approach is essential with generalized grade 1 and grade 2 NHL.

Generalized grade 1 NHL

In 1974 collaborators in the BNLI were unimpressed with reports suggesting that combination chemotherapy was essential in the management of these lymphomas. Pilot studies carried out from 1970 to 1974 indicated that similar effects could be obtained with chlorambucil, combinations of cyclophosphamide, vincristine and prednisone (COP), or with total body irradiation. It was decided to compare chlorambucil with COP. The study was interrupted in 1977, and then recommenced using a tighter protocol. In this second study, a 3-month review was made mandatory. If, after 3 months of treatment in either arm neither complete response nor progressive improvement had occurred the patient was switched into the other arm of the study (Hayhoe, 1981). This study is now complete, and includes more than 300 patients. Both the survival and recurrence-free survival curves are identical. This confirms that the better initial treatment for the patient with generalized grade 1 NHL is chlorambucil. If there is progression, or failure to achieve at least progressive improvement by 3 months, chlorambucil is stopped and the patient commenced on COP. The value of chlorambucil has been confirmed by others (Portlock *et al.*, 1976, Lister *et al.*, 1978).

It has been known for many years that successfully treated generalized grade 1 NHL relapses almost inevitably, although it may be a matter of years before this happens. With the increasing appreciation of the dangers of 'unnecessary' cytotoxic drug therapy, and the apparently incurable nature of this type of disease, it has often been suggested that active treatment should be avoided until essential. The BNLI has undertaken a study to evaluate this point. Patients with generalized grade 1 NHL are first classified as having non-aggressive or aggressive disease. Aggressive disease is defined as the presence of one or more of three factors:

(1) Systemic symptoms
(2) Involvement of vital organs
(3) Measurable progression of disease over a 3-month period of observation.

Patients with non-aggressive disease are randomized for immediate chlorambucil or delayed chlorambucil, when the drug is used only on the appearance of one or more of the above three factors. Patients in the delayed chlorambucil group may receive low dose symptomatic radiotherapy (LDSRT) to eliminate any node masses which may be distressing them. The irradiation technique with LDSRT varies with the lymph nodes being treated, but whatever the site or volume, the general principles differ from those used in localized grade 1 NHL. With strictly localized grade 1 NHL the aim is cure, and the affected nodes receive a radical dose which is

Table 8.3 CHOP regimen

Cyclophosphamide	750	mg/m^2	Days 1 and 8
Hydroxydaunorubicin	25	mg/m^2	Days 1 and 8
Oncovin	1.4	mg/m^2 (max 2 mg)	Days 1 and 8
Prednisone/prednisolone	50	mg/m^2	Days 1 – 8

Repeat course every 28 days from day 1. Clinical reassessment should be made before each course. Patients not showing progressive improvement after the first course and complete response after the third course are unlikely to be controlled by CHOP and should be considered for other treatment. Patients achieving complete response by the third course should continue to a total of six.

considered sufficient for this purpose. This may be up to 4000 cGy in 4 weeks. With LDSRT the aim of treatment is to control local disease and relieve local symptoms until such time as it may be necessary to treat the widespread disease which is already present when the patient is first seen. Doses of 1500–2000 cGy in 2 weeks given with small fields are usually quite sufficient. This is one of the few occasions when orthovoltage 250 kV irradiation may be perfectly acceptable. For example, a patient may be troubled by enlarged superficial nodes in one side of the neck or in one axilla. Using a 250 kV machine, a single direct field may be used to deliver 300 cGy on five occasions, the whole 1500 cGy being spread over 5–10 days. Treatment interferes very little with the patient's normal life, producing almost no side-effects, and enlarged lymph nodes usually respond satisfactorily.

Patients with aggressive disease were randomized originally for immediate chlorambucil or immediate total body irradiation. The total body irradiation arm proved unsatisfactory and the BNLI comparison is now between initial chlorambucil (to be followed by CHOP in 3 months at the latest if the response is unsatisfactory) and initial CHOP. The results to date are interesting. Because of the arrangement of the study, groups of both aggressive and non-aggressive cases are receiving initial chlorambucil. There is a marked difference in their response and survival, the former being worse than the latter, confirming that the BNLI criteria used to define aggressive disease are appropriate. There is no difference in survival or quality of life between the two arms of the study of non-aggressive disease, using either immediate or delayed chlorambucil.

Generalized grade 2 NHL

The original BNLI study compared total body irradiation with modified CHOP (*Table 8.3*). Total body irradiation was found to be inelastic and there was a statistically significant difference in favour of CHOP when the difference in stage distribution between the two groups was taken into account (Pettingale, 1981). Various pilot studies were then undertaken by the BNLI without the discovery of any drug combination offering an obvious improvement over CHOP. The BNLI decided to continue with this drug combination, and have acumulated more than 400 cases. A very important point is that the probability of cure can be related to the rapidity of complete response. Almost all cured patients achieve complete response by the third course at the latest — and many do so earlier.

Although many patients who achieve complete response are cured, failure to achieve complete response or relapse after, occurs with distressing frequency and salvage therapy with routine cytotoxic drug combinations is rarely successful. In these cases, if the bone marrow is not infiltrated with lymphoma, the bone marrow may be harvested and replaced after very high dose chemotherapy. This new technique is at present under investigation in many centres, including some collaborating in the BNLI. It is as yet too early to evaluate this procedure.

Surgery

The importance of the initial biopsy cannot be overemphasized. Rebiopsy of suspected relapse or persistence of disease may be equally valuable. Repeated biopsies kill less frequently than repeated treatment. Extranodal NHL may be discovered only after an operation. Sometimes planned surgery is part of the management programme. This is seen typically in gastrointestinal lymphomas. Successful treatment with cytotoxic drugs or irradiation may lead to perforation; surgical removal is safer by far.

Splenectomy is rarely performed as part of a diagnostic laparotomy, but it may still be necessary because of haemolysis or hypersplenism, or because a huge painful spleen will not respond to other measures.

Palliation

Palliation may be defined as the relief of symptoms without expectation of cure. Obviously much of the management of NHL involves palliative treatment only, but many patients who are incurable live long satisfying lives, interrupted as little as possible with judicious palliation. Painless enlarged nodes are not necessarily an indication for treatment unless they distress a patient or relatives. Painful lesions always require active treatment of some type.

Radiotherapy has a very important part to play in the palliation of lymphomas, and a patient who is managed only by cytotoxic drugs may be grossly disadvantaged. The often exquisite radiosensitivity of many lymphomas makes it possible to provide dramatic, rapid relief from symptoms, with minimal side-effects which are infinitely less than those produced by many cytotoxic drug combinations. Any area of localized symptomatic involvement by HD or NHL should be considered for palliative radiotherapy, the dose of radiation can be somewhat less than that used in radical treatment.

Conclusions

(1) Localized NHL may be cured by irradiation, and this does not preclude the possibility of chemotherapy later if necessary. Chemotherapy may be preferred because of technical reasons which make radiotherapy difficult (e.g. primary gut NHL) or because the lymphoma morphology suggests early widespread

dissemination (e.g. diffuse poorly differentiated NHL of the mediastinum in young persons).

(2) Generalized grade 1 NHL is best treated with chlorambucil. An inadequate response is followed by COP combination chemotherapy.

(3) Generalized grade 2 NHL must be treated with aggressive combination chemotherapy. Failure to respond by the third course at the latest indicates a 90% chance of death within 2 years, and is an indication for more aggressive treatment such as bone marrow harvesting followed by very high dose chemotherapy or total body irradiation.

BNLI collaborators: past and present

Ashe, D., Ashford, R., Atkinson, R. S., Backhouse, T. W., Bagshawe, K., Bain, B., Barley, V. L., Barnard, D. L., Barrett, D., Bellingham, A. J., Benton, F. M., Berry, R. J., Bingle, J. P., Birchall, L. A., Black, A. J., Blecher, T. E., Bleehen, N. M., Bodger, W. A. H., Bodkin, P. E., Bolger, J. J., Bradfield, J. W., Bradshaw, J. D., Brinkley, D., Broad, A. F., Brock, J. E. S., Buchanan, R., Bullimore, J. A., Cade, I. S., Campbell-Robson, L., Cartwright, S. C., Child, J. A., Close, H. J., Corbett, P. J., Coulter, C., Cowley, N., Dalby, J. E., Das, R. N., Davies, S., Dawson, W. B., Deutsch, G. P., Dickson, R., Dische, S., Drake, S. R., Edelstyn, G., El-Sharkawi, A., Fairhead, S., Fenner, M. L., Fermont, D. C., Firth, L. A., Fletcher, J., Folkes, A., Friend, J. H., Gajek, W. R., Galton, D. A., Gamble, D., Garrett, M. J., Golding, P., Goldman, J. M., Goolden, A. W., Grosch, E., Hancock, B. W., Hayhoe, F. G., Hope-Stone, H., Howell Evans, I., Hovenden, A. L., Hutchinson, R. M., Ivey, J. R., Jackson, A. W., Jelliffe, A. M., Jones, W., King, G. M., Kingsley-Pillers, E., Kok, D' A., Koriech, O. M., Lambert, J., Leslie, J., Leyland, M. J., Lillicrap, D. A., Lindup, R., Madden, F., Mahy, D. J., Mantell, B. S., Martindale, J. H., Matthews, E., Matthews, J. H., McKenzie, C. G., Moir, D., Monypenny, E. R., Mott, T. J., Murrell, D. S., Neal, F. E., Newsholme, G. A., Newland, A. C., Newlands, C., O'Connor, D., O'Shea, J. P., Ostrowski, M. J., Owen, J. R., Penn, C. R., Pettingale, K. W., Phillips, D. L., Pratt, W. R., Rees, J. K., Roberts, C. I., Robertson, J. H., Ross, W. M., Rostrom, A. Y., Ryall, R. H., Sambrook, D. K., Saunders, M., Scoble, J. E., Shepherd, J., Shepherd, R. T. H., Simmons, A. V., Sobolewski, S., Spittle, M. F., Sterndale, H., Stevenson, P. A., Stewart, J., Stone, J., Strickland, P., Szur, L., Tappin, J. A., Taylor, C. G., Toghill, P. J., Topham, C., Trask, C. W., Tyrrell, C., Watkins, S., Wiltshire, C. R., Winter, M., Worthy, T. S.

Central organization

Honorary director Jelliffe, A. M.; Deputy director Vaughan Hudson, G.; Present pathology panel Bennett, M. H., Henry, K., Lampert, I., MacLennan, K.; Statistics and computing Easterling, M. J., Haybittle, J. L., Vaughan Hudson, B.; Secretaries Bonner J., Alladine Butt, M.

References

AISENBERG, A. C. (1965) Lymphocytopenia in Hodgkin's disease. *Blood*, **25**, 1037

ARTHUR, J. J., BENNETT, M. H., JELLIFFE, A. M., KENDALL, B. K., MILLETT, Y. L. and TUCKER, A. K. (1970) Small round cell tumours of bone. In *Symposium Ossium*, edited by A. M. Jelliffe and B. Strickland, pp. 136–140. Edinburgh and London: Livingstone

BENNETT, M. H., FARRER-BROWN, G. and HENRY, K. (1973) A classification of non-Hodgkin's lymphomas. *Presented at the Workshop on Classifications on Non-Hodgkin's Lymphomas*. Chicago: University of Chicago

BENNETT, M. H., FARRER-BROWN G., HENRY, K. and JELLIFFE, A. M. (1974) Classification of the Non-Hodgkin's lymphomas. *Lancet*, **2**, 405–406

BENNETT, M. H., MacLENNAN, K. A., EASTERLING, M. J., VAUGHAN HUDSON, B., JELLIFFE, A. M. and VAUGHAN HUDSON, G. (1983) The prognostic significance of cellular subtypes in nodular sclerosing Hodgkin's disease. *British Journal of Radiology*, **44**, 497–501

BENNETT, M. H., MacLENNAN, K. A., EASTERLING, M. J., VAUGHAN HUDSON, B., JELLIFFE, A. M. and VAUGHAN HUDSON, G. (1985) Analysis of histological subtypes in Hodgkin's disease in relation to prognosis and survival. *Proceedings of an International Symposium on the Cytobiology of Leukaemias and Lymphomas*, edited by D. Quaglino and F. G. J. Hayhoe. New York: Raven Press (in press)

BENNETT, M. H., TU, A. and VAUGHAN HUDSON, B. (1981) Analysis of grade I Hodgkin's disease (BNLI Report No. 6). *Clinical Radiology*, **32**, 491–498

BNLI (1976) Initial treatment of stage IIIA Hodgkin's disease. Comparison of radiotherapy with combination chemotherapy, (BNLI Report No. 3). *Lancet*, **2**, 991–995

BONADONNA, G., CASTELLANI, R., NARDUZZI, C., SPINELLI, P. and RILKE F. (1978) Pathological staging in adult previously untreated non-Hodgkin's lymphomas. In *Recent Advances in Cancer Research. Lymphoid Neoplasm II. Clinical and Therapeutic Aspects*, edited by G. Mathe, M. Seligmann and M. Tubiana , pp. 41–50. Berlin, Hiedelberg, New York: Springer-Verlag

BONADONNA, G., FONATI, V. and DeLENA, M. (1978) MOPP vs MOPP plus ABVD in stage IV Hodgkin's disease. *Proceedings of the American Association for Cancer Research*, **19**, 363

BROWN, R. S., HAYES, H. A., FOLEY, H. T., GODWIN, H. A., BERARD, C. W. and CARBONE, P. P. (1967) Hodgkin's disease. Immunological, clinical and histological features of 50 untreated patients. *Annals of Internal Medicine*, **67**, 291–302

BUNTING, J. C. (1914) The blood picture in Hodgkin's disease. *Bulletin of John Hopkins Hospital*, **25** , 177

CARBONE, P. P., KAPLAN, H. S., MUSSHOFF, K.,

SMITHERS, D. W. and TUBIANA, M. (1971) Report of the committee on Hodgkin's disease staging classification. *Cancer Research*, **31**. 1860-1861

CARR, I., HANCOCK, B. W., HENRY, L. and WARD, A. M. (1977) *Lymphoreticular Disease*, pp. 93–100. Oxford and London: Blackwell Scientific Publications

CHABNER, B. A., JOHNSON, R. E., CHRETIEN, P. B. *et al.* (1975) Percutaneous liver biopsy, peritoneoscopy and laparotomy: an assessment of relative merits in the lymphomata. *British Journal of Cancer*, **31**, (Suppl II), 441–449

COLLABORATIVE STUDY (1976) Survival and complications of radiotherapy following involved and extended field therapy of Hodgkin's disease Stage I and II. *Cancer*, **38**, 288–305

CRAVER, L. F. (1964) Hodgkin's disease. In *Practice of Medicine*, vol 6 edited by F. Tice and E. M. Harvey, pp. 1017–1063. Hagerstown, Md.: W. F. Prior

CROWTHER, D. A., and BLACKLEDGE, G. (1978) Gastrointestinal lymphomas. *British Journal of Radiology*, **51**, 75

DeVITA, V. T., SERPICK, A. and CARBONE, P. P. (1970) Combination chemotherapy in the treatment of advanced Hodgkin's disease. *Cancer*, **35**, 98–110

EASSON, E. C. and RUSSELL, M. H. (1963) The cure of Hodgkin's disease. *British Medical Journal*, **1**, 1704–1707

EBSTEIN, W. VON. (1887) Das chronische Ruchfallsfieber, eine nev infectionskrankheit. *Berline Klinische Wehnschrift*, **24**, 564–568

GILBERT, R. (1939) Radiotherapy in Hodgkin's disease (malignant granulomatosis): anatomic and clinical foundations; governing principles; results. *American Journal of Roentgenology*, **41**, 198–241

GLATSTEIN, E. (1977) Radiotherapy in Hodgkin's disease — past achievements and future progress. *Cancer*, **39**, 837–842

GLATSTEIN, E., FUKS, Z., GOFFINET, D. R. and KAPLAN, H. S. (1976) Non-Hodgkin's lymphoma of stage III extent: is total lymph node irradiation appropriate treatment? *Cancer*, **37**, 2806–2812

GLATSTEIN, E., GUERNSEY, J. M., ROSENBERG, S. A. and KAPLAN, H. S. (1969) The value of laparotomy and splenectomy in the staging of Hodgkin's disease. *Cancer*, **27**, 709–718

GLEES, J. P., BARR, L. C., McELWAIN, T. J., PECKHAM, M. J. and GAZET, J. C. (1982) The changing role of staging laparotomy in Hodgkin's disease: a personal series of 310 patients. *British Journal of Surgery*, **69**, 181–187

GOFFINET, D. R., GLATSTEIN, E., FUKS, Z. and KAPLAN, H. S. (1976) Abdominal irradiation in non-Hodgkin's lymphomas. *Cancer*, **37**, 2797–2805

GOLDMAN, J. M. (1981) Combination chemotherapy for Stage IV Hodgkin's disease (BNLI Report No. 14). *Clinical Radiology*, **32**, 531–536

GOWING, N. F. C. (1976) Malignant lymphoma of the testicle. In *Pathology of the Testis*, edited by R. C. B. Pugh, pp. 334–355. Oxford, London and Edinburgh: Blackwell

HANCOCK, B. (1985) In Press

HAYBITTLE, J. L., HAYHOE, F. G. J., EASTERLING, M. J. *et al.* (1985) Review of British National Lymphoma Investigation studies of Hodgkin's disease and development of prognostic index. *Lancet*, **1**, 967–972

HAYHOE, F. G. J. (1981) Chemotherapy in the management of stage III/IV Grade I non-Hodgkin's lymphomas. *Clinical Radiology*, **32**, 547-552

HELLMAN, S., CHAFFEY, J. T., ROSENTHAL, D. S., MALONEY, W. C., CANELLOS, G. P. and SKARIN, A. J. (1977) The place of radiotherapy in the treatment of non-Hodgkin's lymphomas. *Cancer*, **39**, 843–851

HENRY, K. (1975) Electron microscopy in the non-Hodgkin's lymphomas. *British Journal of Cancer*, **31**, (Suppl II), 73–93

HENRY, K., BENNETT, M. H. and FARRER-BROWN, G. (1978) Classification of the non-Hodgkin's lymphomas. In *Recent Advances in Histopathology*, edited by P. P. Anthony and N. Woolf, pp. 275–302. Edinburgh, London, New York: Churchill Livingstone

HEUBLEIN, A. C. (1932) Preliminary report on continuous irradiation of entire body. *Radiology*, **18**, 1051

HOOGSTRATEN, B., OWENS, A. H., LENHARD, R. E. *et al.* (1969) Combination chemotherapy in lymphosarcoma and reticulum cell sarcoma. *Blood*, **33**, 370–377

HOPE-STONE, H. F. (1969) The treatment of the reticuloses. *British Journal of Radiology*, **42**, 770–793

HOPE-STONE, H. F. (1981) The place of radiotherapy in the management of localised Hodgkin's disease. *Clinical Radiology*, **32**, 519–522

HRESHEHYSHIN, M. M., SHEEHAN, F. R. and HOLLAND J. F. (1961) Visualisation of retroperitoneal lymph nodes. Lymphangiography as an aid in the measurement of tumour growth. *Cancer*, **14**, 205–209

JELLIFFE, A. M. (1965) The present place of radiotherapy in the cure of Hodgkin's disease. *Clinical Radiology*, **16**, 274–277

JELLIFFE, A. M. (1975) Diagnostic laparotomy in non-Hodgkin's lymphoma. *British Journal of Cancer*, **31**, (Suppl II), 248–251

JELLIFFE, A. M. (1979) Hodgkin's disease — the pendulum swings. *Clinical Radiology*, **30**, 121–127

JELLIFFE, A. M. and THOMSON, A. D. (1955) The prognosis in Hodgkin's disease. *British Journal of Cancer*, **9**, 21–36

JELLIFFE, A. M. and VAUGHAN HUDSON, G. (1985) Diagnostic laparotomy in Hodgkin's disease. In *Hodgkin's Disease*, edited by T. J. McElwain and T. Selby. Oxford: Blackwell Scientific Press (in press)

JOHNSON, R. E. (1975) Management of generalised malignant lymphomas with systemic radiotherapy. *British Journal of Cancer*, (Suppl II), 450–455

KAPLAN, H. S. (1962) The radical radiotherapy of regionally localised Hodgkin's disease. *Radiology*, **78**, 553–561

KAPLAN, H. S. (1966) Evidence for a tumoricidal dose level in the radiotherapy of Hodgkin's disease. *Cancer Research*, **26**, 1221–1224

KAPLAN, H. S. (1972) *Hodgkin's Disease*. Boston, Mass.: Harvard University Press

KAPLAN, H. S. and ROSENBERG, S. A. (1966) Extended-field radical radiotherapy in advanced Hodgkin's disease: short-term results of two randomised clinical trials. *Cancer Research*, **26**, 1268–1276

LAMB, D. S., VAUGHAN HUDSON, G., EASTERLING, M. J., MacLENNAN, K. A. and JELLIFFE, A. M. (1984) Localised Grade 2 non-Hodgkin's lymphoma: results of treatment with radiotherapy (BNLI Report No. 24). *Clinical Radiology*, **35**, 253–260

LEE, Y. T. M. and SPRAT, J. S. (1974) *Malignant Lymphomas: Nodal and Extranodal Diseases*. Modern Surgical Monograph. New York: Grune and Stratton

LEVITT, W. M. (1952) *Handbook of Radiotherapy*. London: Herney and Blythe

LIPTON, A. and LEE, B. J. (1971) Prognosis of stage I lymphosarcoma and reticulum cell sarcoma. *New England Journal of Medicine*, **284**, 230–233

LISTER, T. A., CULLEN, M. H., BEARD, M. E. J. *et al.* (1978) Comparison of combined single agent chemotherapy in non-Hodgkin's lymphoma of favourable histological type. *British Medical Journal*, **1**, 533–537

LUKES, R. J. and BUTLER, J. J. (1966) The pathology and nomenclature of Hodgkin's disease. *Cancer Research*, **26**, 1063–1081

LUKES, R. J. and COLLINS, R. D. (1975) New approaches to the classification of the lymphomata. *British Journal of Cancer*, **31**, (Suppl 2) 7

McELWAIN, T. J., TOY, J., SMITH, I. E., PECKHAM, M. J. and AUSTIN, D. E. (1977) A combination of chlorambucil, vinblastine, procarbazine and prednisone for treatment of Hodgkin's disease. *British Journal of Cancer*, **36**, 276–280

MacLENNAN, K. A., BENNETT, M. H., TU, A., EASTERLING, M. J., VAUGHAN HUDSON, B., VAUGHAN HUDSON, G. and JELLIFFE, A. M. (1985) The prognostic significance of cytologic subdivision of nodular sclerosing Hodgkin's disease; a study of 1156 patients. In *Proceedings of the Second International Symposium on Malignant Lymphomas,* edited by F. Cavalli, (in press)

MacLENNAN, K. A., VAUGHAN HUDSON, B., EASTERLING, M. J., JELLIFFE, A. M., VAUGHAN HUDSON, G. and HAYBITTLE, J. L. (1983) The presentation haemoglobin level in 1103 patients with Hodgkin's disease (BNLI Report No. 21). *Clinical Radiology*, **34**, 491–495

MacLENNAN, K. A., VAUGHAN HUDSON, B., JELLIFFE, A. M., HAYBITTLE, J. L. and VAUGHAN HUDSON, G. (1981) The pretreatment peripheral blood lymphocyte count in 1100 patients with Hodgkin's disease: the prognostic significance and the relationship to the presence of systemic symptoms (BNLI Report No. 19). *Clinical Oncology*, **7**, 333–339

MEDINGER, F. G. and CRAVER, L. F. (1942) Total body irradiation. *American Journal of Roentgenology*, **48**, 651

MILLETT, Y. L., BENNETT, M. H., JELLIFFE, A. M. and FARRER-BROWN, G. (1969) Nodular sclerotic lymphosarcoma. A further review. *British Journal of Cancer*, **23**, 683–692

NATIONAL CANCER INSTITUTE (1982) NCI sponsored study of classification of non-Hodgkin's lymphomas; summary and description of a working formulation for clinical usage. *Cancer*, **49**, 2112–2135

NICE, C. M. and STENSTROM, K. W. (1954) Irradiation therapy in Hodgkin's disease. *Radiology*, **62**, 641–653

PAPA, G., MAURO, F. R., ANSELIMO, A. P. *et al.* (1984) Acute leukaemias in patients treated for Hodgkin's disease. *British Journal of Haematology*, **58**, 43–52

PECKHAM, M. J., McELWAIN, T. J. and BARRETT, A. (1982) Hodgkin's disease. In *Treatment of Cancer*, edited by K. E. Halnan, pp. 691–793. London: Chapman and Hall

PEL, P. K. (1887) Zu symptomatologie der sogenannten Pseudoleukämie. II. Pseudoleukämie oder chronisches Rüchfallsfieber. *Berlin klinische Wochenschrift*, **24**, 644–646

PETERS, M. V. (1950) A study of survivals in Hodgkin's disease treated radiologically. *American Journal of Roentgenology*, **63**, 299–311

PETERS, M. V. and MIDDLEMISS, K. C. H. (1958) A study of Hodgkin's disease treated by irradiation. *American Journal of Roentgenology*, **79**, 114–121

PETTINGALE, K. W. (1981) The management of generalised grade 2 non-Hodgkin's lymphomas (BNLI Report No. 18). *Clinical Radiology*, **32**, 543–556

PHILLIPS, D. L. (1981) Radiotherapy in the treatment of localised non-Hodgkin's lymphomas (BNLI Report No. 16). *Clinical Radiology*, **32**, 543–546

PORTLOCK, C. S., ROSENBERG, S. A., GLATSTEIN, E. and KAPLAN, H. S. (1976) Treatment of advanced non-Hodgkin's lymphomas with favourable histology: preliminary results of a prospective trial. *Blood*, **47**, 747–756

PROSNITZ, L. R., HELLMAN, S., VON ESSEN, C. F. and KLIGERMAN, M. M. (1969) The clinical course of Hodgkin's disease and other malignant lymphomas treated with radical radiotherapy. *American Journal of Roentgenology*, **105**, 618–628

PUSEY, W. A. (1902) Cases of sarcoma and Hodgkin's disease treated by exposures to X-rays: a preliminary report. *Journal of the American Medical Association*, **38**, 166–169

RAPPAPORT, H. (1956) *Tumours of the Haemopoietic System.* Washington: Armed Forces Institute of Pathology

ROBB-SMITH, A. H. T. (1938) Reticulosis and reticulosarcoma: a histological classification. *Journal of Pathology and Bacteriology*, **47**, 457–480

ROBINSON, T., FISCHER, J. J. and VERA, R. (1971) Reticulum sarcoma treated by radiotherapy. *Radiology*, **99**, 669–675

ROSENBERG, S. A. (1966) Report of the committee on the staging of Hodgkin's disease. *Cancer Research*, **26**, 310

ROSENBERG, S. A. and KAPLAN, H. S. (1970) Hodgkin's disease and other lymphomas. *California Medicine*, **113**, 23–38

SHIELS, R. A., STONE, J., ASH, D. V. *et al.* (1984) Priorities for computed tomography and lymphography in the staging and initial management of Hodgkin's disease. *Clinical Radiology*, **35**, 447–449

SPRY, N. *et al* (1986) Submitted for publication.

STEWART, J. R., COHN, K. E., FAJARDO, L. F., HANCOCK, E. W. and KAPLAN, H. S. (1967) Radiation induced heart disease — a study of 25 patients. *Radiology*, **89**, 302–310

TAYLOR, C. R. (1977) *Hodgkin's disease and the lymphomas*. Lancaster: Eden Press

TRUEBLOOD, H. W., ENWRIGHT, L. P., RAY, G. R., KAPLAN, H. S. and NELSON, T. S. (1970) Preservation of ovarian function in pelvic irradiation for Hodgkin's disease. *Archives of Surgery*, **100**, 236–237

TUBIANA, M., ATTIE, E., FLAMANT, H., GERARD-MERCHANT, R. and HAYAT, M. (1971) Prognostic factors in 454 cases of Hodgkin's disease. *Cancer Research*, **31**, 1801–1810

VAUGHAN HUDSON, B., MacLENNAN, K. A., EASTERLING, M. J., JELLIFFE, A. M., HAYBITTLE, J. L. and VAUGHAN HUDSON, G. (1983) The prognostic significance of age in Hodgkin's disease: examination of 1500 patients (BNLI Report No. 23). *Clinical Radiology*, **34**, 503–506

WERF-MESSING, B. VAN DE (1968) Reticulum cell sarcoma and lymphosarcoma. *European Journal of Cancer*, **4**, 542–557

WESTLING, P. (1965) Studies of the prognosis of Hodgkin's disease. *Acta Radiologica*, Suppl. 245, 5–125

WORTHY, T. S. (1981) Evaluation of diagnostic laparotomy and splenectomy in Hodgkin's disease. *Clinical Radiology*, **32**, 523–526

9

Gynaecological radiotherapy

M. L. Sutton

The emergent clinical discipline of radiotherapy experienced its earliest and most easily identifiable curative successes in the treatment of gynaecological malignancies, notably in cancer of the uterine cervix. Gynaecology remains one of the most rewarding areas in which radiotherapists are engaged, and it provides them with opportunities to collaborate closely with surgical colleagues, with mutual benefit to all, most importantly the patient.

Approximately 15% of female cancer deaths are caused by genital tract malignancies, a relatively small proportion, which reflects the high curability of some gynaecological malignancies in their earlier stages. Until recently, ovarian cancer accounted for nearly one-half of these deaths, but chemotherapy now appears likely to reduce the mortality from this increasingly common disease, which will leave cancer of the cervix as the major single gynaecological cause of death from malignant disease in women.

Cancer of the cervix

Introduction: the continuing problem

Cancer of the cervix is the commonest radiocurable gynaecological malignancy. It has many epidemiological features which strongly suggest that it is a sexually-transmitted disease with a long incubation period (Kessler, 1976). Hypothetically, invasive disease can now be prevented by exfoliative cytological mass screening, but the general British experience is that even energetically pursued screening programmes have had little or only transient impact on the incidence of invasive cancer, which still kills more than 2000 women annually in the UK. There are indications that this figure is continuing to rise.

The incidence of carcinoma *in situ* is much higher than that of invasive cancer, which also has an older age-specific incidence. This suggests that (at least) two factors are involved in the development of invasive cancer (Doll, 1979). The first factor, influential in early adulthood, causes cervical intraepithelial neoplasia (CIN), graded I–III, while the second factor, active in later life, causes or promotes the development of invasion in a proportion of women with carcinoma *in situ*. Neither of these hypothetical factors has yet been identified, but the circumstantial evidence implicating Herpes hominis virus type 2 has been persuasively presented (Thomas; 1984).

In most regions of the world, including the UK, exfoliative cytology is failing badly in achieving eradication of invasive cervical cancer, but it might be expected that the repeated examination of large numbers of symptomless women would lead to invasive cancer being detected earlier: so steep is the gradient of curability stage by stage that earlier detection ought inevitably to lead to improved overall survival, but even this reasonable expectation has not yet been realized. In 1982, 90% of cervical cancer deaths in England and Wales occurred in women over 40 years old (Imperial Cancer Research Fund, 1984), and there is central government pressure to limit screening to women over 35. However, in one UK clinic 77% of patients with CIN grade III were under 35, as were no less than 47% of the patients with established, invasive cancer (Garry, 1984). There are growing perceptions that (1) CIN is becoming more common in even younger women, (2) the transition from CIN to invasive cancer can be very swift in younger patients, making the suggested screening intervals unrealistic, and (3) that the disease itself is often histologically more anaplastic and clinically more aggressive in younger women.

From the foregoing, it seems very likely that cervical cancer will remain a continuing challenge to gynaecological radiotherapists for many years and, accordingly, a large part of this chapter is allocated to its treatment: the technology of this is currently undergoing rapid change, and there is a need to develop more effective strategies to deal with the large number of patients who will foreseeably continue to present with stage IIb and stage III disease.

Histology

It used to be stated that adenocarcinoma of the cervix was inherently less radiocurable than squamous cell carcinoma (SCC), which constitutes 95% of cases. Most major centres find no difference in radiocurability, at least in early stage disease, so that the 5% of cervical cancer patients with adenocarcinoma are, at some centres, no longer referred for surgery. However, it remains important to differentiate between true adenocarcinoma of the cervix, and endometrial cancer presenting as a cervical growth, as their management is very different. SCC is graded I–III, but there is in reality very little evidence of epidermal origin in many grade III lesions.

SCCs are thought to originate at the squamocolumnar junction (which in multiparous women may lie some distance from the apparent external os, due to eversion), whereas adenocarcinomas arise from endocervical glandular tissue, so that many barrel-shaped cervical cancers are adenocarcinomas (*see below*).

Presentation and morphology

The gross morphological characteristics of the tumour to some extent influence the mode of presentation, which may in turn influence the clinical management, particularly in respect of the order in which certain radiotherapeutic and surgical procedures are employed.

Exophytic tumours

These are usually soft diffuse outgrowths, their friability predisposing to presentation with abnormal bleeding, especially postcoitally. While still technically early stage disease, they can be very bulky, so that external irradiation may be required before intracavitary treatment. Serious and continuing blood loss from such tumours may necessitate emergency haemostatic intracavitary radiation treatment on presentation: 'haemostatic' treatments are particularly effective when the lesion is exophytic. When blood loss is controlled, the planned external radiation is carried out, and the remaining intracavitary component is added at its conclusion.

Ulcerative tumours

By definition, these are partly necrotic, are invariably infected, often with anaerobic organisms, and accordingly present with a sero-sanguinous discharge, with or without spontaneous or postcoital bleeding. Destruction of the cervix, the central lower uterine segment, and fornices renders such tumours particularly prone to perforation during instrumentation, usually into the peritoneal cavity, less commonly into the bladder: the destruction may also make successful identification and cannulation of the remaining uterine cavity impossible. Perforation and non-cannulation can alter both the prognosis and the overall treatment strategy.

Infiltrative tumours

Such tumours commonly invade the cervix and its anatomically related structures with little or no representation on the surface of the cervix, and consequently vaginal bleeding may be a late or absent feature. Silent parametrial extension can result in obstruction of the upper urinary tracts and in the lymphatic and venous drainage of lower limbs. Ulcerative and infiltrative lesions are more likely than exophytic lesions to present with disease involving the bladder, and less commonly the rectum and the pelvic nerve plexuses.

Clinical assessment

For convenience, the familiar UICC recommendations for the staging of cervical cancer are summarized briefly in *Table 9.1*. In some ways this classification is insufficiently discriminatory, particularly in respect of the fairly common lack of correspondence between the technical stage of the disease and its apparent volume. Rectal assessment of parametrial spread is imprecise, since the contribution of pelvic inflammatory disease cannot be known. (Some patients are known to have been down-staged following antibiotic treatment.) Computerized axial tomographic (CT) scanning has been unhelpful in this respect, and is not always available. Transrectal ultrasonographic probes may in future provide supplementary information on the extent and volume of disease, which is helpful in individualizing treatment planning, and in assessing responses to new treatments.

Whatever the demerits of the currently employed staging criteria, there is a steep and progressive fall in curability from stage I to stage IV: it is probably realistic to regard most if not all long-term survivors of stage IIIb disease as having been over-staged by virtue of pelvic inflammatory disease. Since staging (always performed under an anaesthetic — EUA) carries important prognostic and therapeutic implications, it should be performed by a radiotherapist, who sees many more cases than most referring gynaecologists, or ideally by a combined assessment.

Table 9.1 IUCC staging recommendations for carcinoma of the cervix

Tis		Carcinoma in situ
T1		Confined to cervix
	T1a	Microinvasive
	T1b	Invasive
T2		
	T2a	Extension to vagina excluding lower third
	T2b	Extension to parametrium short of pelvic wall
T3		
	T3a	Extension to lower third vagina
	T3b	Extension to pelvic wall
T4		Extension to bladder (not bullous oedema) or rectum, or beyond true pelvis
M1		Distant organs

Many gynaecologists fail to record adequately their findings on rectal examination, and few perform cystoscopies, even when bladder symptoms or advanced disease are present.

In all cases intravenous urography should be included in the clinical assessment, but routine pedal lymphography is useless, since: (1) it fails to opacify the nodes of immediate relevance; (2) when truly positive it usually indicates incurable disease; (3) the frequent presence of sepsis makes interpretation difficult; and (4) the result rarely carries therapeutic implications. CT scanning up to now has not provided any more useful information.

Treatment of cervical cancer

In the UK, radiotherapy is fairly widely accepted as the initial method of treatment. Irradiation and surgery yield very similar cure rates in stage I and stage II disease; but the complication rate from radical surgery is notably higher. In North America, surgeons continue to press for access to the young, prognostically favourable, medically fit cases and the Wertheim hysterectomy is more widely employed than in the UK: inevitably, histological examination of the surgical specimen results in a proportion of these patients receiving postoperative irradiation, with a consequential further increase in the incidence of complications.

Stage 0 disease

Radiation has no place in the management of this stage, which was formerly treated and diagnosed by cone biopsy. More recently, diagnosis has been by colposcopy-directed multiple biopsies, and treatment by diathermy or laser vaporization. All three methods conserve ovarian function in the many young patients with CIN, but the new techniques have advantages when subsequent pregnancy is contemplated or deemed likely. Life-long cytological supervision is essential.

Early disease: stages I and II

Intracavitary radiation is employed as the sole method of treatment for early disease in several major centres, and they all recognize the need for supplementary external irradiation for the more advanced case. However, there is considerable variation in practice over the stage at which supplementary external treatment is introduced, and the extent to which it supplants the intracavitary component at each stage. The practice at the UK's largest institute for gynaecological therapy (The Christie Hospital and Holt Radium Institute, Manchester) will be described, with reference to the more commonly encountered variations where appropriate. Central to the rationale for this empirically derived treatment policy are that (1) almost invariably, properly executed intracavitary treatments provide complication-free permanent local control in stage I and stage IIa disease, and (2) tolerance doses of external pelvic radiation frequently fail to control more advanced disease. Accordingly, for potentially curable disease, heavy stress is laid on the intracavitary component. Many UK radiotherapists use the Manchester radium system (Tod and Meredith, 1938), or one of its variants. More modern treatment techniques attempt to mimic this system, at least in terms of the dose–distribution pattern and the manner in which radiation doses are expressed and prescribed, so consideration of its fundamentals remains pertinent.

The Manchester system

Following the early recognition of the curative potential of intracavitary radium, development proceeded in two similar but importantly different directions, now described as the Stockholm method (Forsell, 1917), and the Paris method (Regaud, 1926). Both were intended to encompass the disease within a volume of high-dose radiation achieved by placing radium in the uterine cavity and lateral vaginal fornices: the dose was expressed as the product of milligrams of radium used and the total duration in hours of the insertion(s), in each case amounting to 7000–8000 mg-hours for early disease. The essential differences between the two methods were that the Stockholm treatment was relatively intense (up to 180 mg radium), short (total time 48h), and fractionated (two treatments 21 days apart), whereas the Paris method was less intense (up to 70 mg radium), protracted (120 h), and unfractionated.

The present Manchester radium system most

resembles the Paris method, retaining the low dose rate protracted treatment (total time 140 h), and the use of two independent intravaginal sources. Treatment is given in two fractions, of 70 hours duration each, the second beginning 7 days after the commencement of the first. The innovative features of the Manchester development were:

(1) The doses were expressed in contemporary units of absorbed radiation, (formerly Roentgens, presently cGy)
(2) The dose was specified at a point (known as point A) which was considered relevant to the avoidance of serious late radiation damage (*see below*)
(3) The configurations, dimensions and radium content of the individual intracavitary components were designed so that the dose rate at point A remained almost constant, whatever combination of applicators was employed.

Dose rate is now known to be an important determinant of tissue responses (*see* Chapter 1), and the advantage of a standardized dose rate at the specified critical point A is itself an important justification for the continuing validity of the notion of this point, as many remote afterloading systems involve substantial increases in dose rate, a change likely to result in increased normal tissue damage.

Point A lies 2 cm lateral to the uterine canal, 2 cm rostral to the upper lateral fornix, in the plane of the uterus (*Figure 9.1*). In health, point A roughly corresponds to the conjunction of the uterine artery and the ureter, but this is not always the case even in early stage disease, and is frequently not the case in late-stage disease. However, the dose calculated at point A correlates quite well with the incidence of severe morbidity in the paracervical tissues, that is, a dose-effect relationship is demonstrable. Despite the obvious shortcomings of expressing a predetermined dose at point A in the presence of distortion and assymetry, so doing results in an internal consistency in dosimetry which has permitted several important prospective clinical trials to be successfully executed (Easson, 1973). A 7500 cGy dose to point A is achieved in 140 hours by a dose rate of 53.5 cGy/hour, during a 'standard' insertion. This insertion is one in which a central uterine tube, 4 or 6 cm long, is combined with a transversely disposed pair of lateral forniceal ovoids with an interposed washer ('zero' separation) or spacer (10 mm separation). This arrangement is designed to produce a high dose volume isodose curve resembling a forwardly flexed dependant pear flattened inferiorly. The 4 cm uterine tube contains 10 mg radium in the endocervical canal, and 15 mg in the cavity of the corpus. In the case of longer uterine cavities requiring a 6 cm tube, the extra fundal 2 cm carries an additional 10 mg of radium: the workings of the inverse square law and increasingly oblique self filtration combine to result

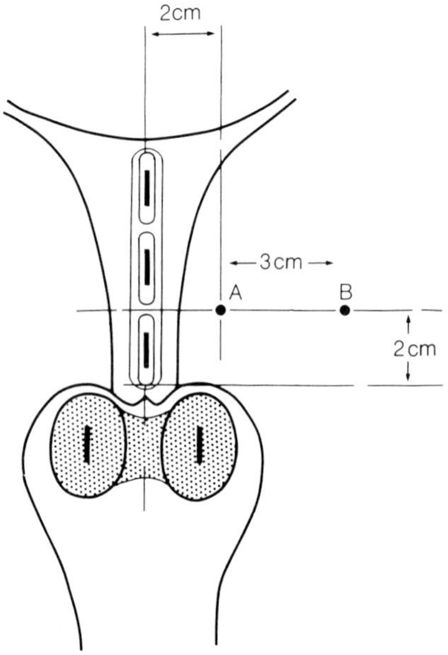

Figure 9.1 Positions in the coronal projection of Manchester points A and B. Within the point A isodose curve (100%) dosage is markedly inhomogeneous, very high doses being received by the surfaces in direct contact with the applicators

in both 4 and 6 cm tubes delivering very close to 34.2 cGy/hour at point A. The shape of the Manchester ovoids is designed so that the external surface of the ovoid describes a three-dimensional isodose curve for its contained radium. Three sizes are available, the smallest containing 17.5 mg radium. In order to maintain the point A dose rate approximately constant at 18–19 cGy/hour, the medium and large ovoids contain an additional 2.5 mg and 5 mg radium respectively. The shape as well as the size of the point A isodose curve (the dependent pear) is influenced by the size of the components used; the larger vaginal components naturally make the pear more broad-based.

'Standard' insertions can be achieved in most patients, the most common exceptions being as follows:

(1) When insufficient space is available to mount even the small ovoids transversely, necessitating their placement longitudinally down the vagina (in tandem). This renders the pear-shape less broad-based, and reduces the dose rate at point A by approximately 8%. Experienced radiotherapists commonly choose to compensate for this by increasing the duration of the insertion, as there is no increased incidence or severity of proctitis.
(2) When the uterine canal cannot be identified at

the first attempt at intracavitary treatment. There are several options for dealing with this latter circumstance: (i) an 'ovoids-only' insertion of standard duration can be carried out, in the often realized anticipation that this will cause sufficient resolution of disease to permit successful cannulation 1 week later. A standard insertion may then be performed, with the intention of performing a third insertion 1 week later, again of standard duration, but with a uterine tube only. Alternatively, if a third anaesthetic is considered undesirable, a 'double strength' uterine tube can be used with standard ovoids: a truly double strength source doubles the dose rate at point A, which receives approximately two-thirds of its dose from the uterine source, and to avoid increased morbidity, the loading of 'double strength' tubes is actually somewhat less than twice that of standard tube. If the 'ovoids-only' treatment fails to facilitate successful cannulation at the second attempt, radical surgery, if feasible, offers the best option for cure, although external radiation could be considered.

The conduct of intracavitary therapy

The extension of cervical cancer is predominantly into paracervical tissues, the upper vagina, and lower uterine segment. Vesical and rectal extension are much less common and, when present, often preclude an intracavitary component to the treatment, because cure is unlikely, whereas fistula formation would be swift. The cervix, uterus and vagina are very tolerant of high surface doses of radiation, whereas the rectum and bladder are very vulnerable to permanent damage. Accordingly, particular attention is paid to minimizing the dose to the rectum and bladder base. This is facilitated by carrying out the insertion with the patient in the knee–chest position. Patients in lithotomy for EUA can often be turned into the preferred knee–chest position while still partly unconscious, or can otherwise be returned to the ward for treatment on another occasion. So great are the advantages of the knee–chest position that an extra general anaesthetic is justified: modern anaesthesia is much less hazardous to the patient than failure to achieve an optimum insertion. The most important advantages of the knee–chest position are that:

(1) It greatly facilitates the placement of moist partly radiopaque gauze packing ribbon behind the ovoids
(2) Atmospheric distension of the vagina gives an accurate and the best impression of the size of the largest ovoids that can comfortably be accommodated across the vault. The larger vaginal components increase the breadth of the volume subtended by the squat base of the pear, and the extra 10 mg radium in the distal 2 cm of the largest uterine tube maintains the point A dose rate; in concert, the larger and more heavily loaded radium applicators broaden the base and mutually deliver more dose to point B. (*See below* — treatment of late stage disease)
(3) Perforation into the peritoneal cavity is signalled by the audible aspiration of air, and accordingly never goes unrecognized
(4) The manipulation and precise placement of the applicators is facilitated by elimination of the need for a second (or even third) retractor, and individual applicators tend to lie gravitationally in their intended ultimate situations, without the need for mechanical constraint during the remainder of the insertion
(5) Having packed the applicators optimally into position with respect to each other and with respect to the anatomical configuration of the vault, the entire radium assembly can be securely fixed in the mid-pelvis by appropriate packing of the vagina. In lithotomy it is difficult to do more than apply fold after fold of transversely disposed layers of continous gauze, whereas in the knee–chest position succeeding long loops of packing can be tracked up and tucked well in, a manoueuvre made simple and safe by the interposition of thin non-space occupying L-shaped retractor between the vaginal walls. Longitudinally placed packing is less likely to be dislodged by the patient's movements than transverse packing.

The knee–chest position is unsuitable for some patients, for example the very elderly, the very fat and those unable to flex the hip or knee joints. If the need for an EUA and/or cystoscopy predicates the lithotomy position (adequate EUA and cystoscopy being impossible in the knee–chest position), the patient should either be turned or given an extra anaesthetic (*see above*). Good manners, a small and sympathetic staff, appropriate gowning and rigid exclusion from the theatre of inessential servitors, invariably overcome the reluctance experienced by some women in adopting what they evidently feel is a somehow degrading posture. If the patient is not to flop about during anaethesia, or even less helpfully gradually to decant into the prone position, it is neccessary that her upper thighs are tightly bound to upright supports on each side of the operator's end of the treatment table. It is reassuring for the patient when this binding is performed by fellow-females, and reassuring for the operator when it is performed by sturdy ones. It should be noted, however, that many centres in the UK practise intracavitary insertions in the lithotomy position and do not necessarily have any increased morbidity. Indeed, at the London Hospital where this latter technique has been used for 21 years, fistula and local pelvic morbidity rate has been negligible while retaining a very high cure rate (Hartgill and Hope-Stone, 1985 personal communication).

A self-retaining urinary catheter is introduced before instrumentation is begun. This avoids urethral compression during subsequent packing, and to some extent reduces ward staff radiation exposure, as the catheter bag can be changed more swiftly than a bed pan can be introduced. The bowel is emptied by an enema before the patient goes to theatre and the bowels thus are not opened for the duration of the insertions.

Not all departments possess in-theatre screening facilities, so that the emplacement of the applicators is checked by anteroposterior and lateral radiographs taken in an adjacent or perhaps even remote X-ray diagnostic facility: this increases radiation exposure generally, and the patient may have recovered from her anaesthetic before it is recognized that her insertion is not ideal, and can possibly be improved. These disadvantages can to some extent be avoided if systematic readings of the rectal dose rates are taken using a rectal probe ensheathed in a disposable examination glove. Such readings correlate poorly with the subsequent occurrence of late radiation effects on the lower bowel, but they do frequently lead to recognition that an unsatisfactory insertion has probably occurred while the patient is still anaesthetized and on the operating table. In this eventuality, the pack is removed, the applicators are visually inspected, adjusted if necessary, the system is repacked, and the rectal probe readings are repeated. Dose rates are recorded at five points. First, with the probe lightly in contact with the anterior rectal wall, a reading is taken at the point where the dose rate is highest, which is usually immediately behind and between the ovoids, in the midline. The probe is then pressed firmly toward the ovoids; if this increases the dose rate by more than a few cGy/hour, the posterior fornix is insufficiently firmly packed and the pack is likely to flatten during the course of the insertion, with the risk of late rectal complications. Readings are then systematically taken at four points superior, inferior and lateral to the point of maximum dose rate. The pattern of distribution of the dose-rate readings about the maximum may indicate: (1) rotation of the ovoid couplet during packing; (2) inadequate packing behind one or both ovoids; (3) slippage of the central tube from the uterine canal toward the vault (signalled also by very high maximum readings); or (4) the uncommon posterior perforation, usually occurring in lithotomy position.

Maximal rectal dose-rate values of 25 cGy/hour or less are usually obtainable (compared with 53 cGy at point A). When two or more insertions are planned, the final cumulative rectal mucosal dose should not exceed 4500 cGy, and the temptation to accept high readings on the first insertion should be resisted, as the intention to compensate by especially low read-

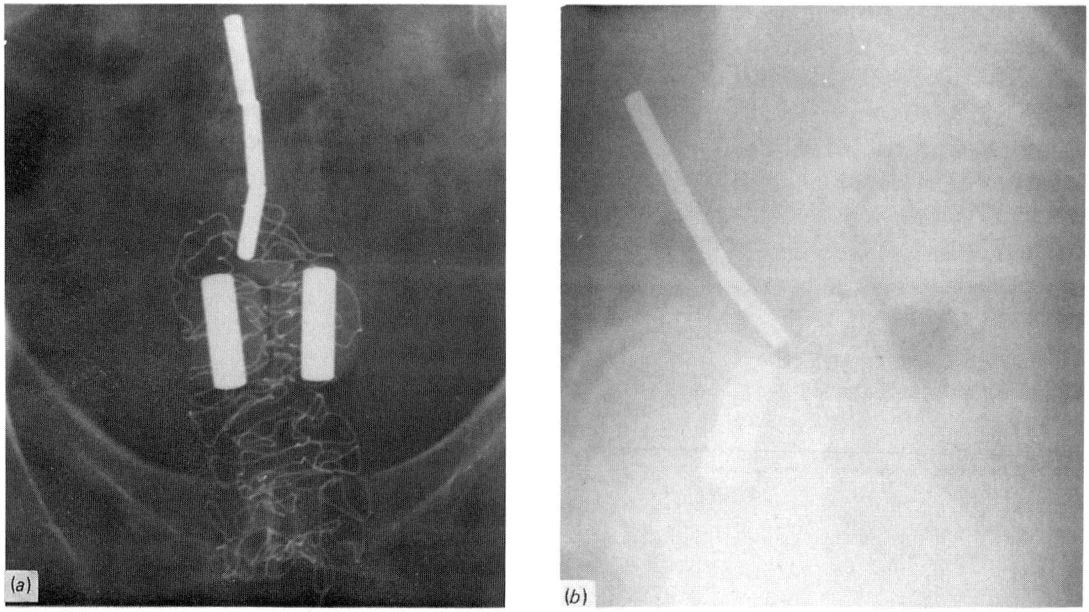

Figure 9.2 Radiographs taken shortly after insertion, in a patient with early stage disease and undistorted anatomy: (a) posterior view, (b) lateral view. The gauze packing contains a radiopaque thread. Note: (1) Adequate posterior packing. (2) Symmetrical disposition of components — no rotation of ovoid couplet during packing. (3) Absence of gap between ovoid couplets and intrauterine tube; such a gap usually occurs when such a packing lies above rather than behind the ovoids, the common result of the selection of too large ovoids. (4) Absence of slippage of the central source from the uterine cavity into the vagina

ings on the second insertion is not often attainable.

Critical inspection of anteroposterior and lateral radiographs (*Figure 9.2*) provides information which correlates far better with late radiation bowel damage than do rectal dose-rate readings. Particular attention is paid to the following:

(1) The adequacy of packing behind *both* ovoids and in the posterior fornix

(2) The absence of a gap between the ovoid couplet and the lowest extent of the endocervical tube (which is usually caused by the use of ovoids too large for the vault anatomy)

(3) Whether the spatial inter-relationships of the three radium applicators is the best that can be achieved, having due regard to the known anatomical circumstances of the patient.

Further practical guidance in the conduct of intracavitary treatments is offered in the subsequent section on afterloading.

Radioactive afterloading

Introduction

Many intracavitary insertions using independent applicators are not geometrically ideal (*Figure 9.3*).

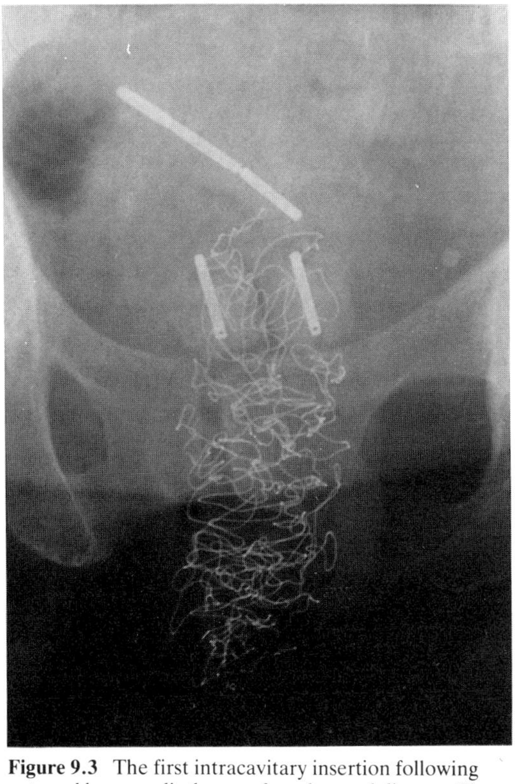

Figure 9.3 The first intracavitary insertion following external beam radiotherapy for advanced disease. The combination of previous inflammatory and present neoplastic disease has deviated the uterus to the right, with a consequential underdosage of the left paracervical tissue and overdosage on the right

In such cases, failure to achieve ideal distribution of sources is due to anatomical distortion caused by disease. In the example illustrated, the paracervical tissues on the right are underdosed, possibly leading to failure to control disease, whereas on the left side there is overdosage, with the risk of radiation-induced morbidity. The hypothetical advantages of using a rigid intracavitary assembly to impose a dose distribution closer to the ideal have long been apparent. However, the dominant impetus for the commercial development of fixed intracavitary assemblies has arisen from the wish to reduce the radiation exposure of hospital staff; gynaecological intracavitary therapy is the biggest single contributor to staff exposure (Fleishman, Notley and Wilkinson, 1983), although in most hospitals only a small proportion of the staff are affected. The few individuals habitually engaged in radium theatre work, doctors, nurses, and sealed-source laboratory staff, generally take a sanguine view of the supposed risks of protracted low dose radiation exposure, regarding 'arms-length' handling of sealed sources, dexterity, and swiftness as conferring sufficient protection.

Ward nurses are usually young women of as yet unexpressed reproductive potential and their exposure has traditionally been minimized by siting patients with radioactive sealed sources *in situ* in those locations which are least frequented by the nursing staff, (that is at the end of the ward furthest from its entrance) and by distributing such patients as widely as possible on different wards. Growing public awareness of the real and imagined hazards of ionizing radiation is making these practices increasingly unworkable. In particular, the more informed ancillary and nursing staff of today are now reluctant to supervise patients containing radioactive sources, and their fears gain credence from the clear intentions of the legislature to impose stringent conditions which will make remote afterloading virtually obligatory in the near future.

In spite of the foregoing, pressure for reduction of exposure to hospital staff comes not only from medical and nursing personnel, but also, more importantly perhaps, from non-medical sources, principally physicists. In the UK, pressure for reduction in radiation exposure originates principally from the National Radiation Protection Board (NRPB), the relevant agency concerned with the protection of the public.

The pressure for reduction in staff dose coincides with the obsolescence of the ageing radium stock in the UK. Radium sources were originally provided by the Radium Commission, and radium sources legally still belong to the successors of that no longer extant body. Deterioration in the platinum encapsulation of radium sources poses an increasing chance of an escape of radon gas, and enforced withdrawal of radium sources of all kinds is imminent. These two circumstances accelerated the conversion from traditional radium treatments, firstly to the use of caesium and cobalt sources for manual insertions and subsequently to afterloading systems, using these alternative radioisotopes.

The speculative extrapolations of the NRPB and similar bodies elsewhere are likely to make RAL systems virtually compulsory, irrespective of their questioned ability to confer cure as effectively as traditional radium methods. Several RAL systems have initially been associated with significant increase in morbidity, and the responses to this have been either to:

(1) Increase fractionation, and/or
(2) Reduce the administered dose (*see* Chapter 1).

The hasty conclusion in both instances has been that changes in dose rate have alone determined the increased morbidity; the extensive experience of one RAL system indicates that such simplistic assumptions may be erroneous (The Manchester Selectron experience, *see below*).

Afterloading refers to the practice of inserting hollow non-radioactive guides into the uterus and vagina (*Figure 9.4*), which are subsequently loaded with radioactive sources. As the applicators are inert, their insertion can proceed at a leisurely pace, and necessary adjustments to the assembly and its packing can be carried out before the system is activated, so that technically optimal insertions are relatively easy to achieve; also training of junior staff can be carried out carefully, slowly and without any radiation hazard. In general, the UK preference has been for metal source-guides, as they are durable, are not degraded by radiation, are easily sterilized, and their relative and absolute relationships are easily seen on radiographs. In addition, their rigidity permits the operator some degree of control over the prevailing anatomy; for example a uterus lying naturally to the left, in contact with the sigmoid colon, can often be induced to occupy a midline position by counter clockwise torsion on the other end of the applicator; similarly, a naturally retroverted uterus is carried safely away from the sigmoid colon by the fixed anteverted central tube. (Damage to the sigmoid colon was a new and serious complication of early RAL treatments (Sherrah-Davies, 1985).)

When optimal distribution and placement of the sources have been achieved and the patient has recovered from her general anaesthetic and has confirmed that her insertion is comfortable, the applicators are activated, either manually or by remote control. Manual afterloading was a logical step in the development of RAL, but its benefits are exclusively limited to theatre staff. Irrespective of the newly expressed fashion of the NRPB to place greater emphasis on the personal rather than the genetic effect of radiation, it is common sense to regard the ward staff as the group for which reduced radiation exposure has the highest priority.

The irradiation of young women must be regarded as wholly undesirable, and in the hospital context this means that RAL is an inevitable development. Since manual afterloading does not provide reduction in ward-staff exposure, its employment might be considered appropriate only in departments dealing with small numbers of patients. Sensitivity, expertise, and experience are crucial to the effective conduct of intracavitary therapy, and these qualities are unlikely to persist in departments which engage in intracavitary therapy on a semi-occasional basis, thus manual afterloading is destined for early demise, at least in the UK.

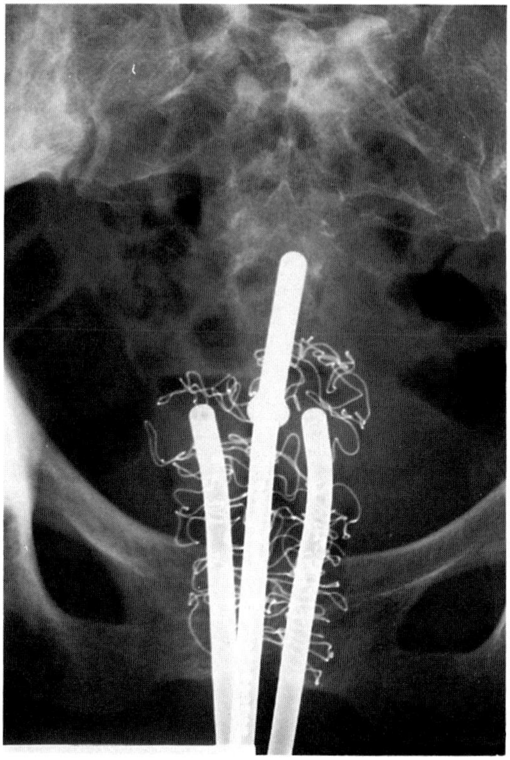

Figure 9.4 Intracavitary radiation employing rigid source guides (Selectron applicators shown). The spatial interrelationships of the three activated ends of the applicators are fixed, although the central tube can be rotated in either direction to impose a more 'ideal' geometry. A gold-seed marker in the substance of the cervix permits recognition of subsequent slippage of the assembly relative to the cervix

Remote afterloading systems (RALS)

The requirements of afterloading are that the radioactive sources are mechanically impelled into the active ends of the applicators with no necessity for radiation exposure of any but the patient herself. This is achieved by carrying out treatments in shielded suites. Staff protection is complete, and the irradiation of other adjacent ward patients undergoing treatment can also be eliminated; (this last requirement is one of the recent recommendations of the NRPB but is felt by some radiotherapists to indicate the extent to which that body has lost touch with the realities of cancer treatment). In the UK the systems most commonly used are the Selectron, Cathetron and Curietron (*see below*).

Although the main emission energy of radium is only marginally higher than the ideal for intracavitary use, it requires an envelope to contain radon and it is not feasible to produce perfect spheres of radium in encapsulated form. Both caesium-137 and cobalt-60 are cheap, easily and safely machined, solid, and have stable decomposition products; both have adequately long half-lives and can be produced in high specific activity, especially cobalt-60. The fact that very high specific activity could be obtained no doubt strongly influenced the decision to produce early RALS which delivered unprecedentedly high dose rates. When RAL was first introduced it was assumed that the patients would be unlikely to tolerate transvaginal dependance on semi-rigid source-lines for periods of up to 3 days, but this anticipation is now known to have been wrong. High activity sources permitted treatments to be carried out in a matter of minutes, often indeed on an outpatient basis.

It was anticipated that major increases in dose rate would enhance normal tissue responses and intricate attempts were made to estimate the magnitude of the reduction in total dose rate which would be required before the very high dose-rate technique using a Cathetron entered service. The conclusions of Liversedge and Dale (1978) resulted from particularly ingenious experiments and suggested that high dose-rate treatments involving small numbers of fractions could be compared with established low dose-rate treatments by the relationship $N = t/4$, where N is the number of high dose-rate treatments, and t is the time in hours taken for the low dose-rate treatment. Many Cathetron users now give up to six intracavitary treatments with a fraction size around 500 cGy, and the overall treatment time has been increased. These changes occurred progressively as increased morbidity from Cathetron treatments became apparent. The assumption underlying these changes was that the increased morbidity was solely attributed to changes in dose-rate; it was not until the Manchester experience, using an alternative method of RAL, that it became apparent that physical factors inherent in the construction of the afterloading applicators themselves could have very important effects (*see below*). Departments in which Cathetrons were originally installed seemed content to continue to use them, having derived what are evidently satisfactory treatment regimens (giving excellent results) by a progressive process of making frequent alterations in treatment policy determined by experience gained on relatively few patients (Joslin and Peel, 1982). Very little of the development of high dose-rate RALS has taken place in the context of controlled clinical trials, and much of the early assessment took place in the context of relatively non-critical preoperative treatments, where the sub-radical radiation doses employed might well have obscured serious deficiencies in this method.

The inconveniently short half-life of cobalt–60 (5.3 years) determined the Manchester option for caesium–137 (half-life 30.5 years), especially as high specific activity was irrelevant to the requirements of the projected studies, which were intended to be at dose-rates comparable to those obtained in the Manchester radium system. The use of apparatus which exactly duplicated the radium system dose rate would be logistically impossible in a centre dealing with 700 insertions annually, since the cost of providing sufficient numbers of RAL apparatus, and the cost of constructing adequate shielded treatment suites, would have been very high. Accordingly, caesium–137 was chosen as the alternative radionuclide best suited to the Manchester requirements. Radium tubes are rigid and of fixed length, and their replacement by small spheres which could at will be interspersed with inactive pellets offers the potential ability to improve dose distributions. The best-engineered apparatus commercially available which most closely conformed to the Manchester requirements was the Selectron, and a pellet strength of 1500 MBq (40 mCi, equivalent to 5 mg of radium) was chosen, so that average treatment times fell from 70 hours to around 20 hours, thus two 6-channel installations could simultaneously treat four patients daily. The effects of a modest (× 3.5) increase in dose rate were not known, but as there was a possibility that reparative mechanisms might be overwhelmed by this increase in the rate at which the cells were experiencing radiation damage, it was considered essential that a prospective randomized trial of radium versus Selectron treatment be instituted, with equal numbers of Selectron patients receiving one of two different doses. This approach generated two points on the dose–response curves for both tumour control and morbidity; interpolation or limited extrapolation permitted the Selectron treatments to be compared with that of radium; both having equivalent morbidity.

Features of the Selectron apparatus

Caesium-137 has a gamma emission of 0.6 MeV and accordingly is relatively easily shielded so that the radiation safe and its associated control mechanisms are fairly small and light, and can be moved around on castors by one person. Assortment of active and inactive pellets, once programmed, is computer controlled. During treatments of up to 20 hours' duration it is necessary to interrupt the patient's solitude to provide food and nursing care and in order to check that there has been no apparent movement of the applicators. Treatments are readily interrupted by remote control and in the last resort by safety interlocks at the entrance to the treatment suite, and the pellets are rapidly returned pneumatically to the radiation safe. A computer automatically adjusts the overall treatment time to account for any interruptions which may have occurred, and terminates the treatment when the specified dose has been delivered. Even when the rigid applicators have been clamped in such a way as to alter the natural disposition of the uterus, insertion times of the order of 20 hours remain comfortable and patients are unaware of the alteration imposed on the geometry of their pelvic organs.

If applicators are suspected of movement within the patient, check radiographs are taken and the position of the applicators relative to an inert gold grain inserted into the cervix at the time of the emplacement of the applicators is compared to the relationship demonstrated on the films which were taken immediately after the insertion.

The recommendations of the NRPB notwithstanding, in Manchester it was decided to site two patients in each Selectron suite, in order to lessen the sense of isolation which many patients might otherwise experience, and to reduce the cost of the of the procedure, since two patients can be treated at the same time by one machine.

The Curietron

The advantages and correctness of altering only one variable at a time were recognized in departments that opted to maintain point A dose rates at levels with which they were already familiar. A successful and to date complication-free low-dose rate system suitable for installation in departments dealing with comparatively small numbers of patients has been evaluated at The London Hospital (Hope-Stone *et al.*, 1981). The system, known commercially as the Curietron (CGR, France), is relatively inexpensive in respect of its purchase price, maintenance costs, and staffing requirements, but now requires the construction of a special protected treatment room in order to comply with the latest NRPB regulations. Its engineering simplicity is associated with a very low mechanical failure-rate, and for its operation it does not depend on sophisticated, and therefore vulnerable, control and safety mechanisms. Manually operated control buttons initiate mechanically-propelled drive-cables which are automatically and independently retracted at preset times. Many simple and therefore reliable safety devices are incorporated, which is particularly important, since the Curietron was originally designed for use in ordinary ward side-rooms rather than in specially protected isolated treatment suites (*see above*). Each Curietron is loaded from a 'mother' safe via a mobile transit safe with up to four source trains, although only three are commonly used. The relatively low activity of the system's caesium-137 glass beads, shielded in the depleted uranium safe of each satellite Curietron, results in very low exposure at the Curietron surface.

At The London Hospital, an average reduction in staff exposure of 50% was achieved (Hope-Stone *et al.*, 1981), the range being from 40–70% reduction, and the main beneficiaries being the ancillary staff and nurses, particularly those nurses working on the wards. At that time at The London Hospital at least 40% of the cases were still being treated with manual caesium insertions.

Staff exposure levels are now so low in the UK that a 50% reduction is a major achievement, and should not be taken as an indication of only half-success of RALS, because background exposure is irreducible and some additional exposure of hospital personnel comes from sources unconnected with intracavitary treatments. However, gynaecological intracavitary treatments remain the single most important cause of potentially avoidable staff exposure, (Fleishman, Notley and Wilkinson, 1983), and further improvements are to be expected. This has now been achieved at The London Hospital with the acquisition of a third Curietron so that almost no manual caesium insertions are carried out and staff exposure is negligble (Hope-Stone, 1985, personal communication).

In many departments, RALS have not totally supplanted manual loading because access to RALS equipment is logistically not yet possible for all patients, or manual loading is required for some patients because RALS are being prospectively and randomly compared with established pre-loading techniques. Occasionally patients will refuse the insertion of a rigid applicator system.

The applicators and ancillary equipment of the Curietron are different from those employed in the Selectron and Cathetron systems. In its London Hospital application the Curietron has a flexible PVC intrauterine catheter, in contrast to the metal tubes of the other two systems, and the equivalents of the 2.0 and 2.5 cm diameter Manchester ovoids, are carried as pairs in a single perspex vaginal applicator with two source-channels. Insertions are carried out in the lithotomy position. Inherent protection of the anterior rectal wall is provided by a posteriorly directed globular extension of the perspex of the applicator, so that posterior forniceal packing is not required. The source channels are shielded, reducing the rectal dose to 70% of the unshielded value. A single in-line system incorporating a uterine tube and vaginal sources is also available for patients with a very narrow vagina. The system has provision for differential loading and independent treatment times in each source train.

The low dose rate delivered by the Curietron means that the treatment times are prolonged well beyond the 18–20 h of the Selectron, and accordingly secure fixation of the applicator assembly within the pelvis is essential. Of practical importance is the reported acceptability by patients of a smooth and appropriately curved and shielded perineal bar, which is securely and snugly tucked up against the perineum by attachment to a harness described as a corset, but which in published figures more resembles a somewhat discouraging suspender belt. Corsets locate around the waist and the London Hospital garment is carefully designed to exert consistent counter-traction on the perineal fixing bar by its 'suspender-belt' location over both iliac crests, which makes it an ideal fixation device for averagely built and slender patients. The perineal bar has two midline apertures for the transmission of the applicator stalks, with appropriate location and locking devices. The whole assembly is held snugly against a soft perineal melolin pad by fixing tapes from the 'corset'. The intracavitary assembly is fixed to the perineal obturator in the theatre while the patient is unconscious; the assembly is first pushed 'as high into the vagina as possible' (Hope-Stone *et al.*, 1981), which means as firmly as knowledge and respect for the elasticity of pelvic tissues permit. The fact that the triple-component assembly is clamped before this manoeuvre takes place guards against the excessive stretching and thinning of the uterine fundus, which are believed to be major sources of bowel morbidity in the early Selectron-treated patients in Manchester (*see below*), because the lateral forniceal components prevent undue penetration of the central source. Dummy sources are loaded for radiographic purposes, but rectal dose-rate readings are not performed. The design of the vaginal applicator (a single unit with two independent source guides) does not always allow it to locate as high in the vagina as would a couplet of two independent ovoids, and to avoid underdosage at the level of the cervix, the intrauterine source train can be lengthened to extend from the external os to the level of the upper ends of the vaginal applicator sources.

In the recent review after a further 4 years' experience with the Curietron, no excess pelvic morbidity has been noted and the fistula rate remains at less than 0.5%. Patients seemed able to tolerate the presence of these applicators for periods of up to 72 hours (Hartgill and Hope-Stone, 1985, personal communication).

The Christie Hospital Selectron experience

Following an inadequate pilot study, a prospective randomized clinical trial in stage I and stage IIa cervical cancer started in late 1980. As argued in Chapter 1, it was considered essential that the novel treatment be carried out at two dose levels, so randomization was (and continues to be) on the basis of a three-way split, equal numbers of patients being assigned to (1) manually loaded treatment, initially with radium, latterly with caesium, (2) higher-dose Selectron treatment, and (3) lower-dose Selectron treatment.

It was originally thought that the preferred Selctron applicators would permit close mimicry of antecedent radium treatments, at least in terms of dose distribution, and so the trial was designed on the scientifically correct premise that only one variable, namely dose rate, was being altered. Within 2 years it became apparent that this assumption was wrong (*see below*).

On the mistaken belief that patients would not readily comply with the requirement to remain attached by flexible tubing to a computer-activated, pneumatically operated, bed-side radiation safe for 70 hours, a pellet strength of 40 mCi (equivalent to 5 mg radium) was chosen. This decision resulted in treatment times of the order of 20 hours or less, which it was correctly anticipated most patients would tolerate. Traditional radium treatments for early disease extended over approximately 240 hours, whereas the novel treatment was some 50 hours less: it was considered unlikely that this reduction would, *per se*, necessitate a dose modification in the Selectron arms of the trial, and in the absence of reliable clinical and radiological guidance, no attempt was made to correct for it.

Ingenious and specifically commissioned radiobiological experiments (Wilkinson, Hendry and Hunter, 1980) indicated that a 3.5 increment in dose rate would necessitate a 33% reduction in absolute dose, from 7500 cGy (radium) to 4650 cGy (caesium). Previous experience of the fallibility of laboratory derived non-human data to predict accurately clinical consequences led to the unanimous rejection of the notion of such a radical reduction in dose; two out of three potentially curable patients (three-way randomization, *see above*), were considered to have been put at risk of underdosage. The data from which the recommendation of a point A dose of 8000 R was drawn (Tod, 1947) seemed to indicate the presence of a plateau for local control at higher doses, and 8000 R was considered to represent the start of this plateau. Expressed differently, it was felt that 8000 R was well within the tolerance of the critical paracervical tissues. These considerations greatly influenced the initial decision concerning the two-dose levels in the Selectron arms of the trial. Further, overdosage would hypothetically declare itself within a few months of treatment, whereas underdosage, leading to failure of local control, might take much longer to become apparent. Accordingly, the laboratory-derived recommendations were disregarded, and the higher of the two Selectron doses was set at 7500 cGy. Dose-effect differences are clinically rarely detectable below a 5% difference in dose, and because dose–response curves for local control are so steep, dose differences greater than 10% are ethically unacceptable. It was therefore decided to set the lower of the two Selecton doses at approximately 7% less than the higher dose, that is, at 7000 cGy. The prediction that overdosage would declare itself early proved to be correct, and in May 1982, the dose range in the Selectron arms of the trial was reduced to 7000 and 6500 cGy respectively. At the time of this change there was pressure for the randomization to be changed to a two-way split, with patients being allocated in equal numbers to radium (7500 cGy) or Selectron (6750 cGy). Even large regional institutions experience some difficulty in recruiting statistically adequate number of patients into trials, and where only small differences between two treatments are anticipated, as in this case, a three-way randomization might be thought to represent a 'waste' of patients. On the other hand, adoption of a single Selectron dose would have presupposed that it was exactly equivalent to the 7500 cGy radium dose; the results of prospective clinical trials should not be assumed in advance and, accordingly, the present author strenuously and successfully resisted the adoption of a two-way randomization. A second reduction in the dose-range (6000 and 6500 cGy) occurred in November 1982), due to continuing excessive morbidity in Selectron-treated patients. This morbidity was to some extent novel in its nature and distribution, and may have been the result of extraneous factors other than dose rate: this continuing uncertainty underlined the need for a two dose-level study. It seems likely that the Manchester trial will ultimately make a unique contribution to knowledge about the clinical significance of changes in dose rate: so far as the author is aware, no comparable trial using two dose-levels in the afterloading arms is being carried out. (Low dose-rate caesium sources have now replaced radium in the 'radium' arm of the trial, but their physical properties and the dose rate delivered are for practical purposes identical.)

The early and striking increase in morbidity in the Selectron arms of the trial, and the emergence of treatment-associated mortality therein, may be thought solely attributable to insufficient reduction in dose to allow for the 3.5 increase in dose rate. The trial had been designed to alter only one variable, that is dose rate, but painstaking analysis (Sherrah-Davies, 1985) indicated that a number of quite separate variables had been inadvertently and unexpectedly introduced. There are obvious differences between the independent radium applicators and the inflexible Selectron applicators which, when clamped, have fixed spatial relationships: it might reasonably be expected that by imposing a more 'ideal' geometry to the insertion, the rigid applicators would actually reduce the incidence of local high-dose zones, and would therefore be associated with a reduced incidence of complications. The converse was unfortunately true.

The differences occurring in the treatments actually received by the early patients in the radium/Selectron trial are summarized below. As noted above, these differences were unforeseen and unintentional. It is not yet clear to what extent any have contributed to the excess morbidity in the Selectron-treated patients, but practical recommendations to eliminate these variables are now in operation. The continuing widespread adoption of rigid afterloading systems means that nationally, increasing large numbers of young patients are at serious risk of morbidity from the modern version of what used to be an extremely successful and complication-free treatment (although there has been little morbidity using the Curietron). Radiotherapists contemplating the use of rigid afterloading devices should be thoroughly familiar with the excellent analysis of the inherent disadvantages of the Selectron (Sherrah-Davies, 1985).

Differences in the methods of treatments between radium and Selectron techniques

(i) Component size

Traditionally, the largest ovoids and the longest intrauterine tube permitted by the local anatomy were regarded as desirable; this increased the dose at point B, and broadened the base of the pear to subtend the preferential routes of extension of disease. This teaching appears unconsciously to have influenced the conduct of Selectron insertions. The ease of manipulation of the rigid applicators, and the control they confer in their own placement, has resulted in a marked tendency for Selectron treatments to be executed using components larger than those used in radium-treated patients. In particular, the use of long (6.5 cm) intrauterine applicators was 87% in Selectron patients, and only 56% in the radium patients; 95% of Selectron patients with serious irradiation-induced bowel damage were treated with long tubes. Some operators were consistently disposed to use long tubes more often than others; the same operators were also more commonly included to use larger ovoids in conjunction with the long tubes. This suggests that respect for the elasticity and compliance of the uterus and vaginal vault differs widely between individuals. Initially, no provision was made in the Selectron treatment options to reproduce exactly the ovoids-in-tandem situation, which occurred in 12% of the radium-treated patients. Patients who would have had radium ovoids in tandem in the Selectron arms of the trial often received treatment with two half-ovoids, resulting in more distension of the vault. The leverage inherent in the use of long, rigid ovoid supply lines permits distension of the vault of which the operator may be insensible. Having achieved apparently satisfactory placement of the half-ovoids, adequate (i.e. 1 cm minimum) packing of the posterior fornix was frequently not achieved. Of patients with low proctitis (generally settling with conservative management), 85% had been treated with small or half-ovoids, and were commonly postmenopausal, and hence likely to have a small vaginal vault. The occurrence of vaginal tears in the Selectron-treated patients (almost unknown in radium patients) is thought to result from the combination of unconscious selection of larger components than the tissues will comfortably accommodate, and conscious determination to pack adequately.

(ii) Component loading

To elimiate the need for three sets of ovoid supply tubes, all ovoids were and still are loaded identically. The choice of active caesium pellets closely equivalent to 5 mg of radium predicates that all caesium ovoids contain 20 mg radium equivalent (compared with 17.5, 20 and 22.5 in the radium system), and point A doses are adjusted for ovoid size by varying the time for which the ovoids are actively loaded. The assumption that the small changes in dose *rate* at point A would have negligible effect is almost certainly still justified, but the relative overloading of the small and half-ovoids (20 mg radium-equivalent, versus 17.5 mg), raises their surface dose and hence the vault mucosal dose, to 26 000 cGy. This very high dose (compared with less than 15 000 cGy for conventional large radium ovoids), acting in concert with ischaemia from overdistension, is thought to have contributed to the occurrence of delayed vault healing and fistula formation in the first groups of Selectron-treated patients. (In early stage disease, fistula formation is unknown following conventional radium treatments.)

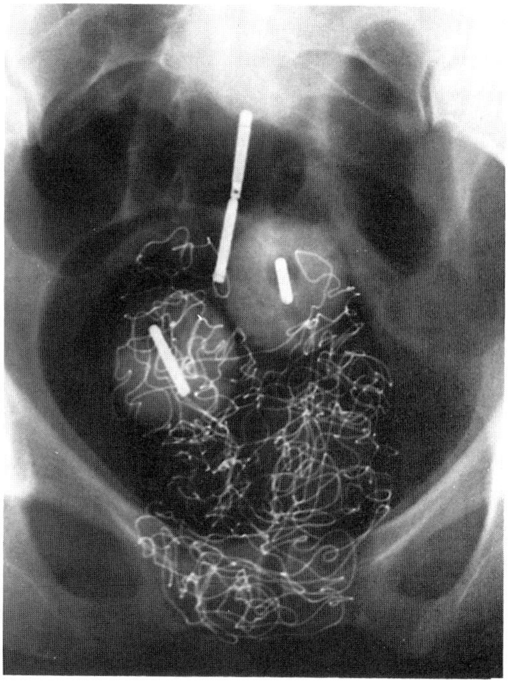

Figure 9.5 An apparently inexpert insertion of pre-loaded sources. In fact, the disposition of the three components is such as to give the closest approximation to the prevailing distorted vault anatomy. Since the surface of the ovoid describes an isodose the orientation of the ovoid does not influence either the point A dose or the vault mucosal dose, but as much of the ovoid surfaces as possible should be in contact with neoplasm

(iii) Component distribution

The surface of the radium ovoid was designed to describe a three-dimensional isodose, so that the actual disposition of the ovoid in the lateral fornix had no influence on the dose-rate at point A. Some insertions (*Figure 9.5*) look less expertly performed than others (*see Figure 9.2*), and such unglamorous examples are rarely chosen to illustrate textbooks: however, the arrangement of sources shown in *Figure 9.5* is that which allowed the snuggest fit of the applicators to the presenting anatomy. Inexperienced radiotherapists might be inclined to tamper with the radium assembly, hoping to obtain check radiographs more closely resembling their idealized notions of a 'perfect' insertion: more experienced colleagues will resist this temptation, recognizing the practical importance of 'covering the ground' as closely as possible. Conventional ovoids, being 'elipses of revolution', can be arranged to conform neatly with a very wide range of anatomically-determined situations, thereby permitting some degree of individualization of each patient's treatment. The long axis of the Selectron ovoid is fixed in relation to the long axis of the vagina (at 60° in the case of the currently employed applicators). The inability to individualize each insertion may be a serious deficiency of the Selectron system, particularly since the absence of graded options generally results in the use of larger rather than smaller components, and this is associated with more frequent and sometimes novel complications.

The length of the long axis of Selectron ovoids is standardized at 3 cm, corresponding to the long axis of the medium radium ovoid. This standardization eliminates the need for additional sets of ovoid carriers corresponding to 2.5 cm (small) and 3.5 cm (large) conventional ovoids. However seemingly appropriate the choice of Selectron ovoids is, whenever small ovoids are used, there is certain to be less space behind them for packing than would have been available if conventional ovoids were used. Similarly, large Selectron ovoids permit rather more posterior (and anterior) packing than their radium counterparts, and this may partly explain why their use has not been associated with late complications. In summary:

(1) Long (6 cm) Selectron tubes are associated with serious damage to the sigmoid colon
(2) Small and Selectron half-ovoids are associated with vault distension, delayed healing, and even fistula formation
(3) In each case, there is a marked trend toward the use of larger components than would have been possible if conventional applicators had been used. The adoption of the recommendations below resulted in an immediate and dramatic fall in the complication rate; in particular, no case of sigmoid colon damage has occurred in patients treated during an experimental period when the use of long (6 cm) intrauterine tubes was suspended altogether.

Further suggestions for the conduct of intracavitary therapy, with particular reference to rigid afterloading systems are:

(1) As serious bowel damage is associated with a high dose zone at the tip of the uterine tube, the top two positions should be occupied by inert pellets
(2) Stretching, thinning and tenting of the uterine fundus can occur without perforation and without the knowledge of the operator; in the recommended knee–chest position, the weight of the intrauterine applicator counteracts slow elastic recoil in the undiseased upper uterus. Tough, fibrous cervices may require considerable force in dilatation; the grip of the cervix transmits considerable resistance, making it difficult to sense when the additional resistance of the fundus is encountered. Dilatation should be slow, deliberate, and proceed no further than the minimum required for the insertion of the central tube; each increment of dilatation should be singular; to and fro thrustings are unnecessary and contribute to tenting of the fundus and the selection of an inappropriately long central tube
(3) *Fixed* washers or collars at the external os prevent inadvertent further protrusion of the central tube into the uterus during the subsequent manipulation and packing of the other components
(4) The angle between the uterine and vaginal segments of the central tube should be 40° or more; smaller angles unnaturally approximate the uterine source to the sigmoid colon. Anteverted and anteflexed intrauterine applicators are not used, as the pressure exerted on the uterus to hold it forward is concentrated at the tip, causing fundal thinning predisposing to small bowel damage
(5) Distention of the vault must consciously be avoided; it is most likely to occur when the vault is contracted by disease, old age, or antecedent X-ray treatment. The natural capacity of the vault is best assessed in the knee–chest position. The provision of an in-line vaginal applicator is essential to contend with situations in which tandem ovoids would have been employed — historically one insertion in eight
(6) When the fixed-angle ovoids project into the space vacated by erosion of the posterior cervix, packing must extend into the posterior fornix, to displace the otherwise very proximate sigmoid colon
(7) When space is available, the anterior fornix is packed; this protects the bladder base should the lateral check radiographs subsequently suggest that the active pellets should be pulled forward away from an inadequately protected rectum by the interposition of one or more extra inert pellets; in the Selectron system, such an anterior displacement of the active sources increases the dose to the adjacent bladder mucosa by up to 30%.

In the UK real expertise in intracavitary procedures now exists only in a very few individuals. If the training of future specialists is not to result in the eclipse of such treatments, those responsible for training need to be aware of the already identified hazards of fixed-applicator systems, and to make their trainees alert to the possibility of their hithertofore unrecognized hazards. Inadequately trained therapists ought to be particularly aware of the pitfalls, all of which are more likely when the lithotomy position is used.

The Cathetron

The high specific activity which can be achieved with cobalt–60 has made treatments of very short duration feasible. For reasons discussed in Chapter 1 under 'Dose-rate effects' these treatments have tended to become increasingly far removed from traditional fractionation practices. For the treatment of early stage disease, six to eight insertions may be performed over a period of several weeks. An advantage of this approach is that many patients can be treated on an outpatient basis, and they seemingly do not require general anaesthesia for the insertion of the intracavitary components, mild sedation apparently being sufficient (particularly for carcinoma of the body of the uterus). A major advantage of this approach is that due to the very short treatment times involved large numbers of patients can be treated with one Cathetron. Also, anaesthetists are not always required and staff exposure is negligible. The disadvantages are that skilled staff are needed on several occasions per patient, and that the overall treatment time for each patient is considerably prolonged. Acceptable fractionation schedules have been developed by a process of progressive adjustment, and early and late normal tissue effects are now said to be comparable with those formerly achieved by traditional low-dose rate treatments. There has been no controlled trial of this method and the true equivalence of morbidity with low-dose techniques has only been loosely established.

The Cathetron (TEM Instruments Ltd, UK), first described by O'Connell (1967), transmits high activity cobalt–60 sources from a static storage safe through hollow flexible tubes into stainless steel catheters which end in three independent components corresponding to the Manchester central tube and two ovoids. The applicator stalks are metal and rigid, but a feature which may be of importance is that the individual components are independent of each other, each being separately clamped in its optimal position to a rigid structure connected to the treatment couch itself, rather than to the other components of the assembly. Thus the sources can be allowed to conform to the prevailing anatomy in a way not permitted by the Selectron system, nor by the Newcastle-style vaginal applicator used at The London Hospital.

The high activity of the cobalt–60 sources and the larger number of insertions per patients predicate that a specially protected treatment suite must be constructed (itself an expensive procedure), with suitable radiographic facilities for checking that the physical distribution of the applicators is the best which can be achieved; because multiple insertions are carried out over several weeks, tumour resolution during the course of treatment can permit progressively more 'ideal' insertions to be achieved.

Authoratative users of the Cathetron now claim that the treatment schedules which have been evolved are equivalent in terms of local control and complications to antecedent manually-loaded techniques, and whereas this is undoubtedy true, the comparisons are historical (Joslin and Peel, 1982).

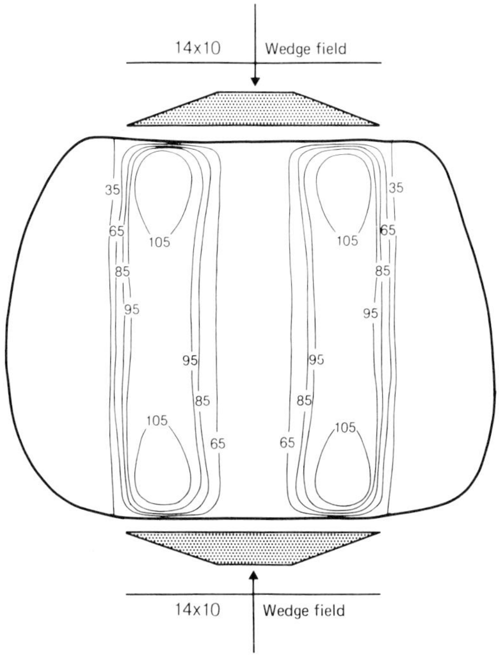

Figure 9.6 Inhomogeneous external pelvic irradiation: an anteroposterior parallel opposed pair using 4 MeV photons with a central wedge filter. Point A receives 50% of the dose at point B, a gradient that is reversed during subsequent intracavitary treatment, leading to a very approximate summation of dose across the central pelvis. Point B will receive a summated dose of 3250 cGy in 16 daily fractions

The treatment of advanced disease

With increasing stage of disease, greater emphasis is placed on the external, rather than internal, contribution of radiation dose, since parametrial extension of disease beyond the point A isodose curve becomes increasingly rapidly underdosed. There is lack of agreement about precisely when external pelvic irradiation should be introduced, and about the degree to which it should supplant intracavitary treatment. External pelvic irradiation reduces the tolerance for subsequent intracavitary irradiation. Radiotherapists impressed with the results of intracavitary treatment in early disease and disappointed with the results of external radiation in late disease, incline to the view that external irradiation should be minimized, in order not to compromise the component of total dose derived from intracavitary treatment. Techniques for pelvic irradiation fall into two categories:

(1) Those which acknowledge the steeply-falling dose-gradient across the pelvis from midline to pelvic side wall, which results from the intracavitary treatment with which they are designed to harmonize
(2) Those which ignore this gradient, and which accordingly are designed to deliver a uniform dose to the whole pelvis.

Central shielding

In the Manchester radium system, point B is defined as lying 3 cm lateral to point A, and in this situation it receives 30–40% of the point A dose from intracavitary sources. The midline structures (bladder, and rectum) determine the radiation tolerance when external and intracavitary treatments are mixed. Intracavitary treatment is seldom indicated in intrapelvic stage IV disease because of the almost inevitable production of fistulae, and in such cases the pelvis should be uniformly irradiated. However, when emphasis is laid on the importance of intracavitary treatment after external radiation (that is in stages II

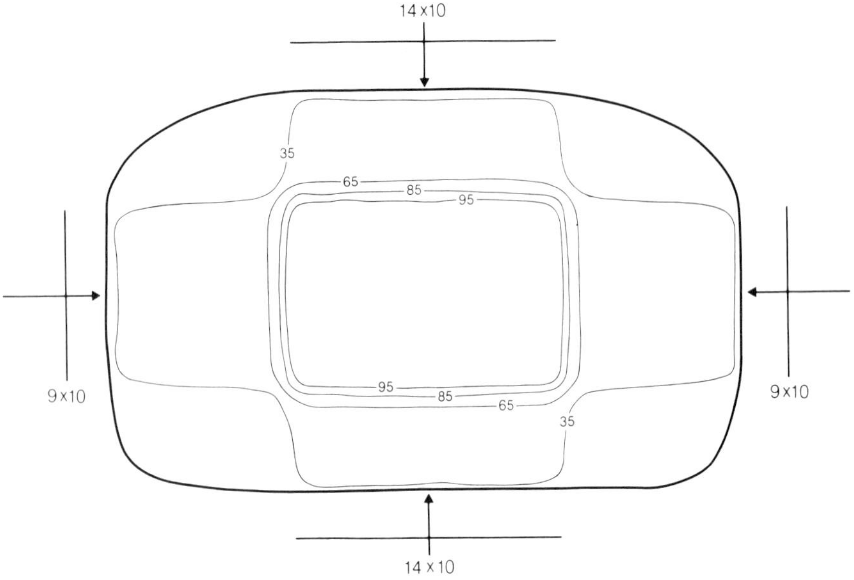

Figure 9.7 Homogeneous pelvic irradiation, commonly referred to as a pelvic 'brick'. Each of the two parallel opposed pairs can give equal contribution to the dose at either the midpoint of the pelvis, or in the subcutaneous tissues. Dose to the femoral necks is less in the latter circumstance. The tumour dose can be 4250 cGy in 16–20 daily fractions

and III), the midline may be shielded; this can be with a simple lead block, or a more complex wedge designed to compensate for the steep fall-off in parametrial dose from the intracavitary sources (*Figure 9.6*). At the Christie Hospital a wedge is used which gives 50% of the point B dose at point A, uniformly irradiating the parametria. In view of the very similar results reported in stage II and stage III disease from different centres, it would appear that no one shielding technique is superior to any other. Midline shielding in advanced cervical cancer is unique in that in no other radiotherapeutic context is the primary tumour centrally shielded during the first weeks of treatment. Many centres overcome this problem by not shielding the midline and giving subsequently a single lower dose with intracavitary radiation (2500–3500 cGy at point A).

It is generally assumed that the survival benefit conferred by parametrial irradiation derives from the eradication of nodal disease within the pelvis; a contrary view is that in advanced disease the effect on local nodal metastases is minimal, and that the benefit derives from shrinkage in the primary tumour, permitting its outermost extensions to fall within tumoricidal isodose levels resulting from the subsequent intracavitary treatment. The volume of irradiated tissue imposes dose limitations on pelvic treatments, and in many centres the parametrial dose given is one which commonly fails to control nodal metastases of squamous cancer at other sites, but which frequently causes partial or total regression of the primary tumour.

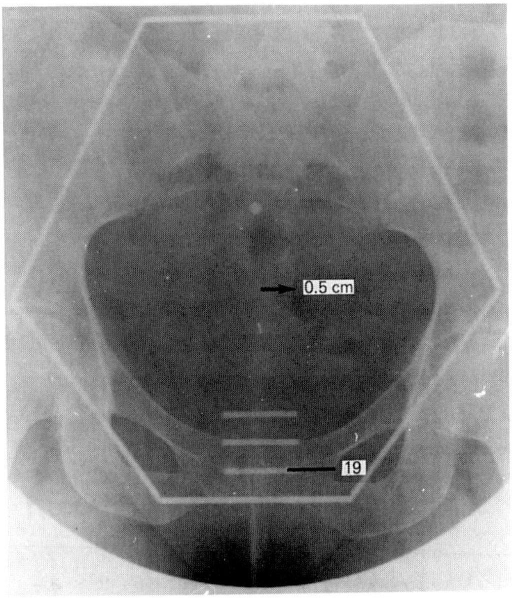

Figure 9.8 Homogeneous irradiation extending beyond the true pelvis to encompass disease in the common iliac and lower para-aortic regions, Anterior and posterior hexagonal fields are employed in conjunction with a parallel opposed pair of lateral fields subtending identical upper and lower limits. A tumour dose of 4000 cGy in 16 daily fractions is given

Table 9.2 Three representative treatment policies for potentially curable advanced cervical cancer

	Pelvic X-ray dose (cGy)	*Duration (weeks)*	*Fraction number*	*No. of intracavitary treatments*	*Interval between last pelvic X-ray treatment and first intracavitary treatment (weeks)*	*Cumulative intracavitary therapy dose at point A (cGy)*
Treatment policy 1	6000 (homogeneous)	6	30	1	2	2500
Treatment policy 2	4000 (homogeneous)	4	20	2	1	4000
Treatment policy 3	3250 (point B)	3	16	2	0	6000

Note 1 Most centres now agree that intracavitary treatment should follow external pelvic X-ray treatment

Note 2 Volumes for pelvic X-ray treatment differ considerably between centres

Note 3 No account of para-aortic radiation taken in

Note 4 Intracavitary doses administered in the range of approximately 60 cGy/hour

Uniform pelvic irradiation

The predilection for lateral and downward spread of cervical cancer, and the apparent rarity of presacral nodal involvement, have resulted in the development of external beam techniques which uniformly irradiate the central pelvis from side wall to side wall. An elementary four-field technique suitable for disease limited to the pelvis is illustrated in *Figure 9.7*; the larger treatment volume required when extensive nodal disease is known or suspected to be present is better administered by a technique such as the hexagonal (*Figure 9.8*), which has as its upper limit the fourth to fifth lumbar vertebral interspace, and where the four shielded corners minimize the volume of irradiated bowel. There are two (anterior and posterior) hexagonal fields, supplemented by a lateral parallel pair subtending a mid-section of the pelvis similar to that illustrated in *Figure 9.7*. A lower intracavitary contribution to the dose at point A is given following homogeneous pelvic irradiation than following centrally-shielded treatments. There are in use many gradations between the three representative treatment policies summarized in *Table 9.2* , and most appear to generate very similar incidences of cure and complication.

Late cervical cancer as a model in clinical radiobiological research

The 5-year survival results of treatment for true stages IIb and III cancer of the cervix are between 30 and 40%, and are obtained in many institutions employing a wide variety of techniques. Cervical cancer is very curable in its early stages, is common in its later stages, has relatively low potential for distant (i.e. non–lymphatic) dissemination, has been demonstrated to be hypoxic, and is easy of access for repetitive studies during treatment. Accordingly, advanced cervical cancer has been used to test some long-lived and still current hypotheses about the causes of treatment failure (*see* Chapters 1 and 2) in which the failure of hyperbaric oxygen and misonidazole are discussed.

High linear energy transfer radiation

The oxygen effect is proportionately of less influence when densely ionizing radiation is used. External beam fast neutron therapy actually worsens the therapeutic ratio in locally advanced cervical cancer (Morales, Hussey and Maor, 1981). The radioisotope californium-252 emits both gamma rays and fast neutrons (mean energy 2.3 MeV) and has been used as a substitute for caesium-137 in intracavitary therapy. When used in conjunction with high-dose fractionated pelvic X-ray treatment in stage IIIb, californium-252 achieved 54% 5-year survival, compared with only 12% 5-year survival in conventionally-treated patients (Maruyama *et al.*, 1985). Three considerations cast doubt on the validity of these results:

(1) Patient numbers in this prospective randomized study were small (total 36)
(2) The 54% 5-year survival figure for californium-252 appears to indicate that *all* patients without

distant metastases were cured, an astonishing circumstance

(3) Fast neutron brachytherapy appears to confer benefit only when given before external pelvic irradiation, an unexpected finding, since tumour shrinkage and reoxygenation resulting from pelvic irradiation would be expected to minimize the absolute numbers of hypoxic cells, and to concentrate them centrally in the pelvis, within range of the poorly-penetrating 2.3 MeV fast neutrons emitted by californium.

In summary, despite diligent efforts, the treatment of advanced cervical cancer has generated very little or no support for the notion that hypoxic clonogenic tumour cells are a major cause of radiotherapy treatment failure.

Complications of treatment

Conventional intracavitary treatment of early disease is virtually free of serious consequences (Easson, 1973). Occasional tiresome acute reactions almost always settle within 2 months of the conclusion of treatment. Although in most human tissues there is a poor correspondence between the severity of late and early reactions, the transient and generally mild nature of the acute response is matched by a correspondingly low incidence of grievous late effects. The foregoing statements presuppose that in all cases intracavitary insertions are performed ideally; when this is not the case, some increase in morbidity is inevitable. Both the early and late normal tissue sequelae of radiotherapy are worsened by adverse general and local factors, such as diabetes, hypertension, previous transperitoneal surgery, previous pelvic inflammatory disease, and co-existent conditions such as pelvic infection and diverticular disease. The last mentioned condition is quite common amongst older patients with cervical cancer whereas many younger patients have or have had identifiable episodes of pelvic inflammatory disease.

Acute complications of treatment, including those arising during treatment

In many institutions, early stage low volume disease is treated by intracavitary means alone. Self-limiting proctitis and cystitis of mild degree are almost universal, and require short-term symptomatic treatment in some 20% of patients. Troublesome or threatening acute reactions generally occur only in patients undergoing combined external and internal irradiation. Severe acute reactions are best described in terms of the structure affected:

(i) Uterus

Perforation of the uterus occasionally occurs during the instrumentation which precedes the introduction of intracavitary sources; it occurs more commonly when attempts are made to cannulate formerly massive central disease which has previously been treated by external pelvic irradiation. In these circumstances, the tissues presenting at the vaginal vault frequently have the consistency of soft cheese; the ulcerated, deficient anatomy of the vault may give little clue as to the natural situation of the remaining endocervical canal, and perforation can occur with minimal instrumentation. In the knee–chest position, perforation is always recognized. It is not necessary to abandon definitive treatment if perforation occurs, because although insertion of a cental uterine tube in this circumstance would be reckless, lateral forniceal ovoids can safely be positioned in the frequently realized expectation that successful cannulation of the uterine cavity may take place 1 week later. It is the routine practice in Manchester to give broad-spectrum antibiotics to women who have sustained a perforation, and subsequent peritonitis almost never occurs. It has not been found necessary to give drugs active against the anaerobic organisms which frequently contaminate the lower genital tract of women with cervical cancer; perhaps even more surprisingly, carcinomatosis peritonei almost never occurs following instrumental perforation into the peritoneal cavity. Pyometritis is not uncommon in cervical cancer, and while it is not strictly a complication of treatment, its presence may modify treatment. Small pyometria in previously afebrile patients may be disregarded, the intracavitary insertion proceeding as planned; a sample of the uterine pus is sent for culture and broad-spectrum antibiotics are given and discontinued when, as is usually the case, the pus is shown to be sterile. Larger pyometria, associated with uterine cavities greater than 6 cm in length, require drainage, (dilatation to a minimum of Hegar 8), and a week or so is allowed to elapse to permit the uterus to contract in size; a distended uterus may have a very thin wall, with the risk of high dose effects on the small or large bowel.

(ii) Rectosigmoid colon

Some degree of diverticular disease is very common in older patients with cervical cancer and may be associated with enhanced acute lower bowel reactions. Proctitis is almost invariable following intracavitary treatments, but is mild and self-limiting provided the insertion had been technically satisfactory. When pre-exisiting disease or technical failure produce unusually severe or prolonged proctitis, prednisolone suppositories or retention enemas of prednisolone are helpful. Radiation reactions in the lower bowel are minimized if the stools are rendered bulky and soft by the use of methyl cellulose taken by mouth from the onset of treatment. Constipation should be corrected before intracavitary treatment is commenced, as it is associated with worse acute morbidity in the lower colon and rectum.

(iii) Ileum

The symptoms of large bowel irradiation (tenesmus, mucus and/or blood per rectum) differ from those of small bowel irritation (fluid diarrhoea, with or without colicky abdominal pain), although they may coexist. As a complication of intracavitary treatment alone, ileitis was virtually unknown until the introduction of rigid high-dose rate afterloading systems (*see above*). Ileitis now most commonly occurs when external pelvic irradiation is combined with intracavitary treatment. Its incidence increases with total dose, dose per fraction, and volume of irradiated tissue. Previous transperitoneal surgery, particularly when sepsis was involved, increases the incidence and severity of small bowel reaction, presumably by incarcerating segments of the normally mobile small gut within the irradiated volume. Increased dose rate also worsens small bowel acute damage, since intestinal epithelial stem cells have broad shoulders on their single-dose survival curves, implying an unusually high capability for the repair of sublethal damage (*see* Chapter 1). Higher dose rates and increased fraction size have disproportionately greater effects on the intestinal epithelium than on other adjacent tissues, and accordingly small bowel damage, both early and late, emerged as a significant complication of the first high dose rate intracavitary treatment regimens (*see* Cathetron above).

Acute radiation ileitis is the commonest cause for interruption or abrogation of the planned treatment regimen. Some patients can be 'nursed' through their course of pelvic irradiation until the intended total dose has been absorbed, by resting them from treatment periodically for one or more days, depending on the frequency of their diarrhoea or the reported severity of their small bowel colic. Stretching the overall treatment time in this manner may have radiobiological consequences for tumour control.

Occasionally, severe ileitis occurs early during the proposed course of treatment, in which circumstance radical surgery should be considered. Most small bowel reactions can be managed by the same agent given to minimize the reaction in the large bowel, that is methyl cellulose. This gives form to what otherwise tends to be rather fluid faeces, and appears to alleviate the severity of colic pain. Drugs such as Loperamide (Imodium) are used in more severe cases, provided that glaucoma is not present, in which case simple measures using kaolin or codeine phosphate can be used.

(iv) Bladder

Urgency, frequency, nocturia and dysuria are very common consequences of treatment. Patients have usually experienced multiple and recent instrumentation of the lower urinary tract and, accordingly, these symptoms sometimes arise from infection rather than from irradiation. Routine weekly mid-stream specimens of urine should be collected for culture and appropriate antibiotic therapy may be required. Following correctly-executed intracavitary insertions, radiation cystitis is mild and transient. The very unpalatable mist. potassium citrate appears to have a marginal benefit in reducing bladder irritability, but tablets of Effercitrate (3 twice daily) which are quite tasteless, are equally effective. Cetiprin can sometimes be helpful.

(v) Vagina

The acute desquamative reaction in the vaginal vault can swiftly result in the formation of occlusive adhesions, although it otherwise does not generate symptoms. Vault stenosis can lead to subsequent pyometrium, uncertainty as to disease-free status at follow up, and sexual difficulties. The manufacturers of the commercially available vaginal dilators, intended by virtue of daily insertion to prevent the formation of adhesions, are apparently unaware that the vagina is most capacious at its upper end, and patients are best advised to procure their dilators from less conventional sources.

It may take up to 3 months before the vault epithelium is fully reconstituted, and it is customary to advise sexually active women to defer intercourse until 6 weeks after the conclusion of treatment. Some women experience intense burning feelings after ejaculation, and the present author recommends the use of a sheath for 3–4 months after treatment, or until the vault mucosa appears to be intact. Local applications of oestrogen creams may help when the natural vaginal lubrication is reduced from ovarian failure (*see below*). Sexual intercourse should be encouraged to prevent the 'vicious circle' associated with vaginal adhesions.

(vi) Parametrium

Acute parametrial reactions from radiation *per se* are not recognized, but the frequent coexistence of pelvic inflammatory disease may lead to exacerbations of sepsis, including tubo-ovarian abscess. Parametritis is painful, and reduces radiation tolerance; the responsible microorganisms are rarely identified, but commonly include anaerobic species. A combination of oral metronidazole and trimethoprim almost always controls the manifestations of such infections. (The commonly used combination of metronidazole and co-trimoxazole is irrational, as the sulpha-drug component of co-trimoxazole is antagonistic, rather than synergistic, to the trimoxazole).

Late complications, including radiation-induced malignant disease

Late complications of radiotherapy for cervical cancer usually manifest within 6–24 months of treatment, although some effects, particularly bowel stenosis, malabsorption syndromes, and carcinogenesis can appear after many years. In harmony with the classification used in discussion of acute reactions, late complications are described by reference to the affected tissue or organ, listed approximately in order of frequency and consequence. There is no widely acknowledged definition of what constitutes an unacceptable complication of irradiation for cervical cancer, but many would accept that changes resulting in a requirement for surgical correction represent serious morbidity, and indeed occasionally result in mortality.

(i) Rectum

Anterior rectal wall ulceration, usually occurring immediately below and behind the cervix 6–18 months after treatment, is the commonest serious manifestation of late radiation damage in this context. It almost always follows an intracavitary insertion or insertions in which posterior forniceal packing had been inadequate, or in which caudal slippage of the intrauterine tube was not corrected or was unrecognized when the post-insertion radiographs were scrutinized (*see Figure 9.2*). Routine systematic readings of the rectal dose rate should render this tiresome complication (painful defaecation, tenesmus, rectal bleeding) obsolete, but it persists, usually as the legacy of insufficiently experienced operators.

When it causes severe and persistent symptoms, this complication (pseudocarcinoma, the intrinsic reaction of Todd, 1938), is best managed by permanent defunctioning colostomy; simultaneous or subsequent attempts to remove the affected rectum carry high risk of ureteric and vesical fistula formation. Pain and rectal blood loss are usually relieved by defunctioning colostomy, but mucus discharge may persist.

In the absence of surgical intervention, rectovaginal fistulae are rare, and are usually the consequence of massive central disease or unusually extensive vaginal involvement by the original disease. Such fistulae should not be regarded as complications of treatment as they are more consequences of the tumour itself, and this is also true of many vesicovaginal fistulae. If such fistulae are uncritically regarded as ‘radionecroses’, inappropriate conclusions may be drawn about what constitutes pelvic radiation tolerance.

(ii) Sigmoid colon

Stricture, ulceration leading to perforation, and occasionally fistula formation, may occur from between 6 months to many years following treatment, especially when the uterus was retroverted, or when rigid afterloading applicators have held the uterus in close apposition to the sigmoid colon. The consequences are those of lower bowel obstruction or less commonly perforation, and specialist operators skilled in the surgery of the irradiated large bowel may be able to excise the affected segment with ultimate restoration of the continuity of the bowel.

(iii) Bladder

Telangiectasia of the bladder base mucosa may cause repeated and usually self-limiting episodes of haematuria. If clots form in the bladder, antifibrinolytics may be required to stop the bleeding, and cystoscopic evacuation of clot is sometimes necessary. Fulguration of a prominent and identifiable source of bleeding is often successful, but instillation of sclerosants such as formaldehyde or silver nitrate solutions may be required to control blood loss.

Vesico-vaginal fistula (VVF) is usually the result of previous involvement of the bladder mucosa by tumour, or recurrent disease. VVF may be precipitated by multiple biopsies taken to exclude residual or recurrent disease. Even when inoperable central disease is known to exist, ileal loop diversion may provide many months free from the personal and social misery of perpetual incontinence.

(iv) Small bowel

Of patients who have had combined external pelvic and intracavitary irradiation 10–15% suffer from persistent or intermittent attacks of diarrhoea, usually accompanied by abdominal pain. This complication was virtually unknown following low-dose intracavitary treatment alone. Its incidence increases with previous laparotomy and pelvic inflammatory disease. The most severely affected segment is usually the terminal ileum, which in health is responsible for the entero-hepatic circulation of the bile acids, and the absorption of vitamin B_{12}. Mucosal damage causes conjugated bile salts to pass into the caecum, where they are deconjugated with the subsequent production of compounds which interfere with salt and water absorption in the colon, causing diarrhoea. The binding resin cholestyramine sequesters colonic bile salts and prevents their deconjugation, with symptomatic improvement in the diarrhoea of bile salt malabsorption.

A less common form of small bowel diarrhoea is caused by bacterial contamination of the normally sterile ileal contents with bacteria derived from the colon. This diarrhoea responds to broad-spectrum antibiotics and can be differentiated from malabsorptive diarrhoea by isotopic studies (Ludgate and Merrick, 1985).

Haematologically significant vitamin B_{12} malabsorption is rare, and usually manifests many years after treatment, but measurable defects of absorption are demonstrable in approximately 10% of patients (Ludgate and Merrick, 1985). Most patients presumably have liver stores of B_{12} able to last many years. Occasionally, localized strictures of the small bowel are formed, usually corresponding to an ileal segment held in close apposition to the uterine fundus by peritoneal adhesions. Such strictures are usually discovered after a prolonged period of morbidity, often after previous fruitless attempts to confirm their suspected presence radiologically; generally, by-pass is safer than excision.

(v) *Ovary*

Premenopausal patients undergo premature ovarian failure following treatment, the oestrogen-deficiency aspects of which are often symptomatic within 3 months. Replacement doses of ethinyloestradiol (100–300 μg daily) usually abolish the symptoms of early and abrupt menopause (vasomotor instability, vulvitis and vaginitis), but in view of the potential dangers of unopposed oestrogen stimulation, oestrogen/progesterone triphasic replacement may be safer, and is more physiological.

(vi) Ureter

Hydronephrosis appearing for the first time following treatment is usually due to recurrent disease, but can occasionally be due to fibrosis. Fistula formation is rare, but is a considerable risk if later 'salvage' surgery is undertaken.

(vii) Vagina

Occlusive stenosis and the formation of adhesions in the vaginal vault invariably occur in sexually inactive women, and may make assessment of the primary site difficult. Younger patients can be provided with dilators (*see above*).

(viii) Skin

Radiotherapists obliged to use cobalt–60 beams for pelvic irradiation commonly use anteroposterior opposed pairs, as the indifferent penetration of such beams precludes their use in lateral opposed pairs. Patients with anteroposterior diameters greater than 16 cm are at increasing risk of subcutaneous fibrosis, which in extreme cases can be uncomfortable or even painful.

Radiation-induced second malignancy

Treated cervical cancer patients are an ideal population in which to study the possibility of induction of second malignancies by therapeutic irradiation because:

(1) There are large numbers of survivors
(2) There has traditionally been long and adequate follow-up of survivors after treatment
(3) The radiation dose received by other organs can be estimated with some accuracy from data on the intracavitary and external beam dose-contributions
(4) A 'control' group of patients exists who were treated by surgery alone.

The International Agency for Research on Cancer has accumulated data on over 600 000 women-years in patients who previously received radiation treatment, and 180 000 of the 600 000 women-years were accummulated 10 and more years after treatment (WHO, 1983). The ratio of observed/expected (O/E) second primary cancer has been calculated for most important sites and organs in the body, and overall, the O/E ratio is 1.1 in both surgically and radiotherapeutically treated groups. However, this over-all equivalence obscures significant differences in the organ-specific O/E ratios: and excess of second cancers in lung, bladder, and to a lesser degree, rectum, is fortuitously balanced by a relative paucity of second cancers in breast, corpus uteri, and ovary. These trends are roughly the same in the radiotherapy and surgery groups, with some obvious and expected variations — for example cervix patients treated by hysterectomy have very low incidence of subsequently diagnosed corpus cancer (O/E 0.1), and as the ovaries are commonly removed at hysterectomy, there is a relative lack of second ovarian cancer (O/E 0.5) in the surgery group. On the other hand, radiation seems genuinely protective for breast cancer (O/E 0.7), possibly by inducing prema-

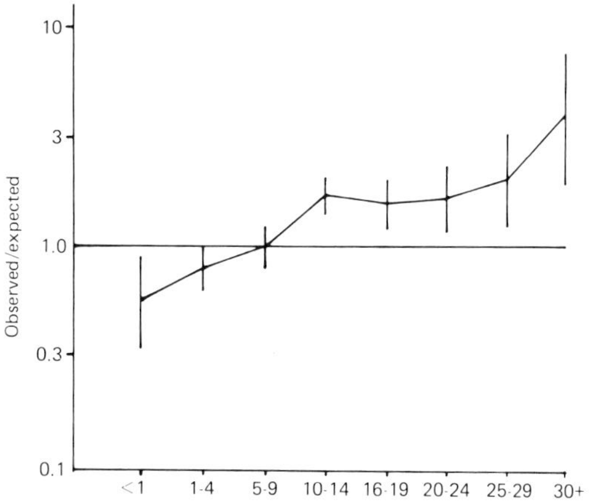

Figure 9.9 The ratio of observed to expected incidence of rectal carcinoma as a function of time after successful radiation treatment of cervical cancer (IARC, 1983). Radiation appears to demonstrate a carcinogenic potential in a shorter time than is commonly thought to be the latent interval for carcinogenesis, and there does not appear to be an inflection in the curve — again in contrast to widely-held dogma

ture ovarian failure in premenopausal patients as the effect is concentrated in that group of patients under 40 years old.

Further clues to the possible role of radiation in the production of second malignancies have been obtained by plotting data to show how many years must elapse after exposure before the O/E ratio deviates from 1, and comparing the resulting curves with similar curves derived for surgically treated patients. *Figure 9.9* shows that from about 5 years after treatment, there appears to be an increase in carcinoma of the rectum attributable to radiation, and the same is true for bladder. From 15 years after treatment, there may be radiation induced carcinogenesis in the ovary, but 80% confidence limits in this case are wide. For all other sites, radiation appears to have no carcinogenic effect, perhaps a surprising finding in, for example, colon and stomach. There is a fivefold increase in O/E lung cancers, concentrated in the first few years, suggesting that these 'bronchial neoplasms' were in truth pulmonary metastases from the cervical primary. Or alternatively patients with carcinoma of the cervix are often heavy smokers which will of course induce a higher incidence of both lung and bladder cancer.

Results of radiotherapy and surgery are periodically reported by the International Federation of Gynaecology and Obstetrics. The 18th Report (1982) covers the years 1973–1975 inclusive, and contains data submitted from 120 centres throughout the world. The striking features of this report, in so far as it concerns cervical cancer, are:

(1) There are considerable differences between centres in the stage-related 5-year survival figures, e.g. 97.2% for stage I from one hospital in Brño, Czechoslovakia, versus 38.9% for one London teaching hospital
(2) There is less difference between centres treating large numbers of patients than between centres dealing with relatively few patients
(3) The pooled figures from major institutions show stage by stage survival generally to be somewhat lower than is commonly perceived and taught; comparisons of the results with earlier reports indicate that in the best institutions there has been a consistent trend towards increased survival for at least two decades.

The figures given below are those which should be achieved in centres where competent staging and radiotherapy are performed:

Stage	*5-year survival* (%)
Ia	90–95
Ib	80–85
II	60–65
III	30–35
IV	0–15

Cancer of the uterine corpus

Although the treatment of endometrial cancer has recently been described as non-controversial (Joslin and Peel, 1982), there is more diversity in the treatment methods currently employed than in any other gynaecological malignancy. This probably reflects the prejudices and preferences of individual gynaecologists, rather than as is commonly supposed, that no one approach is superior to any other. The many well-established clinical and pathological feature of this disease in fact clearly indicate how it is best managed.

Clinical features determining treatment policy

(1) Stage

Endometrial cancer is the only important internal malignancy to present overwhelmingly with early stage disease. That it should do so is the result of several factors. Although the disease is itself associated with late menopause, 75% of patients are postmenopausal at presentation, and spontaneous postmenopausal bleeding is recognized as aberrant more immediately than is intermenstrual or postcoital bleeding, particularly in this group of patients, who tend to have better social and educational backgrounds than do patients with carcinoma of the cervix. Of all endometrial cancers 90% present as dysfunctional uterine bleeding, 75% are in stage 1, and only 12% have involvement beyond the uterus at presentation.

(2) Differentiation

Endometrial cancer is predominantly a well-differentiated disease, possibly because it commonly arises from pre-existing hyperplasia resulting from unopposed oestrogen stimulation of the endometrium. Three grades are recognized, well differentiated (G1), moderately differentiated (G2), and poorly differentiated (G3). Four-fifths of all cases are either well or moderately differentiated (Jones, 1975), and the grading dominates the other allegedly prognostically significant features of the disease, especially the degree of myometrial penetration, and the propensity for pelvic or distant metastasis. The conjunction of low grade and early stage confer a survival rate of 75–80% in stage 1 disease, 50% in stage 2, and an overall 5-year survival of 66%.

(3) Spread

Extrauterine extension is present in only 12% of new cases. Spread is predominantly within the uterine cavity and into the myometrium. True stromal invasion of the cervix provides access to the cervical lymphatics, and when well established it is associated with a 33% incidence of pelvic node involvement. Fractional curettage, an indispensible part of the evaluation of this disease, readily identifies spread of disease to the endocervical canal (which has no prognostic or therapeutic implications), but it must often fail to identify true myometrial invasion which can usually only be identified with certainty by examination of the removed uterus. Spread via tubal lymphatics to the ovaries is sufficiently common for bilateral salpingo-oophorectomy to be an essential component of the surgical management of this condition. Ovarian and serosal involvement, which are uncommon, permit transperitoneal spread. An important route of extension is via submucosal lymphatics to the upper vagina, which ultimately occurs in about 12% of unirradiated postoperative cases. Subsequent spread to involve the lower half of the vagina is not common, but may be curable; such involvement on presentation is always associated with advanced intrapelvic disease, and cure in these circumstances is unlikely. One half of cases with involved pelvic nodes also have para-aortic node involvement, which is a late feature.

(4) Fitness

The group characteristics of patients with this disease may have very important influence on the treatment policy for individual patients. There is a well established association of endometrial cancers with specific circumstances which have in common the feature of chronic exposure of the endometrium to oestrogens in the absence of progesterones (Gusberg, 1976), including prolonged exogenous oestrogen administration, oestrogen-secreting ovarian tumours, and polycystic disease of the ovary, although these conditions account for only a small proportion of all endometrial cancers. Of more immediate relevance to the aetiology of the disease in the majority of patients is that in obesity there is increased conversion of endogenous androgens to oestrogens. Many patients with endometrial cancer are obese, and also diabetic, hypertensive and arteriopathic. The age-specific incidence for endometrial cancer is approximately 10 years older than that for cervical cancer, and the combination of advanced age, diabetes, hypertension and arteriopathy precludes surgery for many patients, while co-existent obesity makes surgery difficult and sharply increases the postoperative complication rate. The low parity and late menopause characteristic of these patients are further examples of the action of excessive or prolonged unopposed oestrogens.

(5) Age

Although age will to some extent determine the fitness of patients with endometrial cancer, it has an independent influence on treatment policy, as younger patients tend to have more well differentiated, less advanced disease.

Preoperative radiotherapy

(a) Intracavitary treatment

The results of initial surgery are consistently, though sometimes only marginally, superior to those of radiotherapy alone, and when the general condition of the patient is suitable, treatment should be by abdominal hysterectomy and bilateral salpingo-oophorectomy, which will be curative for most patients. This then invalidates the routine use of preoperative intracavitary radiotherapy, which continues to be sought by many gynaecologists; the only well established achievement of preoperative radiotherapy is marked reduction in the later incidence of vault recurrence, and this can be achieved equally effectively by postoperative treatment. Postoperative radiotherapy can be given on a selective basis to patients at high risk of vault recurrence, who can be identified by careful histological examination of the hysterectomy specimen. Endometrial cancer is a relatively common disease, so there are obvious advantages, economic and otherwise, in avoiding the unnecessary over-treatment of relatively large numbers of patients.

Preoperative treatment usually takes the form of one or more intracavitary insertions; the technique is exactly that described below for inoperable cases, but the radiation doses are reduced, casting further doubt on the validity of this approach. Lower doses may nonetheless prejudice effective postoperative X-ray treatment in those cases where the operative or pathological findings indicate that the disease was more extensive than had been expected. In such cases, the doses received by the bladder and rectum must be taken into account when the subsequent pelvic X-ray treatment is planned. The present author does not think it practical to compensate for high midline doses by employing wedges such as those used in the treatment of intermediate stages of cervical cancer, as these are designed to dove-tail with differently shaped central dose-distributions (but many centres do indeed use midline shielding with great success). The practice of carrying out vaginal rather than abdominal hysterectomies following intracavitary treatment, as advocated in some major American centres, is deplorable, as it squanders the opportunity to gain confirmatory evidence at laparotomy that the tumour was indeed confined to the uterus.

In summary: preoperative intracavitary treatments prolong patients' duration of hospitalization, are inappropriate and ineffective, and may occasionally preclude subsequent potentially curable X-ray treatment.

(b) Preoperative X-ray treatment

The prognostic significance of the length of the uterine cavity in endometrial cancer is uncertain. Earlier indications that longer cavities are associated with increased probability of extrauterine spread have been authoritatively challenged (Decker and Malkassian, 1979), but some centres continue to use this criterion as a basis for administering preoperative whole-pelvis irradiation when the cavity exceeds 8 cm in length (Rutledge *et al.*, 1976). The best guide to the presence of extrauterine spread is the degree of differentiation of tumour; routine preoperative treatments based on the dubious premise that cavity length is important represent over-treatment for the majority of patients, as extrauterine spread at presentation is so uncommon. Such treatment may obscure the subsequent identification at laparotomy of pathological features which have prognostic and therapeutic importance. The only rational basis for preoperative X-ray treatment is when advanced disease is known to exist on clinical grounds, and where treatment might subsequently enable curative surgery to be performed; such hopes are seldom realized.

Primary radiotherapy for corpus cancer

Advanced age, obesity, hypertension, diabetes and vascular disease consign a poor surgical risk group to radiotherapy as the primary method of treatment, as may coincidental conditions such as chronic lung disease. These patients lack the benefit of accurate staging at laparotomy, so a proportion are certain to be assigned on clinical examination to earlier stages than would be appropriate if all the relevant data were known. The overall 5-year survival of endometrial cancer is approximately 66%, whereas that of stage III is only 30%, so that understaging will have an adverse effect on the results of radiotherapy. However, the impact of understaging is considerably reduced in practice, because only 10 – 15% of new cases are stage III, and stage IV tumours are unlikely to be mistaken for anything else, even on exclusively clinical assessment. Allowing for the shorter life expectancy of patients rejected for surgery, all published data indicate the inferiority of radiotherapy compared to surgery. This inferiority is sometimes marginal in early cases, but is usually quite substantial in the later stages of the disease. A very important consideration is that excessive morbidity and mortality from surgery is immediate, whereas increased mortality from failure of radiotherapy is usually considerably deferred, so that even uncured patients often enjoy prolonged survival free of distressing local symptoms, and this makes the somewhat poorer long-term results of radiotherapy acceptable.

In view of the usually multiple adverse features that patients referred for radiotherapy have, treatment is generally limited to intracavity irradiation, as few surgical rejects will tolerate pelvic X-ray treatment in addition. There is, however, a group of patients who are inoperable not by virtue of poor general condition, but by virtue of clinically apparent extensive pelvic disease; such patients receive whole-pelvic irradiation, following which they are assessed for either supplementary intracavitary treatment or surgery, although in practice few are ever operated upon.

There is more variation in the technical aspect of uterine corpus intracavity applications than in cancer of the cervix, some systems dispensing with lateral forniceal applicators altogether. A major disadvantage of some techniques which seek to overcome the supposed deficiencies of the Manchester system (*see below*), is that they are not readily adaptable to remote afterloading, since multiple transcervical source-guides are not at present feasible. Accordingly, the development of remote afterloading for corpus uteri cancer is likely to proceed along lines dictated by the need to retain a single central intrauterine source carrier, which is a feature of the Manchester system; this system, once considered obsolescent by many, is therefore reviewed.

The Manchester system for carcinoma of the corpus uteri

As the extent of myometrial and cervical invasion is unknown in these patients, treatment is designed to irradiate the whole myometrium, the cervix, the inner paracervical tissues, and the vaginal vault. Experience with radium has shown that in spite of very heavy central tube loading, bowel morbidity is virtually non-existent, and that, as in the case of carcinoma of the cervix treatments, the paracervical tissues are the relevant critical radiovulnerable structures, and consequently the concept of expressing dose at point A is retained.

In order to treat the vaginal vault, ovoids identical to those used in the cervical system, are placed in the lateral fornices. The ovoids are disposed transversely so that the otherwise cylindrical pattern of dose distribution along the uterine axis is inferiorly flattened anteroposteriorly, to maintain the dose at point A, and yet offers relative protection to the bladder and bowel. Nulliparity and age not uncommonly oblige that the ovoids be placed in tandem. In this situation, an 8% increment in insertion time is applied to compensate for reduction in dose at point A; when tandem ovoids are used to treat the postoperative vault, no such correction is made, as it is the surface dose rather than the point A dose which determines tolerance.

The cervical central tube is modified to meet the special requirements of intrauterine growths:

(1) Longer tubes are required, from 6 to 12 cm, in 2 cm increments
(2) Heavy fundal loading is necessary to create a cylindrical isodose pattern around the upper uterus
(3) The segment of the uterine tube closest to point A is identically loaded to a cervical tube, as the heavy fundal loading contributes significantly to the point A dose, in spite of the inverse square law and oblique self-filtration
(4) Radium sources are encased in a thick plastic tube of external diameter 0.6 cm to limit radionecrosis to the inner myometrium while simultaneously extending the reference isodose outwards. The strongest available radium tube contains 30 mg radium, and this amount cannot be increased, so its effective strength is augmented by reducing the platinum filtration from 5 mm (standard tubes) to 1 mm, which increases its fragility and the risk of radon gas release.

All the above modifications must be consistent with maintaining the constancy of the central tube's dose-rate contribution at point A.

Figure 9.10 shows how these several requirements are met in practice. The differential distribution of radium is the best that can be achieved with the commercial sources which were originally available. Unavoidably, the cervical segment of the tube is consistently loaded with two 10 mg sources, which are not quite strong enough to extend the reference isodose laterally to point A, so consequently this receives 6 – 8% less dose than the volume of tissues bounded by the reference isodose. In many experimental and clinical situations, dose-effect differences are detectable when doses differ by 7%. Since the dose tolerance of point A is known, at least at certain dose rates, the replacement of radium by other radioactive sources such as caesium–137, especially in pellet remote afterloading systems, offers an opportunity to overcome this imperfection.

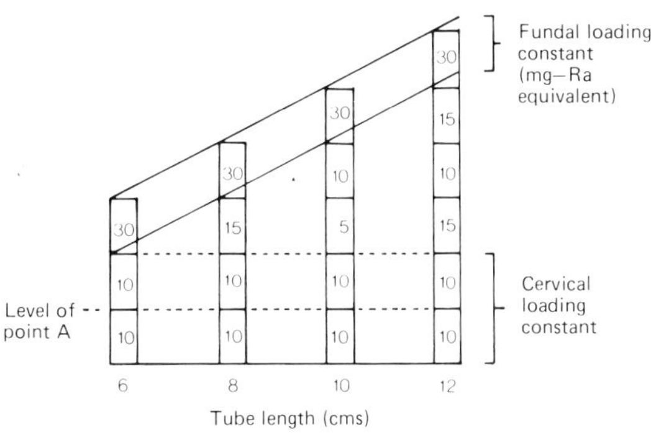

Figure 9.10 The differential loading required for intrauterine tubes used in the treatment of body carcinoma shown here in milligrams of radium. Note that this not quite ideal distribution need not be precisely followed in remote afterloading systems employing a central source

In terms of dose distribution, the system results in a cylinder of 4 cm diameter along most of the axis of the uterus, the cylinder being flattened and widened inferiorly below a slight waist at the level of the point A; all tissues encompassed by this isodose receive not less than 7500 cGy, which is administered in two equal 55 hour insertions 1 week apart. (Dose rate at point A approximately 64 cGy/hour.)

In hypothetical terms, the main deficiency of this system is that disease extending deeper than 2 cm into the myometrium, or into one or both cornua, falls outside the reference isodose, as would the base of any solid element of tumour more than 2 cm thick. The fact that local control is frequently obtained in spite of this apparent inadequacy of method may be due wholly or in part to the following:

(1) The uterine cavity itself is curretted free of tumour and evacuated before intracavitary treatment takes place
(2) The cornual recesses are partly effaced as the uterus assumes the sausage-shape typical of endometrial cancer
(3) Clinically evident thickness in the uterine walls may be the result of persistent oestrogenic stimulation, rather than tumour infiltration
(4) A proportion of endometrial cancers may be curable at doses below 7500 cGy.

More likely, however, in a proportion of cases the shrinkage of tumour and uterus which occurs between the first and second insertions has an important effect on disease inadequately irradiated during the first insertion, that is, it comes to occupy a situation some way inside the reference isodose. In this situation it will receive a far higher dose than 3750 cGy (half the total dose). Because of the operation of the inverse square law the dose on this second insertion could be as high as 7500 cGy, which would itself be curative. All the above criteria would apply if manual insertion were carried out using cobalt–60 or caesium–137 sources.

Remote afterloading (RAL)

In early cancer of the cervix, ideal radium insertions produce almost guaranteed local tumour control, virtually free of serious morbidity. Logically, the intention has been to use remote afterloading systems to reproduce as closely as possible the dose-distribution characteristics of radium insertions. The requirement for close reduplication of this latter system is absent when RAL is applied to the treatment of endometrial cancer, because it is not an ideal one. Thus RAL offers an opportunity to improve on the antecedent technique. The constraints on innovation are that:

(1) The inferior aspect of the uterocervical treatment volume must be flattened anteroposteriorly to protect the bladder and rectum
(2) The dose tolerance at point A is probably 7500 cGy.

The dose actually received at point A from treatment using radium for corpus uteri is 7000 cGy (93% × 7500, *see above*). If lateral forniceal ovoids are to be retained as a means of flattening the inferior aspect of the treatment volume, and to treat the vault, there is inevitably a contribution from these ovoids to the point A dose. Thus it is clear that any modification in the loading of the uterine portion of the central tube must be such that the resultant effect on the dose at point A is limited to an increase of 500 cGy. An attempt to reduce the contribution to point A from the ovoids reduces the flatness of dose distribution between the bladder and rectum, and so is self-defeating.

Experience with RAL as the only form of radiotherapy in endometrial cancer will accrue slowly. Since only limited improvements can be expected from RAL, many departments are anticipating the impending withdrawal of manually loaded sources by combining external X-ray treatment with a minor RAL-delivered component given subsequently. An interval between the external and internal modes of treatment allows the uterus to shrink, which minimizes the disadvantages in dose distribution inherent in intracavitary treatment alone. Whole-pelvis X-ray treatments are widely advocated, with the recommendation that the dose given be reduced below tolerance by an amount considered to be appropriate to the magnitude of the intracavitary contribution. As noted elsewhere, notions of pelvic X-ray tolerance vary widely; the acceptable normal tissue end-points are difficult to define, and are rarely stated in clinical reports. The elderly obese patients commonly referred for radiotherapy often also have a degree of colonic diverticular disease, and as individuals cannot always accept whole-pelvis irradiation dose levels which are well short of 'tolerance'. (In this context it may be noted that clinical radiobiologists are accustomed to regard the *late* effects of radiation as the relevant end-points, but in this group of patients it is usually the *acute* effects that cause serious harm.) Unrealistic expectations generate unacceptable morbidity; elderly obese patients with a multiplicity of associated medical problems are best served by radiation treatments whose limited objective is the attainment with minimum radiation toxicity of what would otherwise have been achieved by simple hysterectomy.

This objective is feasible if X-ray treatment is restricted to the uterus, upper vagina, and their immediate environs, and is followed by a single intracavitary RAL treatment after the uterus has shrunk to normal or near normal size. Such treatments can conveniently be delivered by three field techiques (*Figure 9.11*), rotational techniques, (*Figure 9.12*) or by modification of the four field brick technique (*see Figure 9.7*).

Postoperative radiotherapy

With the exception of tumour grade, the major determinants of survival can only be established following adequate surgery. Adverse factors include:

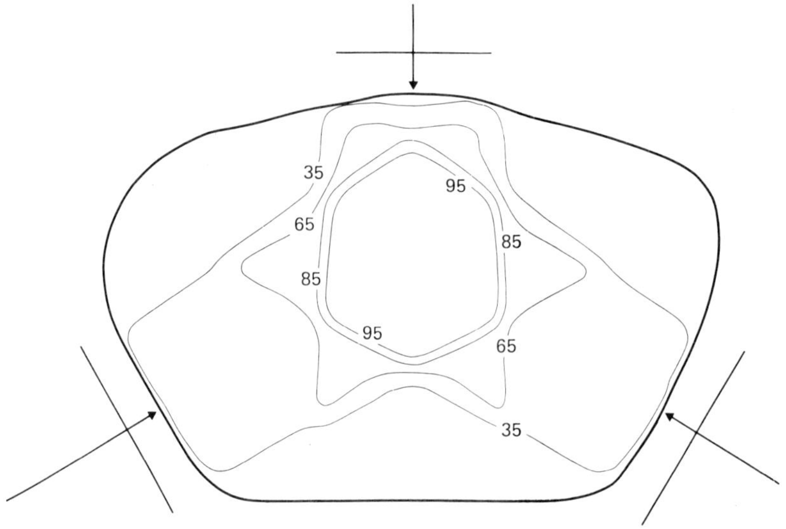

Figure 9.11 External pelvic irradiation. A three field technique for the treatment of corpus carcinoma which can be modified for the treatment of vaginal tumours. A dose of 4250 cGy in 15 daily fractions is given

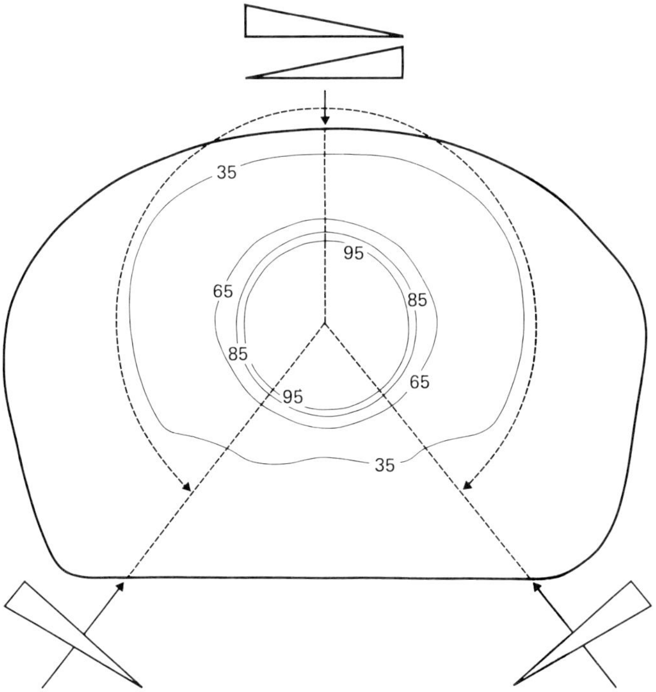

Figure 9.12 A rotation technique suitable for treating central pelvic disease in the body, cervix or vagina. A dose of 4500 cGy in 16 daily fractions is given

(1) Deep myometrial penetration
(2) Cervical stromal infiltration
(3) Extrauterine extension, most common in the ovaries and pelvic lymph nodes.

Opinion differs as to when the degree of myometrial penetration becomes seriously threatening, but since penetration is never uniform throughout the uterine wall, it is reasonable to regard penetration greater than half the thickness of wall over more than a small proportion of its total surface as being significant. Cervical segment invasion is very significant, being associated with up to 33% pelvic nodal involvement. Transverse section of the hysterectomy specimen may indicate the desirability of pelvic node sampling, or even limited lymphadenectomy, if the pelvic nodes are obviously involved. Extrauterine extension limited to the adnexae is a special case, surgical cure being claimed in up to 80% of cases (Bruckman, Bloomer and Marck, 1980), but in all other cases extrauterine extension carries a risk of pelvic local recurrence. The magnitude of this risk has never been determined in controlled studies. As it has long been almost universal practice to give radiotherapy to patients considered to be at high risk of pelvic recurrence, there are no recent data on the post-surgical natural history of the disease, and accordingly the effectiveness of radiotherapy in controlling postoperative recurrence is unknown. Retrospective analysis of exclusively surgical series cannot provide convincing data about the true incidence of postoperative recurrence because the antiquity of such studies means that there is paucity of detail concerning matters which are now recognized as being of importance in assessment.

Also, there are uncertainties about the completeness and consistency of the surgical procedures employed. Although the risk of postoperative pelvic recurrence is not precisely known, consideration of survival data suggests that the risk is 30 – 50% in 'high risk' cases with no macroscopically evident postoperative residual disease. In the absence of controlled prospective studies, the contribution to cure of postoperative radiotherapy is somewhat conjectural, except in the prevention of vault recurrence. The rationale for postoperative X-ray treatment rests somewhat on the success of intracavitary treatment in early stage disease, which unequivocally demonstrates the radiocurability of endometrial cancer, and also on a few historically controlled studies. One such recently reported study of postoperative cases with less than half myometrial penetration indicates that the addition of external irradiation to intravaginal therapy improves the 6-year survival from 76 to 100% (Joslin and Peel, 1982). Having regard for the age-range in which endometrial cancer arises, the 100% survival figure is clearly actuarially derived, but even so, total 6-year survival implies that the X-ray treated patients had extraordinarily well differentiated tumours with remarkably low potential for distant metastasis: this may not have been so in the 24% of the historical controls who failed to survive following intracavitary treatment alone; indeed, the 76% survival figure in this latter group accords rather well with known figures for distribution between grades — 35% grade II, 20% grade III. (In cervical cancer, pelvic irradiation is mostly associated with cure when it is sequentially combined with a large intracavitary component, and its curative capability when used alone is undoubted but unquantified; the same is true for endometrial cancer.)

(a) Intracavitary postoperative radiotherapy

Approximately 12 – 15% of patients who have undergone apparently curative surgery for intrauterine disease subsequently develop recurrence at the surgical vault, and this figure can be reduced to 1 – 2% by routine intracavitary irradiation of the healed surgical vault. One advantage of postoperative treatment is that in the absence of the uterine cavity, only intravaginal applicators are required, so that the intracavitary assembly requires very considerably less radium or radium substitute (45 mg versus 135 mg at the extreme) and this is an advantage in departments not yet employing afterloading systems. Postoperative treatment is also more convenient for the patient, as it can be carried out as a single insertion of shorter duration (96 hours for radium) than preoperative treatment, thereby reducing overall duration of hospitalization, and reducing the load on inpatient facilities. Further, in the postoperative situation much more is known with certainty about each patient's disease, permitting an element of selection of patients requiring treatment. Many centres now limit treatment to certain well-defined categories whose pathological data indicate special vulnerability to vault recurrence. Very few low risk patients go on to develop such recurrence, and provided follow-up supervision is adequate, the recurrence is identified early, when it is curable by vault treatments identical to those used prophylactically (*see below*). The contrary philosophy that routine treatment of all patients reduces the obligations of follow-up is wrong, as patients continue to need follow-up to detect recurrent disease other than that in the vault, and it is as improper to subject unnecessarily large numbers of patients to a treatment not entirely free of tiresome complications (proctitis, vault stenosis), as it is to squander health care resources.

Postoperative vault treatments are indicated when grade I and grade II tumours have infiltrated beyond half the thickness of the uterine wall, but are still well clear of the serosa, and when disease encroaches on the cervical canal. (Grade III lesions meeting either or both of these criteria should receive pelvic irradiation, *see below*.)

The technique of prophylactic vault treatment is simple. In Manchester, two standard (cervix) ovoids are used, usually transversely disposed. Surgical closure of the upper vagina may result in a small-volume vault, as may advanced age and nulliparity, in which cases the ovoids are placed in tandem. No correction is made to the treatment time to account for ovoids-in-tandem situation, (*see* Treatment of cervical cancer), since the dose at point A is irrelevant, as the intention is to give a high surface dose (10 000 cGy in two insertions) to the vaginal mucosa; for the same reason, there is no stringent requirement to use much packing. The function of the latter in this situation is merely to hold the radium assembly in place, and not to protect the anterior rectal wall and bladder base.

Prophylactic postoperative vault treatments are seldom followed by later development of submucosal spread to the lower reaches of the vagina, (sub-urethral recurrence is described below). The routine use of in-line sources is not justified, as the incidence of rectal complications and vaginal stenosis is thereby increased.

Intravaginal treatments can be carried out using afterloading systems, although the absence of an anteverted uterine tube deprives the assembly of a valuable element of its stability within the pelvis. Low dose-rate afterloading systems which require attachment to the patient for many hours carry the risk that the sources may become downwardly displaced away from the intended treatment zone. This undoubtedly occurred during the early development of afterloading, particularly in North America, where there is greater experience of this method in the postoperative situation. (The transatlantic ratio of corpus vault treatments to intracavitary cervix treatments is roughtly 3:1, virtually the reverse of the situation in the UK.) Careful packing, as described in the section on cervix afterloading, helps to maintain the sources in the intended position. Although apparently barbaric, stitching the vulva over the pack is well tolerated by patients, or alternatively harness arrangements can be employed, as with the Curietron.

(b) Postoperative external irradiation

Treatment of the vault alone is inappropriate when there is known to be residual pelvic disease, and when it is considered that extravaginal recurrence is likely, as when:

(1) Tumour approaches or involves the serosa
(2) Extrauterine disease involving lymph nodes or ovaries is present
(3) When the cervix is involved.

Additionally, grade III tumours irrespective of apparent extent of spread, are likely to generate pelvic recurrence, and in any case have rarely penetrated less than half the uterine wall by the time that hysterectomy is performed.

All the above circumstances indicate the need for irradiation of the whole pelvis, using techniques identical to those used for advanced cervical cancer (*see above*, Treatment of late stage disease). Postoperatively, radiation tolerance is reduced; for a 3-week 16-fraction treatment, the Manchester dose is 4250 cGy, although doses as low as 3000 cGy are employed elsewhere; some centres employ 4-week 20-fraction treatments giving 4000 cGy, while others regularly prescribe 5000 cGy in 25 fractions over 5 weeks. If nothing else, these values indicate that 'pelvic tolerance' is indeed an elastic concept.

It is almost universal practice to follow pelvic X-ray treatment with intracavitary vault treatment, suitably reduced in strength to compensate for the expenditure of part of the radiation tolerance of the bladder and the bowel during external irradiation. As a Wertheim hysterectomy is rarely used in the initial treatment of endometrial cancer, the risk of fistula formation to the bladder and ureters is very small compared with when comparable treatments are carried out following radical surgery for cervical cancer. Thus at the conclusion of external irradiation, the Manchester preference is to proceed directly to the intravaginal insertion (48 hours, surface dose 8000 – 11 000 cGy); occasionally, following an unusually pronounced bowel reaction, treatment is deferred for 2 weeks, and may be omitted altogether in particularly frail patients. Other centres give a single surface dose of 4000 cGy.

Adjuvant hormone therapy

Prophylactic treatment with progesterone has many advocates for early cases (methyprogesterone acetate 100 mg three times a day). The evidence for this has never been proven by a random controlled trial, nor is it certain for how long the drug should be given. In advanced cases the drug has been given with the occasional anecdotal good response.

Carcinoma of the vagina

These tumours are uncommon, accounting for less than 2% of all gynaecological malignancies. Presentation is with abnormal vaginal bleeding, often postmenopausal, usually accompanied by offensive discharge. The thinness of the rectovaginal septum and the proximity of the urethra and bladder base result in symptoms of urinary tract and lower bowel irritability being quite common, and urethral involvement can cause urinary retention. In older neglected patients faecal or less commonly urinary fistulae may be the presenting features.

Table 9.3 Staging recommendations for vaginal carcinoma in use at the Christie Hospital, Manchester

Stage	
1	Tumour limited to vaginal wall
2	Subvaginal extension short of the pelvic wall
3	Extension to pelvic wall
4	Involvement of bladder, rectum, or structures beyond the true pelvis

As surgery would often need to involve partial or total pelvic exenteration, and as vaginal cancer occurs in predominantly older women, there is a strong bias in favour of treatment by radiotherapy. Larger tumours are known to have a high incidence of nodal involvement, but as the nodes of immediate relevance are very difficult to assess by any means, most institutions employ staging systems based on FIGO recommendations, rather than on those of the UICC. The staging practised at the Christie Hospital, Manchester is shown in *Table 9.3*.

Although vaginal carcinoma *in situ* is often multicentric, invasive tumours are usually solitary. In older women they are usually fairly well-differentiated squamous cell carcinomas; they can occur at any site, but the posterior fornix and sites associated with chronic ulceration from ring pessaries worn to control prolapse, are especially likely to give rise to these tumours.

Adenocarcinoma of the vagina is very rare in the UK and when it occurs in older women it usually arises in the lower two-thirds of the vagina. Submucosal lymphatic metastases from adenocarcinoma of the endometrium are much commoner than primary vaginal adenocarcinomas, so diagnostic curettage is an indispensible part of the investigation of patients suspected of having primary vaginal adenocarcinoma.

The long-abandoned practice of giving diethylstilboestrol for threatened abortion is associated with the subsequent development of vaginal (usually upper third) adenocarcinoma in the female issue of such pregnancies, the tumours becoming manifest in the teens and early adolescence. The at-risk population in the UK was never very great, and this cohort is about to pass through what appears to be the period of maximum risk.

Treatment

In many UK centres, surgery is reserved for young patients with stilboestrol-associated adenocarcinoma, for patients with small introital tumours, and occasionally, for patients in whom radiation has failed to control the disease, especially in the inguinofemoral nodes.

(a) Small lesions

A variety of techniques is employed to treat small stage I or stage II tumours, choice being largely determined by the location of the tumour within the vagina. Disease in the upper third, which commonly involves the posterior fornix, can be treated with identical applicators to those used for intracavitary treatment of cervical cancer, with the ovoids placed in tandem if necessary to cover the entire lesions with at least 1 cm of normal mucosal margin. More accessible lesions in the lower two-thirds of the vagina can be treated by interstitial implantation with caesium needles or iridium wire. Small superficial lesions respond well to permanent implantation of radioactive gold seeds (*Figure 9.13*; *see* Chapter 16).

Carcinoma *in situ* is often multicentric and is by definition superficial, so it may ideally be treated by a cylindrical applicator extending from the vault to the introitus, the diameter of the cylinder (2.5 – 3.0 cm) and the duration of the insertion being chosen to

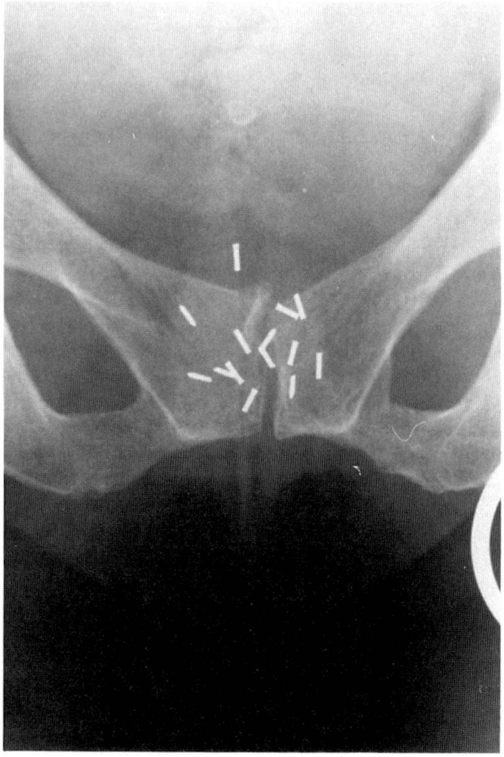

Figure 9.13 A permanent implant of Au^{198} seeds for a small superficial lesion at the introitus

deliver a surface dose of 7500 cGy in approximately 80 hours. Following such treatment, vaginal stenosis and occlusion are common, but by virtue of age are of little consequence to the majority of patients with this condition. Patients who wish to remain sexually active, or for whom adequate assessment at follow-up is considered particularly desirable, are given vaginal dilators which are inserted into the full length of the vagina at least twice daily until the mucosal radiation reaction has subsided.

(b) Large lesions

Most stage II and stage III lesions require external irradiation in addition to some form of internal treatment. The long axis of the vagina diverges from the long axis of the trunk by almost 45°, so that the anteroposterior diversion of the treatment volume must be great enough to subtend the relevant portions of the vagina; the placement of inert gold seeds at the upper posterior and lower anterior limits of the tumour as determined at EUA facilitate radiographic verification that treatment portals are adequate. The use of two posterior-oblique fields to counterbalance an anterior field spares much of the circumference of the rectum (*Figure 9.11*). In Manchester, 4750 cGy are administered in 15 fractions over 3 weeks; after a 2-week gap, during which the rectal reaction usually subsides, the patient is reassessed and commonly proceeds to an intracavitary treatment by a line-source cylindrical applicator giving a mucosal dose of 6000 cGy over approximately 60 hours. This treatment is associated with a marked tendency to subsequent adhesive obliteration of the vagina.

Stage IV disease

Many patients with stage IV disease are better left untreated, especially if very aged, uraemic, or already possessing a fistula. Patients in reasonable general condition should be considered for faecal or urinary diversion. The results of treatment for stage IV disease are so poor (5-year survival 0–5%) that pelvic irradiation should be minimized to that which alleviates symptoms: an intracavitary component to the treatment almost always results in early fistula formation.

Results

Approximately 75% of stage I vaginal cancers are cured by radiotherapy, approximately 60% of stage II, but only 20–25% of stage III.

Carcinoma of the vulva

Vulval cancer has a low incidence similar to that of vaginal carcinoma, and its victims are generally older than is the case for any other group of gynaecological malignancies. Whereas the vaginal mucosa is unusually tolerant of radiation, the vulval mucosa is much less so, and vulval radiation reactions are much more symptom-producing than vaginal reactions. These circumstances place radiotherapy in a role very much subservient to that of surgery in the curative situation, and greatly limit the usefulness of radiotherapy in the palliative situation. As radiotherapists have a restricted contribution to make to the management of this disease, the complex TNM staging recommendations are of no consequence to radiotherapists, and they will not be tabulated or discussed.

A wide variety of chronic vulval dystrophies predispose to the development of invasive cancer, and these conditions are frequently neglected or concealed by the predominantly elderly women in which they arise, and the duration of frank malignant change is often impossible to determine from the history. In older patients, field-change occurs, so that carcinoma *it situ* is often, if not usually, multifocal, and local excisions are commonly followed by serial recurrences, or more properly, by subsequent primary tumours. For these reasons, radical vulvectomy has become the preferred surgical approach, with simultaneous or subsequent bilateral inguinofemoral lymphadenectomy. Simple vulvectomy may be adequate for carcinoma *in situ*, and for small superficial tumours, but necessitates regular and indefinite follow-up.

Self-neglect and concealment cause many of these tumours to be advanced on presentation, and one-third have positive inguinal nodes. Nearly all lesions cause chronic sepsis in the surrounding tissues, making assessment of the true extent of the primary difficult, and the assessment of the regional lymphatics uncertain. Nearly all vulval cancers are squamous cell carcinomas, although malignant melanoma, basal cell carcinoma, intraepithelial carcinoma, and adenocarcinoma (from Bartholin's gland) may rarely occur. Even elderly patients withstand radical vulvectomy quite well, but postoperative morbidity and mortality rise sharply when bilateral groin dissection is also performed, usually due to sepsis. In North America, eligible patients with histologically verified inguinal node involvement also undergo pelvic lymphadenectomy, but this is rarely contemplated in the UK.

Radiotherapy is indicated in a few rather restricted circumstances:

(1) When small postoperative recurrence(s) occur, commonly around the introitus
(2) When surgically curable lesions arise in medically unfit patients
(3) When posteriorly placed lesions exist where surgery would compromise the anus.

The requirements of these situations are usually best met by interstitial treatments with needles, as the needles confer a degree of rigidity to the implant. Gold seed implants are particularly suitable for some introital recurrences (*see* Chapter 16). Many vulval cancers arise on the inner surface of the labium majus, where a single plane implant may be an ideal treatment (*Figure 9.14*). A practical upper limit for implantation is 6 cm maximum diameter: thick lesions requiring two-plane implants are best treated by placing the second plane superficially in the contralateral tissues. The poor quality of the surrounding tissues in most patients with vulval cancer, and the limited tolerance of the vulval mucosa itself, determine that the recommended dose limits are, in this situation, lower than is desirable from a tumour-control view point: 5250 cGy in 7 days for a single plane implant is close to tolerance, and two-plane implants should deliver not more than 5250 cGy midplane, 5000 cGy being a safer dose. Apart from averting or preventing ulceration in inguinal nodes, teletherapy is rarely useful in vulval carcinoma: wide-field irradiation of disease, inoperable by virtue of local advancement, generally causes more misery than it alleviates. But local palliative irradiation with a direct electron or 300 kV field may help to alleviate the misery of a fungating locally recurrent tumour. 4500 cGy in 15 daily fractions will suffice.

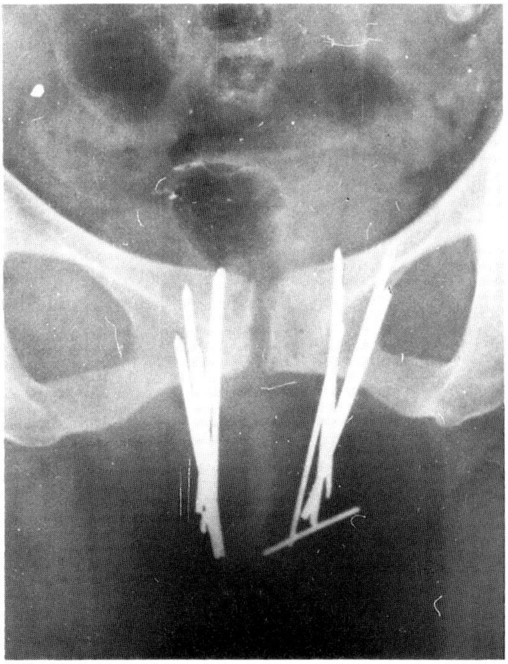

Figure 9.14 A two-plane needle implant for vulval carcinoma. Dose 5500 cGy at 0.5 cm in 168 hours

Ovarian cancer

Although radiotherapy now has a subordinate role in the management of ovarian cancer, it is still of some value. This disease (or more correctly this group of diseases) is responsible for approximately 4000 deaths annually in the UK, and the incidence appears to be steadily rising. Some features of ovarian malignancy are unlikely to change, especially its late presentation, as the symptomatology and clinical findings often mimic those of other intra-abdominal conditions, offering no realistic prospect of early diagnosis. It was never possible to submit rational guidance about X-ray treatment in this group of malignancies, since reported results have been critically stage dependent, whereas the staging itself has been hopelessly lacking in uniformity and degree of thoroughness. The unwieldly staging recommendations for ovarian cancer are fortunately rapidly becoming as irrelevant as they were unworkable; not many general surgeons and only a few gynaecologists record sufficient detail of their laparotomy findings to enable oncologists retrospectively to stage adequately the patients referred to them. Depending on interpretation, there are at least 13 subgroups in the recommended FIGO classification, and their therapeutic implications and prognostic significance are uncertain. Fortunately, the evolution of truly effective chemotherapy, and the identification of reliable ovarian tumour markers, seem likely to make traditional staging concepts redundant. Clinical assessment of the extent of malignant disease and its reponse to treatment is probably nowhere more unreliable than in the case of these tumours, and this provides a charitable explanation for some optimistic reports of the efficacy of various radiotherapeutic methods of treatment for ovarian cancer. Despite the histological diversity of ovarian tumours, most secrete identifiable antigens which are measurable in serum. The properties of the antigen designated CA 125 have been most widely exploited in the UK (Canney *et al.*, 1984). CA 125 has a conveniently short half-life (5 days), and it can therefore be used as a rapidly responsive indicator of the effectiveness of treatment, where it is of established reliability. Presumably as a result of tumour lysis, patients destined to respond well to chemotherapy experience an acute elevation of CA 125 shortly after the inception of their treatment, so the assay has early prognostic significance. CA 125 is not specific for ovarian cancer but in practice this does not diminish its usefulness as an indicator of disease in established ovarian malignancy; 84% of ovarian tumours secrete CA 125, and all mucinous and undifferentiated variants do so. Only two-thirds of endometroid growths secrete, but these are relatively uncommon tumours.

The lack of specificity of the hithertofore identified ovarian antigens limits their potential in screening asymptomatic women, and ovarian cancer will forseeably continue to present as advanced disease. In the UK ovarian cancer accounts for 25% of all gynaecological malignancies, but until recently it has been responsible for 50% of the deaths. Although drug treatment is likely to reduce this percentage in the short and intermediate term, it is not at present clear whether or not definitive cure is being achieved in ovarian cancer as has apparently occurred in testicular teratomas, with the aid of tumour markers. Nearly all malignant ovarian tumours are of epithelial origin, and irrespective of their gross and minute characteristics, 70% seem completely responsive to present-day combination chemotherapy. Susceptibility to ovarian cancer rises steadily from the age of 40 years and its age-specific incidence plateaus at 60 years so that many patients by virtue of age or infirmity will be judged unable to withstand the demands of radical chemotherapy. Such patients are now often referred for radiotherapy, under the mistaken impression that this represents a less taxing option. The radiocurability of some ovarian tumours is established; 30% of patients known to have residual local tumour survive 5 years following postoperative pelvic radiotherapy (Dalley, 1969), but it is difficult to be sure of the role of radiation treatment under the present rather fluid circumstances, and the following advice is offered somewhat tentatively.

Most hormonally inert ovarian tumours are advanced at the time of their diagnosis, both in terms of local pelvic extension and transcoelomic spread; fortuitously discovered and unfortunately uncommon stage 1 disease is associated with retrohepatic deposits in up to 15% of cases, and it is realistic to regard these diseases as being invariably transperitoneal. Radiation treatments which purport to subtend the entire peritoneal cavity are now less widely employed and the diminished role of radiotherapy seems confined to the high-dose low-volume treatment of localized pelvic disease. Confirmation of the diagnosis of ovarian cancer is necessarily surgical, and it has long been the practice to remove the maximum possible amount of tumour during the course of the initial laparotomy. The more radical the exenteration, the more likely are postoperative complications; as chemotherapy is now so effective, it is no longer clear that major extirpations are necessary, but for the present it seems prudent to recommend that the initial surgical attack should, where possible, involve removal of the uterus and its appendages on both sides.

Omentectomy is now seldom performed in the major centres, while abdominopelvic CT scanning, and the estimations of tumour markers, have rendered 'second-look' laparotomies as unnecessary as they are unrewarding.

Irradiation

(a) Wide field

Wide field radiotherapy designed to cover the whole peritoneal cavity is in eclipse, partly because of chemotherapy, and partly because whereas such treatments generally acknowledge the essentially transperitoneal nature of the disease, they fail to acknowledge the predilection to produce bulky lymphatic involvement, which may extend into the mediastinum. Radiation nephropathy is inevitable unless the kidneys are shielded after their cumulative dose has reached 2000 cGy, and even this modest dose is probably too high in circumstances where platinum drugs have either already been, or may subsequently be given. Whole abdominopelvic irradiation is rational only when the entire peritoneum is potentially diseased, so kidney shielding inevitably involves tumour shielding. Lastly, high radiation doses are incompatible with large treatment volumes, especially for patients who frequently have multiple sites of small bowel involvement (Jackson 1976); so low is the irradiation dose commonly achieved under these circumstances that patients with widespread abdominal disease frequently perish from it in less time than it would have taken for radiation nephropathy to develop. From the foregoing, it is clear that 'whole abdomen' irradiation is a poor treatment option, but it may justifiably be employed as a palliative venture in women with widespread disease unresponsive to chemotherapy, in an attempt, for example, to control ascites; convincing evidence of benefit is rarely seen.

Technically whole abdomen treatments require linear accelerators which can provide sufficiently long focus skin distances to give fields extending from the xiphisternum to below the pelvic floor. The posterior field can be treated through the couch on many machines, but depending on the shielding provisions on individual machines, it may be better to treat the patient prone, in order to facilitate kidney protection; in the presence of ascites or large abdominal masses, some patients may be unable to lie prone. The kidneys are shielded from both anterior and posterior beams when their cumulative dose has reached 2000 cGy; their position having been determined by a marker IVP towards the middle of the third week of treatment. Systemic radiation side-effects generally preclude weekly increments greater than 750 cGy, and haematological collapse may impose interruptions, so that the intention to give 3000 cGy midplane dose in 20 fractions often takes longer than the 4 weeks planned, especially when, as is now frequently the case, chemotherapy has previously been given. As implied previously, patients not considered fit enough for chemotherapy can seldom endure a full course of abdominopelvic radiation.

(b) Moving strip techniques

These were developed (and later abandoned) in Manchester in an attempt to reduce acute radiation morbidity by not irradiating the whole of the small bowel at once. The most successful recent application appears to have been at the Princess Margaret Hospital in Toronto, (Dembo *et al.*, 1979).

In view of the remarkable results claimed, the technique is described in some detail, although it is understood that it is no longer in use in Toronto.

At the start of treatment 2250 cGy are delivered to the pelvis in 10 fractions; the second phase of treatment follows immediately with the irradiation of a strip of upper abdomen and thorax so placed as to subtend both domes of the diaphragm; in practice this means that the upper border of the abdominal field starts at or close to, the nipple line. The field below this upper border is divided into strips 2.5 cm in depth, extending downwards to cover the lowest extent of the pelvic floor. On days 1, 2 and 3 of the second phase of treatment, the top two strips, 5 cm in depth, are irradiated as an anteroposterior parallel opposed pair, both fields being treated daily. A third strip is added on treatment days 4 and 5, and a fourth strip is added for days 6, 7 and 8. Thereafter, the four strips, total 10 cm long, are moved inferiorly by 2.5 cm every other treatment day. In this way most of the 2.5 cm strips receive 10 fractions of 225 cGy midplane dose; the most superior strip receives eight fractions only, and the most inferior strip receives seven or eight fractions, depending on the number of 2.5 strips in the total length of the field, as the depth of the moving strip is reduced to 7.5 cm and 5 cm over the last few days of treatment. The ultimate dose to the pelvis will be 2250 plus 2250 (4500 cGy) in 20 fractions. In a report of a large series of patients with stages Ib, II and III ovarian cancer who had previously undergone total abdominal hysterectomy and bilateral salpingo-oophorectomy, Dembo *et al.* (1979), stated that the addition of abdominal irradiation (2250 cGy in 10 fractions) to pelvic irradiation alone (4500 cGy in 20 fractions), raised the actuarial 5-year relapse-free survival from 44 to 77%. The abdominal component of this treatment delivered doses well below that required for eradication of micrometastatic disease in other locations; perhaps the same biological peculiarities of ovarian tumours which confer drug sensitivity also confer unusual radiosensitivity, but this speculation seems weakened by the disappointing performance of X-rays in the treatment of known bulk disease in the pelvis.

The Toronto authors suggested that their results were particularly good because (1) the upper limit of their treatment volume was higher than is usual in moving-strip treatments, and (2) liver shielding was omitted. The striking benefit from abdominal strip irradiation has not subsequently been confirmed elsewhere.

(c) Restricted field

Irradiation limited to the pelvis is still appropriate in

some circumstances:

(1) Where it seems likely that chemotherapy has eradicated all disease with the exception of some residuum at the primary site
(2) In elderly patients whose disease seems confined to the pelvis, and who are thought unsuitable for serious combination chemotherapy or wide-field radiation
(3) In patients who have tumours of borderline or low potential malignancy imcompletely removed from the pelvis. Serial estimations of tumour markers in patients known to be antigen secretors are of considerable assistance in the selection of those patients who may require pelvic treatment, especially in conjunction with serial CT scanning. A four-field pelvic treatment technique similar to that described for advanced cervical cancer is often suitable for these patients (*see Figure 9.7*), although a pair of parallel and opposed fields might well suffice. So far those patients heavily pretreated with drugs do not seem to have shown increased severity in either their acute or late reactions to high-dose pelvic irradiation (in Manchester 4250 cGy in 16 fractions over 3 weeks, in many centres elsewhere 4500–5000 cGy in 20–25 fractions over 5 weeks).

It is unclear whether or not patients who have apparently achieved complete remission of their disease through drugs should receive irradiation to the pelvic site or origin of their previously identified bulk disease. There is already a disconcertingly high incidence of second malignancies in patients with lymphoma treated by sequentially combined chemotherapy and radiation (*see* Chapter 8); marker-secreting patients who have persistently normal levels following chemotherapy could therefore be kept under review, and should not receive routine pelvic irradiation.

It is sometimes necessary to undertake palliative treatments, when for example, lymphatic and venous obstruction to a lower limb is causing clamant symptoms: in these circumstances the extent of disease within the pelvis is frequently such that a simple

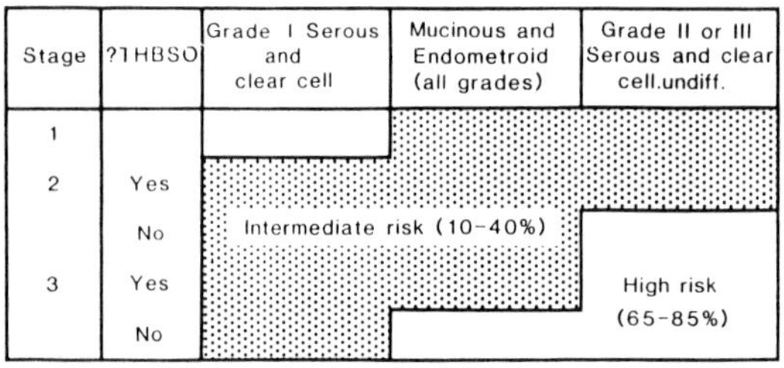
Stage
?1HBSO
Grade I Serous and clear cell
Mucinous and Endometroid (all grades)
Grade II or III Serous and clear cell.undiff.
1
2
3
Yes
No
Yes
No
Intermediate risk (10–40%)
High risk (65–85%)

Figure 9.15 The risk of recurrence within the irradiated abdomino-pelvic volume by stage, histology and grade. (After Dembo, 1985)

anteroposterior parallel pair is most appropriate, giving midplane doses of 3500 cGy in 16 fractions in 3 weeks.

The peculiarities of organization of cancer treatment in the UK are such that at present many victims of ovarian cancer are treated by general surgeons and gynaecologists, a large number of whom by training and temperament are not well suited to the rapidly changing requirements of ovarian cancer treatment: in particular, it is still not widely known that even modest treatment with oral alkylating agents always precludes subsequent potentially curative treatment with the really effective drugs (Canney, Moore and Wilkinson, 1984), which are hydroxydaunorubicin, etoposide, the platinum compounds and bleomycin. Nevertheless, in older patients, the use of single alkylating agents, such as treosulphan, may be the best form of chemotherapy. Special units for the centralization of ovarian cancer treatment are desirable to consolidate and extend the recent gains: in such units anticoagulation is now routine, following the recognition that up to 25% of deaths in women with bulky pelvic disease are due to pulmonary embolism (Canney *et al.*, 1984). The avoidance of embolism as an immediate cause of death is likely to improve short-term survival figures, and true comparison of competing chemotherapy regimens will be best achieved in special units, where such 'extraneous' factors are standardized. In view of the toxicity of the effective regimens, recent claims that ultra-high dose progestogens can produce sustained responses in nearly 50% of patients need urgent confirmation.

Results

The impact, if any, of chemotherapy on long-term results previously obtained by combined surgery and irradiation is at present unknown; indeed it is not yet clear whether chemotherapy and abdominopelvic irradiation are complementary or competitive. Accordingly, precise statements about prognosis after treatment are difficult to make. It has been convincingly argued, (Dembo, Bush and Brown, 1982) that by classifying according to histological findings (pathological subtype, grade of lesion I–III) as well as by stage and size of residual disease, patients can be confidently assigned to an intermediate or low risk group.

The largest diameter of the largest residual lesion is a strong prognostic indicator in stages I, II and II disease, there being few 5-year survivors when the residuum is 2 cm or more in diameter.

Figure 9.15 shows the classification in use at the Princess Margaret Hospital, Toronto (Dembo, Bush and Brown, 1982); following abdominopelvic irradiation (moving strip or open-fields) 75% of the intermediate risk group survive 5 years, but only 30% of the high-risk group do so. Survival in stage IV disease is very poor, 5–15%, but may be influenced by modern chemotherapy.

Addendum

It is now increasingly clear that 'total responders' to ovarian chemotherapy commonly relapse within 6–9 months of cessation of aggressive chemotherapy; the roles or oral maintenance chemotherapy and adjuvant X-ray treatment in such patients are currently being investigated.

References

BRUCKMAN, J., BLOOMER, W. and MARCK, A (1980) Stage III adenocarcinoma of the endometrium: two prognostic groups. *Gynaecological Oncology*, **9**, 12–17

CANNEY, P. A., MOORE, M., WILKINSON, P. M. and JAMES, R. D. (1984) Ovarian cancer antigen CA 125; a prospective clinical assessment of its role as a tumour marker. *British Journal of Cancer*, **50**, 765–769

DALLEY, V. M. (1969) Radiotherapy in malignant disease of the ovary. *Proceedings of the Royal Society of Medicine*, **62**, 359–361

DECKER, D. G. and MALKASSIAN, G. D. Jr. (1979) In *Advances in Medical Oncology, Research and Education Volume VIII, Gynaecological Cancer*, edited by N. Thatcher, Oxford: Pergamon Press

DEMBO, A. J. (1985) *Cancer*, **55**, 2285–2290

DEMBO, A. J., BUSH, R. S. and BROWN, T. C. (1982) Clinico-pathological correlates in ovarian cancer. *Bulletin of Cancer*, **69**, 292–297

DEMBO, A. J., VAN DYKE, J., JAPP, B. *et al.* (1979) Whole abdominal irradiation by a moving-strip technique for patients with ovarian cancer. *International Journal of Radiation Oncology, Biology and Physics*, **5**, 1933–1942

DISHE, S., SEALY, R. and WATSON, E. R. (1983) Carcinoma of the cervix — anaemia, radiotherapy and hyperbaric oxygen. *British Journal of Radiology*, **56**, 251–255

DOLL, R. (1979) Epidemiology of cervix cancer. In *Advances in Medical Oncology, Research and EducationVolume VIII, Gynaecological Cancer*: edited by N. Thatcher, pp. 175–183. Oxford: Pergamon Press

EASSON, C. (ed) (1973) *Cancer of the Uterine Cervix*. London: W. B. Saunders Co., Ltd

FLEISHMAN, A. B., NOTLEY, H. M. and WILKINSON, J. M. (1983) Cost benefit analysis of radiological protection: a case study of remote after-loading in gynaecological radiotherapy. *British Journal of Radiology*, **56**, 737–744

FORSELL, G. (1917) Uetserischt uber due Resultate die Krebsbehandling am Radiumhemm et Stockholm 1910–1915. *Forstchimft a.d. Geb.d. Roentgenstrohlen*, **25**, 142–149

GARRY, R. (1984) Letter *British Medical Journal*, **289**, 1225

GUSBERG, S. B. (1976) The individual at high risk for endometrial cancer. *American Journal of Obstetrics and Gynecology*, **126**, 535–542

HOPE-STONE, H. F., KLEVENHAGEN, S. C., MANTELL, B. S., MORGAN, W. Y., SCHLOMICK, S. A., (1981) Use of the Curietron at The London Hospital. *Clinical Radiology*, **32**, 17–23

INTERNATIONAL FEDERATION OF GYNAECOLOGY AND OBSTETRICS (1982) 18th Report

JOSLIN, C. A. F. and PEEL, K. R. (1982) Uterus. In *Treatment of Cancer*, edited by K. E. Halnan, p. 568. London: Chapman and Hall

KESSLER, I. I. (1976) Venereal factors in human cervical cancer. *Cancer*, **39**, 1912

LIVERSEDGE, W. E. and DALE, R. G. (1978) Dose-time relationships in irradiated weevils and their relevance to mammalian systems. *Current Topics in Radiation Research*, **13**, 97–187

LUDGATE, S. M. and MERRICK, M. V. (1985) The pathogenesis of post-irradiation chronic diarrhoea: measurement of SeHCAT and B_{12} absorption for differential diagnosis determines treatment. *Clinical Radiology*, **36**, 275–278

MARUYAMA, Y., KRYSCIO, R., VAN NAGELL, J. R. *et al.* (1985) Neutron brachytherapy is better than conventional radiotherapy in advanced cervical cancer. *Lancet*, **1**, 1120–1122

MORALES, P., HUSSEY, D. H., MAOR, M. H. (1981) Preliminary report of the M.D. Anderson Hospital randomised trial of neutron and photon irradiation for locally advanced carcinoma of the uterine cervix. *International Journal of Radiation Oncology, Biology and Physics*, **7**, 1533–1540

O'CONNELL, D. (1967) The treatment of uterine carcinoma using the Cathetron; part I — technique. *British Journal of Radiology*, **40**, 882–887

REGAUD, C. (1926) Traitment des cancers du col de l'uterus par les radiations: idee sommaire des methodes et des resultats: indications therapeutiques. *Rapport VIII-ieme Congresse de La Societe Internale Chirugique*, **1**, 35

RUTLEDGE, F. N., FLETCHER, G. H., SMITH, J. P. *et al.* (1976) *Gynaecological Cancer in Cancer Patient Care*, edited by R. L. Clark and C. D. Howe, Chicago: Year Book Medical Publishers Inc.

SHERRAH-DAVIES, E. (1985) Morbidity following low-dose-rate Selectron therapy for cervical cancer. *Clinical Radiology*, **36**, 131–139

THOMAS, D. B. (1984) The epidemiology of cervical cancer: the herpes virus question. *Contemporary Issues in Clinical Oncology*, Volume 2; *Gynaecological Cancer*, edited by A. A. Forastire, pp. 33–46. Edinburgh: Churchill Livingstone

TOD, M. C. (1947) Optimum dosage in the treatment of cancer of the cervix by radiation. *Acta Radiologica*, **28**, 1

TOD, M. C. and MEREDITH, W. J. (1938) A dosage system for use in the treatment of cancer of the uterine cervix. *British Journal of Radiology*, **71**, 809–824

TODD, T. F. (1938) Rectal ulceration following radiation treatment of carcinoma of the uterine cervix. *Surgery, Gynecology and Obstetrics*, **67**, 617–622

UICC (1978) *TNM Classification of Malignant Tumours*, 3rd ed. Geneva: UICC ICRF (1984)

WILKINSON, J. M., HENDRY, J. H. and HUNTER, R. D. (1980) Dose-rate considerations in the introduction of low dose-rate afterloading intracavitary techniques for radiotherapy. *British Journal of Radiology*, **53**, 890–893

WORLD HEALTH ORGANIZATION (1983) *Second Cancer in Relation to Radiation Treatment for Cervical Cancer*, edited by N. E. Day and J. D. Boice, Jr. Lyons: International Agency for Research on Cancer Scientific Publications

10

Tumours in children

P. N. Plowman

Paediatric cancer is rare and afflicts approximately one in 10 000 children; a large proportion of these tumours, perhaps 50% of the total, occur in the first 5 years of life. The commonest childhood malignancy is acute leukaemia, comprising 30% of the total, being usually acute lymphoblastic leukaemia. Central nervous system tumours are the commonest solid tumours in children and account for 20% of the total. Less common malignancies are malignant bone tumours and sarcomas (14%), lymphomas (10%), neuroblastomas (8%), Wilms' tumour (6%).

The management of paediatric cancer represents one of the most challenging and interesting subjects in medicine. First, a close understanding rapport with the whole family is essential to forestall the catastrophic reaction which may follow the diagnosis; this is particularly necessary where there is a chance of cure — but only by a long and arduous treatment programme. Second come the scientific and intellectual challenges of annihilating tumour with minimal normal tissue morbidity and psychological sequelae in a growing child. This task is different from adult cancer management in that childhood tumours often respond better to therapy and, while some normal tissues (e.g. bone marrow) seem more resilient to the acute side-effects of therapy, the potential for damage to developing childhood organs is great; as always, the search is for the optimal therapeutic ratio. Lastly, the terminal care of the slowly dying child together with the enormous psychosocial trauma for the family is a major project for the whole management team, clinicians and nurses — both hospital and community — social and other paramedical workers.

This chapter reviews current concepts concerning systemic cancers in children; brain tumours are reviewed in Chapter 15. Radiotherapy details are expounded fairly fully and it will be noted that 'conventional fractionation' of external megavoltage beam therapy for children is in the region 850–900 cGy per week, tumour dose, in five daily fractions. Empirically, this slightly lower fraction size has not resulted in lesser tumour control and spares normal tissues; the greater weighting now given to the fractional exponent in isoeffect formulae for late tissue damage (Ellis, 1969; Sheline, 1980), or high beta/alpha ratio (Thames *et al.*, 1982) is mathematical 'lip-service' to this empiric observation. Virtually all paediatric radiotherapy is delivered using megavoltage apparatus and, in radical plans, every field is treated daily. Chemotherapy strategies are broadly outlined in this review. Noteworthy are the established use of adjuvant chemotherapy in the paediatric practice and the extreme wariness of chemotherapy–radiotherapy interactions (e.g. the actinomycin-radiation recall phenomenon).

One particular and practical radiotherapeutic problem is the need for the unsupervised child to remain completely still in the intimidating surroundings of a treatment room for the duration of the day's therapy. Turning of the head, for example, could lead to irradiation of an uninvolved eye and missing the tumour. With children beyond the age of 2, friendly persuasion and gentle restraining procedures together with adequate television monitoring and two way vocal communication systems for mother to child dialogue, usually allow treatment to proceed without sedation. In the more fractious child, oral trimeprazine (up to 4 mg/kg stat dose) is administered half an hour prior to treatment. In very young children, a short-acting anaesthetic is required. It is essential that a trained anaesthetist be present for the duration of the anaesthetic and a fully equipped paediatric anaesthetic trolly is based in the radiotherapy department. Ketamine is currently employed at St Bartholomew's Hospital; this drug produces short-lasting 'dissociative anaesthesia', with a latency of onset of 3 minutes after intramuscular injection and a duration of 5–20 minutes. The child is supervised in hospital until fully recovered which may take a futher 1–2 hours.

The anaesthetist must monitor the child from a distance and this creates its own problems. A colour television camera with zoom lens and microphone assist to some degree but the circuitry on a linear accelerator interferes with the electronic stethoscope and an apnoea monitor is too crude a device for sensitive monitoring. At St Bartholomew's Hospital a simple instrument has been brought into routine use to monitor both audibly and visually the gas flow at the nose and mouth of babies and sedated children. A facial strap positions one thermistor over the mouth and one over the nostrils; temperature changes during the respiratory cycle are sensed and accurately reflect the respiratory pattern (Langford, O'Connor and Smith *et al.*, 1984).

Acute lymphoblastic leukaemia (ALL)

Acute lymphoblastic leukaemia is the commonest childhood malignancy. In approximateley 70% of cases the cells bear the unique 'common ALL antigen' (cALLA), regarded as a stem-cell marker. Approximately 15% of cases are T-cell ALL and 2% are B-cell ALL, while 13% bear no distinguishing markers (null cell ALL). T-cell, B-cell and null cell ALL have a poorer prognosis than cALLA positive disease. Other prognostic factors in childhood ALL include the initial white cell count (a presenting white count in excess of $100 \times 10^9/\ell$ being particularly adverse), age at diagnosis (children less than 2 years and older than 10 years being less easily cured), significant masses in nodal or extranodal sites, early CNS disease, certain karyotypic changes and male sex (slightly adverse).

Systemic treatment of childhood ALL is commenced with weekly intravenous vincristine with oral prednisolone with L-asparaginase and/or hydroxydaunorubicin (adriamycin). All patients should be placed on allopurinol and those with high initial counts pre-hydrated and alkalinized. This induction scheme results in a 93% remission rate, usually by 4 weeks. A four drug and more intensive chemotherapy induction (and consolidation) scheme is currently being explored in many centres for high risk patients. For standard risk patients (e.g. cALLA positive patient with low presenting white count and no other adverse features) subsequent maintenance therapy might be daily oral 6-mercaptopurine, weekly oral methotrexate and monthly vincristine and prednisolone, continued for 2–3 years.

Such systemic therapy has been employed for well over a decade and it was recognized early that subsequent CNS/leptomeningeal relapse was common, (up to 50%), even though the chemotherapy had produced sustained marrow remission. The work from St Jude Children's Research Hospital (Hustu *et al.*, 1973) showed that the risk of CNS leukaemia could be greatly reduced by either neuraxis radiotherapy to 2400 cGy conventionally fractionated, or by combination of intrathecal methotrexate and cranial radiation (similarly to 2400 cGy). The latter method was widely adopted as CNS prophylaxis in most of the ALL treatment programmes, the cranial radiotherapy taking place after induction of marrow remission — usually at weeks 4–7.

Despite reports of any early and transient somnolent period following radiotherapy, which does not seem to augur late effects, and of minor late neuropsychological sequelae and subclinical growth hormone secretory deficits, the survival advantages amply justified this CNS prophylaxis programme in all children over 2 years of age. More recently it has been demonstrated that the dose of cranial radiotherapy can be reduced to 1800 cGy in 10 daily fractions without a significant increase in CNS relapse (Nesbit *et al.*, 1981). It may be that children with the most favourable prognostic factors at diagnosis can be safely managed with a course of intrathecal methotrexate only or intrathecal methotrexate and cytosine arabinoside. However, this is not the present author's current recommendation, and chronic intrathecal chemotherapy is not necessarily less toxic than low dose equivalent radiotherapy.

In the situation of isolated CNS relapse following standard therapy, the current recommended management is as follows: intrathecal injections of methotrexate are given twice weekly until the blast cells are cleared from the CSF, whereupon neuraxis radiotherapy is given to a tumour dose of 2400 cGy in 15 fractions in 19–21 days. Intrathecal methotrexate is not administered during this retreatment irradiation, and is not used again immediately afterwards — as methotrexate and radiation together increase the risk of brain damage in this situation. The American Children's Cancer Study Group data and our own data from the Hospital for Sick Children, London demonstrate that a substantial proportion of these children will be salvaged by this approach (Pinkerton and Chessells, 1984).

CNS radiation technique

The target volume for cranial radiotherapy includes the meningeal coverings of the brain, following the contours of the anterior, middle and posterior cranial fossae, the dural sleeve of the optic nerve and, by convention, extending caudally to C2. The patient is planned at simulation when individually tailored cerrobend blocks or standard lead block shapes are manipulated to ensure maximal coverage of all essential areas, while protecting the eyes and other struc-

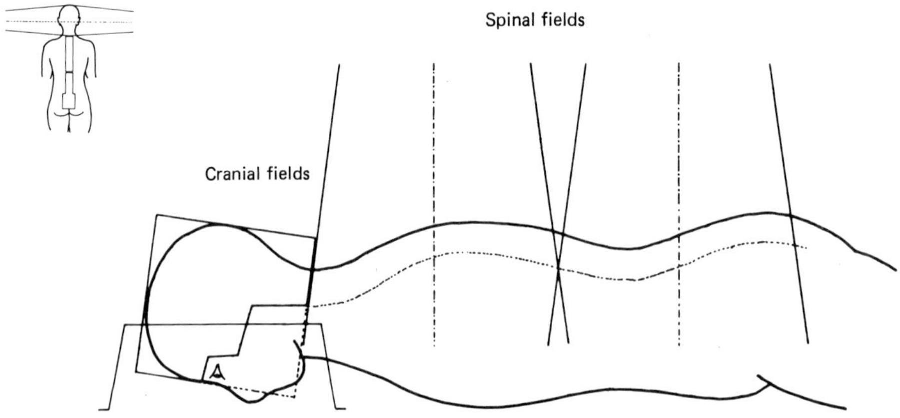

Figure 10.1 Linear accelerator portals for craniospinal (neuraxis) radiotherapy. Note the critical gap region — a calculated gap between the spinal portals prevents overdosage due to divergence of the beams. The plane of the cranial portals matches the angle of divergence of the upper spinal portal

tures. The patients lie on their sides with the head straight, so that the two eyes lie in one vertical plane. This is vital if overdosage to the eyes is to be avoided; if head movement occurs, the child needs sedation or an immobilizing head shell. 'Set up vagaries' are a more important cause of enhanced ocular dosage than deficiencies in the physics of the treatment beam. Nevertheless, field centring over the lateral orbital margin or five degrees posterior angulation of both lateral portals are two techniques aimed to overcome the beam divergence problem affecting the contralateral eye. Ocular dosage should not be greater than 10% of the total and, at this level, later cataracts have not been encountered. Opposed lateral megavoltage photon portals are employed and both fields are treated daily, currently to 1800 cGy midplane dose in 10 fractions over 12 days.

Craniospinal radiotherapy is delivered to the prone patient immobilized in an individually cast head shell. The two lateral cranial portals are as described above, but coming caudally as far as the C4–5 level. The inferior borders of the lateral cranial portals are at a gantry angle of *x* degress, where *x* degrees is the angle of divergence of the superior border of the posterior spinal field (*Figure 10.1*). By this means, it is theoretically possible to abut the lateral cranial and posterior spinal field margins at their surface marking. However, a surface gap of 0.5 cm is employed for safety and is marked on the shell. As in all craniospinal treatments, the therapist is under obligation to ensure that double dosage at the junction of fields does not occur.

The spine is treated in one or two strips depending upon the length of field obtainable from the linear accelerator. The treatment depth is obtained from scrutiny of lateral simulator films of the entire spinal canal and an average depth is usually taken for a modal dose prescription; (but the maximum tumour dose, usually in the upper thoracic region, is always contemplated and documented). If two strips are required, there will be a surface gap between the two portals which must be carefully calculated, unless overlap wedges are used (*see also* Chapter 15). There is an argument for a widening of the spinal portal in the L4–S2 region to encompass the greater breadth of root dural sleeves.

Another important sanctuary from systemic chemotherapy is the testis and 15% or more of boys completing standard ALL therapy are at risk of leukaemic relapse at this site, usually soon after completion of chemotherapy. It is now recommended that all boys have bilateral and multiple wedge biopsies of the testes at the end of ALL chemotherapy. Occult testicular disease is recognized by perivascular aggregates of lymphoblasts. Such children are treated by bilateral testicular radiation as for overt testicular relapse — 2400 cGy TD in 12–15 fractions over 16–21 days. A single, anterior portal encompasses the entire scrotum and both inguinal canals (*Figure 10.2*). Bone marrow relapse often follows testicular relapse, but by the combined use of testicular irradiation and re-introduced systemic therapy, at least one-third of patients survive.

Thus, compared to the 7% survival of children with marrow relapse of ALL, the diagnosis of isolated CNS or testicular relapse is associated with a 30% or more chance of survival following local radiotherapy and the recommencement of chemotherapy. The treatment strategies for marrow relapse are unsatisfactory, and only total body irradiation to a dose beyond haemopoietic death, followed immediately by marrow grafting, currently holds out promise; details of this technique are beyond scope of this discussion, (*see* Chapter 11).

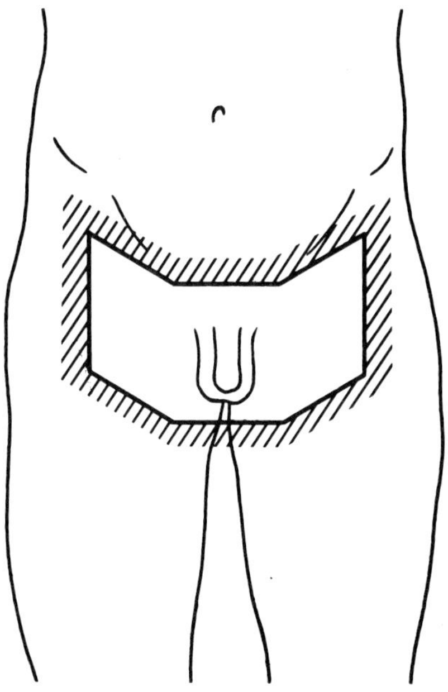

Figure 10.2 Anterior MeV electron portal for testicular radiotherapy in acute lymphoblastic leukaemia

Childhood non-Hodgkin's lymphoma (NHL)

Childhood NHL may present as local lymphadenopathy and apparently localized disease, or as disseminated disease. Using the Rappaport histological classification, the majority of these tumours are diffuse lymphoblastic, diffuse undifferentiated (Burkitt or non-Burkitt type) or occasionally diffuse histiocytic (rarely of true histiocyte lineage). Nodular and cutaneous lymphomas comprise less than 2% of the total. 'Surface marker' analysis has shown that lymphoblastic lymphomas, which are cytologically indistinguishable from ALL are usually T-cell in origin whereas the others are usually of B-cell lineage. Patients presenting with mediastinal masses or cervical lymphadenopathy are likely to have T-cell disease, whereas abdominal primaries are almost always B-cell in origin; mediastinal and abdominal primaries constitute the vast majority of presenting sites. Both T- and B-cell types of disease have a high propensity for CNS dissemination and B-cell disease is the fastest growing of all childhood malignancies. With the cytological identity of T-cell NHL and T-cell ALL, it is necessary to have a working, albeit arbitrary distinction for marrow positive cases. Patients are classified as NHL when the blasts in the bone marrow are less than 25% and there are no abnormal cells in the peripheral blood. Leukaemic relapse ultimately occurs in the majority of progressive T-NHL cases.

Table 10.1 **Staging of paediatric non-Hodgkin's lymphoma**

Stage I	A single tumour (extranodal) or single anatomic area (nodal) except: mediastinum or abdomen
Stage II	A single tumour (extranodal) with regional node involvement Two or more nodal areas on the same side of the diaphragm Two single and extranodal tumours with or without regional lymph node involvement on the same side of the diaphragm A resectable gastrointestinal tract tumour (usually in the ileocaecal area), with or without involvement of associated mesenteric nodes only
Stage III	Two single tumours (extranodal) on opposite sides of the diaphragm Two of more nodal areas above and below the diaphragm Primary intrathoracic tumours Unresectable abdominal disease Paraspinal and epidural tumours
Stage IV	Any of the above with initial involvement of CNS or bone marrow, or both

The Ann Arbor staging system has been replaced by a classificiation specifically for childhood NHL (*Table 10.1*). Using a staging system such as this, one finds that stages I and II are favourable prognostic groups and comprise approximately one-third of all cases, while stages III and IV are unfavourable. Radiotherapy might be curative alone for stage I disease but is usually combined with adjuvant chemotherapy. Modern therapy for stage II disease comprises fairly aggressive chemotherapeutic induction with vincristine, prednisolone and usually cyclophosphamide, perhaps with other drugs (e.g. methotrexate, hydroxydaunorubicin). Maintenance chemotherapy is along ALL lines and often comprises 6-mercaptopurine and methotrexate. Involved field radiotherapy has historically been a part of most treatment schemes and alone historically cured some children. Although some workers have dropped the radiation in trial chemotherapy protocols, it is still to be recommended for children being treated outside trials — to a dose of 2500–3000 cGy conventionally fractionated, usually sandwiched into the chemotherapy.

Stage III/IV NHL is a very dangerous disease and treatment (chemotherapy) is not currently satisfactory. At present T-cell disease is treated along the lines for high risk ALL, with vincristine, prednisolone and asparaginase induction, early cytosine arabinoside and VM26 with maintenance 6-mercaptopurine and methotrexate. B-cell disease is treated with high doses of multiple agents — cyclophosphamide, vincristine, prednisolone, hydroxydaunorubicin with intrathecal and systemic cytosine arabinoside and methotrexate. The courses are condensed in time. Current treatment strategies attempt to 'pack in' high total doses of drugs in the first 6 months of treatment to achieve 'early cure', and the emphasis is no longer on prolonged maintenance. The question of radiation CNS prophylaxis is academic until durable complete remission is achieved.

Overall, there is an 85% chance of survival in stage I/II disease, but a progressively smaller chance as more of the adverse prognostic features of higher stage disease are present.

Hodgkin's disease

Hodgkin's disease (HD) accounts for approximately 5% of paediatric cancer, occurring as frequently as NHL and with an annual incidence of approximately 7×10^{-6} per year. The disease is rare below the age of 5 years and there is a male predominance (M:F, 1.7:1.0) which is most prominent in the younger ages. Supradiaphragmatic, particularly neck, disease is the commonest presenting site, as in the adult practice — usually as painless lymphadenopathy. Lymphocyte predominant histology is commoner than in adults, although the majority of cases still fall into nodular sclerosing or mixed cellularity subtypes; lymphocyte depleted Hodgkin's disease is rare in children.

The Ann Arbor staging system maintains its relevance for paediatric Hodgkin's disease. Staging procedures echo the adult practice, although the 'pick up rate' from bone trephine biopsy is very low indeed and the interpretation of lymphograms is difficult in children due to the frequent occurrence of lymphoid hyperplasia. The staging laparotomy alters the staging in approximately 30% of cases (Donaldson, 1980) and a risk of post-splenectomy sepsis. Standard, megavoltage, extended field radiotherapy (mantle, inverted Y and total nodal irradiation) for stage IA, the mother, nevertheless, abdominal pain and inverted Y and total nodal irradiation) for stage IA, IIA, (IIIA) disease gives high relapse-free survival figures, but significant growth stunting occurs in the axial skeleton. Many UK centres prefer to avoid the laparotomy and splenectomy in children, and accept clinical staging (*see* Chapter 8).

Childhood Hodgkin's disease has a better overall prognosis than the adult form and, in recent years, many workers have attempted to decrease the intensity of first therapy. Such workers argue that with very effective modern salvage chemotherapy, relapse after conservative therapy matters less than the infliction of extra morbidity by 'overtreatment' of the majority of patients who would never relapse. The argument runs counter to the 'traditional approach to cancer management' (absolute necessity for disease-free survival in order to obtain high overall survival), but the good salvage capacity of chemotherapy in childhood Hodgkin's disease is an exceptional situation. The consequence of these arguments has been to move towards involved field radiotherapy, but usually supplemented by chemotherapy, (Sullivan *et al.*, 1982; Tan *et al.*, 1983). In recent years, the St Bartholomew's/Royal Marsden Children's Solid Tumour Group has also explored chemotherapy combined with less than radical dose, involved field radiotherapy for early stage Hodgkin's disease, with excellent disease-free and 95% overall survival rates. The logic of systemic therapy is of course greatest in a clinically staged population. However, as chemotherapy has an unquantifiable late morbidity (e.g. possible infertility and second malignancy), some groups have returned to a therapeutic recommendation from the past for pathologically staged I–IIA disease — involved field radiation and careful follow-up only (Tan *et al.*, 1983). This real challenge to 'the traditional approach to cancer' may have more proponents in the future. The techniques of involved field radiotherapy are described in Chapter 8.

Chemotherapy alone is employed for children presenting with more advanced stages of disease and MOPP (mustine, vincristine, procarbazine, prednisolone) remains the most commonly used regimen, although vinblastine substituting vincristine, and chlorambucil substituting mustine represent minor variants. Such chemotherapy causes complete remission in 80% of patients of whom two-thirds will enjoy prolonged disease-free remission; relapse after chemotherapy is serious as second line chemotherapy regimens are not as effective as had been hoped (*see* Chapter 8). The possibility that another drug combination, (hydroxydaunorubicin bleomycin, vinblastine, DTIC), which contains no alkylating agent, might be equally effective and less liable to induce second tumours, may alter the first choice chemotherapy strategy in the future.

Wilms' tumour

Wilms' tumour occurs with a fairly constant incidence throughout the world (7.5×10^{-6} children) and in the UK comprises approximately 6% of paediatric malignancies. It occurs equally in both sexes and tends to present at a young age. Twelve per cent of cases present in the first year of life and 75% by the age of 5 years; the mean and median age at diagnosis is 3 years. The disease is uncommon after the age of 8 years. There may be associated hamartomas, naevi, hemihypertrophy, ocular defects (particularly of iris or lens), microcephaly, visceromegaly, and facial dystonia. One-fifth of nephrectomy specimens containing Wilms' tumour also contain other renal abnormalities (e.g. hamartomas).

Wilms' tumour arises from the renal pelvis or parenchyma, although rare cases of extrarenal primary Wilms' tumours have been reported. The tumour is bilateral in 5% of cases. The cell of origin is uncertain but is best considered as a pluripotential embryonic cell, perhaps derived from metanephric blastema, capable of differentiating not only into renal elements but also into connective tissue and muscle; thus Wilms' tumour frequently appears as a mixture of renal epithelial and mesenchymal structures. (The infantile mesoblastic nephroma — curable by nephrectomy — must be considered an entity distinct from Wilms' tumour.)

Wilms' tumours having focal or diffuse anaplasia, sarcomatous histology, or demonstrating rhabdoid or clear cell features are now known to carry a poor prognosis, this effect being independent of age and stage. Indeed, in a recent American National Wilms' Tumour Study (NWTS), these unfavourable histology cases, accounted for 52% of the deaths although comprising only 11% of the cases; these findings were almost exactly echoed in the second Medical Research Council (MRC) trial. The recognition of unfavourable histology cases has been a recent advance in Wilms' tumour (Beckwith and Palmer, 1978; Breslow *et al.*, 1978).

Although the most common presenting clinical feature is an abdominal mass, usually discovered by the mother, nevertheless, abdominal pain and haematuria are not uncommon presenting features, and fever and hypertension will also be found in a significant minority of children on their presentation physical examination. The abdominal mass is usually firm, irregular, fixed and, unless massive, lateralized. At presentation, the children are often well-nourished and happy, except those with advanced disease.

The diagnosis will be suspected in the majority of children from the history and examination, but an abdominal grey-scale ultrasound scan is extremely useful in demonstrating a solid or multicystic renal swelling and other possible attendant complications, for example bilateral Wilms' tumours or tumour in the inferior vena cava.

An intravenous urogram (IVU) is also an important investigation to demonstrate an abnormality in the kidney and to delineate the contralateral kidney. A leg injection of contrast is occasionally used to demonstrate the patency of the inferior vena cava. Both tests can confuse an upper pole Wilms' tumour with a locally invasive adrenal neuroblastoma and a negative test for urinary vanillylmandelic acid is important. There is no reliable serum marker for Wilms' tumour although chondroitin sulphate is occasionally detectable in the serum. A chest X-ray is an essential investigation at the time of initial work-up as the lungs are the commonest site of extra-abdominal metastases.

In the absence of extra-abdominal metastases, and unless the abdominal tumour is so enormous as to make surgery hazardous, the diagnosis is made and staging and first phase of treatment are performed at surgery. An anterior abdominal incision is chosen so that a thorough laparotomy may be performed. This will include a careful examination of the other kidney, the liver, the peritoneum and palpation of the inferior vena cava for tumour. The usual definitive procedure is radical nephrectomy with complete removal of tumour extensions as far as is possible. Unresectable tumour is clipped with radiopaque markers. Where the Wilms' tumour is localized within a kidney, a partial nephrectomy may be a safe procedure. Staging is finally decided when the histopathological review of the resected specimen and biopsied tissues is known. The staging of Wilms' tumour is shown in *Table 10.2*.

Recently the TNM classification has been introduced and may supplant the current staging system. The pTNM, post-surgical histopathological classification is set out in *Table 10.3*.

Analyses of patients treated in the 1940s by radical nephrectomy only, suggested that the overall survival rates were not in excess of 30% and that 15–25% was probably the true figure. In the 1950s, the use of radiotherapy postoperatively to the tumour bed led to survival figures of approximately 40%, and in recent years the addition of chemotherapy has improved the results yet further, doubling survival again. The main prognostic variables for Wilms' tumour patients are histology, stage and age, and these three variables now determine the 'strength' of therapy.

Radiotherapy is mainly employed in conjunction with chemotherapy to reduce the risk of relapse in the region of the primary, but the abdominal fields may be opened up to encompass almost the whole abdomen in cases with diffuse peritoneal contamination. NWTS trials have indicated that radiotherapy to the primary tumour bed adds insignificantly to survival in favourable histology stage I cases. This may also hold true for favourable histology stage II cases but this is, as yet, less well established, except for children less than 2 years of age in whom it is probably safe to omit

Table 10.2 Staging of Wilms' tumour

Stage I	Tumour limited to the kidney and completely resected, the renal capsule being intact
Stage II	Tumour extending locally outside the kidney but completely resected (i.e. excision margins clear microscopically)
Stage III	Tumour spread within the abdomen or retroperitoneum that is not completely resected at operation — this includes microscopic tumour at the margins or resection, rupture of the tumour into the abdomen at operation or established abdominal metastases and any abdominal lymph node involvment
Stage IV	Haematogenous metastases
Stage V	Bilateral Wilms' tumours

Table 10.3 Post-surgical histopathological TNM staging classification of Wilms' tumour

Tumour	*Nodes*	*Metastases*
pT1 Intrarenal tumour, completely encapsulated. Excision complete and margins histologically clear	pN0 No evidence of tumour found on histological examination of regional nodes	M0 Absent
pT2 Tumour with invasion beyond the capsule or renal parenchyma. Excision complete	pN1 Evidence of invasion of regional nodes. (Suffix a or b denotes complete or incomplete resection respectively)	M1 Present
pT3 Tumour with invasion beyond the capsule or renal parenchyma. Excision incomplete or with evidence of preoperative or operative rupture pT3a: Evidence of microscopic residual tumour confined to the tumour bed pT3b: Evidence of macroscopic residual tumour or spillage and/or malignant ascites pT3c: Unresectable tumour		
pT4 Bilateral tumours		

abdominal radiotherapy. Stage III cases all require radiotherapy to the tumour bed. In stage IV cases, most workers would tend to use chemotherapy first with delayed surgery with or without radiotherapy later, and the management of stage V is individualized. Following primary tumour bed radiotherapy, analysis of the subsequent relapsers on the first NWTS chemotherapy programme showed that the primary bed is the first site of relapse in 10% of favourable histology cases and 25% of unfavourable histology cases — thus the majority of subsequent relapses are due to systemic metastases.

Low dose whole lung radiotherapy is an important part of salvage therapy in patients relapsing with pulmonary metastases, following a modern chemotherapy programme.

The response rate of Wilms' tumour to single chemotherapeutic agents are: vincristine 71%, hydroxydaunorubicin 60%, actinomycin 45%, cyclophosphamide 33%. Various clinical trials over the last two decades have examined the relative benefits of single versus multiple courses of chemotherapy. The NWTS demonstrated clearly that the two drug combination of actinomycin D and vincristine gave better survival figures in stage II and III disease and that a single course of chemotherapy was insufficient. In a later NWTS trial, triple drug chemotherapy, (hydroxydaunorubicin added to the other two drugs), gave superior results, and patients with stage III and IV disease now usually receive these three drugs, as do patients with unfavourable histology (comprising 11% of the total Wilms' population). At the other end of the scale, a child with a favourable histology stage I tumour probably will only need a short course of adjuvant vincristine. The exact details of the chemotherapy regimens differ between different centres and are not described in detail here; they rarely exceed 9 months in length past complete remission. The side-effects of chemotherapy mainly apply to the combination regimens and include early nausea after administration, alopecia, dose-dependent myelosuppression and vincristine neuropathy.

Radiotherapy technique

For postoperative abdominal radiotherapy, megavoltage photons are employed to treat parallel opposed, anterior and posterior abdominal portals, both fields daily, treatment beginning within 10–14 days of surgery. The portals are simulated and a recent IVU film, demonstrating the position of the surviving kidney, must be available at planning if the portals have to be simulated without a simultaneous IVU.

The volume to be irradiated must include the renal or tumour bed with adequate, at least 2 cm, margins. The medial border comes far enough over the midline to encompass the whole width of the vertebral bodies, such that any growth stunting is symmetrical, but not the contralateral kidney in uncomplicated cases. Indeed, this border may be penumbra trimmed to reduce any contribution to the other kidney. The lateral border of the radiation field frequently extends to the tapering lateral loin margin and the potential 'hot spot' here is reduced by a tangential body wall shield (*Figure 10.3*). There is little evidence that, in the absence of gross residual disease *in situ*, doses in excess of 2000–2500 cGy conventionally fractionated (800–1000 cGy weekly) add to the local control rate and a common prescription for the

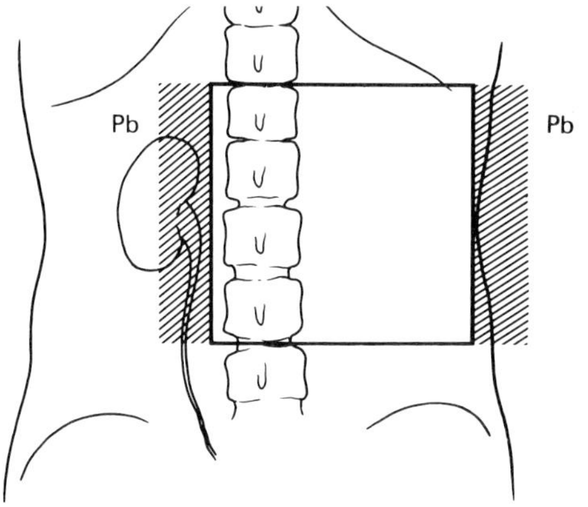

Figure 10.3 Megavoltage photon portal for Wilms' tumour bed radiotherapy

portals just described would be 2000 cGy midplane dose (calculated on the separation at the field centre), in 10 or 11 daily fractions over 2 weeks.

Where there is residual disease left *in situ* a midplane dose of 3000 cGy in 20 daily fractions in 4 weeks is prescribed. Doses to infants are reduced by 50%. Where there is stage III disease, wider portals are often necessary; if the surviving kidney lies within the radiation portal then it should be shielded from the posterior portal throughout treatment — this shielding being carefully planned with an IVU performed at simulation; the dose to the surviving kidney must not exceed 1500 cGy fractionated over 3–4 weeks.

Whole abdominal radiotherapy is only required for gross tumour spill or dissemination. Not only is the surviving kidney partially protected (as above) but the femoral heads are also shielded and, if possible, at least one ovary in girls. Prescriptions of the order of 2500 cGy midplane dose in 4 weeks are given with a 500 cGy boost to sites of bulk disease (conventional, daily fractions).

Both actinomycin D and hydroxydaunorubicin are sensitizers to the biological effects of radiation and may elicit 'recall phenomena' in recently irradiated tissues; for this reason, the concurrent or temporally adjacent administration of radiotherapy and these agents is avoided. Vincristine can be safely administered, however, and is given weekly during radiotherapy in most protocols. The concurrent or adjacent use of the sensitizers with radiation takes on particular importance in patients with right-sided tumours; the radiation portal often encompasses much of the liver and hepatopathy, with disturbed liver function tests and thrombocytopenia, may occur. Other side-effects of abdominal radiotherapy are usually the nausea and enteritis attending small bowel irradiation.

Pulmonary irradiation may play a part in the management of patients with lung metastases which are either slow to disappear with chemotherapy alone or are manifestations of relapse during or after chemotherapy. The entire thoracic cavity is treated through simulated, anterior and posterior, MeV photon portals with the humeral heads shielded, both fields treated daily. The prescribed dose is 1200–1500 cGy midplane in 8–10 daily fractions, the total dose varying with age and the salvage chemotherapy regimen. Individual metastases may be boosted through postage stamp portals up to a further 1000 cGy, or resected. Patients who relapse 'off therapy', particularly those relapsing some time 'off therapy', stand a reasonable chance of 'salvage', with re-introduction of chemotherapy and lung irradiation. Overall, the long-term disease-free survival in an unselected group of Wilms' patients, treated in specialist centres is over 80%; higher risk patients can now often be defined at diagnosis and treatment intensified in these. The three major prognostic factors are age at diagnosis (children less than 1–2 years having a better outlook), stage at diagnosis, and histology (*see above*). The period of relapse risk is greatest in the first year and uncommon after 2 years off therapy. Follow-up checks, at first monthly with a routine physical examination and chest X-ray, are gradually spaced with periodic grey-scale ultrasound imaging of the tumour bed and surviving kidney. The blood pressure is monitored at each follow-up.

Neuroblastoma

Neuroblastoma accounts for 8% of malignant tumours in children in the UK, with an annual incidence of 1.8×10^{-6} per annum. In one autopsy series of children dying from other causes, the incidence of neuroblastoma was 40 times that expected; further, neuroblastoma has the highest spontaneous regression rate amongst malignant tumours — these data suggesting a much higher incidence of occult and spontaneously regressing tumours. There is geographic variation, for example, the tumour is uncommon in Africa. In a minority of patients there is a familial link (e. g. von Recklinghausen's disease). There is a slight predominance of males.

Neuroblastoma can rarely present at birth and one-half of all cases present within the first 2 years of life.

Three-quarters of all cases present by 4 years and the disease becomes much less common in the older age groups.

The tumours are soft, often apparently encapsulated and possess rich vasculature; there are not infrequent areas of haemorrhage, calcification or necrosis. Microscopically, closely packed, small round sympathogonia are seen, sometimes growing as solid sheets with many mitoses visible; other areas may show cellular groupings into rosette structures. In yet other areas of a single tumour, young ganglion cells may be identifiable and in parts the tumour cells may demonstrate a positive chromaffin reaction; electron microscopy may demonstrate storage vesicles. Thus both differentiation pathways may be represented within the same tumour and this explains the potential to mature into a benign ganglioneuroma (comprising ganglion cells and nerve fibres) or phaeochromocytoma (comprising phaeochromocytes with the potential to store and secrete catecholamines). Neuroblastoma-specific monoclonal antibodies have recently been used to help in the diagnosis of poorly differentiated small round cell tumours.

Neuroblastoma originally derives from neural crest tissue and may arise anywhere in the sympathetic nervous system. Abdominal primaries account for two-thirds of all cases (60% adrenal origin) and the chest, usually the posterior thoracic sympathetic chain, accounts for 15%. A minority, perhaps 5%, arise in the head and neck region and approximately 15% are of unknown origin.

The clinical presentation varies, but in contradistinction to Wilms' tumour, the child is likely to appear ill with malaise and weight loss; anaemia and fever may be present. An abdominal lump or pain is the presenting feature in one-quarter of all cases and bone pain in 15%. Symptoms from catecholamine excess (e.g. palpitations, headache), and rarely from vasoactive intestinal polypeptide (e.g. diarrhoea), multisite lymphadenopathy (particularly cervical), spinal cord compression (classically from the extension of a paraspinal primary tumour through the root canals to cause extradural pressure), and symptomatic bony metastases are all recognized presentation features in a minority of patients. Distant effects of neuroblastoma are rare and not understood, but include an acute cerebellar encephalopathy. Many patients present with symptoms due to metastases and the propensity of this tumour to spread to bone and particularly to the skull accounts for some well-known clinical features of neuroblastoma such as bone pain, proptosis, and many of the systemic features of the disease.

Diagnosis is made by biopsy, bone marrow aspirate or by the demonstration of excessive urinary excretion of catecholamine catabolites, particularly vanillylmandelic acid and homovanillic acid. Staging follows diagnosis and will include imaging appropriate to the primary tumour as well as a bone scan and bone marrow examination. The Evans staging system has usually been employed up to the present with a subdivision of stage II (Evans, D'Angio and Randolph, 1971; Ninane *et al.*, 1982) (*Table 10.4*). Evans *et al.* (1980) established convincingly that the special pattern of widespread neuroblastoma designated IVS and occuring in infants, is associated with a much better prognosis than stage IV and merits its special staging. The alternative, post-surgical, histopathological pTNM classification (*Table 10.5*) gives a clear weighting to the recently acknowledged prognostic implication of regional node involvement.

Table 10.4 Staging of neuroblastoma

Stage I	Tumour confined to the organ or structure of origin
Stage II	Tumour extending in continuity beyond the organ of origin but not crossing the midline Stage IIA if ipsilateral lymph nodes negative, stage IIB if positive (NB Some groups have subdivided into IIA —fully resectable, IIB—not fully resectable
Stage III	Tumour extending in continuity beyond the midline or contralateral regional node involvement
Stage IV	Distant metastases present
Stage IVS	Infants who would be in stage I or II were it not for liver, skin or bone marrow involvment are placed in this special, good prognosis group

The treatment of neuroblastoma depends on the age of the patient (young children, particularly those under the age of 1 year, do well) and on the stage (patients with more extensive disease do badly). Surgery, radiotherapy and chemotherapy all have their place in neuroblastoma management, although the emphasis on the different modalities varies between centres, a reflection of unsatisfactory treatment results.

In general terms, the treatment of stage I or IIA disease in children less than 1 year of age will often be surgery alone with a favourable outlook. In infants with stage II, III, or IV disease, the decision to treat further after biopsy will depend on the clinical status and disease progression. In older children, radiotherapy would often be added to surgery for stage I–IIA disease, although some would choose chemotherapy, and more advanced stage patients would usually receive chemotherapy. When chemotherapy is deemed necessary, it is not always intensive and in infants, for example, low dose cyclophosphamide and vincristine, or cyclophosphamide and prednisolone, may be effective at inducing a remission. In older children, more aggressive systemic therapy is frequently required, but the optimal combination of drugs has yet to be found. Manage-

Table 10.5 Post-surgical histopathological TNM staging classification of neuroblastoma

Tumour		*Nodes*		*Metastases*	
pT1	Excision of tumour complete and margins histologically clear	pN0	No histological evidence of tumour invasion	M0	Absent
				M1	Present
pT2	Not yet designated	pN1	Evidence of regional node invasion pN1a: Involved nodes considered completely resected pN1b: Involved nodes considered incompletely resected	Mx	Patient not assessed for metastases
pT3	Evidence of residual tumour pT3a: Evidence of microscopic residual tumour pT3b: Evidence of macroscopic residual tumour				
pT4	Evidence of multicentric tumour	pNx	The extent of regional node involvement not assessed		

ment of the rare stage IVS cases is conservative if possible.

Radiotherapy

Neuroblastoma is a radiosensitive tumour. In the infant, regression can be induced by low doses of the order of 1800–2000 cGy in 15 daily fractions over 21 days. For older children, prescriptions of the order 2500–3500 cGy in 3–4 weeks, daily fractionation, would be delivered, with opposed fields, the higher doses given to macroscopic residual tumour and this might be boosted to 4000 cGy depending on the normal tissues and the bulk of residual tumour.

During the planning of radiotherapy to abdominal tumours, many of the constraints for radiotherapy in Wilms' tumour also apply. At least one kidney must be screened (perhaps only from the posterior portal) throughout therapy and the liver after 1500 cGy. The whole width of the vertebral column should be encompassed and the femoral heads and gonads should be shielded if at all possible.

In stage IVS patients with rapidly enlarging livers, renal, bowel or pulmonary complications may develop due to mechanical compression from massive hepatomegaly, and occasionally coagulopathy develops. Local radiation treatment to the liver is indicated and a dose prescription of 450 cGy midplane dose in three fractions over 4 days (treating every other day), is delivered through parallel opposed lateral MeV photon portals, avoiding the spinal cord and kidneys, and accepting that the posterior part of the liver may not be encompassed. In the Philadelphia experience, such low dose radiotherapy stands a reasonable chance of halting progression, and subequent spontaneous regression may occur.

Radiation techniques for other sites of neuroblastoma are highly variable but for an incompletely resected mediastinal growth, parallel opposed portals and a dose of 2000–2500 cGy midplane in 12–15 daily fractions would be given in addition to chemotherapy. Radiotherapy has an important role in palliation, particularly bony metastases, using faster fractionation, e.g. 1500–1800 cGy in five to six daily fractions. Radiotherapy is urgently indicated for compressive tumour effects on the nervous system (e.g. the spinal cord, and the optic nerves) and the present author believes in careful fractionation in these situations, commencing with daily 150–160 cGy fractions, and with the co-administration of dexamethasone.

The major prognostic features for a patient with neuroblastoma are age (survival: less than 1 year 82%; 1–2 years, 32%; more than 2 years, 10%), and stage (survival: stage I, 90%; II, 70%; III, 25%; IV, 10%; IVS, 67%). Histology may also bear on prognosis and a ganglioneuroblastoma may behave more favourably than a neuroblastoma, while the highly differentiated ganglioneuroma is benign. In the absence of the urinary excretion of catechol acetic acid, vanil lactic acid and vanil ethanol, a high vanillylmandelic acid: homovanillic acid urinary excretion ratio is prognostically more favourable than a low ratio. However, the histological variants and chemical endocrine data do not yet influence treatment recommendations which are largely based on age and stage.

Rhabdomyosarcoma

Rhabdomyosarcoma is the commonest of the malignant soft tissue growth in paediatric practice with an incidence of 3×10^{-6} in children less than 15 years old; the incidence peaks in the first 5 years of life. The sex incidence is towards a slight excess of males; there is no established link with other diseases.

Green and Jaffe (1978) reviewed the literature and found that the disease was distributed in the following sites: orbit, 9%; extra-orbital head and neck sites, 32%; genitourinary and intra-abdominal sites, 34%;

trunk and extremities, 25%. The predominance of primary lesions in the head and neck and pelvic regions is noteworthy.

Macroscopically, the tumours are usually pink and fleshy masses but the botryoid sarcoma may appear as myomatous, polypoid masses. Microscopically, the majority are embryonal rhabdomyosarcomas; this tumour type comprises highly undifferentiated cells, often spindle-shaped and with eosinophilic cytoplasm that may be PAS (periodic acid Schiff) positive. The cells often exhibit myoblastic proliferation and cytoplasmic fibrils may be demonstrable on electron microscopy. Pleomorphic rhabdomyosarcoma cells may also contain myofibrils or cross-striations in cells of more variable shape than embryonal tumours, often closely packed and again with eosinophilic cytoplasm. Alveolar rhabdomyosarcoma is characterized by the presence of empty 'alveoli' separated by connective tissue trabeculae often containing many tumour cells, sometimes giant cells and again the cross-striations and cytoplasmic fibrils may be distinguishable. The American Rhabdomyosarcoma Group have found prognostic usefulness in focusing on the cytological features within the tumour, rather than the conventional tissue pattern. Those with anaplastic or monomorphous cytological patterns (comprising 20% of all cases) were associated with a poorer prognosis; however, it is interesting that monomorphous cytological features correlated quite closely with alveolar pattern.

Clinical presentation varies with site. The commonest head and neck sites are the orbit, the parotid region, the middle ear regions, where enlarging and otherwise asymptomatic masses are usually the presenting complaints, or the naso- and oropharynx, where dysphagia or failure to thrive may be the presenting complaint. Urethral or vaginal masses may be the presenting complaints of patients with genitourinary rhabdomyosarcomas and painless, enlarging masses are the usual complaints of patients with tumours at other sites. Diagnosis is established by biopsy and staging investigations follow. These include full blood count, chest X-ray, bone scan, bone marrow aspirate and trephine. Other radiological imaging tests depend on the site of the tumour. All these investigations allow the designation of stage (Children's Solid Tumour Group Staging CSTG, Kingston, McElwain and Malpas 1983) (*Table 10.6*).

The recently introduced pathological (i.e. post-surgical) pTNM staging system has certain merits (*Table 10.7*), but few large series of patients have been analysed this way to date.

Table 10.6 Staging of rhabdomyosarcoma

Stage I	Local disease – confined to the tissue of origin A – Completely resected B – Incompletely resected
Stage II	Regional disease A – Disease extending outside the tissue of origin to involve contiguous bone or nerve B – With nodal metastases
Stage III	Generalized disease A – Without bone marrow involvement B – With bone marrow involvement

Table 10.7 Post-surgical histopathological TNM staging classification of rhabdomyosarcoma

Tumour	*Nodes*	*Metastases*
pT1 Tumour limited to organ or tissue of origin. Excision complete and margins histologically clear	pN0 Regional nodes clear of tumour	M0 Absent
		M1 Present
	pN1 Evidence of invasion of regional nodes	
pT2 Tumour with invasion beyond the organ or tissue of origin. Excision complete and margins histologically clear	pN1a: Considered completely resected pN1b: Considered incompletely resected	
pT3 Tumour with invasion beyond the organ or tissue of origin. Excision incomplete pT3a: Microscopic residual disease pT3b: Macroscopic residual disease pT3c: Unresectable primary tumour		

Treatment

Treatment strategies for rhabdomyosarcoma must recognize that these tumour types are highly infiltrative locally and often tend to disseminate rapidly.

Radical surgery was the first successful modality of treatment for rhabdomyosarcoma; for orbital primaries, more than one-third of patients were cured by orbital exenteration and perhaps two-thirds of patients with bladder primaries were cured by radical pelvic surgery. Conversely, parameningeal rhabdomyosarcomas or prostatic primaries were rarely cured by radical surgery. The cure potential of surgery remains important although in the modern multi-modality therapy era, the extent of surgery required is now less.

Radiotherapy also has a well-established potential for tumour sterilization and in tumours with less propensity to disseminate early (e.g. orbital) stands a chance of cure. Radiotherapy contributes to the chance of permanent local control in the majority of rhabdomyosarcomas and often allows less radical surgery to be performed.

Triple drug chemotherapy with vincristine, cyclophosphamide and actinomycin D or hydroxydaunorubicin, usually given as bolus therapy once every 2–3 weeks for more than 1 year, is powerful when used in the adjuvant situation following local therapy to the major tumour burden. Following surgery and/or radiotherapy to stage I–II disease, adjuvant chemotherapy has increased the chance of cure. For stage III cases, responses are usually temporary.

Radiotherapy

Conventionally fractionated, megavoltage photon dose prescriptions to 4500–5500 cGy are commonly precribed for primary rhabdomyosarcoma — the lower dose to small bulk disease and in young children, the higher dose to large bulk primary tumours in areas where the surrounding normal tissues will tolerate this. The target volume tends to be generously wide around the tumour initially, but the portals are usually narrowed around the tumour after 4000–4500 cGy. Radiopaque clips placed at surgical resection and preoperative imaging investigations are two important requirements in radiation planning of rhabdomyosarcoma arising in most sites, together with a lucid operation note. For anterior facial or parotid tumour, a single 10 MeV electron portal may be optimal (*Figure 10.4*). For orbital primaries, a 60° wedge pair of anterior and antero-oblique portals is usually employed in the supine child lying in a shell. The target volume is at least the whole orbital cavity. Posterior peaking of the isodoses towards the pituitary, hypothalamus and brain stem may often cause a change of plan after 4000 cGy. Parameningeal tumours are usually widespread and across the midline; parallel opposed

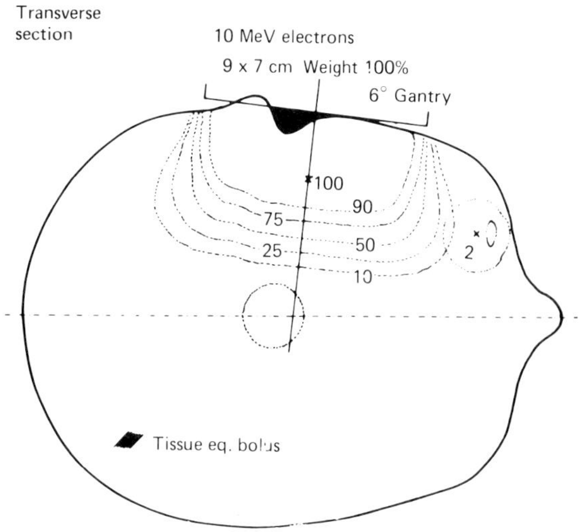

Figure 10.4 Appositional 10 MeV electron portal for localized rhabdomyosarcoma in the parotid region

lateral, MeV photon portals are usually used throughout therapy although these portals are commonly narrowed for the final boost to the primary tumour area. As these parameningeal tumours are rarely resectable, high dose radiation is usually required; adjacent normal structures are often radiosensitive and after a wide field first phase of treatment, the boost may be delivered by electrons, interstitial implants or small and meticulously shaped external beam fields, depending on the individual case. Where there is intracranial extension of the primary tumour, the whole cranium may require radiotherapy together with an intrathecal chemotherapy programme.

Pelvic rhabdomyosarcoma is more amenable to surgery, and radical surgery, which could often mean pelvic exenteration, was standard therapy for these tumours, More recently, it has been possible to obtain local control in many cases with more limited surgery, (perhaps saving the gonads, or rectum). This would be either in conjunction with radiotherapy or by employing the surgery after maximal tumour shrinkage with chemotherapy, omitting radiotherapy altogether. The postoperative radiation target volume is planned from preoperative imaging procedures, the operation report and clips placed at surgery. The portal is shaped appropriately to cover the tumour bed and margins, and tumour doses of 4000–4500 cGy, conventionally fractionated, are delivered. In patients with gross residual disease, an additional boost of 500–1000 cGy may then be delivered through reduced portals, with slightly increased fraction size, or by an implant. An open anterior and two open posterior oblique MeV photon portals might be selected to treat a bladder or prostate tumour bed, and the dose to rectum and hips scrutinized carefully before the acceptance of any plan. If parallel opposed portals are used, they are shaped to avoid the femoral heads if possible and perhaps one ovary (rarely possible). The surgeon must also be mindful of placing any stoma away from a radiation portal and perhaps of displacing bowel from the pelvis (e.g. with the recently available and absorbable polyglactin 910 mesh), when postoperative radiotherapy is used.

Paratesticular tumours require a special mention as the outlook for these patients is good with optimal therapy. A transinguinal orchidectomy with proximal ligation of the spermatic cord and imaging of the retroperitoneal lymph nodes precedes adjuvant therapy in the early stage cases. If the scrotal tissues are infiltrated, postoperative radiotherapy is required, and if the other testis is not at risk of infiltration, it may be translocated to the contralateral groin for the duration of radiotherapy. The radiation portal will encompass the site of the lump with 2–3 cm margins, the scrotum and the inguinal canal; an anterior 6–10 MeV electron portal is usually ideal. A dose of 4000–4500 cGy conventionally fractionated, would be prescribed for microscopic disease. Where para-aortic lymphadenopathy is present, surgical or surgical and radiotherapeutic measures may be employed, treating a para-aortic strip or dog-leg field which encompasses the retroperitoneal nodes and ipsilateral groin and scrotum, to 3500–4000 cGy, conventionally fractionated.

Truncal or extremity tumours are treated by wide local excision and radiation to the tumour bed. It is often possible to deliver safely a higher tumour dose to such sites by a well conceived, individualized plan. As with other limb tumours, a lymphatic corridor is left unirradiated where possible and shrinking field techniques are often appropriate.

Chemotherapy such as described above, plays an important role in all these tumours. If metastases 'break-through' or are present at diagnosis, they are most likely to occur in lung, bone or bone marrow, but failure at the primary site still remains a problem (e.g. parameningeal tumours).

Prognosis

The CSTG data accord with most other investigators that the extent of disease at diagnosis is the strongest prognosticator. Children with tumours confined to the tissue of origin with no evidence of nodal or metastatic spread have a 5-year survival of 85% (Kingston, McElwain and Malpas, 1983). In children with more extensive local disease, the prognosis is less satisfactory and patients with generalized disease have a worse than 20% chance of survival, and less than 10% survival if the bone marrow is infiltrated at presentation. Certain tumour sites are associated with a more favourable outcome (e.g. orbit, bladder, paratesticular, and vagina) than others (e.g. parameningeal, prostate, perineum). A recent large analysis of head and neck rhabdomyosarcomas demonstrated a 91% relapse-free survival for orbital primaries, 46% for parameningeal primaries and 75% for those with other head and neck primaries (Sutow *et al.*, 1982). Embryonal tumours have a better prognosis than those of alveolar or pleomorphic histology, stage for stage and the recently recognized cytological features may also help in prognosis. The vast majority of relapsers will have manifested their relapse within 2 years of presentation.

Bone tumours

Osteogenic sarcoma

This malignant tumour arises from bone mesenchyme and the resulting sarcoma retains the capacity to produce directly osteoid and immature bone to some degree. The paediatric incidence peak is in the second decade and the tumour occurs slightly more frequently in males. Children with familial retinoblastoma have a slightly higher risk of developing osteogenic sarcomas; trauma is not currently recognized as a predisposing cause.

Osteogenic sarcoma arises most commonly in the metaphyseal regions of long bones, (e.g. distal femur, proximal tibia, proximal humerus), and the child usually presents with pain and/or swelling (*see* Chapter 6). In the absence of metastases on CT lung scan or metastases at other sites (bone being the next commonest metastatic location), wide resection of the primary lesion is indicated; this usually involves amputation. In some small tumours with little extraosseous spread, limb conservation may be possible, due to the recent introduction of orthopaedic implants. On close microscopic study, the medullary extension of osteogenic sarcoma appears greater than on macroscopic inspection and has been described up to 5–8 cm beyond the macroscopic tumour edge. The level of amputation varies with individual cases but should always be at least 5 cm beyond visible tumour. More distant 'skip' lesions in the bone bearing the primary are thought to be uncommon but a transmedullary operation does carry this risk. Joint spaces are rarely infiltrated due to the resistance of epiphyseal cartilage to invasion.

Analyses of patients treated by radical surgery demonstrate only a 20–40% survival. This large variation has made it difficult to compare more modern series receiving adjuvant chemotherapy with historical series (Lange and Levine, 1982). Further, the wide availability of CT scanning of the chest brings a 'lead time bias' into the diagnosis of pulmonary metastases as this investigation was not available in the historical, surgical series. It remains to be generally accepted that adjuvant chemotherapy is useful although the recent Paediatric Oncology Group Study is persuasive, and adjuvant whole lung radiotherapy is no longer employed. In metastatic disease, there is no doubt that certain drugs are capable of reproducibly effecting partial responses, (Rosen and Nirenberg, 1982). The drugs include methotrexate (in gram dosage, with folinate rescue), hydroxydaunorubicin, cisplatin, actinomycin D and bleomycin. Single pulmonary metastases may be resected, but such surgery is not worthwhile when the CT chest scan demonstrates multiple metastases.

Ewing's sarcoma

Ewing's sarcoma is less common than osteogenic sarcoma and has an annual incidence of 1×10^{-6}. Young people comprise the majority of patients and 80% of presenting cases are less than 20 years old; there is a slight male predominance. The commonest sites of occurrence in diminishing order are: femur, pelvis, tibia, fibula, humerus, rib, scapula. Less frequently, vertebrae, feet and craniofacial bones are affected. Although long-bone Ewing's sarcoma is commonly described as occurring in the mid-shaft, this is not a good generalization and many cases have been encountered situated at the ends of long bones.

Ewing's sarcoma is a malignancy of bone characterized by uniform, densely packed small round cells with large, prominent and rounded nuclei; the exact cell of origin is in doubt. There is very little evidence of stroma within the tumour and PAS staining will usually demonstrate intracellular glycogen.

Worsening pain and swelling usually bring the patient to attention and sometimes accompanying fever and leucocytosis suggest an inflammatory process. The radiology of the affected bone demonstrates a patchy, mottled or 'moth-eaten' appearance of medullary bone destruction; overlying this, the periosteal reaction appears multilamellar on X-ray — the 'onion-peel' reaction (*Figure 10.5*). A large extra-osseous, soft tissue component may be present. As with osteogenic sarcoma, the radiographic appearances can only ever be suggestive, and diagnosis is obtained by biopsy, the site of biopsy carefully considered with regard to subsequent bone strength; pathological fracture occurs in approximately 5% of cases of Ewing's sarcoma (less commonly than in osteogenic sarcoma).

Ewing's sarcoma tends to spread throughout the medullary cavity of the affected bone and thus the entire bone is at risk, although the tumour rarely penetrates epiphyseal plates. Metastatic spread to the lungs is common as is spread to other bones and perhaps one-quarter of all cases have evidence of metastases at presentation.

The treatment strategy depends upon the primary site but certain general principles may be stated: Ewing's sarcoma is more radiosensitive than osteogenic sarcoma and radical radiotherapy stands at 75–80% chance of permanent local control when backed up by modern adjuvant chemotherapy; large tumour masses of presenting diameter 9 cm or over are less likely to be sterilized. Unless the soft tissue component is very large, early surgical resection of the entire tumour bearing bone leads to a higher rate of local control (e.g. rib, fibula, clavicle), and where the soft tissue mass is large at presentation the lesion

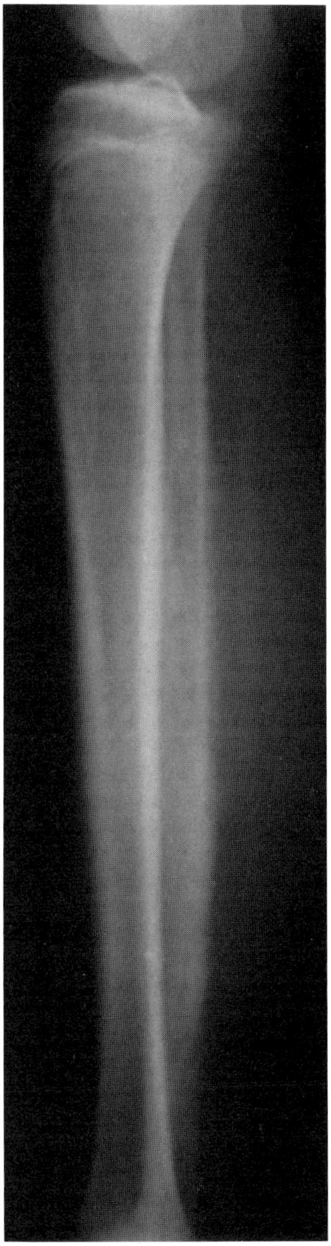

Figure 10.5 X-ray showing onion peel reaction in Ewing's sarcoma

may become operable after several cycles of chemotherapy. Indeed, planned preoperative chemotherapy has many merits. Radiotherapy will need to follow surgical resection where the tumour extended beyond the resection margins. Where resection of the primary bone would lead to functional impairment (e.g. femur and vertebra), radiation is used rather than surgery. An artificial endoprosthesis may be used in other sites following resection of bone bearing the primary tumour. Children with proximal tibial or distal femoral lesions, (particularly if large), who will later have greatly discrepant leg lengths even if radiotherapy is successful, may be best managed by primary amputation. Patients with Ewing's tumour of a foot bone may also be managed better by amputation, as high dose equivalent radiotherapy is not always well tolerated in this region — thus the optimal management of the primary tumour needs to be individually assessed.

Combination chemotherapy with vincristine, hydroxydaunorubicin, cyclophosphamide and/or other drugs (e.g. actinomycin D, methotrexate, bleomycin, BCNU) has proved effective when used in the adjuvant situation. The combination of chemotherapy and radiotherapy has led to early complications in some situations (e.g. bladder and bowel complications following radiotherapy for pelvic Ewing's sarcoma) and late complications (notably an increased incidence of second tumours in the high dose radiation region, particularly osteogenic sarcoma. Nevertheless, it seems clear that the best long-term survival results have come from centres employing thoughtful surgery and/or radiotherapy to the primary tumour together with adjuvant chemotherapy (Rosen *et al.*, 1981), although in most centres the survival results are still below 50%. In patients presenting with overt metastatic disease, the prognosis is worse and few survive.

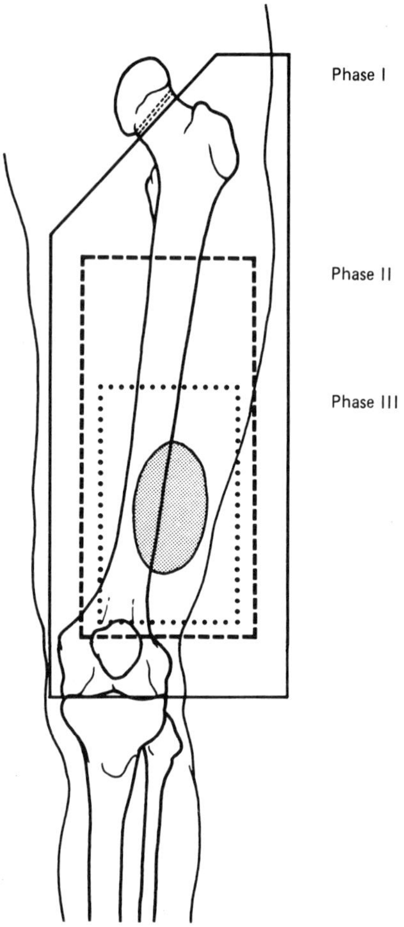

Figure 10.6 Megavoltage photon portal for radiotherapy to a femoral Ewing's sarcoma. Note the three phases of treatment employed — shrinking field technique. Also note the unirradiated skin corridor

Radiotherapy technique

Radiotherapy will frequently be sandwiched into the chemotherapy programme so that the chemosensitivity of the tumour to the regimen is tested on an assessable primary, that some treatment is given early to micrometastatic disease and that radiotherapy is working on a smaller tumour volume. The phase I target volume includes the whole medullary cavity between the two epiphyseal plates of long bones and usually the whole of a flat bone; the treatment portals will be marginally larger. A tumour dose of the order of 4000–4500 cGy in 20–25 fractions over 28–35 days is prescribed, the treatment plan depending upon the site. For long bone primaries, opposed portals are usually employed and a corridor of skin is left unirradiated along one margin — away from the tumour bulk — in order to leave some limb lymphatics unirradiated (*Figure 10.6*). For pelvic primaries it may be possible operatively to displace bowel out of the portal during radiotherapy, for example by the use of absorbable polyglactin mesh (Plowman, Shand and Jackson, 1984). For rib primaries (and others), consideration must be given to the dose received by underlying structures (e.g. lungs). Hydroxydaunorubicin and actinomycin D (both potent radiosensitizers) are not given during radiotherapy, but intermittent bolus cyclophosphamide and vincristine may be continued during radiotherapy unless the bladder is in the field, when the cyclophosphamide is also omitted.

Immediately following the completion of the first phase of radiotherapy, the phase II target volume is carefully planned by simulation and treated, such that only the primary tumour bulk and immediately adjacent tissues receive the phase II prescription of the order of 1500 cGy in eight fractions. The present author sometimes employs three phases of field reduction and has found these 'field shrinking techniques' a useful means of safely achieving a high final tumour dose of 5000–6000 cGy to bulk disease (Suit, 1975). There is general agreement that, where it is safe to do so, prescriptions of over 5000 cGy, conventionally fractionated, are more likely to achieve local control than lower dose equivalents. It is also generally agreed that such radiation must be delivered by accurate and meticulous, megavoltage radiation technique.

Germ cell tumours

Germ cell tumours comprise only a small proportion of paediatric tumours. In the Manchester analysis, the ovary was the commonest primary site followed by the sacrococcygeal region with the testis and intracranial region following in order of frequency (Marsden, Birch and Swindell, 1981). The mediatinum and retroperitoneum were other well recognized sites. Histologically, 60% of tumours were benign teratomas, 24% yolk sac tumours, 11% germiomas and 4% malignant teratomas. Germinoma was encountered in the ovary and intracranial region, but seemed rare in the sacrococcygeal region. Yolk sac features were prominent in the testis and all other sites. Benign teratomas were seen most commonly in the ovary and sacrococcygeal regions, although they also comprised one-half of all the testicular tumours. Histology was often mixed between the histological types and choriocarcinoma was occasionally encountered. Again, in the Manchester experience, the majority of benign sacrococcygeal tumours were diagnosed at birth, usually as a bulging mass in the anococcygeal region, while the majority of yolk sac sacrococcygeal tumours were diagnosed after the first year of life. Testicular germ cell tumours also tended to occur in early life whereas ovarian and intracranial tumours tended to occur around the age of 10 years (Marsden, Birch and Swindell, 1981).

Malignant germ cell tumours secrete α-fetoprotein in at least two-thirds of all cases, and less commonly β-human chorionic gonadotrophin. α-Fetoprotein is a most useful tumour marker as its serum level correlates closely with tumour burden.

The optimal management depends on location and extent of disease as well as histology — germinoma, yolk sac tumour and malignant teratoma are all regarded as having local infiltrative and metastatic potential. The benign sacrococcygeal tumour presenting at birth is optimally managed by an *en bloc* resection of tumour and coccyx either through a posterior approach or, if ultrasound scanning suggests a large pelvic component, an abdominosacral approach; no other treatment is necessary if the histology is favourable. Intracranial (e.g. pineal, third ventricular) germ cell tumours are optimally managed and curable by radiotherapy (*see* Chapter 15) and the radiosensitivity of these tumours at all sites is relevant. With the increasing power of combination chemotherapy against malignant germ cell tumours, radiotherapy is being employed less commonly for extracranial growths. The three-drug regimens cisplatin, vinblastine, bleomycin, or cisplatin, VP16, bleomycin, given as intermittent bolus chemotherapy in doses causing a moderately severe myelosuppression at days 8–14, have largely replaced VAC (vincristine, actinomycin D, cyclophosphamide). When chemotherapy is used in overt disease, there is usually rapid tumour regression with a logarithmic fall in the α-fetoprotein levels. The present author currently recommends three cycles of chemotherapy beyond the achievement of complete remission (often implied from normalization of α-fetoprotein levels). Three adjuvant chemotherapy cycles are also recommended to patients with apparently localized but incompletely resected germ cell tumours which are reported as malignant by the pathologist. Completely resected, localized tumours are treated by surgery and a careful follow-up.

The period of relapse risk is greatest in the early months and all patients should be followed monthly with measurement of α-fetoprotein levels and frequent imaging tests for at least 1 year, before outpatient attendances are spaced. The serial monitoring of α-fetoprotein levels is vital to the modern management of these tumours.

Histiocytosis X

Histiocytosis X comprises a spectrum of granulomatous or infiltrative processes affecting children; there is usually reticuloendothelial system hyperplasia with mononuclear cell infiltration of skin or viscera, often with highly typical lipid-rich histiocytes and an admixture of other immunological cells including eosinophils and lymphocytes. In young children the disease may run an aggressive and perhaps fatal course with skin, lymph node and visceral (liver, spleen, lung and bone lesions in particular) involvement. In other children, the disease presents with lesions in some or all of these sites but runs a waxing and waning course and arrests with age or the passage of time. Sometimes, (radiologically lytic) bone lesions are the dominant site of the disease and the membrane bones of the skull are a common site of involvement, as are the orbit, mastoid and pituitary regions. Soft tissue lesions in these sites may cause important deficits (e.g. exophthalmos, deafness, diabetes insipidus). Sometimes, solitary lesions occur (e.g. eosinophilic granuloma of bone).

In the past, histiocytosis X was regarded as a malignant neoplasm although the remitting tendency seen in many patients has always made this label unsatisfactory. It is currently believed that histiocytosis X is a disease spectrum caused by disordered immunoregulation (Osband *et al.*, 1981). High dose systemic prednisolone or intralesional steroid for bone lesions is often effective therapy. Radiotherapy is also effective but is currently reserved for a minority of dangerously progressing local lesions and is effective in low dose equivalents, e.g. 1000–1500 cGy given by low fraction size (160–175 cGy per fraction) in daily fractions. The chronic administration of potent systemic steroids to children with often spontaneously remitting disease is to be deplored, and the present author has strict indications for systemic steroid therapy: (1) critical visceral involvement; (2) deteriorating general health; and (3) serious skin rash. Cytotoxic chemotherapy may be efficacious but is reserved for these same patient groups if steroid therapy fails.

Table 10.8 Reese staging of retinoblastoma — St Bartholomew's Hospital modification

Stage I	Single or multiple tumours less than 4 disc diameters at or behind the equator. (One disc diameter = 1.5 mm)
Stage IIA	Solitary lesion 4–10 disc diameters at or behind the equator
Stage IIB	Solitary lesion larger than 10 disc diameters at or behind the equator
Stage III	Lesions anterior to the equator
Stage IVA	Multiple tumours, some larger than 10 disc diameters
Stage IVB	Any lesion extending anteriorly beyond the limit of ophthalmoscopy
Stage VA	Massive neoplasms
Stage VB	Vitreous seedlings
Stage VI	Residual orbital disease or optic nerve infiltration

Retinoblastoma

Retinoblastoma is a rare ocular tumour with an overall incidence of one child in 20 000 live births. It occurs sporadically, (approximately two-thirds of all UK cases), or as a familial (autosomal dominant) condition, and has been described in association with mental retardation and a particular karyotypic change (13-D deletion). At presentation, the majority of patients are less than 2 years of age although some sporadic cases present later; the disease is uncommon beyond 4 years of age. Multiple retinal tumours and bilateral tumours are pathognomonic of the familial variety but the hereditary possibility must be suspected in every case, and siblings submitted to regular ophthalmoscopic examinations in early life. Where the basis seems familial, genetic counselling may well be required in later life.

The classical presenting features of retinoblastoma patients are 'the white reflex' (peripheral tumours), a squint (macular tumours), poor vision or glaucoma. Expert binocular indirect ophthalmoscopy with 360° scleral indentation usually allows a firm clinical diagnosis to be made and the disease staged: Reese staging classification — St. Bartholomew's modification (*Table 10.8*). Additional staging procedures include skull X-rays with views of optic foramina and, in more advanced stage disease, technetium diphosphonate bone scanning, bone marrow and CSF examinations for metastases.

Early stage tumours (up to 3 mm or two disc diameters) are best treated by light coagulation (posterior lesions), or cryotherapy (anterior lesions), although external beam radiotherapy may be necessary to treat perimacular tumours. Tumours 3–10 mm diameter are best treated by a cobalt plaque, unless perimacular. Those tumours more than 10 mm diameter or multiple tumours not amenable to other focal therapies, are indications for external beam radiotherapy. Enucleation of the eye is performed only if there is a high risk of local extraocular spread, optic nerve involvement or secondary complications. Enucleation must include excision of the full orbital length of the optic nerve and histological evidence of nerve infiltration or extrascleral extension of tumour are both indications for postoperative radiotherapy to the orbit. Each eye is treated on its own merits.

Each radioactive cobalt plaque or disc is a segment of a sphere of inner radius 11 mm, (which corresponds to the ocular radius of the young child), and of active diameter 5-15 mm. Each disc has a vacuum sealed, platinum casing with projecting lugs for scleral sutures. Within the casing, the radioactive cobalt is arranged in a single annulus or, in the larger sizes, as a central source with one or two concentric annuli (*Figure 10.7a*). The application takes approximately 7 days to deliver the required dose of 4000 cGy to the apex of the tumour. The base of the tumour receives a much higher radiation dose and an endarteritis will occur later; the incidence of cataracts with this technique is less than 5%. The recent interest in ruthenium plaques (whose daughter disintegration products occur with predominantly beta emissions) and iodine plaques has been based on safer handling of these isotopes. The St Bartholomew's Hospital Unit continues to use cobalt plaques at present.

The technique of external beam radiotherapy varies with the individual's disease. The whole retina is at risk either from vitreous seedlings or new primary tumours. Thus one often needs to treat the whole eye — usually with an anterior cobalt field (with the eye open) (*Figure 10.7b*), and a tumour dose of 4000 cGy in 20 fractions in 28 days is delivered. The depth of the dose prescription is obtained from standard tables of ocular size with age. In a child who requires external beam therapy for a single, small perimacular tumour and who is growing out of his age of risk for further tumours, the morbidity associated

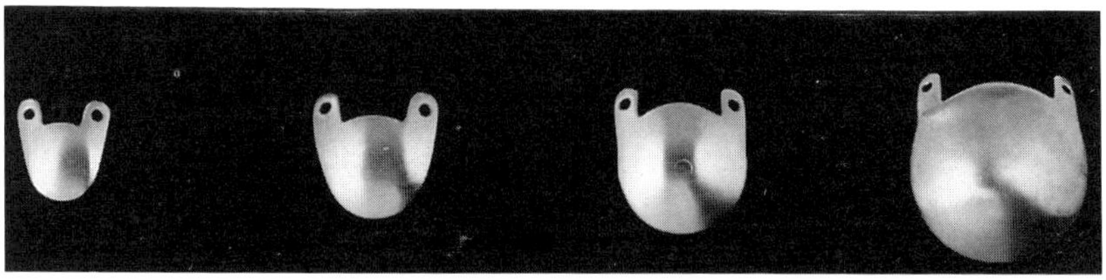

Figure 10.7 (a) Radioactive cobalt discs for retinoblastoma

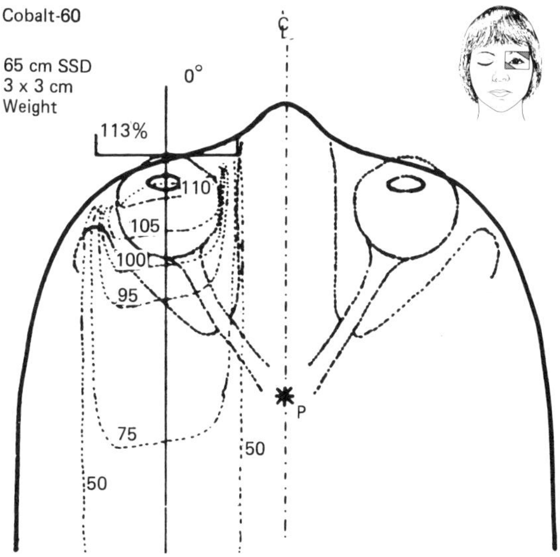

Figure 10.7 (b) Anterior megavoltage photon portal for whole eye irradiation in retinoblastoma. The eyelid is taped open during therapy to spare the anterior ocular tissues. Lacrimal gland and nasolacrimal duct shielding may be possible (inset)

with the anterior field approach (late cataract formation in particular) outweighs the reduced risk of anterior retinal disease. A highly accurate pin and arc set up (from a contact lens) is used to direct a sharply collimated megavoltage X-ray beam from the temporal aspect of the eye (*Figure 10.7c*). This spares the lens and anterior chamber but also screens a little retina anteriorly. Where both eyes require external beam therapy, parallel opposed lateral portals are employed, with attention to lens sparing if possible. Where there is macroscopic disease in the orbit a dose of 4500 cGy, conventionally fractionated, is prescribed.

Cytotoxic chemicals are not highly effective in retinoblastoma and current chemotherapy studies largely comprise the assessment of responsiveness of metastatic disease to single agents and neuroblastoma combination chemotherapy regimens.

Late effects of paediatric cancer therapy

Both radiotherapy and cytotoxic chemotherapy are potential mutagens and carry with their use the risk of late carcinogenesis and mutations in the gametes. These effects are stochastic and difficult to quantify (BEIR, 1980; Plowman, 1982). In the late follow-up of survivors of Ewing's sarcoma who had received

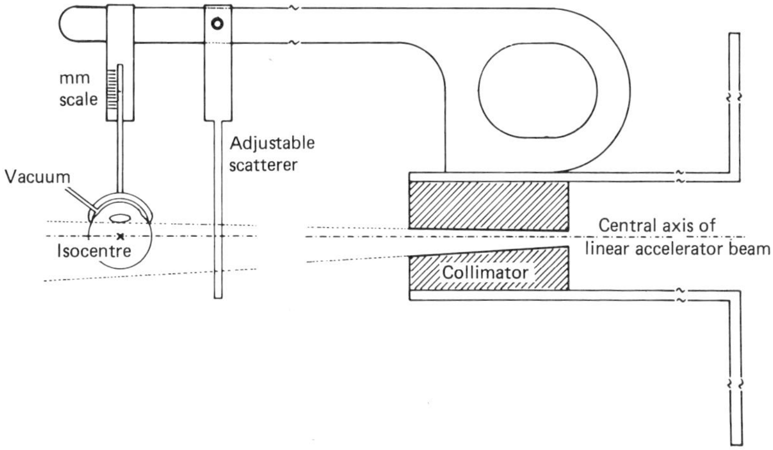

Figure 10.7 (c) Megavoltage photon irradiation of almost the whole retina with lens and anterior chamber sparing. Schipper's method with St Bartholomew's Hospital modifications. (Not to scale)

chemo-radiotherapy, there is now incontrovertible evidence of a small number of second tumours arising within the radiation portals, (notably osteogenic sarcoma and fibrous histiocytoma), although the anecdotal literature reports make it difficult to quantify this risk. In the late follow-up of survivors of combination chemotherapeutic treatment of Hodgkin's disease, there is similarly strong evidence for an increased incidence of second malignancy but, in this situation, acute non-lymphocytic leukaemia is the major hazard with an incidence of perhaps 4%. The alkylating agents and perhaps procarbazine are regarded as the main carcinogens in this drug therapy. These findings in a minority of survivors should be carefully documented in the follow-up of the entire paediatric patient population, and in the future this information may be used to find effective treatment protocols with lesser carcinogenic potential. At the present time, it is rarely possible to reduce the intensity of primary therapy except in a few cases (e.g. stage I Hodgkin's disease — *see above*), and it should be emphasized that here a second malignancy is rare.

Both ionizing radiation and cytotoxic chemotherapy may cause gonadal atrophy or failure, and the alkylating agents are the most commonly incriminated group of drugs. Although it was hoped that the 'resting', pre-pubertal gonads would be more resistant to cancer therapy, in general this has not proved the case and the majority of children surviving aggressive therapy for Ewing's sarcoma and rhabdomyosarcoma will be sterile (Plowman, 1984). Adolescent girls will require hormonal replacement but the Leydig cells of the testis are more resilient than the seminiferous epithelium and boys usually progress normally through puberty. Many survivors of acute leukaemia chemotherapy regimens maintain their fertility and have borne normal children. However, these facts do not refute the stochastic mutagenic potential of many cytotoxic drugs.

The dose of testicular radiation delivered for testicular leukaemic relapse is not only sterilizing but usually also impairs Leydig cell function.

Growth stunting in the musculoskeletal system will occur in the irradiated tissues to a degree inversely related to the child's age at the time of radiotherapy and directly related to the radiation dose. Where craniospinal radiotherapy has been delivered, marked stunting of the growth of the axial skeleton is usual. When a limb bone has been irradiated, there may be late and important growth stunting (e.g. marked leg length discrepancy following conservative therapy of a femoral Ewing's sarcoma). These growth stunting sequelae of radiation are irreversible.

Following radiotherapy to the child's central nervous system, both neuropsychological and neuroendocrine sequelae have been described. After the low dose equivalent cranial radiation prophylaxis with intrathecal methotrexate, such as given in acute lymphoblastic leukaemia therapy, there is a tendency for the children to have slightly lower intelligence quotients than their peers, but these nevertheless fall within the normal range (Chessells, 1983). These studies were performed prior to the radiation dose reduction to 1800 cGy. The data clearly demonstrate that the brains of younger children (less than 2.5 years) are more susceptible to these sequelae. One would expect similar findings in a brain tumour population but these patients are more heterogeneous with regard to dose and volume irradiated. Where the hypothalamopituitary axis has been irradiated to a high dose equivalent, anterior pituitary hormone deficiencies may manifest. Growth hormone deficiency is usually the first to occur followed by gonadotrophin deficiency. Recent data from St Bartholomew's Hospital suggest that the lesion is at the hypothalamic level (Blacklay *et al.*, 1985). ACTH and TSH deficiencies have also been recorded. Circulating prolactin levels may rise. The present author has recently reviewed this subject (Plowman, 1984).

References

BECKWITH, J. B. and PALMER, N. F. (1978) Histopathology and prognosis of Wilms' tumour. *Cancer*, **41**, 1937–1948

BEIR (1980) The effects on populations of exposure to low levels of ionising radiation. *Report of the Committee on the Biological Effects of Ionising Radiations*. Washington: National Academy Press

BLACKLAY, A., GROSSMAN, A., SAVAGE, M. O., PLOWMAN, P. N., COY, D. H. and BESSER, G. M. (1986) Cranial irradiation in children with cerebral tumours — evidence for a hypothalamic defect in growth hormone release. *Journal of Endocrinology*, (in press)

BRESLOW, N. E., PALMER, N. F., HILL, L. R., BURING, J. and D'ANGIO, G. J. (1978) Wilms' tumour: prognostic factors for patients without metastases at diagnosis. *Cancer*, **41**, 1577–1589

CHESSELLS, J. M. (1983) Childhood acute lymphoblastic anaemia: the late effects of treatment. *British Journal of Haematology*, **53**, 369–378

DONALDSON, S. (1980) Paediatric Hodgkin's disease: focus on the future. In *Status and Curability of Childhood Cancers*, edited by J. van Eys and M. P. Sullivan, pp. 235–249. New York: Raven Press

ELLIS, F. (1969) Dose, time and fractionation; a clinical hypothesis. *Clinical Radiology*, **20**, 1–7

EVANS, A. E., CHATTEN, J., D'ANGIO, G. J., GERSON, J. M., ROBINSON, J. and SCHNAUFER, L. (1980) A review of 17 IV-S neuroblastoma patients at the Children's Hospital of Philadelphia. *Cancer*, **45**, 833–839

EVANS, A. E., D'ANGIO, G. J. and RANDOLPH, J. (1971) A proposed staging for children with neuroblastoma. *Cancer*, **27**, 374–378

GREEN, D. M. and JAFFE, N. (1978) Progress and controversy in the treatment of childhood rhabdomyosarcoma. *Cancer Treatment Reviews*, **5**, 7–27

HUSTU, H. O., AUR, R. J. A., VERZOSA, M. S. *et al.* (1973)

Prevention of central nervous system leukaemia by irradiation. *Cancer*, **32**, 585–597

KINGSTON, J. E., McELWAIN, T. J. and MALPAS, J. S. (1983) Childhood rhabdomyosarcoma: experience of the Children's Solid Tumour Group. *British Journal of Cancer*, **34**, 195–207

LANGE, B. and LEVINE, A. S. (1982) Is it ethical not to conduct a prospectively controlled trial of adjuvant chemotherapy in osteosarcoma. *Cancer Treatment Reports*, **66**, 1699–1704

LANGFORD, R. M., O'CONNOR, S. A. and SMITH, R. E. (1984) An instrument to indicate acute airway obstruction in remote anaesthesia. *Proceedings of the Annual Scientific Meeting, Association of Anaesthetists*, UK

MARSDEN, H. B., BIRCH, J.M. and SWINDELL, R. (1981) Germ cell tumours of childhood: a review of 137 cases. *Journal of Clinical Pathology*, **34**, 879–883

NESBIT, M. E., ROBISON, L. L., LITTMAN, P. S. *et al.* (1981) Presymptomatic central nervous system therapy in previously untreated childhood acute lymphoblastic leukaemia: comparison of 1800 rad and 2400 rad. *Lancet*, **1**, 461-466

NINANE, J., PRITCHARD, J., MORRIS-JONES, P. H., MANN, J. R. and MALPAS, J. S. (1982) Stage II neuroblastoma. Adverse prognostic significance of lymph node involvement. *Archives of Disease in Childhood*, **57**, 438–442

OSBAND, M. E., LIPTON, J. M., LAVING, P. *et al.* (1981) Histiocytosis X. Demonstration of abnormal immunity, T-cell histamine H2-receptor deficiency, and successful treatment with thymic extract. *New England Journal of Medicine*, **304**, 146–153

PINKERTON, C. R. and CHESSELLS, J. M. (1984) Failed central nervous system prophylaxis in children with acute lymphoblastic leukaemia: treatment and outcome. *British Journal of Haemalotogy*, **57**, 553–561

PLOWMAN, P. N. (1982) Radiation carcinogenesis — What risk? *Human Toxicology*, **1**, 93–95

PLOWMAN, P.N. (1984) Late effects of cancer therapy. In *Endocrine Problems in Cancer*, edited by R. Jung and K. Sikora, pp. 225–272. London: William Heinemann

PLOWMAN, P. N., SHAND, W. S. and JACKSON, D. B. (1984) Use of absorbable mesh to displace bowel and avoid radiation enteropathy during therapy of pelvic Ewing's sarcoma. *Human Toxicology*, **3**, 229–237

ROSEN, G., CAPARROS, B., NIRENBERG, A. *et al.* (1981) Ewing's sarcoma: ten year experience with adjuvant chemotherapy. *Cancer*, **47**, 2204–2213

ROSEN, G. and NIRENBERG, A. (1982) Chemotherapy for osteogenic sarcoma: an investigative method, not a recipe. *Cancer Treatment Reports*, **66**, 1687–1697

SHELINE, G. (1980) Irradiation injury of the human brain: a review of clinical experience. In *Radiation Damage to the Nervous System*, edited by H. A. Gilbert and A. R. Kagan, pp. 39–58. New York: Raven Press

SUIT, H. (1975) Role of therapeutic radiology in cancer of bone. *Cancer*, **35**, 930–935

SULLIVAN, M. P., FULLER, L. M., CHEN, T. *et al.* (1982) Intergroup Hodgkin's disease in children study of stages I and II. A preliminary report. *Cancer Treatment Reports*, **66**, 937–947

SUTOW, W. W., LINDBERG, R. D., GEHAN, E. A. *et al.* (1982) Three year relapse free survival rates in childhood rhabdomyosarcoma of the head and neck. *Cancer*, **49**, 2217–2221

TAN, C., JEREB, B., CHAN, K. W. *et al.* (1983) Hodgkin's disease in children. *Cancer*, **51**, 1720–1725

THAMES, H. D., WITHERS, H. R., PETERS, L. J. and FLETCHER, G. H. (1982) Changes in early and late radiation responses with altered dose fractionation: implications for dose-survival relationships. *International Journal of Radiation Oncology, Biology and Physics*, **8**, 219–226

11

Haematological malignancy in the adult

G. Mair

Ideally all patients with these conditions should be assessed, treated and followed-up jointly by the haematologist or oncologist and radiotherapist. Where this is impracticable, it is reasonable for the radiotherapist to undertake the management of patients with myelomatosis or chronic lymphocytic leukaemia, but patients with acute leukaemia require the special skills of the haematologist. The emphasis in this chapter has been placed on those aspects of treatment of particular relevance to the radiotherapist.

Acute non-lymphocytic leukaemia

Natural history

This is a fulminant malignancy characterized by infiltration of the bone marrow and other organs by immature 'blast cells' causing progressive marrow failure. Untreated it causes death from haemorrhage or infection within a few months. Central nervous system involvement is found in 6–21% of postmortems but presents clinically in only 10% (Gale, 1979).

Histology

The morphological features of the 'blast cells' are extremely variable. A French, American and British cooperative group (FAB) proposed the following classification (Bennett *et al.*, 1976).

M1 Primitive myeloblasts showing no maturation
M2 Maturation to the promyelocytic stage
M3 Hypergranular promyelocytes with abundant Auer rods
M4 Myelomonocytic leukaemia
M5 Monocytic leukaemia
M6 Erythroleukaemia

Treatment aim

The main aim of treatment is to induce and maintain complete remission resulting in cure. Complete remission is based on the following criteria:

(1) Disappearance of abnormal physical findings
(2) Return to normal of the peripheral blood count
(3) Disappearance of recognizable leukaemic cells from the bone marrow
(4) Less than 5% normal blast cells in a marrow preparation of normal cellularity.

Treatment options

(1) Conventional chemotherapy with or without CNS prophylaxis
(2) Bone marrow transplantation.

Conventional chemotherapy

Complete remission can be achieved in 60-80% of patients using combination chemotherapy. As the most successful single agents are hydroxydaunorubicin and cytosine arabinoside, a combination of these two plus 6-thioguanine is a commonly used induction regimen (Powles *et al.*, 1980).

These same agents are administered for a further two or three courses after complete remission has been achieved as consolidation therapy.

Maintenance therapy remains of unproven value in preventing relapse and prolonging survival but it is used in most centres. A randomized trial in the USA showed no benefit from maintenance therapy with median survival actually better in the unmaintained patients, 76 weeks compared with 56 weeks (Foon and Gale, 1982).

The use of more aggressive chemotherapy (intensification), either following remission induction or during maintenance therapy, may yet prove to prolong survival, although at least 50% of patients still relapse (Bodey, Freirich and McCredie, 1981).

Central nervous system prophylaxis with intrathecal chemotherapy plus or minus cranial irradiation has not been shown to prevent systemic relapse or to prolong survival.

The long-term survival rate with conventional chemotherapy is 15–25%, with most patients dying from leukaemic relapse (Keating *et al.*, 1980). Relapse after 4 years is most uncommon so these patients are probably cured.

Bone marrow transplantation

This procedure was developed in Seattle. The first transplants were performed on patients in haematological relapse with disease refractory to chemotherapy and therefore acutely ill. Despite this, 11% of 54 patients remain in continuous remission 4–7 years after engraftment (Thomas, Buckner *et al.*, 1977).

Encouraged by this, the Seattle group and others began to transplant patients in their first remission following induction chemotherapy. Using allogeneic grafts from the histocompatibility locus antigen-(HLA) compatible siblings, 2-year survival rates of 45–60% have been reported (Thomas *et al.*, 1979; Powles *et al.*, 1980; Blume *et al.*, 1981). Deaths tend to be due to infection, interstitial pneumonitis, and graft versus host disease, with leukaemic relapse extremely uncommon.

Transplantation in second remission using allografting is less successful with a two-year survival rate of 25% (Buckner *et al.*, 1982).

Syngeneic grafts from an identical twin do reduce the incidence of pneumonitis and graft versus host disease, but leukaemic relapse is more common and the two-year survival rate is only 30%. This had led to the suggestion that graft versus host disease may have a significant antileukaemic effect (Weiden *et al.*, 1981).

Treatment policy

At present, the results of bone marrow transplantation appear superior to those of combination chemotherapy. It is therefore the treatment of choice for all patients under the age of 45 years who are in first remission and have an HLA compatible sibling or identical twin. Consolidation therapy with intensification but without CNS prophylaxis is the treatment for all other patients. The gap between the results of these two treatments is narrow and can easily be obliterated by treatment related deaths. Champlin *et al.* (1983) compared patients under the age of 45 years in first remission who had a suitable donor and were transplanted with those who did not and received consolidation therapy. Though the actuarial risk of relapse at 3 years was 22% for transplantation and 63% for chemotherapy, the actuarial 3-year survival rates were 43% and 37%, a difference which was not significant.

Acute lymphoblastic leukaemia

Natural history

This is, in general, similar to that of the disease in childhood (*see* Chapter 10). The prognosis is, however, rather worse. A very variable incidence of CNS involvement has been reported with figures from 7–75% (Wolk *et al.*, 1974).

Histology

The FAB group also proposed a classification for acute lymphoblastic leukaemia with three groups designated L1, L2 and L3 on the basis of certain morphological features and their variability (Bennett *et al.*, 1976). This classification is seldom used.

Treatment aim

The main aim of treatment is to induce and maintain complete remission as previously defined resulting in cure.

Treatment options

(1) Conventional chemotherapy
(2) Bone marrow transplantation.

Conventional chemotherapy

This is less successful in adults than in children with the standard regimens. Complete remission is achieved in only 70% of adults as compared with 90% of children (Lister *et al.*, 1978). Despite consolidation therapy, CNS prophylaxis and maintenance therapy, the median duration of remission is only 20 months and median survival 25–27 months (Lister *et al.*, 1978; Omura *et al.*, 1980).

More encouraging recent results have been reported by Blacklock *et al.* (1981), who found a remission rate of 89% and median survival in excess of 36 months. Similarly the Memorial Sloan Kettering Cancer Center reported an 86% remission rate and 50% of these have survived for 5 years or more (Clarkson *et al.*, 1983).

The benefit of CNS prophylaxis is unclear at the present time. In the USA, a randomized trial showed a reduction in the incidence of CNS relapse from 32% to

10% with cranial irradiation and intrathecal methotrexate but this did not improve survival (Omura *et al.*, 1980). This may be because patients are not surviving long enough to be at risk from CNS relapse. If one looks at long-term survivors only, they do seem at risk. Law and Blom (1977) reported that 50% of their long-term survivors who did not receive CNS prophylaxis developed CNS disease. Once CNS relapse occurred it was difficult to control, and over one-half of these patients had recurrent CNS disease despite appropriate treatment with intrathecal chemotherapy and cranial irradiation.

Bone marrow transplantation

Increasing numbers of patients with disease refractory to chemotherapy are being transplanted in relapse, or in a second or subsequent remission. Using their standard conditioning regimen of cyclophosphamide plus total body irradiation with a single dose of 1000 cGy, the Seattle group reported a 15% survival rate for patients in relapse and 30% for those in second remission (Clift *et al.*, 1982 a, b; Badger *et al.*, 1982). The major cause of death is leukaemic relapse which occurs in 65% of patients, with the central nervous system a common site of relapse.

Two different approaches have been tried to improve the results:

(1) Intensification of the chemotherapy component of the conditioning regimen prior to transplantation. The combination of 6-thioguanine, cyclophosphamide, cytosine arabinoside and hydroxydaunorubicin, instead of cyclophosphamide on its own, reduced the relapse rate to 26% but only 13% of patients survived because of lethal toxicity (Gale *et al.*, 1976).
(2) Higher dose fractionated total body irradiation prior to transplantation. The Seattle group have increased their dose to 1575 cGy administered in seven daily fractions of 225 cGy without an increase in morbidity and with a modest improvement in survival rate (Clift *et al.*, 1982b).

Treatment policy

At present, patients with no additional poor prognostic features other than their age should be treated with conventional chemotherapy. Patients who then relapse should be treated by bone marrow transplantation as, with conventional chemotherapy, they have only a 3% chance of survival.

Patients with additional poor prognostic features such as high blast counts in excess of $100 \times 10^9/\ell$, B-cell markers or T-cell markers should be considered for bone marrow transplantation in first remission as their survival with chemotherapy is poor.

CNS prophylaxis should be given to all patients treated with conventional chemotherapy and this should include intrathecal chemotherapy plus cranial irradiation (*see* Chapter 15 for details).

Technique for bone marrow transplantation

Most transplants are carried out between major histocompatibility complex identical sibling pairs, which means that about 30% of patients will have a suitable donor. Prior to transplantation, patients are treated with high dose chemotherapy and total body irradiation with the twin aims of destroying residual leukaemic cells and producing profound immuno-suppression to permit engraftment.

The standard technique is to administer cyclophosphamide (60 mg/kg) on 2 consecutive days with mesna to prevent urothelial damage. Two to three days later, the patient is given total body irradiation and the following day the donor marrow is infused intravenously.

In most patients, engraftment occurs rapidly and a white cell count of $1 \times 10^9/\ell$ is achieved within 3 weeks. During this 3-week period the patient is kept in protective isolation to prevent infection and will undoubtedly require whole blood and platelets in large quantities. These blood products are normally irradiated prior to administration in order to destroy the donor lymphocytes as they may aggravate graft versus host disease. The products are placed in a perspex box. The remaining space is packed with bolus. A single midplane dose of 1500 cGy is delivered using parallel opposed cobalt-60 fields (*Figure 11.1*).

Total body irradiation

The original technique developed at Seattle used simultaneous radiation from two opposed ^{60}Co

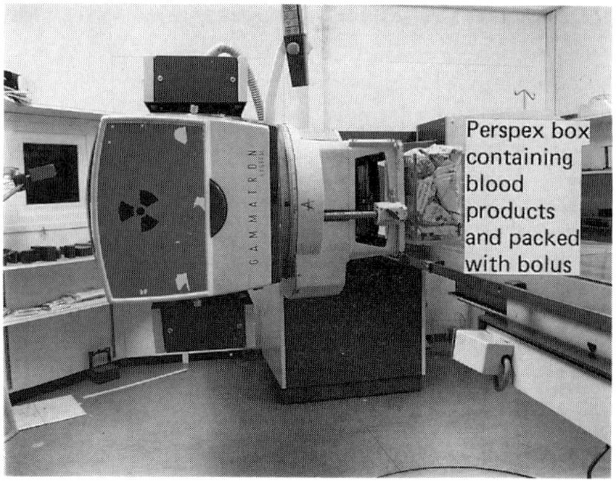

Figure 11.1 Technique for irradiating blood elements

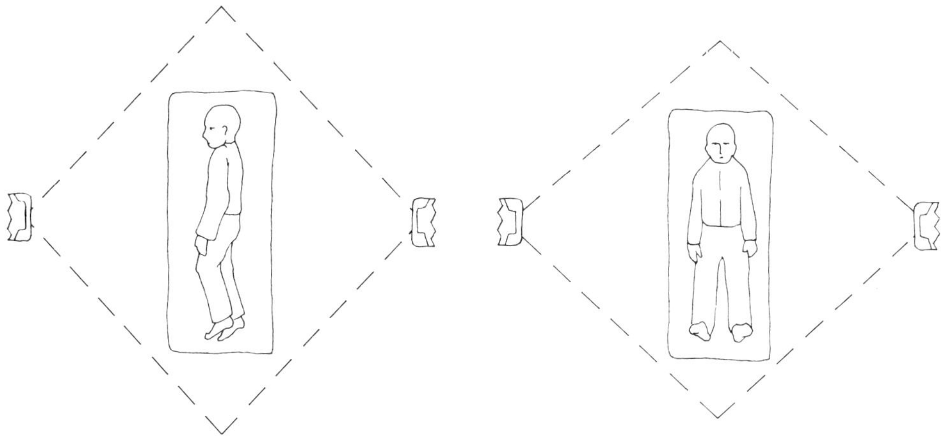

Figure 11.2 Seattle technique for total body irradiation using two opposed cobalt sources

sources to treat anterior and posterior, then two lateral fields (*Figure 11.2*). A total dose of 1000 cGy was administered as a single fraction using a low rate of 5 cGy/minute.

Most centres lack the purpose-built equipment to reproduce this technique and have had to modify it. The University of Minnesota team used two large lateral fields on a 10 MeV linear accelerator. A total dose of 750 cGy was administered as a single fraction with a dose rate of 25 cGy/minute which was considered biologically equivalent to the Seattle dose (Kim *et al.*, 1977).

Fractionated radiotherapy has been used in the hope of reducing toxicity. A single fraction of 1000 cGy was compared with 1200 cGy in six daily fractions. No difference was found in toxicity or antileukaemic effect, but survival was improved slightly with the fractionated treatment (Thomas *et al.*, 1982). Goolden *et al.* (1983) did find reduced immediate toxicity without loss of efficacy by giving a dose of 1200 cGy in six fractions over 3 days.

The London Hospital technique

Prior to treatment, the patient is premedicated with hydrocortisone 200 mg i.v. and domperidone 10 mg i.v. through the Hickman line previously inserted. No attempt is made to sterilize the treatment room, but it does make sense to transfer patients and staff with known infections to other units.

Patients are treated on a 8 MeV linear accelerator at a source-skin (SSD) distance of 4 m. As a wall limits any further increase in SSD, the maximum field size is 135 × 135 cm with a diagonal of 147 cm. This means that adults cannot be treated lying down which would be the most comfortable position. The patient's arms should be by his sides to increase the separation in the thorax thus avoiding the need for a formal compensator to correct the increased transmission through the lungs (*Figure 11.3*). An alternative position for the arms occasionally produces a better dose distribution (*Figure 11.4*).

A lead filter (0.5–2 mm thick) is used to compensate for the reduced separation in the head and neck region. Bolus is packed between and around the legs for the same reason. A perspex screen (1.5 mm thick) immediately in front of the patient provides electron build up ensuring the full dose on the skin surface.

Two large lateral fields are treated consecutively. A total dose of 1200 cGy is administered in six fractions treating twice per day with a gap of 8 hours between fractions and a dose rate of 30 cGy/minute (*Figure 11.3*).

The treatment room is occupied for about 20 minutes for each fraction, with an extra 10 minutes if lithium fluoride dosimetry is performed.

Dosimetry

Rather than attempting to calculate the midplane dose using multiple separations and estimating the effect of varying amounts of lung tissue, a test dose is administered prior to therapy. Lithium fluoride dose meters are attached to both sides of the body at the head, neck, upper and lower chest, waist, hips, knees and ankles. A nominal dose of 100 monitor units is given to each field. From the results obtained, the total monitor setting to give a modal dose of 1200 cGy can be calculated. The test run administers a dose of about 10 cGy to the patient (*Table 11.1*).

The aim is to achieve uniformity of dosage within the range plus or minus 10%, and the results will show whether the thickness of lead or the amount of bolus needs to be altered. The measurements are repeated on the first treatment to ensure a satisfactory distribution of dose.

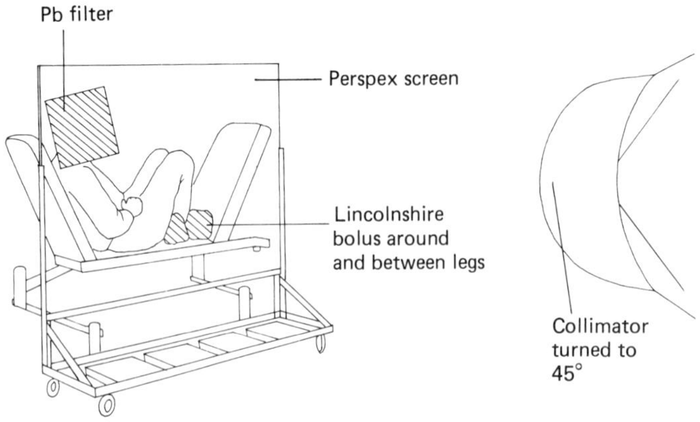

Figure 11.3 London Hospital technique for total body irradiation

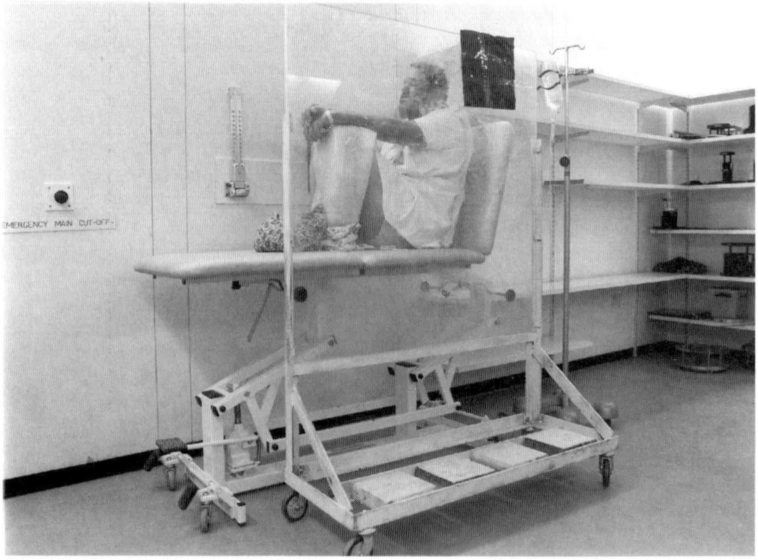

Figure 11.4 Alternative arm position for total body irradiation

Table 11.1 Doses from trial run total body irradiation

Site	*Dose* (cGy) *Left*	*Right*	*Mean dose* (cGy)
Head	9.34	9.91	9.63
Neck	9.44	9.74	9.59
Upper chest	10.89	10.79	10.84
Lower chest	10.35	10.41	10.38
Waist	10.36	10.40	10.38
Hips	9.82	9.98	9.90
Mid-thigh	10.27	10.51	10.39
Knee	10.54	10.33	10.43
Ankles	9.91	9.42	9.67

Overall mean dose = 10.13 cGy (± 4.4%)

Toxicity

It is not possible to separate the side-effects due to total body irradiation from those due to other aspects of the procedure.

Acute side-effects

(1) Nausea and vomiting occur in most patients despite premedication with corticosteroid and antiemetic. If a single fraction is used, vomiting will often occur during therapy causing repeated interruptions.

(2) Fever develops in the majority of patients, but settles within 24 hours.

(3) Parotitis may develop and this takes 2–3 days to subside.
(4) Mucositis of pharynx and oesophagus develops in the majority of patients within 5–6 days. About 50% of patients develop diarrhoea.
(5) Veno-occlusive disease of the liver occurs in less than 10% of patients but is fatal in one-third of these (Woods *et al.*, 1980).
(6) Reversible alopecia will occur in patients not already epilated by induction chemotherapy.

Delayed side-effects

(1) Interstitial pneumonitis

This syndrome, indistinguishable from radiation pneumonitis, was reported in 54% of patients in the initial transplant programme at Seattle. Radiation cannot be the only causal factor as the same syndrome develops in patients who have received cyclophosphamide only and no radiation prior to transplantation (Bortin and Rimm, 1977).

Pneumonitis is more common in patients who receive lung doses in excess of 900 cGy in a single fraction (Keane, Van Dyck and Rider, 1981), in patients receiving dose rates in excess of 5.7 cGy/minute (Bortin *et al.*, 1982), in patients transplanted in relapse (Neimann *et al.*, 1980) and in those who develop graft versus host disease (Keane, Van Dyck and Rider, 1981).

Infective agents such as *Pneumocystis carinii* and cytomegalovirus are found on lung biopsy in 65% of patients with interstitial pneumonitis.

The syndrome can be expected in about 20–30% of patients undergoing allogeneic grafting in first remission.

(2) Gonadal function

Sanders (1982) reported that only 8% of patients had normal menstrual function and only 5% had spermatogenesis following bone marrow transplantation.

(3) Cataract formation

Deeg (1983) found cataracts in 40% of patients within 2 years of transplantation.

(4) Second malignancies

The Seattle group have reported three second malignancies in a group of 300 patients followed up for 1–12 years.

(5) Graft versus host disease

This is a three system disorder causing dermatitis, hepatitis and intestinal disturbance. It occurs in 50–70% of patients receiving allografts despite prophylaxis with methotrexate, and is fatal in 25% of these. The use of cyclosporin A does not reduce the incidence, but does reduce the mortality to about 8% (Powles *et al.*, 1979).

Chronic granulocytic leukaemia

Natural history

Despite its name this is a rapidly progressive malignancy with a median survival in untreated cases of only 19 months (Minot, Buckman and Isaacs, 1924). It is characterized by the proliferation of primitive granulocytes in the bone marrow and other organs, the spleen in particular. These cells are mostly myelocytes and, in the majority of cases, these demonstrate a specific cytogenetic abnormality with the translocation of the long arm of chromosome 23 to chromosome 9. Such cases are called Philadelphia chromosome positive (Ph^1+ve). The infiltration of the bone marrow results in progressive bone marrow failure due to suppression of normal haemopoiesis.

About 80% of patients develop an acute terminal phase called blast transformation or metamorphosis in which the disease becomes refractory to therapy and there is a progressive rise in the white cell count. Immature 'blast cells' start to appear in the peripheral blood and in some cases the appearances are indistinguishable from acute myelogenous leukaemia. Once transformation has occurred, death results within 6 months.

Treatment aims

(1) The complete eradication of all leukaemic cells from the body resulting in cure. This is possible only with bone marrow transplantation.
(2) Symptom relief and maintenance of the peripheral blood count within normal limits. This is the only aim possible in the majority of patients.

Treatment options

(1) Cytotoxic chemotherapy } palliative
(2) Splenic irradiation } palliative
(3) Bone marrow transplantation — ? curative.

Chemotherapy

Oral busulfan has been used for many years and is an effective treatment. It reliably reduces spleen size, reduces the white cell count to normal and maintains the haemoglobin and platelet count in most patients. Median survival is increased to about 40 months (MRC, 1968).

Splenic irradiation

Intermittent courses of splenic irradiation have been the traditional treatment and are equally effective in reducing the white cell count to normal limits. A randomized controlled trial by the MRC found splenic irradiation to be less effective in maintaining the haemoglobin and the overall control was inferior to that achieved with busulfan (MRC, 1968). There is a tendency for the duration of remission to become shorter each time treatment is given until the disease becomes refractory. Median survival is increased to about 30 months.

Bone marrow transplantation

Because of the good results in acute leukaemia, the Seattle group began to transplant patients once blast transformation had taken place. This was not very successful, although 8% of patients receiving allogeneic grafts and 19% of those receiving syngeneic grafts were long-term survivors.

The theoretically attractive idea of cryopreserving the patient's own marrow during the chronic phase for use as an autograft once blast transformation occurs has been assessed. Unfortunately, the duration of the second chronic phase is only 10 weeks and the median survival only 27 weeks (Goldman *et al.*, 1981).

Encouraging results have been reported by Fefer, Cheever and Boyd (1981), who carried out syngeneic graft in 12 patients in the chronic phase. Ten of these patients are alive 9–35 months after engraftment with no Ph^1 + ve cells in their marrow which suggests the disease has been eliminated.

Treatment policy

Patients less than 45 years of age with a HLA-compatible sibling or identical twin should be treated by bone marrow transplantation in the chronic phase as this is the only potentially curative treatment. The remaining patients should be treated palliatively with busulfan which is more effective than splenic irradiation. Splenic irradiation is indicated for patients with symptoms producing splenomegaly resistant to chemotherapy, or patients in whom drug compliance is a problem.

Treatment techniques

Splenic irradiation

This technique was developed when orthovoltage equipment only was available. Anterior and posterior fields, 15 × 10 cm, were given an incident dose of 25 cGy on alternate days. Treatment continued until the white cell count was reduced to $10 \times 10^9/\ell$. No attempt was made to include the whole spleen if this could not adequately be encompassed within a 15 × 10 cm field.

With megavoltage equipment parallel opposed fields are used and a midplane dose of 25 cGy administered daily until the white cell count falls to $10 \times 10^9/\ell$. Treatment should be suspended if the platelet count drops below $80 \times 10^9/\ell$. A total dose of 300–400 cGy is usually required and it is unusual to exceed 800 cGy. It should be remembered that the white cell count and platelet count will continue to drop for 2 weeks after treatment is completed.

Toxicity

The only significant side-effect is thrombocytopenia which can be severe where the platelet count was already low or where previous chemotherapy has been given. The larger the spleen the more rapid the drop in white cell count and platelet count, and such cases require careful monitoring.

Busulfan therapy

This drug is given orally on a daily basis in a dose of 0.06 mg/kg body weight and only rarely should a dose in excess of 4 mg be given. The drug is continued until the white cell count drops to $10 \times 10^9/\ell$. Busulfan should be restarted when the white cell count increases above $25 \times 10^9/\ell$.

Toxicity

(1) Bone marrow suppression especially thrombocytopenia
(2) Skin pigmentation
(3) Amenorrhoea
(4) Pneumonitis causing pulmonary failure (busulfan lung)
(5) Addisonian-like wasting syndrome
(6) Cataract formation.

The last three are uncommon and tend to occur only with prolonged administration.

Bone marrow transplantation

The same technique is used as for the acute leukaemias and the toxicity is identical.

Chronic lymphocytic leukaemia

Natural history

The disease is characterized by the proliferation of lymphoid cells resulting in a massive accumulation of small and large lymphocytes in the bone marrow, peripheral blood, lymph nodes, liver and spleen. Two forms of the disease are recognized:

The *indolent* form occurs in elderly patients,

causes little or no morbidity and progresses slowly. The diagnosis is made as a chance finding on a blood count, requested for other reasons, which shows a moderate lymphocytosis (20–60 × $10^9/\ell$). This is compatible with survival for many years without treatment.

The *aggressive* form is typified by enlargement of the superficial lymph nodes, a lymphocytosis in excess of 100 × $10^9/\ell$ and progressive anaemia. Death occurs within 2 years from the onset of active symptomatic disease as a result of bone marrow failure. About 10% of patients develop secondary haemolytic anaemia. This should be suspected in patients whose severity of anaemia is out of proportion to the degree of lymphocytosis in the peripheral blood.

Treatment aims

There is no known curative therapy and no treatment which reliably prolongs survival. Symptomatic patients need treatment to shrink lymph node masses and to maintain an adequate haemoglobin.

Treatment options

(1) Chemotherapy
(2) Corticosteroids
(3) Low dose total body irradiation
(4) Palliative radiotherapy to symptomatic masses
(5) Splenectomy.

Chemotherapy

Chlorambucil, orally, established itself as the best drug for initial use. Galton *et al.* (1961) reported that 50% of patients achieved complete remission of their disease as indicated by a return to normal of the blood count and regression of the lymph nodes and spleen. These findings were confirmed by Huguley (1977) who found a response rate of 62% in a series of 459 patients. A satisfactory response can be obtained with cyclophosphamide, but this agent appears to have no advantage over chlorambucil.

Corticosteroids

The main indication for these are haemolytic anaemia and haemorrhagic tendency due to thrombocytopenia. In adequate dosage, corticosteroids are lympholytic and will cause regression of the nodes and spleen and reduce the white cell count. Galton *et al.* (1961) reported a 50% response rate in patients resistant to chlorambucil.

Total body irradition

This has been used for decades as a treatment for chronic lymphocytic leukaemia (del Regato, 1974). There has been a resurgence of interest in the technique in North America in recent years. Johnson (1976) reported that one-third of his patients responded to low dose treatment (5 cGy per day) with complete disappearance of symptoms, fall in white cell count to normal levels, disappearance of anaemia, complete regression of lymph nodes and spleen, and reduction of lymphocytosis in the bone marrow to less than 30% of the differential count. The survival of this group of patients appeared better than with other forms of therapy.

Palliative radiotherapy

This is a radiosensitive tumour and rapid shrinkage of symptomatic tumour masses can be achieved with modest doses. It is of little value in treating hypersplenism (Comas, Andrews and Nelson, 1968; Wilson and Johnson, 1971).

Splenectomy

This has no direct effect on the proliferation of lymphocytes. It is the most effective therapy for hypersplenism not responding to corticosteroids.

Treatment policy

Patients with indolent disease require no therapy until symptoms develop. Patients with active disease should be treated with chlorambucil because of the ease of administration and freedom from side-effects. This can be supplemented by the judicious use of corticosteroids and palliative radiotherapy when required. Corticosteroids can be particularly valuable as a means of re-establishing patients on chlorambucil where it has been discontinued because of thrombocytopenia.

Total body irradiation should be considered for patients with disease refractory to chemotherapy or those in whom drug compliance or regular outpatient attendances cause difficulties.

Treatment regimens

Chlorambucil

Galton *et al.* (1961) recommend an initial dose of 0.15 mg/kg daily by mouth and treatment continued until the white cell count returns to normal. In most cases the drug has to be stopped after 4–6 weeks and is then re-introduced in lower dosage. A satisfactory haematological response is usually achieved within 12 weeks.

Toxicity

Neutropenia is the most common side-effect and

treatment should be suspended if the neutrophil count drops below $1 \times 10^9/\ell$. Thrombocytopenia does occur particularly where the platelet count is already low prior to therapy.

Total body irradiation

Since only low doses are being given and the aim of treatment is palliative, a simple technique is adequate. The same basic pattern is used as for bone marrow transplantation. The patient is treated with two large lateral fields to encompass the whole body on the 10 MeV linear accelerator at a SSD of 400 cm. With a dose rate of 25 cGy/minute, a daily dose of 5 cGy is given until the total white cell count returns to normal. A total dose of 170–300 cGy is usually required. No compensators or build up material need be used.

Side-effects

There will be no nausea, vomiting or epilation. The only significant problem is neutropenia and for this reason the blood count should be monitored carefully.

Palliative radiotherapy

Extramedullary deposits can be treated with a single megavoltage or othovoltage beam or a parallel pair. A dose of 500 cGy in two daily fractions or 3000 cGy in 10 daily fractions is sufficient to produce regression.

Corticosteroids

To be effective, prednisolone should be administered in a dose of 30–40 mg daily. Enteric coating may help to reduce the incidence of gastric irritation, cimetidine should be given if there is a history of peptic or duodenal ulcer.

Survival

The median survival for treated patients is 4–6 years from the onset of symptoms. A minority of patients will survive for 10 years or more.

Extramedullary leukaemic deposits

These lesions are not uncommon in all forms of leukaemia. In addition to the definitive treatment, radiotherapy is indicated for rapid symptomatic relief or to eradicate leukaemic cells in sites such as the meninges or testes which are not affected by systemic chemotherapy. For lymphocytic leukaemias a modest dose of 3000 cGy in 10 daily fractions, or its equivalent in a shorter time, will produce complete regression. For myeloid leukaemias, a rather higher dose of 4000 cGy in 15 daily fractions or its equivalent is required (Johnson, 1977; Chak, Sapozink and Cox, 1983). Complete regression of gum deposits in acute myeloid leukaemia with local radiotherapy is shown in *Figures 11.5* and *11.6*.

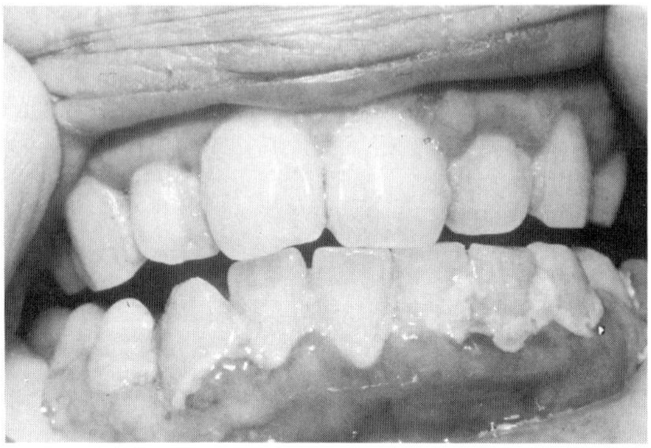

Figure 11.5 Deposits of acute myeloid leukaemia on patient's gums

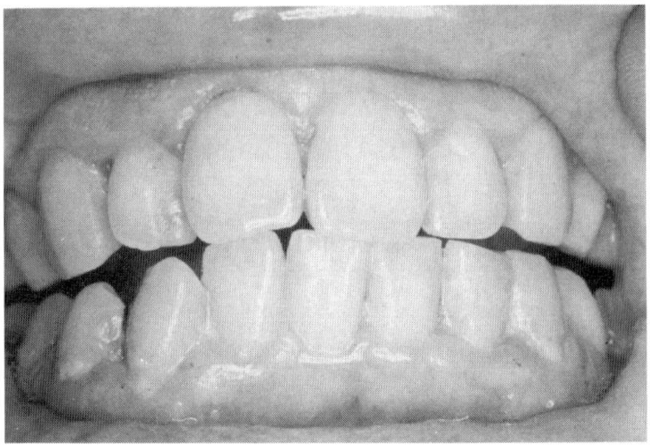

Figure 11.6 Same patient as in *Figure 11.5* showing complete remission with palliative radiotherapy

Chloroma (granulocytic sarcoma)

This is the term used to describe localized subperiosteal leukaemic deposits which may develop in acute or chronic myeloid leukaemia. These contain a green pigment which fades on exposure to light. They commonly occur in the skull, particularly in the orbit where they may cause exophthalmos. As these deposits often involve the skin or conjunctivae, the 'skin sparing' effect of megavoltage beams is a disadvantage. The use of a single orthovoltage beam avoids this problem.

Polycythaemia rubra vera (primary proliferative polycythaemia)

Natural history

This is a chronic disease of insidious onset and unknown aetiology which is characterized by excess production of the formed elements of the blood by a hyperplastic bone marrow. The essential feature is over-production of red cells, but leukocytosis occurs in 75% and thrombocytosis in 65% of patients. It has been shown that the condition results from neoplastic proliferation of a single mutant clone of marrow cells (Adamson *et al.*, 1976).

The disease develops slowly over several years during which there are no symptoms, no abnormal clinical findings and the diagnosis is made as a chance finding on a blood count. This is followed by a proliferative phase in which there is a progressive increase in the haemoglobin, red cell count and venous haematocrit and the typical clinical features develop.

Many patients die during this phase from cerebral thrombosis or haemorrhage, coronary occlusion, congestive cardiac failure and gastrointestinal haemorrhage. These complications are a direct consequence of the increased blood volume, increased viscosity and raised platelet count. In an untreated series of patients, 50% were dead within 18 months of diagnosis (Chievitz and Thiede, 1962).

Patient who survive the proliferative phase enter a 'spent' phase in which the features of polycythaemia disappear and progressive anaemia develops. This is due to the onset of myelosclerosis in which the marrow becomes obliterated by the proliferation of fibrous tissue and the spleen enlarges massively due to extramedullary haemopoiesis. Terminal leukaemia develops in about 1% of untreated cases and this is usually acute myelogenous leukaemia, although chronic granulocytic leukaemia has been reported.

Diagnosis

Polycythaemia rubra vera should be suspected in any male with a persistently elevated venous haematocrit above 0.50, or a female with a value above 0.47. The disease must be distinguished from secondary polycythaemia and relative polycythaemia. Estimation of the red cell mass will eliminate relative polycythaemia since this is normal in this condition, but raised in both polycythaemia rubra vera and secondary polycythaemia. An increase of greater than 25% above his own predicted value for a male or 30% above her predicted value for a female excludes relative polycythaemia.

Polycythaemia rubra vera can be distinguished from secondary polycythaemia by the presence of splenomegaly, leukocytosis, thrombocytosis, raised leucocyte alkaline phosphatase score, and raised serum B_{12} or serum B_{12} binding capacity.

Treatment aim

The main aim of treatment is to prolong survival by the prevention of vascular complications. Studies have shown that the incidence of vascular occlusive events is reduced if the venous haematocrit is maintained at 0.45 and the platelet count below $400 \times 10^9/\ell$ (Pearson and Wetherley-Mein, 1978). Cerebral blood flow is markedly reduced in the untreated case and steadily improves as the venous haematocrit falls to normal levels (Thomas, Marshall *et al.*, 1977).

Treatment options

(1) Venesection or erythropheresis
(2) Myelosuppression with ^{32}P
(3) Myelosuppression with cytotoxic chemotherapy.

Venesection

This is the most rapid method of reducing blood volume and lowering whole blood viscosity. It has no effect on the fundamental abnormality in the bone marrow and little effect on the platelet count if this is markedly increased. It is successful in preventing vascular complications and the median survival is increased to 4–8 years.

This form of treatment causes no unpleasant side-effects although if repeated frequently it can cause iron deficiency. It does not appear to increase the incidence of terminal leukaemia which remains at 1% (Berk *et al.*, 1981).

^{32}P therapy

This was introduced by Lawrence in 1938 (Lawrence, Scott and Tuttle, 1939) and rapidly became the standard treatment. A complete remission (defined as disappearance of all reversible symptoms and a return to normal of the blood picture for 6 months) is obtained in 82% of patients. A partial remission in which the response lasts for less than 6 months is achieved in a further 13%. The median duration of complete responses is 22 months (Szur, Lewis and Goolden, 1959). The 5% who do not respond ^{32}P are those with a white cell count in excess of $25 \times 10^9/\ell$ or splenomegaly greater than 10 cm below the left costal margin (Calabresi and Meyer, 1959). The median survival is increased to 11–13 years (Calabresi and Meyer, 1959; Lawrence, Winchell and Donald, 1968), although repeated doses of ^{32}P will be required.

The acute toxicity of ^{32}P is insignificant. There is no nausea and vomiting, no hair loss, and severe marrow suppression causing neutropenia or thrombocytopenia is extremely uncommon. An increase in the incidence of terminal leukaemia from 1 to 10% has been reported by Modan and Lilienfield (1964). These authors found the incidence of leukaemia to be dose dependent, with patients receiving a cumulative dose of 5–9 mCi showing a 5.2% incidence whereas those receiving greater than 60 mCi had a 30% incidence Lawrence, Winchell and Donald (1969) could find no correlation between dose and the incidence of leukaemia in their patients, and advanced the view that the increased incidence of leukaemia was due to the better survival and therefore more patients were at risk for longer.

Cytotoxic therapy

A variety of alkylating agents has been used to treat patients with polycythaemia rubra vera. They appear to produce a complete remission rate similar to ^{32}P and are effective in reducing an elevated platelet count as well as the haematocrit. The time taken to induce remission is more variable than with ^{32}P but is broadly similar at 3–5 months. If maintenance therapy is not used, then the duration of remission is shorter than with ^{32}P, with 23–25 weeks for chlorambucil and cyclophosphamide, and 65 weeks for busulfan (Gilbert, 1968). The median survival is increased to 7–8 years (Berk *et al.*, 1981).

The acute toxicity is minimal with most single alkylating agents but the incidence of severe marrow suppression is greater than with ^{32}P, particularly if busulfan is used when 38% of patients develop thrombocytopenia (Gilbert, 1968). Hair loss may occur with cyclophosphamide and busulfan may cause skin pigmentation and pulmonary fibrosis.

Initially there were few reports of increased risk of leukaemia but in a recently published report, the Polycythaemia Vera Study Group showed that the incidence of leukaemia in a group treated by chlorambucil was 11% compared with 6% in a group treated with ^{32}P and only 1% in a group treated by venesection (Berk *et al.*, 1981).

Treatment policy

In a randomized trial, the Polycythaemia Rubra Vera Study Group found no difference in survival in patients treated by venesection alone, ^{32}P, or chlorambucil therapy. Venesection or erythropheresis is therefore the treatment of choice since this produces the lowest incidence of leukaemia. This is particularly true for the younger patients since prognosis is inversely related to age. Myelosuppressive therapy should be reserved for patients who required venesection excessively frequently to maintain the haematocrit at 0.45 or those who have persistently elevated platelet counts above 400 × $10^9/\ell$. At present, ^{32}P is probably the treatment of choice for this group since it requires less frequent clinic attendance, produces a longer median remission and has a lower incidence of terminal leukaemia than chlorambucil. Further studies are still required to see whether an agent such as hydroxyurea or 6-thioguanine might be less leukaemogenic. Chemotherapy is indicated for patients unresponsive to ^{32}P.

Treatment regimens

^{32}P therapy

^{32}P is a radionuclide with a half-life of 14.3 days. It is a pure beta particle emitter with a maximum penetration in tissue of 8 mm and a half-path of 2 mm. It can be administered orally but is normally injected intravenously. ^{32}P is concentrated selectively in the hyperplastic bone marrow of patients with polycythaemia. It has been estimated that a 4 mCi dose will deliver a dose of 117 cGy to the bone marrow and 17 cGy to the other tissues.

A number of formulae have been developed to try to calculate the precise dosage required to produce remission. These take into account the patient's height and weight, surface area, or lean body mass and sometimes the haematocrit or red cell mass. There is no evidence that the use of a formula is superior to the empirical selection of a dose between 3 and 7 mCi based on the patient's stature. The simplest formula to apply is that used by the Polycythaemia Vera Study Group who recommend an initial dose of 2.3 mCi/m^2 surface area with an increment of 25% if this is ineffective.

^{32}P is injected intravenously in the radioisotope department where local rules should describe the procedure for administration and the action to be taken in event of spillage. The doctor should wear a gown, mask and gloves to prevent contamination of his hands or clothing, or inhalation due to aerosol formation. A lead or perspex shield can be used to surround the syringe to reduce the external irradiation of the doctor's hands. If the isotope is extravasated into the subcutaneous tissues, irrigation of the area with hyaluronidase will speed absorption into the blood stream. The standard doses described above can be given safely on an outpatient basis and there is no restriction on travel by public transport.

Follow-up

The effect on the platelet count is maximal at 4–6 weeks but the full effect on the haemoglobin and haematocrit is not seen until 3–4 months have elapsed. Blood counts should be performed at 8, 12 and 16 weeks at which time the response is assessed. If the blood picture has returned to normal, the patient should attend 3 monthly for a blood count and further ^{32}P is indicated only if there is a rise in haematocrit not easily controlled by venesection or if the platelet count rises above 400 × $10^9/\ell$. A minimum of 4 months should elapse between injections and a cumulative dose of 30 mCi should not be exceeded. Most patients will require four or five injections during the proliferative phase.

If there is an unsatisfactory response to the initial dose of ^{32}P, a further injection should be given after 4 months with the dose increased by 25%. If this also fails, cytotoxic therapy should be considered.

Cytotoxic therapy

The safest drug and the most effective schedule has yet to be established. Busulfan appears to produce the longest unmaintained remission, but tends to cause amenorrhoea, skin pigmentation and, more rarely, pulmonary fibrosis. Chlorambucil is simpler to administer and has few side-effects, but has been shown to be leukaemogenic.

Busulfan	4 mg daily on alternate months until remission is obtained. No maintenance therapy
Chlorambucil	10 mg daily for 6 weeks continuously then the same dose on alternate months
Hydroxyurea	0.5–1 g daily until remission obtained then the same dose on alternate months.

Venesection

Around 300–500 ml of whole blood are removed through an intravenous cannula on alternate days until the haematocrit drops below 50. Usually a total of 6–8 units of blood are removed to obtain remission. In patients with ischaemic vascular disease, it is advisable to replace the blood removed with a high molecular weight dextran solution.

Erythropheresis

This is essentially the same procedure as venesection except that the patient is connected to a cell separator and packed cells rather than whole blood are removed. This may have an advantage over venesection in reducing the blood viscosity more rapidly.

Supportive management

Patients with high platelet counts should be given agents which prevent platelet aggregation to reduce the high incidence of thromboses. Soluble aspirin 300 mg on alternate days or dipyridamole 100 mg three times a day should be given until the platelet count drops below $400 \times 10^9/\ell$.

Hyperuricaemia is common due to high cell turnover and is particularly likely when myelosuppressive therapy with ^{32}P or cytotoxics is instituted. Allopurinol 300 mg daily should be given as a prophylaxis against renal tubular damage for at least 4 months following ^{32}P and many clinicians continue it indefinitely.

Myelofibrosis (myelosclerosis)

Natural history

This disease is thought to be due to neoplastic proliferation of primitive mesenchymal tissue resulting in progressive fibrosis of the bone marrow. This causes a leuco-erythroblastic anaemia, massive enlargement of the spleen and sometimes liver due to extramedullary haemopoiesis. It is closely related to the myeloid leukaemias and to polycythaemia rubra vera and these conditions are sometimes referred to collectively as the 'myeloproliferative disorders'.

The disease either starts *de novo* or as the end stage of polycythaemia rubra vera. In most patients it runs a slowly progressive course with a median survival of 5–7 years and some patients live for 20 years. About 25% of patients have an acute terminal phase in which acute myelogenous leukaemia develops and is rapidly fatal.

Diagnosis

This condition should be suspected in patients with massive splenomegaly and leuco-erythroblastic anaemia particularly where there is a past history of polycythaemia. Confirmation of the diagnosis can be obtained by carrying out a bone marrow trephine at several sites which will show replacement of haemopoietic tissue by fibrosis. This will also exclude chronic granulocytic leukaemia which may be suspected because of the splenomegaly and primitive white cells in the peripheral blood.

Treatment aims

No curative therapy exists for this condition. The purpose of treatment is to maintain an adequate haemoglobin, to control the discomfort caused by splenic enlargement, to prevent haemorrhage due to thrombocytopenia and to control complications such as hyperuricaemia.

Treatment policy

The mainstay of treatment is blood transfusion along with folic acid supplement because of the high incidence of conditioned folate deficiency. Anabolic steroids are frequently administered to try to stimulate haemopoiesis thus reducing the need for transfusion.

Massive splenomegaly can be treated by cytotoxic chemotherapy, splenic irradiation or splenectomy. Since there is a small mortality rate associated with splenectomy it should be considered only where other measures have failed. No method of treatment has been adequately studied but Bouroncle and Doan (1962) reported 15 good responses in a group of 21 patients treated with busulfan with the response maintained for up to 4 years, whereas only two good responses were found in a group of 15 patients receiving splenic irradiation and these were maintained for 2–6 months.

Splenectomy should be reserved for patients in whom the haemoglobin cannot be maintained despite repeated transfusions, those in whom haemorrhage develops due to thrombocytopenia refractory to folic acid therapy and patients whose splenomegaly cannot be controlled as above. Bouroncle and Doan (1962) reported 14 good responses among 24 patients treated by splenectomy and one-half of these required no further blood transfusions. There were two fatal and seven non-fatal complications in this group.

Treatment regimens

Busulfan

An initial dose of 2–4 mg daily, orally, for 3–4 weeks followed by maintenance therapy with 2 mg two or three times per week is given. The drug is given on an intermittent basis as dictated by the size of the spleen and the suppression of the peripheral blood count. Usually treatment is given for 6–8 months at a time.

Toxicity

As described under chronic granulocytic leukaemia.

Splenic irradiation

A parallel pair of megavoltage fields is the most satisfactory arrangement. It is unnecessary to include the whole spleen within the radiation fields. A midplane dose of 25 cGy per day for a large spleen should be delivered until symptomatic relief occurs. As the spleen is the major site of blood production, a precipitous drop in the white cell count and platelet count can occur. It is usually this rather than the shrinkage of the spleen which dictates when treatment is stopped. A total dose of 300 cGy is commonly given. The blood count must be monitored several times per week.

Toxicity

Neutropenia and thrombocytopenia are the only side-effects.

Anabolic steroids

Oxymethalone is probably the drug of choice and should be given in a dose of 2–5 mg/kg until a response is achieved. Maintenance therapy with 50% of this dose should be continued in responders. If no response is seen after 12 weeks the drug should be discontinued.

Toxicity

(1) Virilization in the female
(2) Weight gain
(3) Hyperuricaemia
(4) Jaundice.

Uricosuric agents

Allopurinol is the drug of choice and should be given prophylactically in a dose of 300 mg daily, and continued throughout treatment.

Multiple myeloma

Natural history

This is a chronic, progressive and ultimately fatal malignancy which is characterized by neoplastic proliferation of plasma cells which infiltrate the bone marrow and other tissues. These plasma cells produce an homogeneous paraprotein which can be detected in serum or urine. Because the paraprotein is homogeneous, it is thought that the disease arises from a single mutant clone of plasma cells.

Clinical features

Bone pain is the commonest presenting symptom and occurs in up to 80% of patients. Typically the pain is in the lumbar or thoracic spine while pain in the skull is uncommon even when multiple deposits are present. Pathological fractures or wedge compression of the vertebral bodies are found in 20–25% of cases due to destruction of cortical bone. This in turn can lead to root pain or spinal cord compression which develops in 10% of patients.

Palpable tumour deposits are not uncommon and may occur in any bone but are most evident in the ribs. Anaemia due to suppression of the normal marrow elements is present in most cases and is severe in advanced cases. Hypercalcaemia is found in up to 40% of cases. This can be severe enough to result in premature death. Lowered resistance to infection is present in the majority of patients due to suppression of the normal immunoglobulins. Hyperviscosity of a degree to produce symptoms is present in 5% of all cases. This can cause visual disturbance, headache, vertigo, coma and bleeding from mucous membranes. Renal insufficiency develops in 50% of all cases but is an uncommon presenting feature.

A detailed description of the clinical findings can be found in a review of 859 cases by Kyle (1975).

Diagnosis

A firm diagnosis of myeloma can be made in the presence of two or more of the following features:

(1) Characteristic 'myeloma' cells in a tumour biopsy or bone marrow trephine
(2) Greater than 10% plasma cells in a bone marrow trephine
(3) An homogeneous paraprotein band on serum electrophoresis
(4) Bence Jones proteinuria
(5) 'Punched out' lytic bone deposits on radiography.

'Myeloma' cells vary in appearance from small, mature, differentiated plasma cells to large immature cells 20–30 μm in diameter. Multinucleate cells, large prominent nucleoli and a perinuclear halo are common findings. These cells frequently constitute 15–30% of the cells in the bone marrow, but the actual percentage is not of prognostic significance.

Increased numbers of plasma cells are found in the marrow of patients with conditions such as aplastic anaemia, rheumatoid arthritis, hepatic cirrhosis, sarcoidosis and secondary carcinoma. These cells are mature, of normal size and rarely exceed 10% of the marrow cells. Plasmacytosis in excess of 10% implies multiple myeloma.

A sharply defined 'M' band is found on cellulose acetate electrophoresis of the serum of 80% of patients with multiple myeloma. The position of this band is usually in the gamma globulin zone although it can be in the alpha or beta globulin zones. No 'M' band is found in 20% of cases.

Immunoelectrophoresis will show that the paraprotein is an immunoglobulin of one to five types: IgG, IgA, IgM, IgD and IgE. Unlike normal immunoglobulin, these tumour products have only one type of light chain (κ or λ). IgG is identified in 50% of patients, IgA in 25% of patients and IgD in 1–2% (Hobbs, 1967).

Sensitive techniques for demonstrating Bence Jones protein (light chains) in the urine will find it in 50–70% of cases with an 'M' band. In the 20% of patient having no 'M' band, light chains are almost invariably present in urine and will be entirely either κ or λ.

The typical X-ray finding on the skeletal survey in myeloma is the presence of multiple, rounded, discrete, 'punched out', lytic lesions with no sclerosis at the edges. Not infrequently myeloma presents with

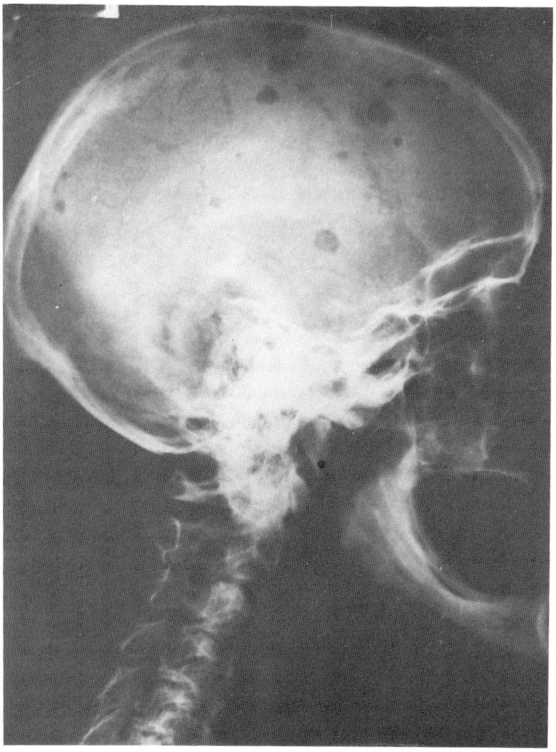

Figure 11.7 Typical bone deposits in the skull in myelomatosis

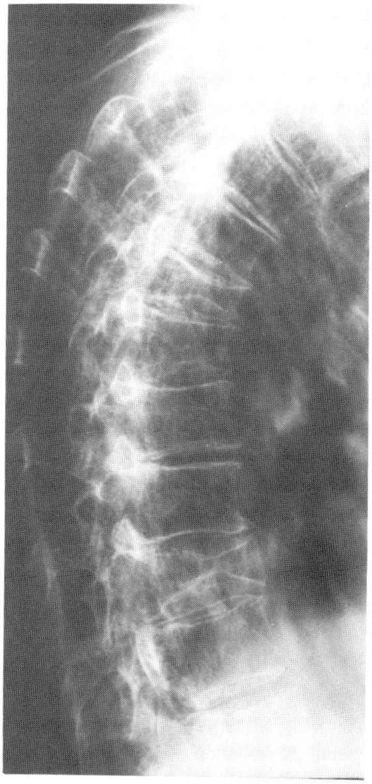

Figure 11.8 Diffuse osteoporosis with wedge compression of vertebrae in myelomatosis

diffuse osteoporosis particularly in the vertebrae where it can cause compression (*Figures 11.7* and *11.8*). This has to be distinguished from senile osteoporosis and hyperparathyroidism. The serum alkaline phosphatase is often of value, as this is usually normal in multiple myeloma, while it is raised in these other conditions. Ten per cent of patients with myeloma have no demonstrable bone lesions.

Staging

Tumour mass has been shown to correlate well with survival and the probability of response to chemotherapy (Salmon and Smith, 1970). The tumour mass can be estimated from easily obtained clinical data and this is the basis of a staging proposed by Durie and Salmon (1975):

Stage I (low tumour mass)

All of the following criteria:

(1) Haemoglobin greater than 100 g/ℓ (1.55 mmol/ℓ)
(2) Serum calcium less than 2.6 mmol/ℓ
(3) Few or no lytic bone lesions on radiography
(4) Low paraprotein levels — IgG less than 50 g/ℓ in serum
IgA less than 30 g/ℓ in serum
Bence Jones proteinuria less than 4 g/24 hours.

Stage II (intermediate tumour mass)

Having the criteria for neither stage I nor stage III.

Stage III

One or more of the following criteria:
(1) Haemoglobin less than 85 g/ℓ (1.3 mmol/ℓ)
(2) Serum calcium in excess of 3 mmol/ℓ
(3) Multiple lytic lesions on radiography
(4) High paraprotein levels — IgG in excess of 70 g/ℓ in serum
IgA in excess of 50 g/ℓ in serum
Bence Jones proteinuria in excess of 5 g/24 hours.

The suffix A or B is used to denote that renal function is normal or impaired as demonstrated by a serum creatinine in excess of 175 mmol/ℓ.

Using these criteria, the South West Oncology Group (1975) found that, in a sample of 482 patients with myeloma, 23% were allocated to stage I, 29% to stage II and 45% to stage III. This correlated well with median survival of 39 months, 27 months and 17 months respectively.

The MRC Working Party (1980b) could find no prognostic significance in paraprotein levels in its third myelomatosis trial and have advocated a slightly different staging:

Stage I (good prognosis)

All of the following criteria:

(1) Blood urea less than 8 mmol/ℓ
(2) Haemoglobin in excess of 100 g/ℓ (1.55 mmol/ℓ)
(3) Minimal or no symptoms.

Stage II (intermediate prognosis)

Having the criteria for neither stage I nor stage III.

Stage III (poor prognosis)

One or both of the following criteria:

(1) Blood urea in excess of 10 mmol/ℓ with restricted physical activity
(2) Haemoglobin less than 75 g/ℓ (1.16 mmol/ℓ) with restricted physical activity.

Using this staging the MRC found 22% of their patients in stage I, 56% in stage II and 22% in stage III. There was again a close correlation between stage of disease and 2-year survival.

If the more commonly used American staging is employed then a higher percentage of patients will be placed in the worst prognosis group than with the MRC staging. This should be borne in mind when comparing treatment results.

Prognostic factors

These have been well reviewed by Alexanian *et al.* (1975) from data accumulated by the South West Oncology Group.

(1) Anaemia. Patients with an initial haemoglobin of less than 85 g/ℓ (1.3 mmol/ℓ) have a shorter remission on chemotherapy and an inferior median survival (15 months).
(2) Hypercalcaemia. Patients with a serum calcium in excess of 3.1 mmol/ℓ had a median survival of 11 months compared with 26 months for those with a calcium less than 2.85 mmol/ℓ.
(3) Type and amount of immunoglobulin. Patients with IgA myeloma had an inferior median survival (17 months) than those with IgG myeloma (25 months) or Bence Jones myeloma (24 months). Patients with paraprotein levels in excess of 50 g/ℓ had a poorer median survival than those with less.

Treatment aims

There is no known curative treatment for multiple myeloma. The purpose of treatment is to prolong survival, to palliate symptoms and to prevent or control complications.

Treatment options

(1) Cytotoxic chemotherapy
(2) Palliative radiotherapy
(3) Plasmapheresis.

Cytotoxic therapy

Cytotoxic therapy is the only treatment which has been demonstrated to prolong survival. The median survival in untreated myeloma is 9–12 months (Korst *et al.*, 1964) which is similar to that of patients who do not respond to chemotherapy (Alexanian *et al.*, 1969). With single agent melphalan or cyclophosphamide the median survival is increased to 24–32 months (Korst *et al.*, 1964; Speed, Galton and Swan, 1964). An MRC trial comparing melphalan with cyclophosphamide found both to be equally effective (Galton and Peto, 1968).

Alexanian *et al.* (1969) reported that a combination of melphalan and prednisone produced an objective response rate of 70% and a median survival of 24 months compared with 35% and 18 months respectively for melphalan. These findings were confirmed by Bersagel (1972) and more recently by the MRC Working Party second myelomatosis trial (1980a). Intermittent melphalan and prednisone thereafter became the standard treatment.

There have been conflicting reports of the value of more aggressive combination chemotherapy. The Memorial Sloan Kettering Cancer Center reported a median survival of 36 months and an objective response rate of 80% with their M2 protocol. Since their experience with melphalan and prednisone was that it produced a median survival of 18 months and an objective response rate of 40%, they decided it would be unethical to set up a randomized trial (Case, Lee and Clarkson, 1977; Lee, Lake-Lewin and Myers, 1982; Lee and Myers 1983).

The South West Oncology Group developed two vincristine containing regimens which produced response rates of 60% and median survival of 30 months. A randomized trial was set up comparing these two regimens with melphalan and prednisone. The objective response rates were found to be similar, but median survival was better in stage III patients who received the combination (Salmon, Alexanian and Dixon, 1979).

The Cancer and Acute Leukaemia Group B reported a randomized trial of intermittent melphalan and prednisone against combination BCNU, cyclophosphamide, melphalan and prednisone. Again improved median survival was found in stage III patients only who received the combination (Harley *et al.*, 1979).

The National Cancer Institute of Canada compared that same combination with melphalan and prednisone in a randomized trial. They found no improvement in median survival or objective response rates but did not report a very high incidence of leukaemia in the patients treated with the combination (Bersagel *et al.*, 1979).

The MRC third myelomatosis trial again compared the same combination with melphalan and prednisone in stage III cases only and found no improvement in survival (MRC Working Party, 1980b).

It is difficult to interpret these results because of the different criteria used for objective remission by different authors. It would be helpful if future trials used the criteria laid down by the Myeloma Task Force of the National Cancer Institute in 1973. All of the following should be fulfilled:

(1) Reduction in size of plasmacytomas, by palpation or X-ray, by 50% or more in the product of the two largest dimensions
(2) A fall in serum paraprotein levels to 50% or less
(3) If urinary paraprotein greater than 1 g/24 hours, a reduction to 50% or less. If urinary paraprotein 0.5–1 g/24 hours, a reduction to less than 0.1 g/24 hours
(4) Definite healing of skeletal lesions.

Maintenance chemotherapy

There is conflicting experimental and clinical evidence as to the value of maintenance therapy for patients who are in remission 1 year from the start of therapy.

It has been shown that, when treatment starts, initially there is a progressive decrease in the estimated myeloma mass. After 3–9 months, a plateau is reached and no further reduction in cell mass can be produced by continuing or even intensifying the chemotherapy. The plateau remains, even in patients on no therapy, until regrowth ends the remission (Salmon and Durie, 1975). This suggests that there would be no point in maintenance therapy.

Salmon (1975) has also demonstrated an increase in the growth fraction following treatment with alkylating agents which suggests that it may be unwise to stop therapy in responding patients in case rapid regrowth ends the remisssion.

On clinical data, the Memorial Sloan Kettering Cancer Center strongly opposes the cessation of therapy in patients who are in remission. They report a 50% death rate within 6 months in their patients in whom this was done. Their policy is to continue the M2 protocol in all patients until relapse occurs.

The South West Oncology Group have reached the opposite conclusion. They randomly allocated patients in remission to continue melphalan and prednisone as maintenance therapy, to change to BCNU and prednisone as maintenance therapy or to no further treatment. The median survival was best in the unmaintained group (South West Oncology Group, 1975). In a subsequent paper from the same group it was reported that patients who relapsed after an unmaintained remission had an 80% chance of responding a second time to melphalan and prednisone (Alexanian *et al.*, 1978). The MRC third myelomatosis trial was likewise unable to demonstrate prolongation of remission or survival with maintenance therapy (MRC Working Party, 1980b).

An Italian group using the M2 protocol were unable to confirm the Memorial Sloan Kettering Cancer Center findings. There were no early deaths in patients whose therapy was stopped after 1 year in continuous remission. On re-introduction of the M2 protocol 82% of patients responded, although the second remission was shorter than the first. More than one-half of the patients who were given a third exposure to the M2 protocol again responded (Paccagnella *et al.*, 1983).

Palliative radiotherapy

Bone pain occurs in 80% of patients with myeloma. Palliative radiotherapy will nearly always produce pain relief (Todd, 1965). Continuing pain despite adequate radiotherapy is strongly suggestive of pathological fracture.

Plasmapheresis

Hyperviscosity causes symptoms in about 5% of patients. Such patients should be treated on the cell separator (Powles *et al.*, 1971). Prompt treatment is required to prevent blindness in patients who complain of deteriorating vision.

Treatment policy

Asymptomatic patients with indolent stage I multiple myeloma require no therapy until symptoms develop or the disease begins to progress. Patients with symptomatic progressive disease should be treated initially with melphalan and prednisone. Although this produces survival inferior to that with combination chemotherapy, it is justified by the ease of administration and freedom from side-effects which give the patient a better quality of life. In patients who are in remission after 12 months on therapy, treatment should be stopped until further progression occurs.

Patients who do not respond to melphalan and prednisolone or who relapse while on this treatment should be given combination chemotherapy. Patients who relapse after an unmaintained remission should be treated with melphalan and prednisolone as there is an excellent chance of a second response.

Palliative radiotherapy is indicated for patients with bone pain.

Internal fixation is indicated for patients with pathological fractures in long bone or as prophylaxis in patients with lytic deposits in weight bearing bones showing 65% or more destruction of cortical bone.

Spinal cord compression develops in about 10% of patients usually as the result of vertebral collapse. The treatment of choice for a patient in good general condition is surgical decompression by laminectomy as this is most likely to prevent infarction of the cord and permanent loss of function. Where this is considered inappropriate, urgent palliative radiotherapy combined with dexamethasone 4 mg four times daily is indicated.

Supportive therapy is of great importance and blood transfusion to treat anaemia is required in most patients. Hypercalcaemia is present in 45% of patients and symptomatic patients should receive urgent treatment with hydration and corticosteroid. Those who fail to respond should be treated with phosphate or calcitonin.

Treatment regimens

Intermittent melphalan and prednisolone

Melphalan 0.15 mg/kg per day orally for 4 days only
Prednisolone 1 mg/kg per day orally for 4 days only.
Cycles are repeated on a 6 weekly basis.

Therapy should be discontinued for patients in remission for 12 months.

The M2 protocol

Cyclophosphamide 10 mg/kg i.v. bolus day 1
Vincristine 0.03 mg/kg i.v. bolus day 1
BCNU 0.5 mg/kg i.v. bolus day 1
Melphalan 0.25 mg/kg orally for 4 days
Prednisolone 1 mg/kg orally for 7 days.
Cycles are repeated evey 5 weeks.

Dose reduction may be required because of myelosuppression or renal failure.

Toxicity

Myelosuppression is the main problem with melphalan and prednisolone in combination and this is uncommon except in advanced disease. Some patients develop dyspepsia and this can be minimized by using enteric coated steroids.

The M2 protocol causes a greater degree of myelosuppression and nausea, vomiting, hair loss and peripheral neuropathy are not uncommon.

The use of chemotherapy has been shown to increase the risk of developing acute leukaemia. The Memorial Sloan Kettering Group report a 2% incidence for patients in the M2 protocol (Lee, Lake-

Lewin and Myers, 1982). Patients entered into the MRC trials have an overall incidence of 2.3% and this rises to 10% in patients surviving more than 4 years (Buckman, Cuzick and Galton 1982). The National Cancer Institute of Canada found an incidence of 17.4% in patients surviving for 50 months or more (Bersagel *et al.*, 1979).

Radiotherapy

A single orthovoltage or megavoltage field or a parallel pair is suitable for most patients. The field size will vary from 15 × 10 cm for spinal deposits to 30 × 40 cm for a pelvic bath. A megavoltage dose of 3000 cGy in 10 daily fractions or its equivalent is recommended and will produce pain relief in 90% of patients with only 6% requiring re-treatment (Todd, 1965; Mill and Griffith, 1980).

Toxicity

Significant side-effects occur only when large volumes are irradiated. Whole body, half body and pelvic bath techniques are likely to cause nausea and vomiting, diarrhoea and bone marrow suppression. This latter side-effect prevents concurrent administration of cytotoxics and these techniques should be used only if essential.

Treatment results

With chemotherapy, an overall median survival of 24–36 months is expected. The median survival for responders is about 4 years, whereas the non-responders have a median survival of 10–12 months. Lee and Myers (1983) report that 22% of their patients have survived for 10 years or more and it is this group who are at risk of developing leukaemia.

Solitary plasmacytoma

There is a group of patients who present with a plasma cell tumour apparently confined to one site. This may be in bone, solitary plasmacytoma of bone, or in soft tissue, extramedullary plasmacytoma. It is not yet clear whether these are separate pathological entities or whether they are simply variants of multiple myeloma.

Solitary plasmacytoma of bone shows many similarities to multiple myeloma. The initial lesion occurs in the bones commonly affected by myeloma. Most patients will develop generalized disease and when this happens it is indistinguishable from multiple myeloma. Bataille and Sany (1981) reported that, although only 23% of patients had multiple deposits at 2 years, these had developed in 85% by 10 years. Yentis (1956) reported that dissemination could occur even 26 years after diagnosis and expressed the view that, provided the patient did not die from other causes, all cases would disseminate eventually.

Extramedullary plasmacytoma shows marked dissimilarity to multiple myeloma. It occurs in a younger age group with many patients in their third and fourth decade. Three-quarters of the lesions develop in the head and neck and dissemination is uncommon with a primary tumour in this site (Dolin and Dewar, 1956; Woodruff, Whittle and Malpas, 1979). In those cases where progression does occur, the new lesions tend to be in lymph nodes or soft tissue and not in bone. These findings have led Wiltshaw (1976) to question the relationship between extramedullary plasmacytoma and multiple myeloma.

Diagnosis

To make a firm diagnosis of solitary plasmacytoma all the following criteria should be met:

(1) Biopsy proven plasma cell tumour in bone or soft tissue
(2) Absence of 'myeloma' cells or less than 10% plasmacytosis in bone marrow from a non-involved site
(3) A normal skeletal survey apart from the involved site
(4) Absent or low levels of paraprotein in serum or urine with disappearance following local treatment
(5) Absence of anaemia, azotaemia or hypercalcaemia.

There is agreement that the presence of paraprotein does not preclude a diagnosis of solitary plasmacytoma, but persistently raised levels following surgery or radiotherapy suggest generalized disease (Corwin and Lindberg 1979; Tong *et al.*, 1980).

Staging

There is no suggested staging for solitary plasmacytoma of bone. A simple staging has been suggested for extramedullary plasmacytoma (Woodruff, Whittle and Malpas, 1979).

Stage I	Disease confined to a single site
Stage II	Spread to regional lymph nodes
Stage III	Generalized disease.

Treatment policy

There is no way in which patients with true solitary plasmacytoma can be distinguished prospectively from those who will develop generalized disease. The initial survival for all patients with apparently localized plasmacytoma is much better than that of myeloma, therefore all patients should receive radical radiotherapy. Chemotherapy should be withheld for use once dissemination occurs. Lymph node involvement in extramedullary plasmacytoma does not preclude radical radiotherapy and is not an indication for cytotoxic therapy (Corwin and Lindberg, 1979; Tong *et al.*, 1980).

Patients with advanced disease may require palliative radiotherapy as well as chemotherapy along with any of the other supportive measures described for multiple myeloma.

Treatment regimens

Radical radiotherapy

For solitary plasmacytoma of bone a single orthovoltage or megavoltage field or parallel pair is usually adequate. There is no advantage in administering a dose in excess of 4000 cGy in 3–4 weeks. Mill and Griffiths (1980) found no local recurrence provided a dose in excess of 3500 cGy was given, whereas Meyer and Shulz (1974) had reported a high risk of local recurrence with doses less than 3000 cGy.

For extramedullary plasmacytoma, particularly in the head and neck region, more elaborate field arrangements similar to those used for epithelial tumours may be required to minimize dose to the eyes, the brain stem or spinal cord. British authors recommend a dose of 4000 cGy in 20 daily fractions or its equivalent (Todd, 1965) (*Figures 11.9 and 11.10*). American authors report recurrences with doses less than 5000 cGy and therefore recommend a higher dose of 5000–6000 cGy in 5 or 6 weeks (Corwin and Lindberg, 1979; Mill and Griffith 1980).

Treatment results

Most reports on solitary plasmacytoma are based on small numbers of patients, rarely exceeding 30. Percentage survival is, therefore, of doubtful significance. In Todd's (1965) series of 30 patients treated prior to the advent of modern chemotherapy, the 5-year survival figure was 60%. In Corwin and Lindberg's (1979) more recent series, the 5-year survival was 75%. Early dissemination and death are

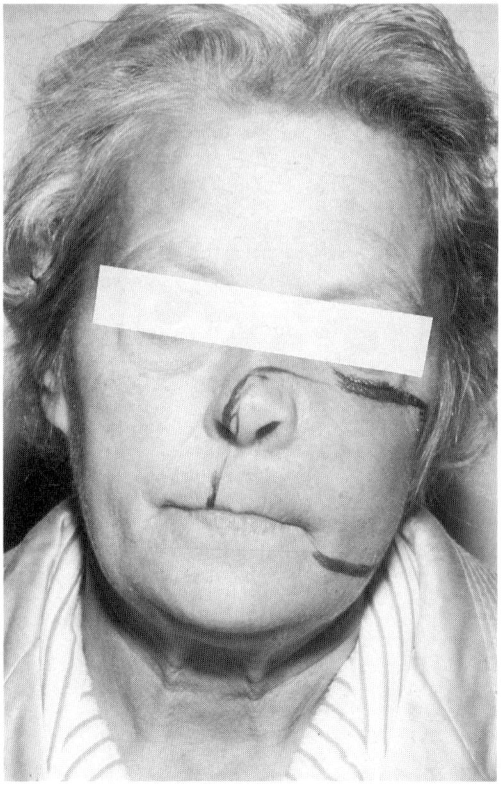

Figure 11.9 Extramedullary plasmacytoma of left maxillary antrum

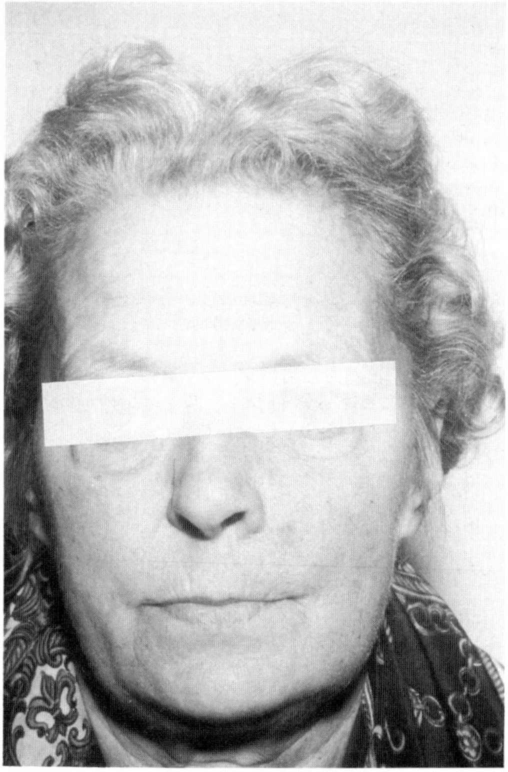

Figure 11.10 Same patient as in *Figure 11.9* with complete regression following local radiotherapy (4000 cGy in 20 fractions)

more common in solitary plasmacytoma of bone than in extramedullary plasmacytoma. Todd (1965) and Tong *et al.* (1980) report a 30% death rate within the first 3 years for solitary plasmacytoma of bone. Long-term survival is more common with extramedullary plasmacytoma. Corwin and Lindberg (1979) report that six of nine patients at risk for 10 years or more are still alive.

References

ADAMSON, J. W., FIALKOW, P. J., MURPHY, S., PRCHAL, J. F. and STEINMANN, L. (1976) Polycythaemia vera. Stem cell and probable clonal origin of the disease. *New England Journal of Medicine*, **295**, 913

ALEXANIAN, R., BALCERZAK, S., BONNER, J.D. *et al.* (1975) Prognostic factors in myeloma. *Cancer*, **36**, 1192

ALEXANIAN, R., GEHAN, E., HAUT, A., SAIKI, S. and WEICK, J. (1978) Unmaintained remission in myeloma. *Blood*, **51**, 1605

ALEXANIAN, R., HAUT, A., KHAN, A. V. *et al.* (1969) Treatment for multiple myeloma. *Journal of the American Medical Association*, **208**, 1680

BADGER, E., BUCKNER, C. D., THOMAS, E. D. *et al.* (1982) Allogeneic marrow transplantation for acute leukaemia in relapse. *Leukaemia Research*, **6**, 383

BATAILLE, R. and SANY, J. (1981) Solitary myeloma. *Cancer*, **48**, 845

BENNETT, J. M., CATOVSKY, D., DANIEL, M. T. *et al.* (1976) Proposals for the classification of acute leukaemia. *British Journal of Haematology*, **33**, 451

BERK, P. D., GOLDBERG, J. D., SILVERMAN, M. N. *et al.* (1981) Increased incidence of acute leukaemia in polycythaemia vera associated with chlorambucil therapy. *New England Journal of Medicine*, **304**, 441

BERSAGEL, D. C. (1972) Plasma cell myeloma — an interpretive review. *Cancer*, **30**, 1588

BERSAGEL, D. E., BAILEY, A. J., LANGLEY, G. R., McDONALD, R. N., WHITE, D. F. and MILLER, A. B. (1979) Chemotherapy of plasma cell myeloma and the incidence of acute leukaemia. *New England Journal of Medicine*, **301**, 743

BLACKLOCK, H. A., MATHEWS, J. R. D., BUCHANAN, J. E., OCKELFORD, P. A. and HILL, R. S. (1981) Improved survival in acute lymphoblastic leukaemia in adolescents and adults. *Cancer*, **48**, 1931

BLUME, K. G., SPRUCE, W. E., FORMAN, S. J. *et al.* (1981) Bone marrow transplantation for acute leukaemia. *New England Journal of Medicine*, **305**, 101

BODEY, G. P., FREIRICH, E. J. and McCREDIE, K. (1981) Prolonged remission in adult acute lymphoblastic leukaemia following late intensification and immunotherapy. *Cancer*, **47**, 1937

BORTIN, M. M., KAY, H. M., GALE, R. P. and RIMM, A. A. (1982) Factors associated with interstitial pneumonitis after bone marrow transplantation for acute leukaemia. *Lancet*, **1**, 437

BORTIN, M. M. and RIMM, A. A. (1977) Severe combined immunodeficiency disease. Characterisation of the disease and results of transplantation. *Journal of the American Medical Association*, **238**, 591

BOURONCLE, B. A. and DOAN, C. A. (1962) Myelofibrosis. Clinical, haematologic and pathologic study of 110 patients. *American Journal of Medical Science*, **243**, 697

BUCKMAN, R., CUZICK, J. and GALTON, D. A. G. (1982) Long term survival in myelomatosis. *British Journal of Haematology*, **52**, 589

BUCKNER, C. D., CLIFT, R. A., THOMAS, E. D. *et al.* (1982) Allogeneic marrow transplantation for patents with acute non lymphoblastic leukaemia in second remission. *Leukaemia Research*, **6**, 395

CALABRESI, P. and MEYER, O. O. (1959) Polycythaemia rubra vera II. Course and therapy. *Annals of Internal Medicine*, **50**, 1203

CASE, D. C., LEE, B. J. and CLARKSON, B. D. (1977) Improved survival times in multiple myeloma treated with M2 protocol. *American Journal of Medicine*, **63**, 897

CHAK, L. Y., SAPOZINK, M. D. and COX, R. S. (1983) Extramedullary lesions in non-lymphocytic leukaemia. Results of radiation therapy. *International Journal of Radiation Oncology, Biology and Physics*, **9**, 1173

CHAMPLIN, R., ZIGHELBOIM, W., HO, S. *et al.* (1983) Treatment of acute myelogenous leukaemia: bone marrow transplantation versus consolidation therapy. *Proceedings of the American Society of Clinical Oncology*, **2**, 180 (abstract C701)

CHIEVITZ, E. and THIEDE, T. (1962) Complications and cause of death in polycythaemia vera. *Acta Medica Scandinavica*, **172**, 513

CLARKSON, B., ARLIN, T., GEE, R. *et al.* (1983) Improved survival of acute lymphocytic leukaemia in adults. *Proceedings of the American Society of Clinical Oncology*, **2**, 180 (abstract C703)

CLIFT, R. A., BUCKNER, C. D., THOMAS, E. D. *et al.* (1982a) Allogeneic marrow transplantation using fractionated total body irradiation in patients with acute lymphoblastic leukaemia in relapse. *Leukaemia Research*, **6**, 401

CLIFT, R. A., BUCKNER, C. D., THOMAS, E. D. *et al.* (1982b) Allogeneic marrow transplantation for acute lymphoblastic leukaemia in remission using fractionated total body irradiation. *Leukaemia Research*, **6**, 509

COMAS, F. V., ANDREWS, G. A. and NELSON, B. (1968) Spleen irradiation in secondary hypersplenism. *Radiology*, **104**, 668

CORWIN, J. and LINDBERG, R. D. (1979) Solitary plasmacytoma of bone v extramedullary plasmacytoma and their relationships to multiple myeloma. *Cancer*, **43**, 1007

DEEG, H. J. (1983) Acute and delayed toxicity of total body irradiation. *International Journal of Radiation Oncology, Biology and Physics*, **9**, 1933

del REGATO, J. A. (1974) Total body irradiation in the treatment of chronic lymphocytic leukaemia (Janeway Lecture). *American Journal of Roentgenology*, **120**, 504

DOLIN, S. and DEWAR, J. P. (1956) Extramedullary plasmacytoma. *American Journal of Pathology*, **32**, 83

DURIE, B. G. M. and SALMON, S. E. (1975) A clinical staging for multiple myeloma. *Cancer*, **36**, 842

FEFER, A., CHEEVER, M. A. and BOYD, C. (1981) Clinical and cytogenetic complete remission in chronic myelogenous leukaemia after chemoradiotherapy and identical twin bone marrow transplantation. *Proceedings of the American Society of Clinical Oncology*, **22**, 492 (abstract C622)

FOON, K. A. and GALE, R. P. (1982) Controversies in the therapy of acute myelogenous leukaemia. *American Journal of Medicine*, **72**, 963

GALE, R. P. (1979) Advances in the treatment of acute

myelogenous leukaemia. *New England Journal of Medicine*, **300**, 1189

GALE, R. P., FEIG, S., OPELZ, G. *et al.* (1976) Bone marow transplantation in acute leukaemia using intensive chemotherapy. *Transplant Proceedings*, **8**, 611

GALTON, D. A. G. and PETO, R. (1968) A progress report on the MRC therapeutic trial in myelomatosis. *British Journal of Haematology*, **15**, 319

GALTON, D. A. G., WILTSHAW, E., SZUR, L. and DACIE, J. V. (1961) The use of chlorambucil and steroids in the treatment of chronic lymphatic leukaemia. *British Journal of Haematology*, **7**, 73

GILBERT, H. S. (1968) Problems relating to the control of polycythaemia rubra vera – the use of alkylating agents. *Blood*, **32**, 500

GOLDMAN, J. M., JOHNSON, S. A., CATOVSKY, D., WAREHAM, N. J. and GALTON, D. A. G. (1981) Autografting for chronic granulocytic leukaemia. *New England Journal of Medicine*, **304**, 700

GOOLDEN, A. W. G., GOLDMAN, J. M., KAM, K. C. *et al.* (1983) Fractionation of whole body irradiation before bone marrow transplantation for patients with leukaemia. *British Journal of Radiology*, **56**, 245

HARLEY, J. B., PATAK, T. F., McINTYRE, O. R. *et al.* (1979) Improved survival of increased risk myeloma patients on triple alkylating agent therapy. *Blood*, **54**, 13

HOBBS, J. R. (1967) Paraproteins. Benign or malignant? *British Medical Journal*, **3**, 699

HUGULEY, C. M. (1977) Treatment of chronic lymphocytic leukaemia. *Cancer Treatment Reviews*, **4**, 261

JOHNSON, R. E. (1976) Total body irradiation of chronic lymphocytic leukaemia: relationship between therapeutic response and prognosis. *Cancer*, **37**, 2691

JOHNSON R. E. (1977) Role of radiation therapy in the management of adult leukaemia. *Cancer*, **39**, 852

KEANE, T. J., VAN DYCK, J. and RIDER, W. D. (1981) Idiopathic interstitial pneumonitis following bone marrow transplantation. The relationship with total body irradiation. *International Journal of Radiation Oncology, Biology and Physics*, **7**, 1365

KEATING, M. J., SMITH, T. L., GEHAN, E. A. *et al.* (1980) Factors related to length of complete remission in adult acute leukaemia. *Cancer*, **45**, 2017

KIM, T. H., KERSEY, J., SEUCHAND, W., NESBIT, M. E., KRIVITT, W. and LEVITT, S. H. (1977) Total body irradiation with a high dose rate linear accelerator for bone marrow transplantation in aplastic anaemia and neoplastic disease. *Radiology*, **122**, 523

KORST, D. R., CLIFFORD, G. O., FOWLER, W. M., LOUIS, J. and WILSON, H. E. (1964) Multiple myeloma. *Journal of the American Medical Association*, **189**, 758

KYLE, R. A. (1975) Multiple myeloma. A review of 869 cases. *Mayo Clinic Proceedings*, **50**, 29

LAW, I. P. and BLOM, J. B. (1977) Adult acute leukaemia: frequency of CNS involvement in long term survivors. *Cancer*, **40**, 1304

LAWRENCE, J. H., SCOTT, K. G. and TUTTLE, L. W. (1939) Studies on leukaemia with the aid of radioactive phosphorus. *International Clinics*, **3**, 33

LAWRENCE, J. H., WINCHELL, H. S., and DONALD, W. G. (1969) Leukaemia in polycythaemia vera. *Annals of Internal Medicine*, **70**, 763

LEE, B. J., LAKE-LEWIN, D. and MYERS, J. E. (1982) Intensive treatment of multiple myeloma. In *Controversies in Oncology*, edited by P. H. Wiernik, pp. 61–79. New York: J. Wiley and Sons

LEE, B. J. and MYERS, J. E. (1983) Long term survival in multiple myeloma. *New England Journal of Medicine*, **309**, 243

LISTER, T. A., WHITEHOUSE, J. M. A., BEARD, M. E. J. *et al.* (1978) Combination chemotherapy for acute lymphoblastic leukaemia in adults. *British Medical Journal*, **1**, 199

MEDICAL RESEARCH COUNCIL WORKING PARTY (1968) Chronic granulocytic leukaemia. A comparison of radiotherapy and busulfan therapy. *British Medical Journal*, **1**, 201

MEDICAL RESEARCH COUNCIL WORKING PARTY (1980a) Second myelomatosis trial. *British Journal of Cancer*, **42**, 813

MEDICAL RESEARCH COUNCIL WORKING PARTY (1980b) Third myelomatosis trial. *British Journal of Cancer*, **42**, 823

MEYER, J. E. and SCHULZ, M. D. (1974) Solitary myeloma of bone. *Cancer*, **34**, 438–440

MILL, W. B. and GRIFFITH, R. (1980) The role of radiation therapy in the management of plasma cell tumours. *Cancer*, **45**, 647

MINOT, J. B., BUCKMAN, T. E. and ISAACS, R. (1924) Chronic myelogenous leukaemia — age, incidence, duration and benefit from irradiation. *Journal of the American Medical Association*, **82**, 1489

MODAN, B. and LILIENFIELD, A. M. (1964) Leukaemogenic effect of ionising radiation treatment in polycythaemia. *Lancet*, **2**, 439

MYELOMA TASK FORCE, NATIONAL CANCER INSTITUTE (1973) Guide lines for protocols. *Cancer Chemotherapy Reports*, **4**, 145

NEIMANN. P. E., MYERS, J. D., MODEIROS, E., McDONGALL, J. K. and THOMAS, K. D. (1980) Interstitial pneumonia following marrow transplantation for leukaemia and aplastic anaemia. In *Biology of Bone Marrow Transplantation,* edited by R. P. Gale, pp. 75–81. London: Academic Press

OMURA, G. A., MOFFIT, S., VOGLER, W. E. and SALTER, M. (1980) Combination chemotherapy of adult acute lymphoblastic leukaemia with randomised CNS prophylaxis. *Blood*, **55**, 199

PACCAGNELLA, A., CARTEI, G., FOSSER, V. *et al.* (1983) Treatment of multiple myeloma with M2 protocol and without maintenance therapy. *European Journal of Cancer and Clinical Oncology*, **19**, 1345

PEARSON, T. C. and WETHERLEY-MEIN, G. (1978) Vascular occlusive episodes and venous haematocrit in primary proliferative polycythaemia. *Lancet*, **2**, 1219

POWLES, R. L., BARRATT, A. J., CLINK, H., KAY, H. E. M., SLOANE, J. and McELWAIN, T. J. (1979) Cyclosporin A for treatment of graft versus host disease in man. *Lancet*, **2** 1327

POWLES, R. L., CLINK, H. M., BANDINI, L. *et al.* (1980) Place of bone marrow transplantation in acute myeloid leukaemia. *Lancet*, **1**, 1047

POWLES, R. L., SMITH, C., KOHN, J. and HAMILTON FAIRLEY, G. (1971) Method of removing abnormal protein rapidly from patients with malignant paraproteinaemia.*British Medical Journal*, **3**, 664

SALMON, S. E. (1975) Expansion of the growth fraction in multiple myeloma with alkylating agents. *Blood*, **45**, 119

SALMON, S. E., ALEXANIAN, R. and DIXON, D. (1979) Non cross-resistant combination chemotherapy improves survival in multiple myeloma. *Blood*, **54**, 207

SALMON, S. E. and DURIE, B. G. M. (1975) Cellular kinetics

in multiple myeloma. *Archives of Internal Medicine*, **135**, 131

SALMON, S. E. and SMITH, B. A. (1970) Immunoglobulin synthesis and total body tumour cell number in IgG myeloma. *Journal of Clinical Investigation*, **49**, 1114

SANDERS, J. (1982) Effects of cyclophosphamide and total body irradiation on ovarian and testicular function. *Experimental Haematology*, Suppl. **11**, 49

SOUTH WEST ONCOLOGY GROUP (1975) Remission maintenance therapy for multiple myeloma. *Archives of Internal Medicine*, **135**, 147

SPEED, D. E., GALTON, D. A. G. and SWAN, A. (1964) Melphalan in the treatment of myelomatosis. *British Medical Journal*, **1**, 1664

SZUR, L., LEWIS, S. M. and GOOLDEN, A. W. G. (1959) Polycythaemia vera and its treatment with radio-active phosphorus. *Quarterly Journal of Medicine*, **28**, 397

THOMAS, D. J., MARSHALL, J., ROSS RUSSELL, R. W., WETHERLEY-MEIN, G., du BOULAY, G. H. and PEARSON, T. C. (1977) Cerebral blood flow in polycythaemia. *Lancet*, **2**, 161

THOMAS, E. D., BUCKNER, C. D., BANEJI, M. *et al.* (1977) One hundred patients with acute leukaemia treated by chemotherapy, total body irradiation and allogeneic marrow transplantation. *Blood*, **49**, 511

THOMAS, E. D., BUCKNER, C. D., CLIFT, R. A. *et al.* (1979) Marrow transplantation for acute non lymphoblastic leukaemia in first remission *New England Journal of Medicine*, **301**, 597

THOMAS, E. D., CLIFT, R. A., HERSMAN, J. *et al.* (1982) Marrow transplantation for acute non lymphoblastic leukaemia in first remission using fractionated or single dose irradiation. *International Journal of Radiation Oncology, Biology and Physics*, **8**, 817

TODD, I. D. H. (1965) Treatment of solitary plasmacytoma. *Clinical Radiology*, **16**, 395

TONG, D., GRIFFIN, T. W., LARAMORE, G. E. *et al.* (1980) Solitary plasmacytoma of bone and soft tissues. *Radiology*, **135**, 195

WEIDEN, P. L., SULLIVAN, K. M., FLUORNOY, M. S., STORB, R. and THOMAS, E. D. (1981) Antileukaemic effect of chronic graft versus host disease. *New England Journal of Medicine*, **304**, 1529

WILSON, J. F. and JOHNSON, R. E. (1971) Splenic irradiation following chemotherapy in chronic leukaemia. *Radiology*, **101**, 657

WILTSHAW, E. (1976) The natural history of extramedullary plasmacytoma and its relationship with solitary myeloma of bone. *Medicine* (Baltimore), **55**, 217

WOLK, R., MASSE, S., CONKLIN, R. and FREIRICH, E. (1974) The incidence of CNS involvement in adults with acute leukaemia. *Cancer*, **33**, 863

WOODRUFF, R. K., WHITTLE, J. M. and MALPAS, J. S. (1979) Solitary plasmacytoma I. Extramedullary soft tissue plasmacytoma. *Cancer*, **43**, 2344

WOODS, W. G., DEHNER, L. P., NESBIT, M. E. *et al.* (1980) Fatal veno-occlusive disease following high dose chemotherapy, irradiation and bone marrow transplantation. *American Journal of Medicine*, **68**, 285

YENTIS, I. (1956) The so-called solitary plasmacytoma of bond. *Journal of Faculty of Radiologists*, **8**, 132

12

Skin malignancy

D. G. Bratherton

The treatment of skin malignancy forms a large part of the work of any radiotherapy department, skin cancer being second only to lung cancer in its frequency. As many of the tumours are small and easily curable they tend to be regarded as insignificant. There is thus a danger that a standard treatment may produce a cosmetic result which falls short of the best obtainable. There are many ways of treating skin cancer and this is an area where consultation between dermatologist, radiation oncologist and surgeon can be most fruitful.

Aetiology

Sunlight

Ultraviolet radiation plays a large part in the production of skin cancer. In Australia, where white skins are exposed to high levels of sunlight, the frequency is the highest in the world (Doll, 1977), and in Queensland, 20% of men may expect to develop skin cancer before the age of 75. Fortunately, the population is well aware of this fact and seeks treatment at an early stage. The face, being more often exposed, is the commonest site for basal and squamous cancer. An increase in skin cancer may be expected with the rise in popularity of sun bathing and the use of sun lamps in the home. This increase has already been seen in melanoma (Bakos and McMillan, 1973; Retsas, 1982).

Ionizing radiation

Many of the early pioneers working with X-rays developed skin cancer on the hands and face, some of which proved fatal. X-ray induced cancer is now seen in patients treated many years ago for benign disease.

Epilation of the scalp for ringworm was a very useful treatment before the development of the fungicides. X-rays were very effective in reducing the pain and stiffness of ankylosing spondylitis and, before the danger of leukaemia was appreciated, multiple courses were sometimes given. These frequent repeated small doses were followed many years later by basal cell carcinoma in a small proportion of cases. These malignancies differ in no way from spontaneous malignancies and are equally sensitive to radiation which can be used unless the skin is devitalized or atrophic.

Old scars

Cancer developing in old scars is a clinical rarity and occurs when there has been poor healing and frequent breakdown of the skin. This so-called Marjolin's ulcer is preferably treated with surgery and grafting of healthy skin as radionecrosis is likely after radiotherapy (*Figure 12.1*).

Chemicals

Tar warts progressing to squamous cell carcinoma are well known in the gas and tar industry. Cotton workers in the Lancashire mills worked all day in clothes soaked in mineral oil which was rubbed into the groins as they leant over the looms. Many subsequently developed cancer of the scrotum.

A previous generation used the arsenical Fowler's solution as a tonic for its anaemic and debilitated young, and this has now produced a crop of skin

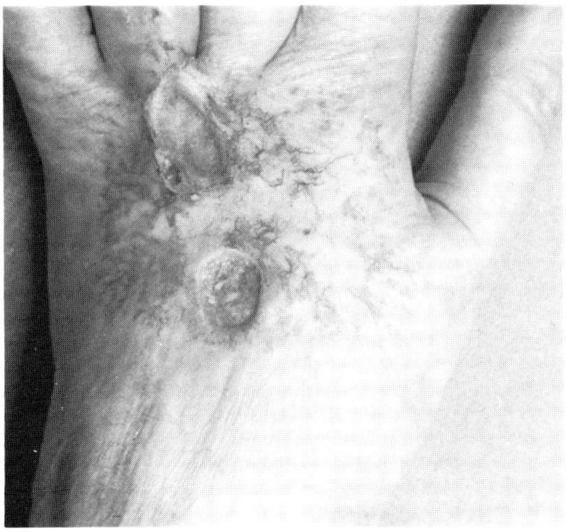

Figure 12.1 Squamous cell carcinoma developing in the scar of a burn received when a child. Treatment 20 years ago by radium mould. Healed for 10 years before becoming radionecrotic after minor injury. Initial plastic surgery would have been preferable

lesions mainly of the intraepidermal or Bowen's type. These are in areas not exposed to sunlight and may be associated with other internal cancers.

Genetic

The albino has a high incidence of basal and squamous cancer in exposed sites. Gorlin's syndrome is an inherited disease with several unusual features. Multiple basal cell lesions develop mainly on the face but also at other sites including the legs, back and perineum. The mandible contains cysts lined with squamous epithelium, and bony abnormalities include frontal bossing, abnormal dentition and bifid ribs. In the skull the falx is calcified and the pituitary fossa bridged over. The hands show pits on the palmar surface. These patients may also develop ovarian tumours or medulloblastoma, a tendency they pass on to their offspring. The sheer number of the lesions poses problems for the radiotherapist and it may be necessary to use fields with square edges where lesions are contiguous.

Xeroderma pigmentosa is a congenital condition in which increased sensitivity to sunlight produces basal and squamous lesions at an early age. Protective barrier creams and sunglasses are essential, prevention being better than cure.

Epidermolysis bullosa has as its main feature large bullae which progress to shedding of the epithelium of both skin and mucous membranes. Squamous carcinoma may develop on these scarred areas which, being devitalized, do not support radiotherapy well.

Anatomy

The epidermis itself is avascular, deriving its nutrition from vascular loops projecting from the dermis. It may well be this avascularity that explains the poor results from chemotherapy in most skin cancer. Mitotic cells are found in the lowest or basal cell layer and in the prickle cell layer from which they pass to the granular layer and finally to the horny layer of keratin. This process takes about a month. The production of cells keeps pace with the rate of desquamation so that the thickness of the epidermis remains constant. The rate of division is reduced by methotrexate, bleomycin and other anticancer drugs.

The basal cell layer also contains melanocytes which increase under the influence of ultraviolet light to produce pigmentation. Basal cell carcinoma develops from the basal cell layer forming clumps of densely staining round cells whereas squamous cell carcinoma is produced from the prickle cell layer. Some of the cells form keratin in the shape of cell nests.

The dermis makes up the greater part of the skin and contains collagen and elastic fibres supporting blood vessels, nerves and lymphatics. The hair follicles are at a depth of 2–3 mm and thus do not escape irradiation with most skin treatment by radiotherapy. Single doses of 500 cGy produce temporary epilation, which is likely to be permanent with a single dose of 1000 cGy or its equivalent in fractionated dosage.

Cell layers superficial to the basal layer are often shed after an injury either from friction, heat, ultraviolet or X-rays. A blister then forms outside the basal cell layer and the superficial layers are shed as moist desquamation. Healing is complete and the final cosmetic result is good. More extensive irradiation with X-rays produces a blister below the basal cell layer in the dermis. Subsequent healing takes place with scarring and a poor cosmetic result.

Pathology

There are a great many different types of skin tumours, the majority being benign and resistant to radiation with X-rays. The radiotherapist therefore sees a selected population of which the most frequent are basal cell carcinomas (60%), followed by squamous carcinomas (30%) and finally melanomas (5%). The remaining tumours are rare and being radioresistant are mainy a surgical problem. They include dermatofibroma protuberans, which may recur locally but rarely metastasizes, and the dangerous angiosarcoma which develops in the oedematous arm after mastectomy. Others such as mycosis fungoides and the lymphomas are very radiosensitive. Keratocanthoma is often confused with squamous

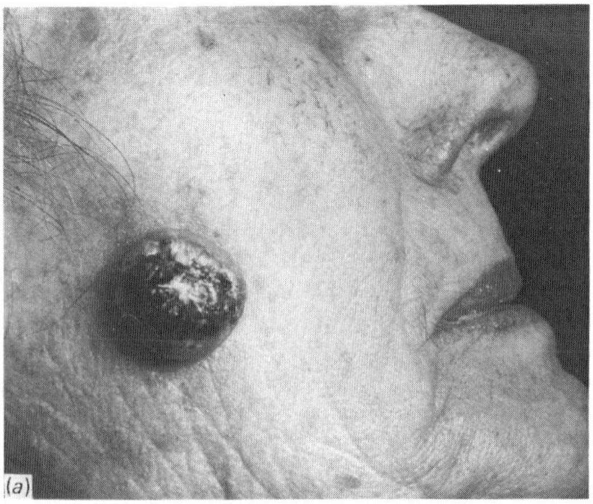

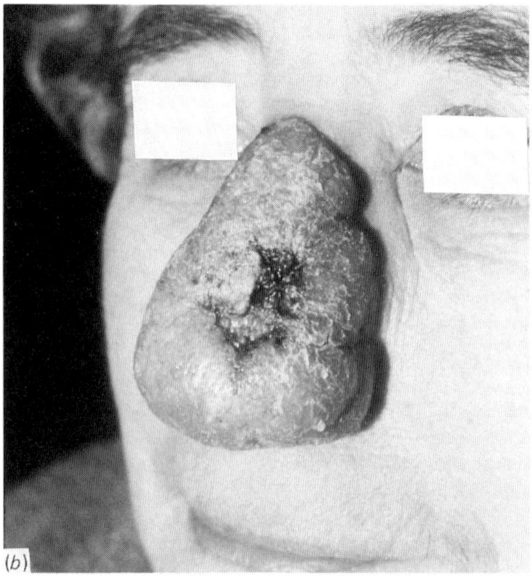

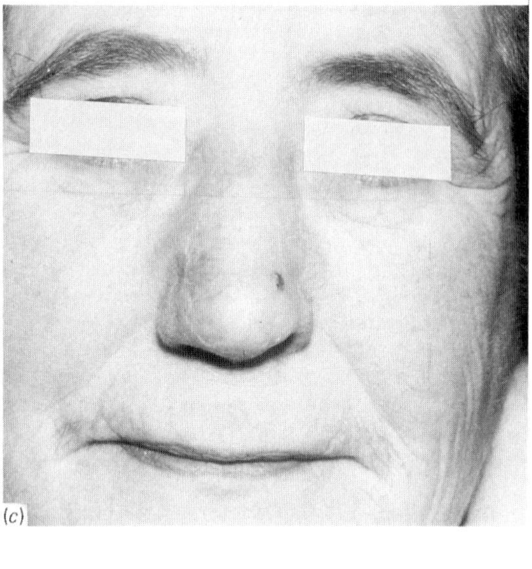

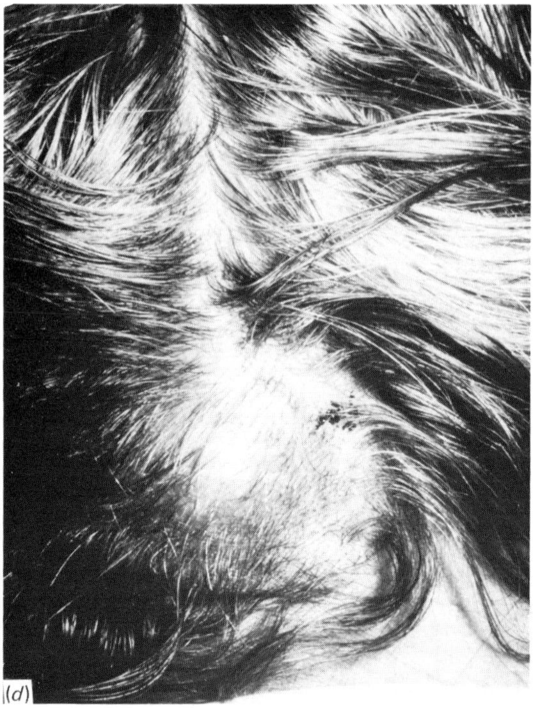

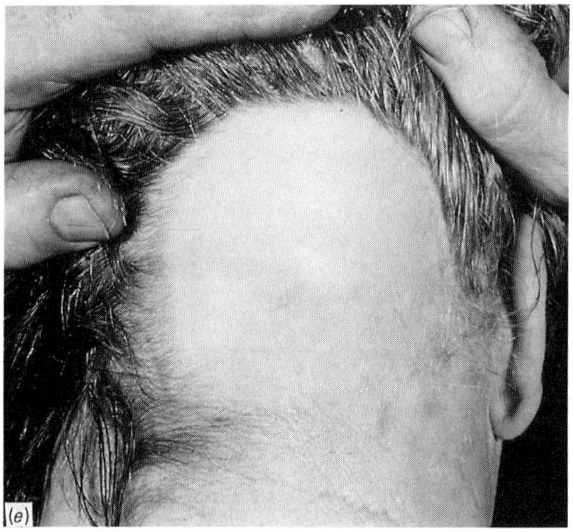

Figure 12.2 (*a*) Keratoacanthoma. Distinguishing features are rapid growth and sharply defined edge and central keratin plug. (*b*) Large keratoacanthoma treated with 5000 cGy 3 weeks (15 daily fractions) 300 kV. (*c*) One year after treatment. (*d*) Skin appendage tumour recurrent after local surgery. Treated with 10 MeV electrons 5500 cGy in 20 daily fractions (*e*) One year after treatment. (Courtesy of Dr H.F. Hope-Stone)

carcinoma especially when atypical. The distinguishing features are the well defined edge of the lesion and the central keratin plug (*Figure 12.2a*). They respond to a dose three-quarters of that required for established carcinoma. If there is any doubt at all about the pathology they should receive full treatment and follow-up as for carcinoma (*Figure 12.2b, c*).

Carcinoma of the sebaceous glands (skin appendage tumours) is more frequently seen on the head and neck. It does not often spread to lymphatic glands and is usually cured by local excision, if recurrent, electron therapy, 5000–5500 cGy in 20 daily fractions will control the condition (*Figure 12.2d, e*). Tumours of the sweat glands appear more often in the axilla, scrotum or vulva, all of which are tissues which tolerate radiation badly. They are again a surgical problem and often require a block dissection of involved regional nodes. Tricoepithelioma and trichofolliculoma arise from hair follicles and are locally malignant responding to local excision.

Premalignant conditions

Solar keratitis

Both X-rays and sunlight produce keratotic changes which may progress through carcinoma *in situ* to full malignancy. The appearances are those of dry atrophic skin, often scaly, with an indefinite edge, sometimes pigmented. These lesions rarely metastasize and it is important not to over treat with X-rays in skin which is already devitalized.

Bowen's disease

This presents as reddened patches with a sharp edge not confined to exposed areas and often multiple. There may be a history of arsenical medication in the past. The changes are limited to the epidermis, but 5% show evidence of invasion in the larger lesions. One-third of these may produce secondary deposits and it is for this reason that the disease must be treated early. There is a tendency for these patients to have malignant disease elsewhere.

Queyrat's erythroplasia

This is an intraepidermal lesion affecting the penis or vulva. Surgical removal is usually effective, irradiation can be used to treat the former (*see* Chapter 3).

Extramammary Paget's disease

This is more common in the female affecting the vulva or perianal skin. It is characterized microscopically by the presence of large clear Paget's cells in the underlying dermis. There is often an underlying carcinoma of apocrine origin especially in the perianal region. Radiotherapy is disappointing due to the presence of infection and the difficulty of keeping the area dry. Therefore surgery is always the treatment of choice.

Staging

The International Union Against Cancer (UICC) classification for verified skin cancer (apart from melanoma) is based on division into six regions (*Table 12.1*).

Table 12.1 The UICC classification for verified skin cancer

Regions

(a)	Eyelid, ear and nose
(b)	Face, scalp and neck
(c)	Upper limb
(d)	Trunk above umbilicus
(e)	Trunk below umbilicus
(f)	Lower limb

Regional nodes to which the above spread are:

(a) and (b)	Cervical (bilateral)
(c)	Axillary and epitrochlear (unilateral)
(d)	Axillary (bilateral)
(e)	Inguinal (bilateral)
(f)	Inguinal and popliteal (unilateral)

T Primary tumour

T1s	Preinvasive carcinoma (carcinoma **in situ**)
T0	No evidence of primary tumour
T1	Tumour 2 cm or less and strictly superficial
T2	Tumour over 2 cm but not more than 5 cm with minimal deep extension
T3	Tumour over 5 cm or with deep dermal extension
T4	Tumour in cartilage, muscle or bone

N Regional lymph nodes

N0	No palpable nodes
N1	Movable homolateral nodes
N1a	Nodes not considered to contain growth
N1b	Nodes considered to contain growth
N2	Movable contralateral or bilateral nodes
N2a	Nodes not considered to contain growth
N2b	Nodes considered to contain growth
N3	Fixed nodes

M Distant metastases

M0	No evidence of distant metastases
M1	Distant metastases or satellite nodules more than 5 cm from primary

Treatment for precancerous skin lesions

Actinic keratosis

Treatment depends on clinical assessment of the thickness of the lesion. Transition to malignancy is often difficult to assess pathologically as the biopsy may not be typical of the whole lesion. Superficial areas may be treated by electrocautery or by the application of 5-fluorouracil ointment. A 5% concentration is applied daily for 3–4 weeks according to the reaction produced.

Bowen's disease

Lesions are mostly superficial but larger areas may have infiltration in the centre. X-rays at 90 kV are used with a single dose of 2000 cGy or with a fractionated regimen, as outlined below, for squamous carcinoma.

Treatment of early basal and squamous carcinoma

Most dermatologists use curettage and electrocoagulation for small basal cell carcinomas. The treatment is quick and can be carried out at one session at which the curettings can be examined immediately under the microscope. This is the preferred treatment for the cystic type of basal cell carcinoma which tends to resolve very slowly after X-ray therapy. The cosmetic result is acceptable if the lesion is not above 3 cm diameter, and the process may be repeated if there is a recurrence.

Radiotherapy

Many small lesions can be successfully treated by a single dose of X-rays and this is a great advantage in the elderly or for people who are geographically isolated. However, the cosmetic result can be vastly improved by fractionation and therefore a compromise must be sought. A weekly treatment gives an acceptable result, but for the young patient with a long life expectancy further fractionation to nine or 15 treatments is desirable. Large or deeply infiltrating lesions also require more fractions. The small growth of 2–3 cm can be treated with X-rays of 90–150 kV according to the depth of infiltration. A short focus skin distance (FSD) of 15 cm will give a high output and short treatment time which is an advantage when dealing with the elderly or with people who are nervous or have difficulty in keeping still. Single doses tend to leave a sharp punched out margin which is often conspicuous. This may be avoided by using a lead shield with a bevelled edge which produces a more gradual fall off of dose at the periphery. A set of these lead shields for circles of various diameters may be made of lead 1 mm thick for 90 kV X-rays and 2 mm thick for 150 kV X-rays. Irregular areas or shielding for complex sites such as the inner canthus may need the specialist services of a mould room.

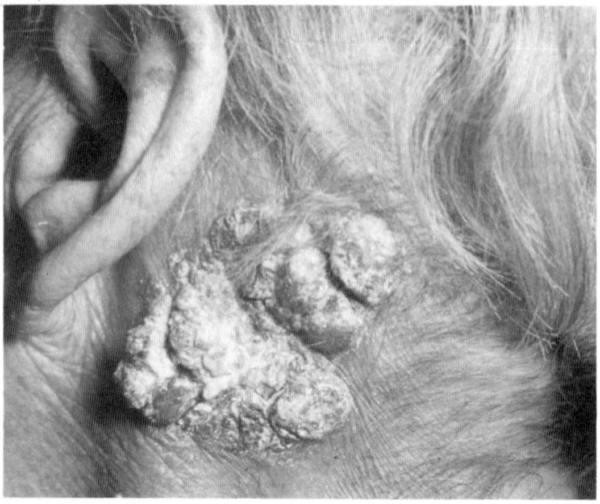

Figure 12.3 (*a*) Rapidly growing squamous cell carcinoma with many mitoses in a woman of 86. Because of age few fractions used

The type of X-rays used will depend on the depth of infiltration but also on the nature of the underlying tissues. Soft radiation is selectively absorbed in bone and cartilage and where these are involved high voltage irradiation with electrons is the ideal. If these are not available 250–300 kV X-rays are preferable to 90 kV, and treatment must be fractionated. Large lesions require five fractions a week for at least 3 weeks whereas smaller lesions may be treated with fewer visits. The doses given below with their equivalent nominal standard doses in rets may be employed.

2000 cGy single dose
900 cGy weekly for 3 weeks—total 2700 cGy (1780 rets)
1000 cGy weekly for 3 weeks—total 3000 cGy (1800 rets) (*Figure 12.3*)
500 cGy 3 times a week for 3 weeks—total 4500 cGy (2000 rets)
4200 cGy in 10 daily treatments.

Larger doses than this are often given and these date from an era when much more advanced and neglected growths were encountered. These doses produce an unacceptably poor cosmetic result in the smaller lesions seen today.

Care must be taken in certain areas which tolerate radiation badly. The anterior abdominal wall is more easily damaged, either by burns or radiation, than the posterior surface. The back of the hand is another danger area because of the underlying tendons and

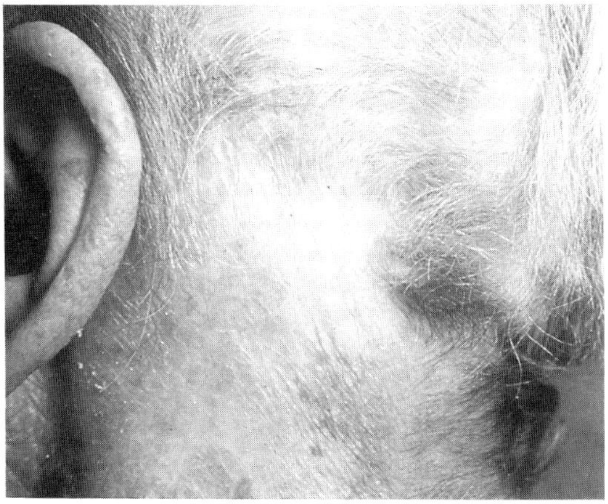

Figure 12.3 (*b*) After 220 kV X-rays, three weekly doses of 1000 cGy (1880 rets, NSD)

the absence of subcutaneous tissue (*see Figure 12.1*).

The skin of the lower limb heals poorly, especially if varicose veins are present, and squamous carcinoma developing in a varicose ulcer demands excision and grafting.

Treatment of advanced disease

Several varieties of basal cell carcinoma are recognized, the most frequent being a raised nodule on the face often with dilated capillaries coursing over the edge. The epidermis over it may be intact with the nodule being palpable as a fibrous plaque. A more superficial type has areas which have healed with a tissue paper scar. These apparently healed areas must be included in the treated zone. The morphoeic type presents as a flat plaque which is slightly raised, while other lesions are pigmented and may be confused with malignant melanoma. Others may be cystic. All these varieties respond equally well to radiation and their distinction is of academic interest only.

The amount of infiltration is, however, of great importance and the clinician must recognize the deeply penetrating or terebrant variety (*Figures 12.4, 12.5 and 12.6*). In this type, infiltration is present

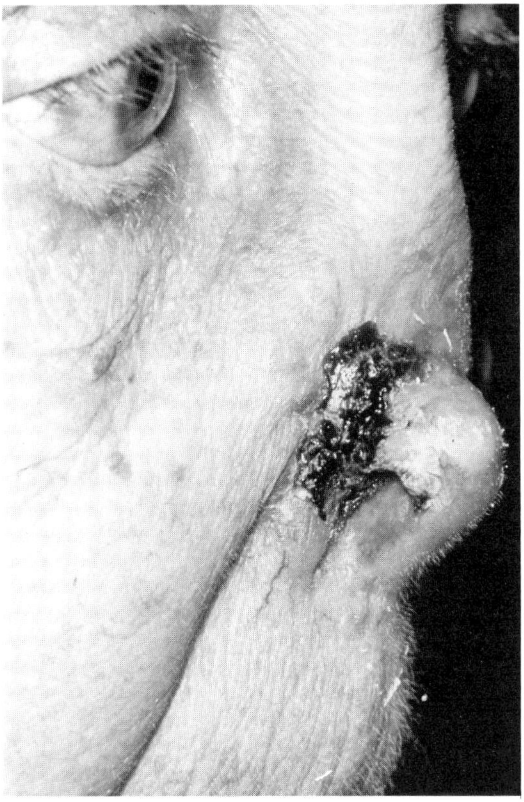

Figure 12.4 (*a*) Penetrating basal cell carcinoma in scar of old lupus in woman of 84 with severe head tremor. Lesion outlined by lead shield using larger field to overcome effect of tremor.

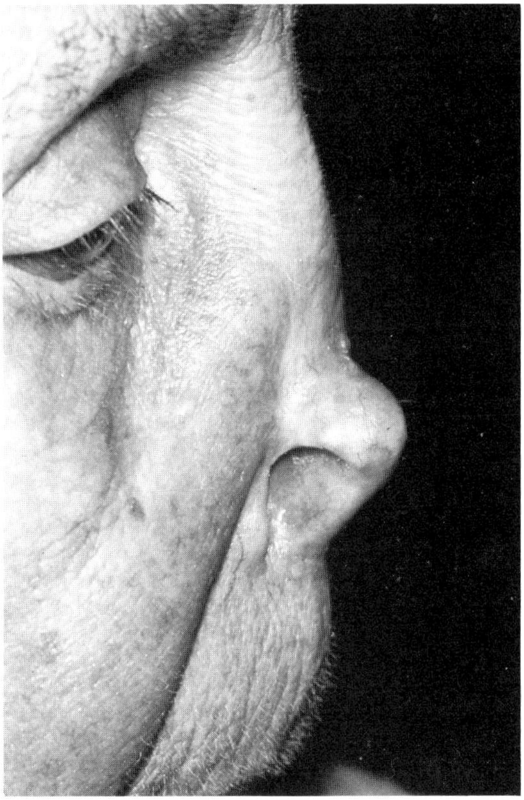

Figure 12.4 (*b*) After electron therapy, 10 MeV, 4050 cGy in nine treatments over 21 days (1700 rets NSD)

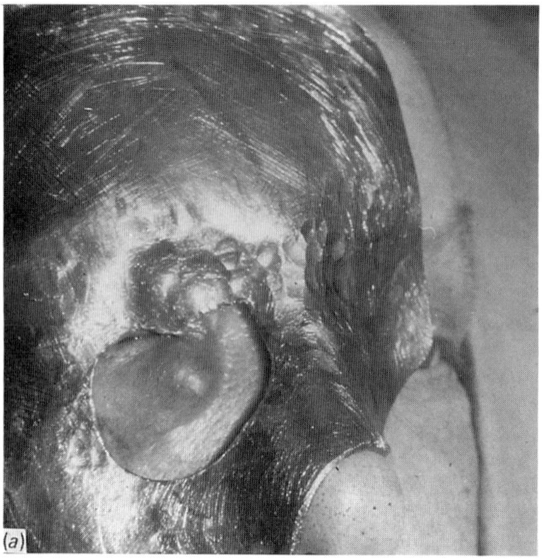

Figure 12.5 (*a*) Penetrating basal cell carcinoma fixed deeply to medial side of orbit. Lead shield 2 mm thick protects eye. Dose 5000 cGy 15 treatments in 18 days of 250 kV X-rays.

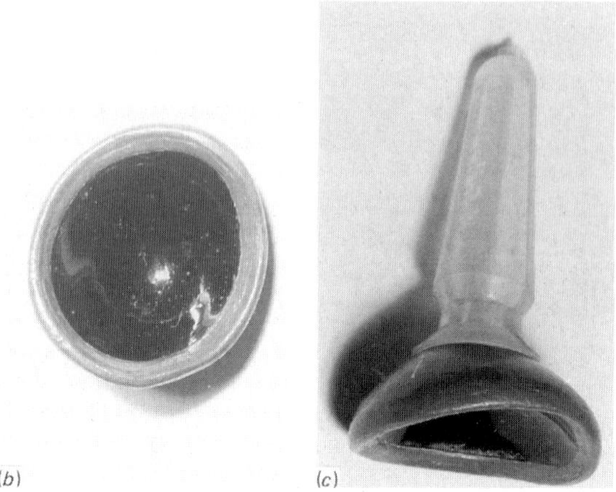

Figure 12.5 (*b*)Contact eye shield. (*c*) Rubber sucker to remove eye shield

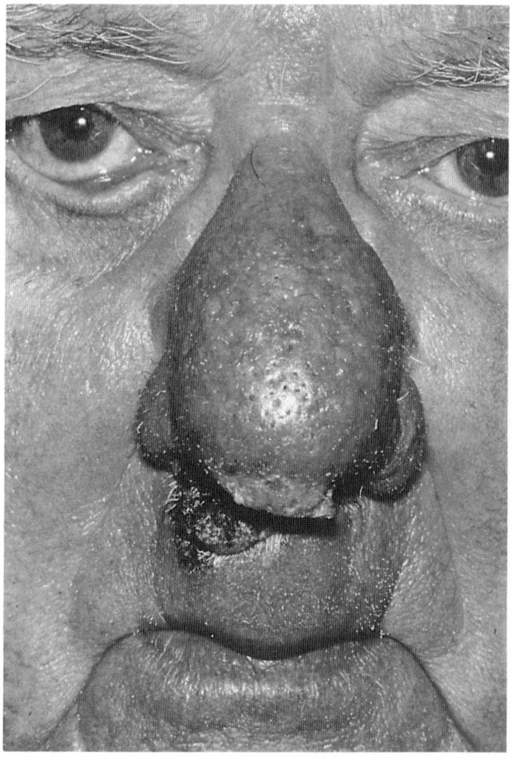

Figure 12.6 (*a*) Squamous cell carcinoma of the nose and columella.

from the start and failure to cure may lead to a fatal conclusion after many ineffective treatments. Here full dosage and fractionation are essential.

In most cases of this type it is necessary to make a lead shield to outline the tumour with a margin of 8–10 mm all around. This is particularly important if the patient has difficulty in keeping still, as even small movements are of significance. The production of lead shields is a precision technique which ideally requires the facility of a mould room. An accurate

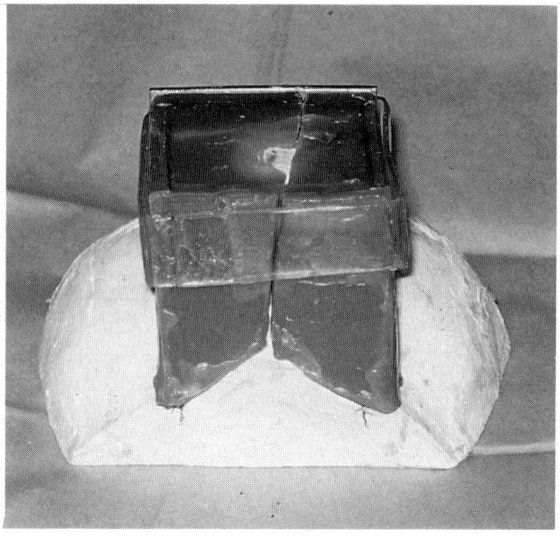

Figure 12.6 (*b*) Wax build up made for 20 MeV electron therapy. Dose 5000 cGy 15 treatments three times a week for 5 weeks. The patient is well to date at 3 years

model of the patient is constructed by the following method. Plaster of Paris bandages are first applied to the region to be treated which has been greased to facilitate removal. When these are set, they are removed to form a mould from which the model is made and on this the exact area to be treated can be drawn. It is then possible to make the lead cut-out (*Figure 12.5*) or to make a wax seating for electron therapy (*Figure 12.6b*).

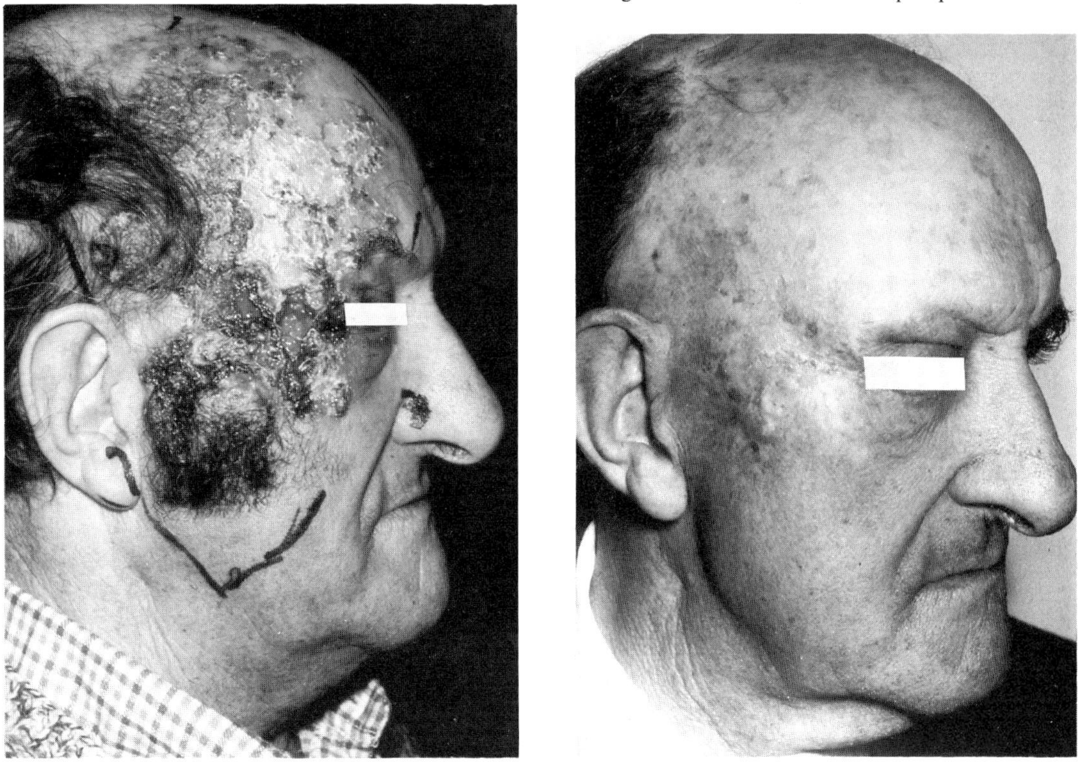

Figure 12.7 (*a*) Neglected basal cell carcinoma in male aged 64.

(*b*) After treatment with electrons at 6 MeV 4500 cGy in nine treatments in 19 days (1990 rets NSD)

Suitable doses are 5000 cGy in 15 daily treatments over 3 weeks (18 days, 2000 rets) or 5500 cGy in 25 daily treatments over 5 weeks (32 days, 1980 rets) using either 250–300 kV X-rays or electrons at 6–10 MeV (*Figures 12.7 and 12.8*).

Special sites

Inner canthus

Stenosis of the tear duct may follow irradiation of this area which may be most troublesome, especially out of doors, or in a strong wind. Attempts to keep it open by probing are rarely successful and the patient must be warned of this possibility if the punctum has to be included in the treatment field. Care must be taken to shield it if it is not involved (*see Figure 12.5a*).

Lower eyelid

The cornea can be protected by a contact eyeshield fitting below both lids made of perspex with a lead backing (*see Figure 12.5b*). These are sterilized in chlorhexidine gluconate solution rather than phenol-based antiseptics which might attack the plastic. They are washed in saline to remove any trace of the solution. The eye is anaesthetized with drops of 1% amethocaine hydrochloride having warned the patient that these sting before producing anaesthesia. After sterile drops of paraffin have been inserted the patient is asked to look down while the shield is inserted below the upper lid, and to look up while it is pushed behind the lower lid. After the treatment the procedure is reversed by pushing the lower lid below the eyeshield to break the contact and allowing it to slip out easily. A small rubber suction pad will facilitate removal (*see Figure 12.5c*). The patient is sent out with an eyepad to protect the eye from dust

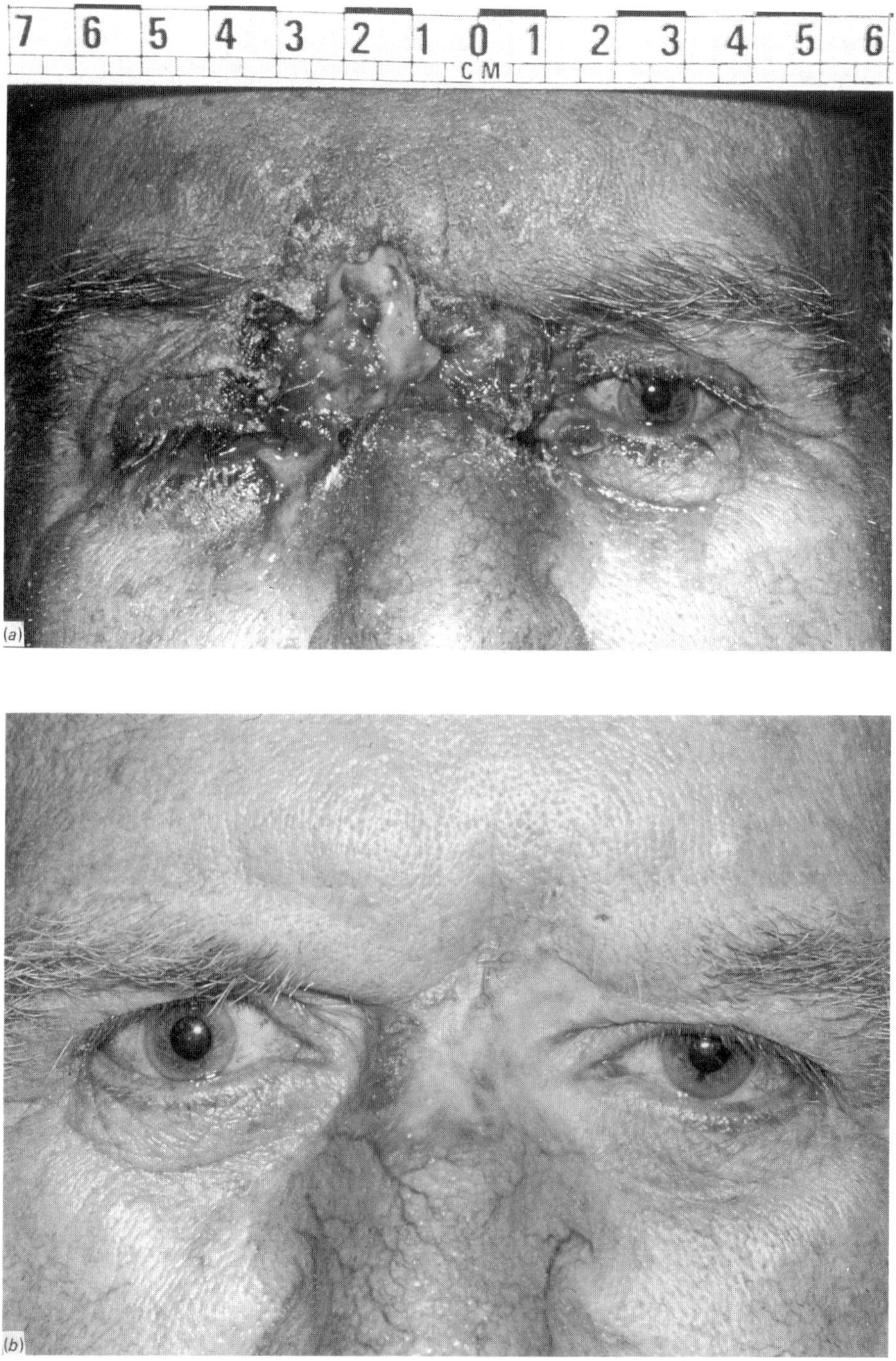

Figure 12.8 (*a*) Extensive basal cell carcinoma. (*b*) After electron therapy 6 MeV, total 4500 cGy in nine treatments three times a week for 3 weeks (1990 rets NSD)

until sensitivity returns to the cornea. If this type of eyeshield is used the upper lid must be protected by an additional external shield. An alternative to the internal shield is one which is placed between the lids after the upper lid is closed and secured with sellotape. The shield is not then in contact with the cornea and can be a simple polished piece of lead (*Figure 12.9*).

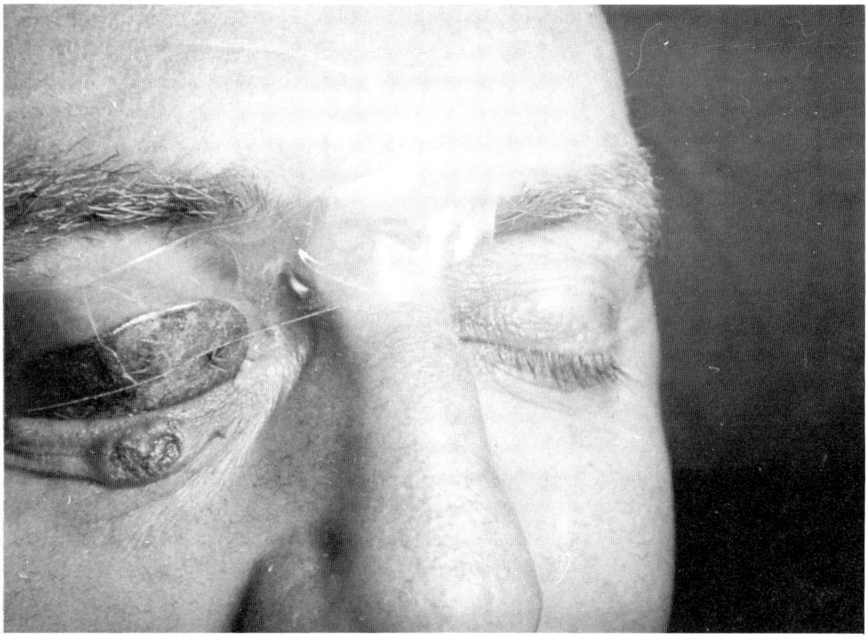

Figure 12.9 Lead shield placed in front of closed upper lid for treatment of basal cell carcinoma of lower lid

Upper eyelid

Small lesions not involving the whole lid may be treated after insertion of an internal eyeshield, but if the whole lid is involved there is a great danger of a dry eye due to absence of tears which may progress to corneal ulceration. Hypermellose drops may help, but surgical removal and grafting may be preferable.

Entrance to auditory canal

This is a difficult site on account of the convolutions and the cartilage immediately below the tumour. Electron therapy is ideal but an alternative is a contact mould of dental wax which can be moulded accurately into the convolutions and contours of the ear. Radioactive gold grains are inserted 5 mm into the mould to give a surface dose of 6000 cGy in 7 days.

Entrance to the nasal cavity

If the columella is involved treatment with a wax mould is indicated using either opposed fields or a platform for electron therapy (*see Figure 12.6*).

Lip

Small lesions are treated with a regimen which allows treatment to be completed before the reaction commences. This avoids handling a painful lip. A suitable shield is made by cutting a semicircular flap in a piece of lead 2 mm thick and bending this back to fit behind the lip and to protect the tongue (*Figure 12.10*). For small lesions, a regimen of seven daily doses of 550 cGy of 90 kV X-rays (total 4950 cGy in 8 days, 1920 ret) is adequate.

Larger or infiltrating lesions (*Figure 12.11a*) require a 3-week course of 250 kV X-rays to a total dose of 5000 cGy in 15 treatments over 18 days (2000 rets). If electrons are used, the lip may be built up with a wax seating and a similar dose given. With prolonged treatment regimens the patient may have difficulties in eating due to the reaction, and a split course regimen is useful such as 2000 cGy in 2 weeks (10 treatments) alternating with 2 weeks' rest to a total dose of 6000 cGy (*Figure 12.11b*).

Carcinoma of the lip may also be treated by a double-mould technique using cobalt-60 sources. The slow dose rate and the lack of a sharp edge to the irradiated area give an excellent cosmetic result. The disadvantage is the need to hospitalize the patient and the exposure of staff to radiation. The cobalt tubes of the inner mould are mounted on a bite block which is secured by a rod to the outer perspex plate, thus ensuring an accurate separation between the two moulds. The mould is worn for 6 – 8 hours a day for 1 week. For a lip thickness of 1 cm, the dose to the skin is 5500 cGy and to the mucosa 6500 cGy giving a central dose of 5000 cGy. The method cannot be used if the lesion extends down to the sulcus inside the

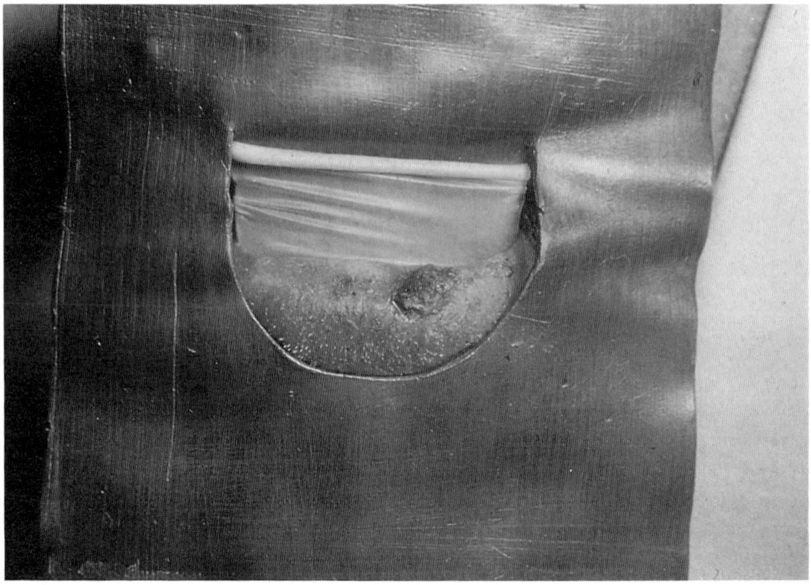

Figure 12.10 Lead shield for the treatment of carcinoma of the lower lip. The semi-circular flap is bent backwards and placed behind the lip to protect the tongue, and is covered with a rubber finger cot

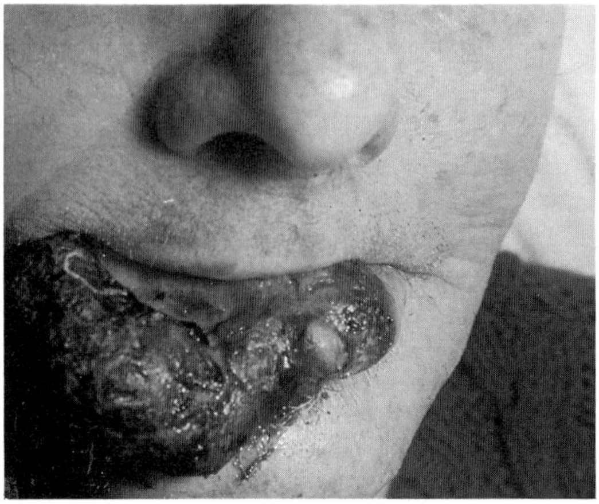

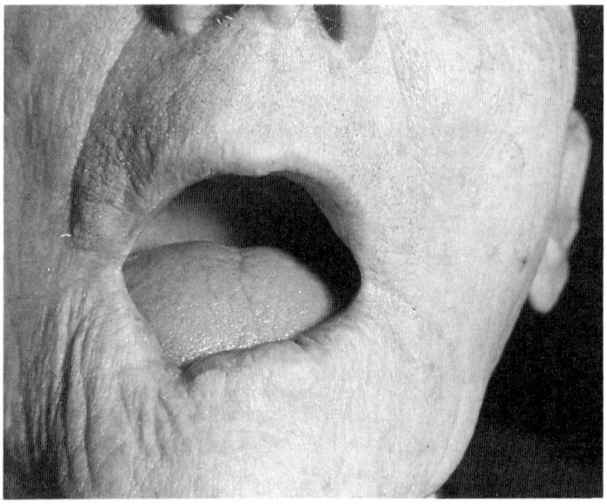

Figure 12.11 (*a*) Squamous cell carcinoma of the lip in male aged 77. Treated as a split course to allow the reaction to settle. Lead shield behind lip

(*b*) After X-rays at 250 kV, seven treatments of 400 cGy in 2 weeks, 2 weeks rest, and a further similar course. Total 5600 cGy in 14 treatments in 47 days

mouth as the inner mould cannot be placed below the tumour.

Pinna of the ear

A lesion often confused with carcinoma is the small ulcerated nodule on the edge of the pinna due to chondritis of the underlying cartilage. It is exquisitely tender especially when the patient sleeps on that side. It requires local excision. Carcinoma of the ear requires high energy radiation on account of the underlying cartilage (*Figure 12.11c,d*). If electron therapy is not available small lesions can be treated by an elastoplast mould, bearing radioactive gold grains, treating at a distance of 0.5 cm. This is worn continuously for 7 days giving a surface dose of 6000 cGy.

Thicker lesions which have not spread on to the side of the scalp are suitable for treatment by a

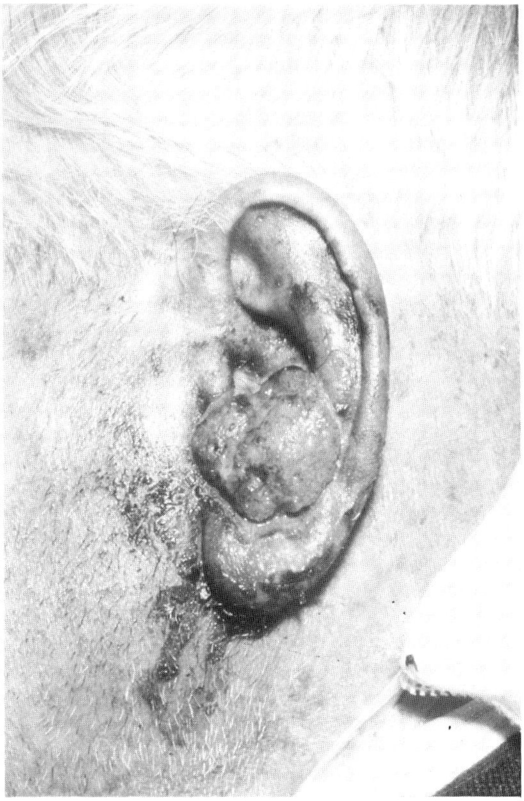

Figure 12.11 (*c*) Squamous cell carcinoma — left pinna

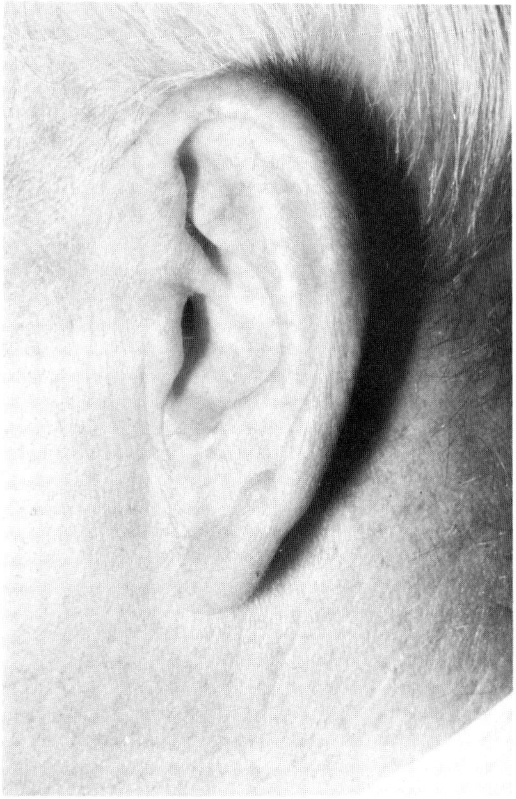

(*d*) After 10 MeV electron therapy — 5500 cGy in 20 daily fractions

double mould calculated to give a combined skin dose from both moulds of 5500 – 6000 cGy in 7 days (*Figure 12.11e,f,g*). If neither mould room facilities nor electrons are available, X-rays at 250–300 kV are preferable to lower voltage radiation, and antibiotics are indicated to control infection. A suitable dose is 5000 cGy in 15 daily treatments over 3 weeks (2000 rets NSD).

Late complications of radiotherapy

Heavy doses of radiation may lead to a gradual reduction of blood supply to the irradiated area due to a slow process of endarteritis in which the intimal cells proliferate to narrow the lumen of the arterioles. This may be of little importance unless there is a sudden call for increased blood supply after trauma, sunburn or infection. The resulting radionecrosis may take months to heal requiring long-term treatment with low dose antibiotics. Plastic surgery will shorten the treatment time. These events are more likely to follow second courses of treatment or the irradiation of tissues whose blood supply has already been compromised by scarring or varicose ulceration (*see*

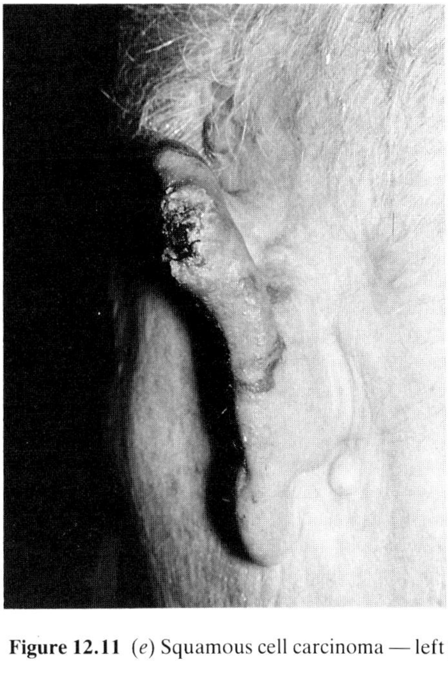

Figure 12.11 (*e*) Squamous cell carcinoma — left pinna

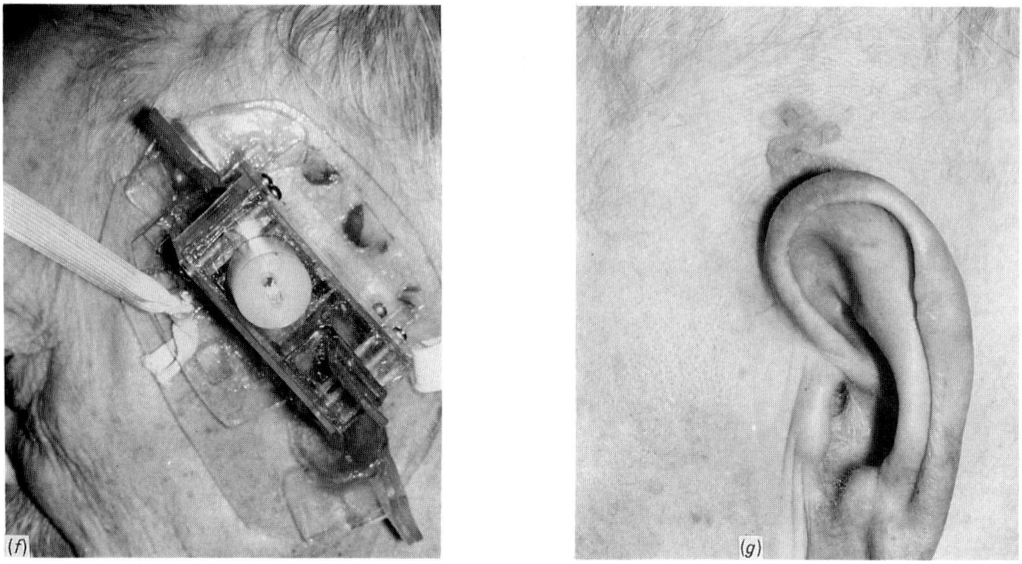

Figure 12.11 (*f*) Double caesium mould. (*g*) After 6500 cGy at midpoint — 7 days' treatment (worn 12 hours daily). (Courtesy of Dr H. F. Hope-Stone)

Figure 12.1). These are better treated by surgery in the first instance.

A second course of radiotherapy can safely be given to a recurrence on the edge of a previously treated area as only a portion of the irradiated area is then retreated.

When skin cancer invades cartilage or bone and especially if there is gross infection, the chances of radionecrosis are high. Infection must be eliminated and if this is not possible surgery may well be considered the treatment of choice.

Melanoma

There has been a steady increase in the mortality of malignant melanoma in all countries for which reliable statistics exist (Jensen and Bolander, 1980). It is thought that ultraviolet light is responsible for the doubling of this mortality over the last 20 years.

However, inconsistencies are seen in that indoor workers have higher mortality rates than farmers or fishermen (Lee and Strickland, 1980), and the incidence is also higher in professional people. Unlike other skin cancers, melanoma is not more frequent on exposed sites and it may well be that intense intermittent exposure to ultraviolet light is more important than cumulative exposure.

Diagnosis

Early diagnosis is the main factor in determining the outcome and it is important that both the medical profession and the general public are aware of the potential malignant change in any pigmented lesion. These are:

(1) Change in shape or size or rapid growth
(2) Frequent irritation
(3) Alteration of pigmentation
(4) Erythema or haemorrhage
(5) Ulceration.

It was considered for many years that biopsy of a lesion suspected of being a melanoma would hasten the onset of metastases but this has been shown to be false. Epstein, Bragg and Linden (1969) compared 115 cases having biopsies with 55 cases who had excision without biopsy and found no difference in survival.

Types of lesion related to prognosis

The depth of infiltration of the growth is the most important factor affecting the prognosis. The common clinical types are:

(a) Superficial spreading

This type makes up 70% of all melanomas and is more frequent in males between the ages of 35 and 45. It extends horizontally for a period which may be several years before invading more deeply, thus raising for the first time the suspicion of malignancy. Clark *et al.* (1969) showed that when the lesion was confined to the epidermis (level 1) a survival of 95–

100% could be expected after excision. This falls to 90% when the dermis is invaded (level 2), and to 65% when the papillary–reticular junction is reached (level 3). Deeper extension to the reticular dermis or the subcutaneous tissue (levels 4 and 5) lowered the survival rates to 54 and 48% respectively.

(b) Nodular

This type occurs more frequently in males often on the trunk and in a slightly older age group. They have a shorter history and penetrate more readily. They are more dangerous than the previous variety with a 5-year survival of the order of 30%.

(c) Lentigo maligna

This is more common in the female after the age of 60 and acounts for 10% of melanomas. Being often seen on the face and areas exposed to sunlight it is frequently removed for cosmetic reasons before deep extension occurs. The margin of excision does not need to be large and block dissection of the glands is not necessary, the prognosis being good.

Node dissection

Nodes over 1 cm which are rubbery or discrete should be removed by block dissection. Larger masses may be debulked by surgery prior to radiotherapy or chemotherapy. The decision to carry out block dissection in the absence of enlarged nodes depends on the probability of their being involved. If the penetration is over 1.5 cm, especially on the trunk in middle-aged men, then block dissection should be performed.

Radiotherapy

Melanoma is a relatively radioresistant tumour and radiotherapy has no part in the primary treatment if surgery is possible. However, patients may be unfit for surgery or the fixation of the growth may make its removal impossible; these cases are then worth treating radically in the hopes of cure although it must be admitted that the main use of radiotherapy is for palliation. Ulceration, bleeding, or the pain of infiltration can all be relieved by doses which range from one-half to three-quarters of a radical dose.

Khan and Ross (1984) analysed 63 cases treated between 1975 and 1980 which had recurred or spread after primary excision. Of these, 42 had spread to regional lymph nodes and 21 had disseminated further. Treatment was given with X-rays varying widely in their penetration and with doses ranging from a palliative 2000 cGy to a more radical 6000 cGy with different time schedules. There was an overall response rate of 73% of which 47% was complete and 26% partial. Deposits in skin and nodes responded better than in bone or brain. These responses compare very favourably with those of chemotherapy. If surgical excision is impracticable and the patient is in good physical condition an attempt should be made to irradiate, preferably with electron therapy, to full tolerance with the hope of cure. There is some evidence that larger individual fractions of the order of 600 – 800 cGy are more effective than smaller doses, but the variation in sensitivity between patients makes statistical evidence hard to find.

Isolated nodules will respond to single doses of 3000 cGy of 90 kV X-rays provided the field is not larger than 1 cm. Larger areas will not heal after this dose. It would seem therefore that palliation of melanoma is effective and can most conveniently be given on a weekly basis using doses of the order of 600 – 800 cGy with the final dose being adjusted according to response.

Melanoma produces brain secondaries more frequently than any other tumour and these are often multiple. Symptoms can readily be relieved by a short course of radiotherapy to the whole brain given by opposed fields using a midline dose of 3000 cGy in 10 fractions over 12 days. Dexamethasone 2 mg three times a day must be commenced before the treatment starts and continued throughout, to prevent cerebral oedema and subsequent headache and vomiting (*see* Chapter 15).

Chemotherapy

Dacarbazine (DTIC) has for some years been the mainstay of therapy with a response rate of 20–30%. These responses are usually short lived and are bought at the expense of severe vomiting and diarrhoea. More recently vindesine, a synthetic alkaloid drug, has given similar results with far less toxicity (Retsas, Newton and Westbury, 1979). This, in combination with DTIC and cisplatin, has achieved longer remissions. For brain secondaries lomustine is an agent capable of crossing the blood–brain barrier and may prolong the effect of radiotherapy. Chemotherapy must be considered a palliative procedure and we await the arrival of more effective and less toxic drugs.

Mycosis fungoides

This is a lymphoma of T-cell origin which remains confined to the skin, only occasionally progressing to invade lymph nodes and viscera. It is twice as common in males with a peak incidence in the fifth decade of life. The typical mycosis cell has a large nucleus but little cytoplasm, and for many years may remain confined to the epidermis or the upper layers of the dermis (*Figure 12.12*). It is at this stage that diagnosis is most difficult and the term premycotic may be used. In due course the lesions thicken and may ulcerate or weep. A characteristic feature is the

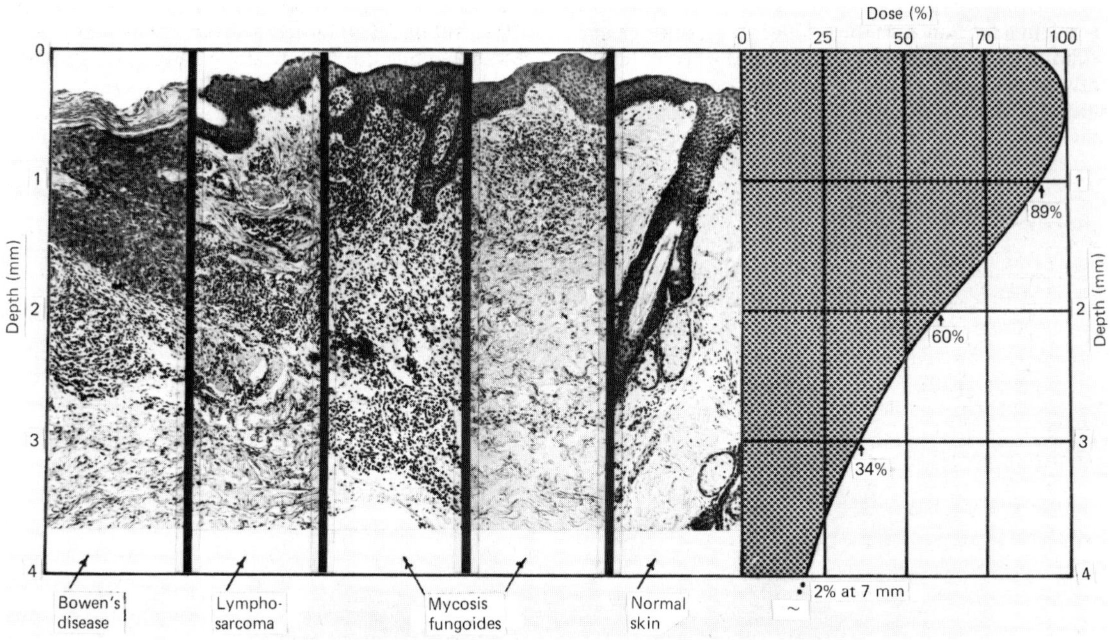

Figure 12.12 Diagram of the penetration of beta rays from strontium-90 in normal skin in which the hair follicles are shown at the 60% isodose level. The infiltration of mycosis cells can be seen in an early case at the 80% level but extending more deeply in a later case

presence of small foci in the epidermis, the micro-abscesses of Pautrier. A later stage is the development of 'tomato tumours' which ulcerate and are very painful. In the 'tumeur d'emblée' type these arise from relatively normal skin.

The classical form of the disease starts with reddened patches on breasts, buttocks or upper thighs. These slowly spread to involve all areas of skin and occasionally mucous membranes. Later, infiltrated plaques form; a process which may take as long as 30 years. The mycosis cell may be found in lymph nodes draining a plaque, but more often the enlargement is dermatopathic and due to chronic infection. It must be said, however, that enlarged lymph nodes from either cause are a bad prognostic sign.

Poikiloderma is often associated with mycosis fungoides; in these cases the skin is atrophic and the disease remains confined to the epidermis for many years with a correspondingly better prognosis.

A rarer form involves the whole skin in a red intensely irritable infiltration. This erythrodermic or 'homme rouge' type may be associated with a spill of mycotic cells into the blood stream, the Sézary syndrome, with a very poor prognosis.

The final stages of the disease can be very distressing, and depression and suicidal tendencies are common. Not only is the patient's social life totally disrupted, but the onset of infection requires frequent dressings and hospital admissions. Septicaemia is a more common terminal event than systemic spread.

Treatment

Mycosis fungoides responds very poorly to chemotherapy in striking contrast to the other types of lymphoma and such remissions as are obtained are partial and of short duration. This may well be due to the avascularity of the epidermis and failure of the cytotoxic agent to reach the site of the disease. However, nitrogen mustard, applied topically, is very effective and often holds the situation for many months, but some patients develop a sensitivity to it. A solution of 10 mg in 50 ml of tap water is rubbed into the entire skin daily by the patient who wears plastic gloves.

In the early stages of the disease simple emulsifying creams and topical corticosteroids are sufficient to control symptoms often for many years. Some patients find that they improve in the summer months, and for them ultraviolet light is beneficial, especially for localized areas.

Therapy with ultraviolet light after the administration of the photosensitizing drug, psoralen (PUVA), may hold up the process of infiltration for a time. This carries a risk of inducing squamous carcinoma (Stern *et al.*, 1984), but at this stage of the disease any effective treatment either by X-rays or chemotherapy carries a similar risk and the possibility can be ignored.

The disease is highly radiosensitive, but any radiation used must be of limited penetration to spare radiosensitive tissues such as the marrow and gut.

The difficulty is to treat the whole body surface and to reach involved areas in the folds of groin, buttock and submammary regions and also in the cavities of the nostril and ear. Fortunately, an abscopal effect is seen and areas which have received less than the optimal dose appear to clear up with the rest (*Figures 12.13* and *12.14*). This may be due to a humoral mechanism.

Electron beam therapy was initially described in 1939, but was developed by Trump and Bagshaw in America (Fuks, Bagshaw and Farber, 1973) and in England by Szur and Bewley (Spittle, 1979). Energies of 2.5, 3 or 3.5 MeV are used with the patient standing 6 m from the linear accelerator. This gives an 80% isodose at between 6 and 12 mm. Doses of 400 cGy are given twice weekly to a total dose of 2400

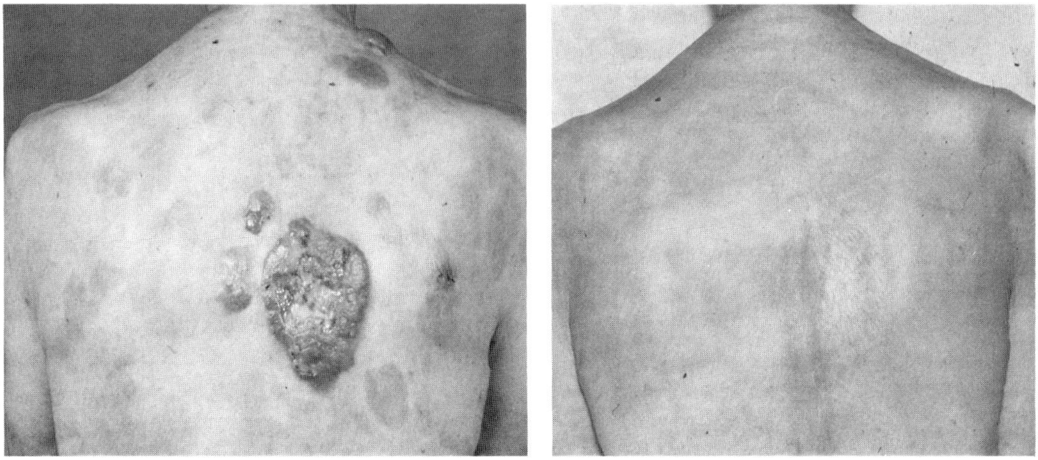

Figure 12.13 Mycosis fungoides treated with beta rays from the strontium-90 unit. Dose 2000 cGy in 10 daily treatments over 12 days. Thicker 'tomato tumours' given additional 250 kV treatment. The patient was well until death from a road accident at 3 years

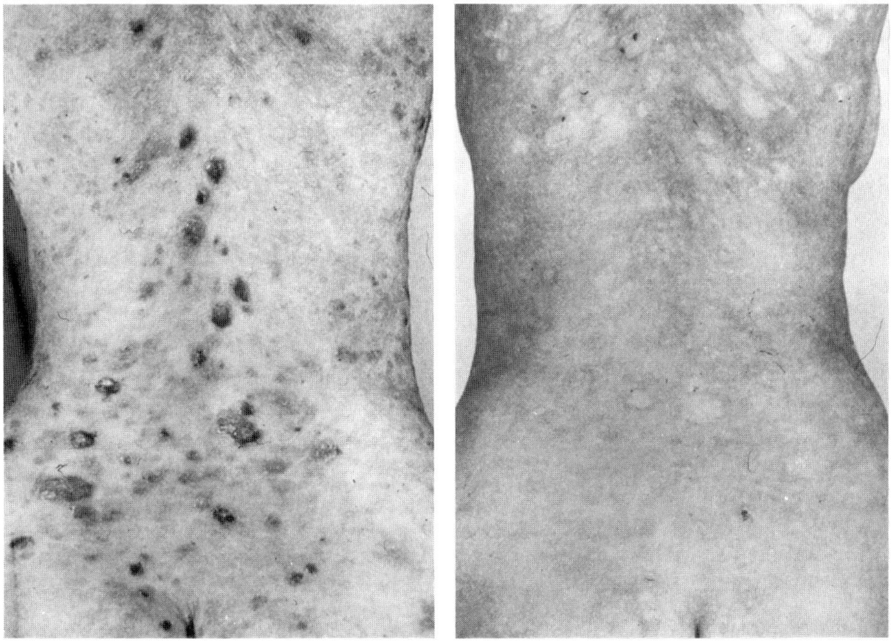

Figure 12.14 Mycosis fungoides treated with beta rays from strontium-90 unit. Dose 2000 cGy in 10 treatments in 2 weeks. Note response of lesions theoretically too thick to respond

to 4000 cGy according to response. Side-effects include temporary peripheral oedema, loss of finger and toe nails and alopecia of short duration.

At Cambridge, treatment is given with beta rays (*Figure 12.15*) from a strontium-90 source (Bratherton, 1972). This contains 60 Ci spread over an area 53 × 2 cm, thus enabling the whole width of the body to be covered as it moves longitudinally over the patient. The measured dose rate at a source skin distance of 40 cm is 123 cGy/minute and the dose delivered in one traverse of the body is 50 cGy. A dose of 200 cGy to one surface of the patient of average length 170 cm requires four traverses taking about 10 minutes. The front, back and one lateral side of the patient can be treated in half an hour. A thin nylon sheet is placed over the patient to supply privacy and some warmth during this time.

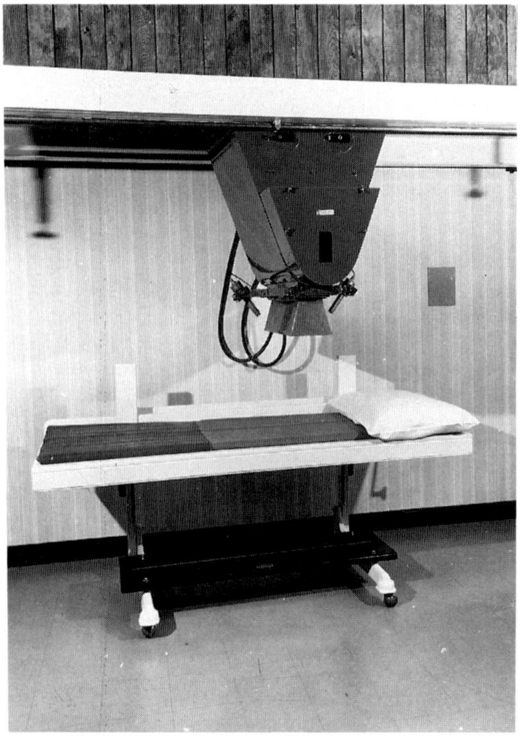

Figure 12.15 Moving strip strontium-90 unit

A study of the structure of normal skin in relation to the depth dose curve (*see Figure 12.12*) shows that the epidermis, including its sensitive basal cell layer, does not extend below 0.5 mm and is in the 100% dose level. The hair follicles extend down to 2.5 mm where the dose has fallen to 50%. Below this level the fall off is extremely rapid with the result that the blood supply of the skin is not affected. This has an important effect on the clinical response and, in the absence of any gamma ray component, there are no systemic symptoms such as nausea or vomiting. Nor is there any damage to the haemopoietic system. Thicker lesions require supplementary doses of 250 kV X-rays (*see Figure 12.13*).

Preliminary tests showed that the lesions would respond at a dose below that needed to produce moist desquamation. The latter would be most undesirable if the whole body surface became denuded, with subsequent loss of plasma. A schedule of 2000 cGy given in 10 daily treatments over 2 weeks has been found to be well tolerated. The anterior and posterior surfaces are treated daily with 200 cGy to a total dose of 2000 cGy. In addition, one lateral surface is given 200 cGy on alternate days and thus receives 1000 cGy over 2 weeks. At the conclusion of the course a brisk erythema develops which settles during the following week. As eyelids are often involved, the eyes are closed during the passage of the source over the face. If there is much ulceration or infection the reaction tends to be more severe, and a split course is given with a rest after the first week to allow the lesions to heal. Many of these cases have received chemotherapy or corticosteroids and are immunosuppressed. Antibiotic cover especially against Pseudomonas infection is often required and transfusion of blood may be indicated. If electron therapy is not available, local lesions can be controlled by a weekly dose of 750 cGy of 90 kV X-rays to a total of 2250 cGy.

It is difficult to assess the value of therapy in a disorder with such a protracted course. The radiotherapist is usually presented with the patient at a stage when many other treatments have been tried and the disease is out of control. In the Cambridge series, few cases with limited disease were seen as they were treated elsewhere usually with a dose of 3000 cGy which caused permanent regression. The non-infiltrating poikilodermic type responds readily and even if generalized may have excellent remissions of long duration.

The radiotherapist is therefore more likely to see cases at the plaque stage with many ulcerated lesions. In these a remission of 6 months to 2 years may be expected, but further treatment is the rule. The treatment course can be repeated and as much as 20000 cGy has been given over a period of years with only minimal skin atrophy.

A total of 233 cases has been treated at Cambridge over the last 23 years. The distribution of the various stages is as follows:

Localized disease	6 cases (3%)
Non-infiltrative	48 cases (21%)
Erythrodermic	22 cases (9%)
Plaque stage	131 cases (56%)
Tumour formation	26 cases (11%)

It will be seen that over one-half of the patients have infiltrated plaques. Presentation of the results in such a protracted disease presents problems as earlier referral can dramatically influence survival, and it is therefore important to present results in a way which shows the whole duration of the disease, both before and after radiotherapy. An attempt to do this giving the age of referral and future progress has been made both for the less serious non-infiltrative type (*Figure 12.16*) and for the more lethal tumour cases (*Figure 12.17*). The other stages of plaques and the erythrodermic type have a prognosis midway between these two extremes with the latter being slightly worse.

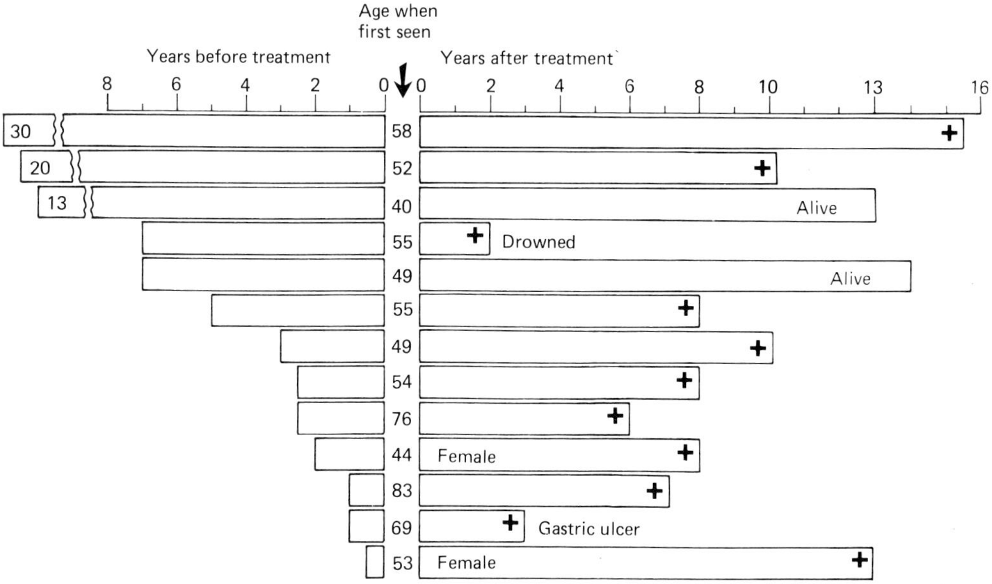

Figure 12.16 Response of 13 patients (between 1962 and 1974) with non-infiltrating stage of mycosis fungoides showing duration of disease before and after treatment with beta rays. + = death

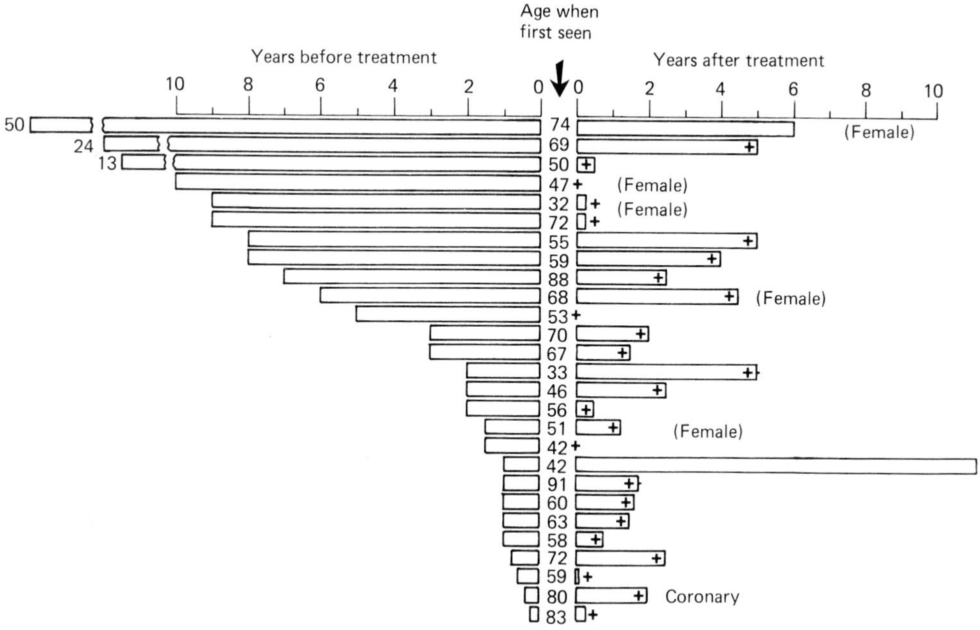

Figure 12.17 Response of 27 patients (between 1961 and 1974) with mycosis fungoides with tumour formation showing duration of diseases before and after treatment with beta rays. + = death

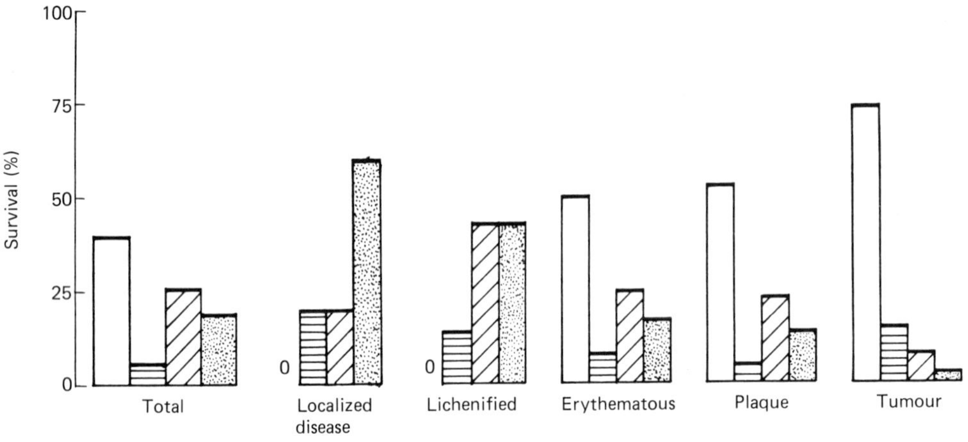

Figure 12.18 Five-year survial of mycosis fungoides after beta-ray therapy. □ Dead from disease; ▤ dead, other causes; ▨ alive, with disease; ▩ alive, free of disease

A summary of all the cases at 5 years (*Figure 12.18*) shows that one-half of the patients will have died of the disease or other causes; only 20% of all patients are free of disease. No patient with localized disease has died but there is only one survivor with tumour formation.

Lymphomatous conditions affecting the skin

Skin lesions are seen in the terminal stages of Hodgkin's disease and other lymphomas. They respond readily to radiotherapy (orthovoltage) with doses of 2000–3000 cGy over 2 weeks, but remissions are much shorter and survival rarely exceeds 1 year.

Kaposi's sarcoma is now seen to be the skin manifestation of the acquired immunodeficiency syndrome (AIDS). The lesions are usually a dusky red colour commencing as nodules which coalesce and later ulcerate. As the progress of the whole systemic disease is of the order of 5 – 10 years it is important to control the local disease which is extremely radiosensitive (*Figure 12.19*). Isolated nodules respond to single doses of 1000 cGy of 90 kV X-rays. It may be necessary to treat the whole limb with 250–300 kV X-rays to a total dose of 3000 cGy over 3 weeks with five

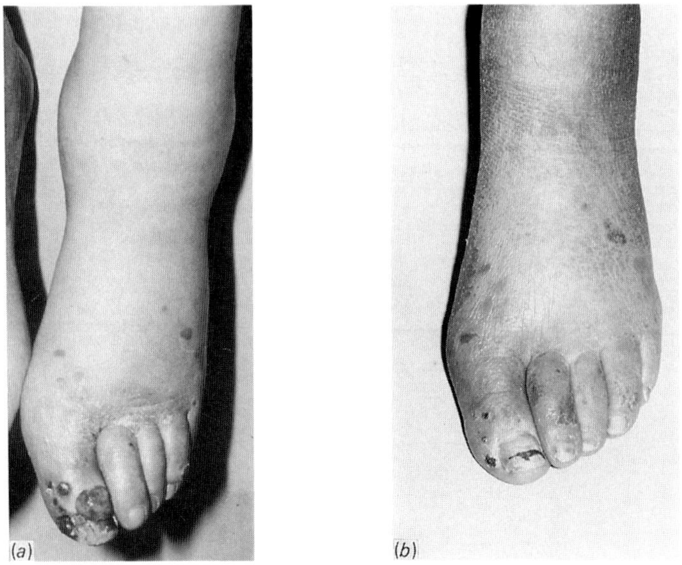

Figure 12.19 Kaposi's sarcoma: (*a*) before treatment; (*b*) after 3000 cGy to whole leg (250 kV) in 15 fractions in 3 weeks

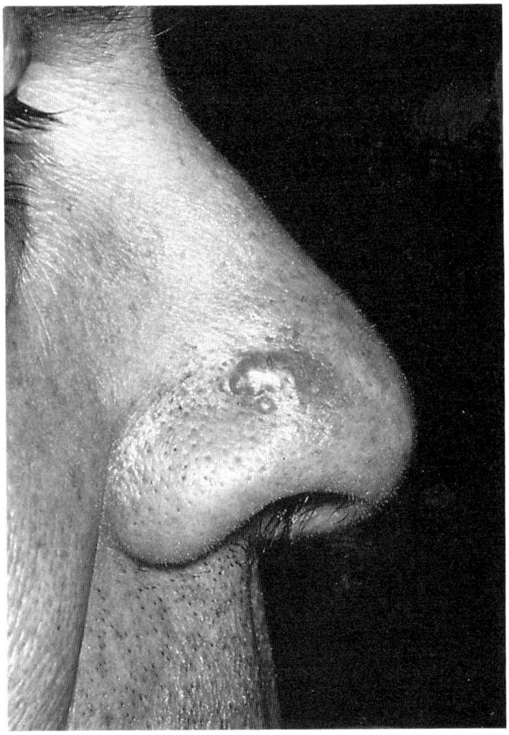

Figure 12.20 Benign lymphoma cutis in male of 61. Recurred twice after curettage and diathermy. Treated with 90 kV X-rays, 700 cGy weekly for three weeks, total 2100 cGy. Clear to date at 2 years

fractions a week. Great care should be taken to see that opposing fields are strictly parallel and that suitable bolus is used to avoid areas of overdosage. If possible a small strip of skin should be left untreated to prevent subsequent lymphatic blockage and oedema of the limb. Chemotherapy is now being used with regimens similar to those used for the lymphomas and the disease is showing some response to interferon.

Benign lymphoma cutis presents as nodules around the face and neck more often in females (*Figure 12.20*). They are radiosensitive and respond to a dose of 2000 cGy of 75 – 90 kV X-rays in five treatments in 2 weeks.

References

BAKOS, L. and McMILLAN, A.L. (1973) Malignant melanoma in East Anglia, England. An 11 year survey by site and type. *British Journal of Dermatology*, **88**, 551–556

BRATHERTON, D.G. (1972) Strontium beam therapy. In *Modern Trends in Radiotherapy*, 2. Ch 13, pp. 176–187. London: Butterworths

CLARK, W.H. JR., FROM, L., BERARINO, E.H. and MIHM, M.C. (1969) The histogenesis of biologic behavior of primary human malignant melanomas of the skin. *Cancer Research*, **29**, 705–726

DOLL, R. (1977) Strategy for detection of cancer hazards to man. *Nature*, **265**, 589–596

EPSTEIN, E., BRAGG, K. and LINDEN, G.J. (1969) Biopsy and prognosis of malignant melanoma. *Journal of the American Medical Association*, **208**, 1369

FUKS, Z., BAGSHAW, M.A. and FARBER, E.M. (1973) Prognostic signs and the management of mycosis fungoides. *Cancer*, **32**, 1385–1395

JENSEN, O.M. and BOLANDER, A.M. (1980) Trends in malignant melanoma of the skin. *World Health Statistics*, **33**, 2–26

KHAN, M.S. and ROSS, W.M. (1984) Management of malignant melanoma; a retrospective analysis of 182 patients. *Clinical Radiology*, **35**, 151–154

LEE, J.A.H. and STRICKLAND, D. (1980) Malignant melanoma; social status and outdoor work. *British Journal of Cancer*, **41**, 757–763

RETSAS, S. (1982) Non-surgical treatment of malignant melanoma. *Hospital Update*, September, 1139–1146

RETSAS, S., NEWTON, K.A. and WESTBURY, G. (1979) Vindesine as a single agent in the treatment of advanced malignant melanoma. *Cancer Chemotherapy and Pharmacology*, **2**, 257–260

SPITTLE, M.F. (1979) Electron beam therapy in England. *Cancer Treatment Reports*, **63**, 639–641

STERN, R.N., LAIRD, N., MELSI, J. *et al.* (1984) Cutaneous squamous cell carcinoma in patients treated with PUVA. *New England Journal of Medicine*, **310**, 1156–1161

13

Tumours of the endocrine system

P. N. Plowman

Thyroid cancer

Although thyroid cancer is relatively uncommon it is, nevertheless, an important malignancy; young people are not infrequently afflicted and, with optimal treatment, the disease is often curable.

The normal thyroid gland is situated in the anterior neck, the two lateral lobes extending from the thyroid cartilage to approximately the sixth tracheal ring. The gland lies within a connective tissue sheath and this pretracheal fascia firmly fixes it to the thyroid and cricoid cartilages so that the thyroid moves up on swallowing. The proximity of the gland to the trachea, vascular bundle, recurrent laryngeal nerves and parathyroid glands (*Figure 13.1*) may all be relevant in the management of a patient with thyroid cancer and the regional lymphatic drainage goes beyond the neck to include the upper mediastinum. The relatively anterior position of the cervical cord in the neck is an anatomical feature which is noteworthy for radiotherapeutic practice (*Figure 13.1*).

The geographical variations in the incidence of carcinoma of thyroid may be related to diet, environment and race. In Iceland the incidence is the highest: 15×10^{-5} (females), 5×10^{-5} (males), but it is also high in Israel and Hawaii. The USA, French, Swiss and Scandinavian incidence rates are intermediate between those of the previously mentioned countries and those with low rates such as the UK (1×10^{-5} (females), 0.6×10^{-5} (males)) Hungary and Romania. The female preponderance of thyroid cancer is present in all races and in all ages, although less pronounced in the elderly. Thyroid cancer is uncommon in childhood. The incidence curves then rises much more steeply in young adult women than men, in whom the incidence rises more gradually with advancing age.

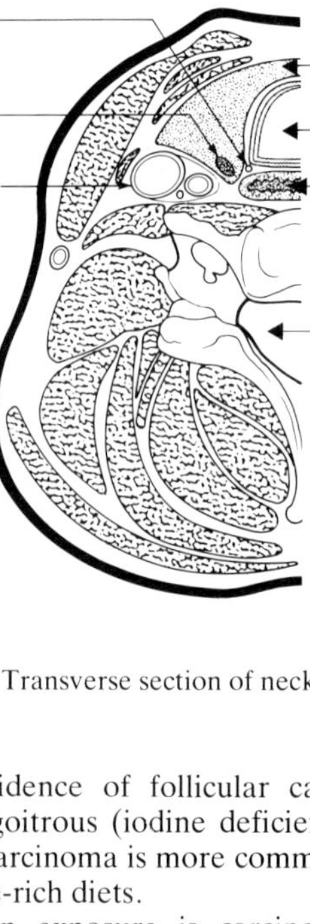

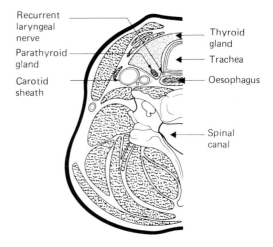

Figure 13.1 Transverse section of neck at level of thyroid gland

The incidence of follicular carcinoma appears higher in goitrous (iodine deficient) areas whereas papillary carcinoma is more common in populations with iodine-rich diets.

Radiation exposure is carcinogenic to thyroid tissue and many cases of thyroid cancer following low dose radiation exposure to the neck in childhood have now been documented (Modan *et al.*, 1974; Maxon *et al.*, 1977), in addition to cases observed in survivors of the atomic bomb explosions. The latency period is 5–40 years with a peak incidence at 15. The increased incidence of thyroid cancer after irradiation is mainly that of papillary carcinoma, but there is also a modest increased incidence of follicular, and anaplastic carcinoma. Following therapeutic radiation to the neck in patients with Hodgkin's disease, hypothyroidism is a well-documented late occurrence. The incidence of thyroid carcinoma following radiation to the thyroid to therapeutic doses — as in mantle radiotherapy for Hodgkin's disease — is increased, but is not as frequent as would be expected if there was a linear, quadratic or linear–quadratic incidence relationship with dose. McDougall *et al.* (1980) concluded that doses in excess of 2000 cGy (megavoltage fractionated radiotherapy) to the thyroid led to a lesser incidence of late thyroid carcinoma than that observed following lower dosages, e.g. by Modan *et al.* (1974). Compensated hypothyroidism is even commoner in this group of patients (that is, serum biochemistry showing a high circulating thyroid stimulating hormone (TSH), but normal thyroxine (T4), free thyroxine index (FTI) and tri-iodothyronine); it has been suggested that the high TSH drive augments the carcinogenic effects of the radiation. The present author has not yet been persuaded to put these patients with normal T4 levels on replacement exogenous T4, but some authorities recommend this as cancer prophylaxis. (Some consider the high endogenous serum TSH in goitrous areas to be a risk factor.)

Hashimoto's thyroiditis predisposes to thyroid lymphoma but not, it is now thought, to other forms of thyroid malignancy.

Inheritance plays a major aetiological role in medullary carcinoma of thyroid (MCT), and this inheritance is by an autosomal dominant trait. Approximately 20% of MCT patients have the familial form, but this figure rises to 80% in patients with multifocal MCT; in patients with familial MCT, the carcinoma may occur alone, together with a phaeochromocytoma or as a part of multiple endocrine neoplasia. Papillary carcinoma of thyroid has been described in several unusual familial syndromes.

Clinical and diagnostic aspects

The majority of patients with thyroid tumours present because of a neck swelling and much can be ascertained from an unrushed consultation by an experienced clinician. The history will already have disclosed the rate of appearance of the swelling and any symptoms due to changes in thyroid hormone status, but specific enquiry may elicit pain, hoarse voice, stridor, dysphagia or even 'symptoms' from metastases.

The general physical examination will establish that most patients with primary thyroid malignancy are euthyroid. Careful palpation of the neck will disclose the tumour/goitre and any local spread with cervical lymphadenopathy. If the lower border of the thyroid has not been identified, retrosternal extension must be suspected. Systemic searches for thyroid bruits and venous changes may be appropriate.

It is the management of the clinically solitary thyroid nodule which is most controversial. The present author recommends that such patients should have an isotope thyroid scan which will demonstrate that 35–50% of cases have a multinodular goitre — almost invariably benign. Of the remaining cases, a minority (5–10%) will have a hot nodule — again almost invariably benign. Patients with a solitary cold thyroid nodule on isotope scan usually require surgical exploration, although a thyroid ultrasound which demonstrated a thin and regular walled thyroid cyst corresponding to the nodule would often allow conservative management.

A chest X-ray (with a thoracic inlet view), CT of the chest and indirect laryngoscopy may all be appropriate in individual patients, as may serum calcitonin measurement.

Classification and pathology

The classification of primary malignant thyroid tumours is shown in *Table 13.1*. It should be noted that papillary, follicular and anaplastic carcinomas are of follicular cell origin.

Table 13.1 Classification of primary malignant thyroid tumours

Follicular cell origin
Differentiated carcinoma
Papillary (WHO type I)
occult
intrathyroidal
extrathyroidal
Follicular (WHO type II)
microangioinvasive
angioinvasive
Anaplastic carcinoma
Parafollicular cell (C-cell) origin
Medullary carcinoma
Lymphoma
Others
Sarcoma
Haemangioendothelioma

Papillary carcinoma

In the large Mayo Clinic series, papillary carcinoma of thyroid (which includes all mixed follicular and papillary tumours) comprised 61% of all primary thyroid carcinomas (Woolner *et al.*, 1961). Approximately 10% of all cases present before the age of 20 years and the mean age at presentation is between 30 and 40 years; the disease is commoner in females (2.4:1, F:M) and usually presents as a thyroid swelling, although cervical adenopathy is the presenting feature in 10%.

Although the basic microscopic papillary structure of these usually well-differentiated growths is the key to the diagnosis, follicular, lobular or trabecular patterns occur and the follicular component may predominate. Irregular plaques of calcium are often present and these may show concentric rings (psammoma bodies). The growth pattern varies; the carcinoma may be long confined by a false capsule (and occult tumours may remain this way), or invade by direct extension or by lymphatic permeation. The frequent occurrence of non-contiguous papillary carcinoma in the contralateral lobe of a surgical specimen resected for this disease is believed to reflect more frequently the multifocal nature of this tumour than metastatic spread. The significance of these often occult second primaries is not known, but one necropsy series suggested that occult papillary carcinoma could be found in as many as 6% of the population (Sampson *et al.*, 1974).

There is an established and prognostically useful distinction between intrathyroidal and extrathyroidal growths. Extrathyroidal growths are more commonly associated with nodal and distant metastases, although, as we shall see, the prognostic import of operable cervical nodes is uncertain. After the regional lymph nodes, the lungs are the next favoured site of metastatic spread.

Follicular carcinoma

Follicular carcinoma accounts for fewer cases of thyroid carcinoma (about 18% of the total), although representing a higher proportion of the cases in an iodine deficient area. The mean age at presentation is approximately 50 years, and thus the disease tends to occur in an older population than papillary carcinoma.The female predominance holds true (2.6:1, F:M), and the prognosis for females is slightly better than for males.

Microscopically, most follicular carcinomas are well or moderately differentiated (itself a prognostically useful distinction), with follicles superficially resembling normal thyroid and with no papillae. (The presence of even a minor papillary component is associated with tumour behaviour consistent with papillary carcinoma and so such tumours are classified as papillary.) The microscopic architecture may be varied: the tumour may be composed of microfollicles comparable to those seen in fetal adenoma, but solid sheets, trabecular patterns or Hurthle cell variants are all recognized. Follicular carcinoma may appear to be well encapsulated or to be infiltrating adjacent glandular tissue. Angioinvasiveness is a prognostically useful pathological observation and the tendency for follicular carcinoma to spread by the blood is a notable feature which probably accounts for the more widespread sites of metastases, notably bones and lungs.

Anaplastic carcinoma

The incidence of anaplastic carcinoma is approximately 15% of all thyroid carcinomas, although its incidence has been reported to exceed that of follicular carcinoma in some series. It tends to occur in a later age group (mean age at presentation 55–60 years) than differentiated follicular cell origin carcinomas and is uncommon below the age of 40 years. Histologically, the tumour exhibits a variety of undifferentiated patterns. There is often extreme cellular pleomorphism, with many spindle and giant cells; a high number of mitoses reflects the rapid growth and invasiveness of this tymour type. Areas of distinguishable follicular cell origin carcinoma may accompany anaplastic carcinoma and some authorities regard the anaplastic growth to have arisen from a more differentiated cancer.

Medullary carcinoma of thyroid (MCT)

MCT accounts for approximately 8% of all cases of thyroid carcinoma, and of these 20–25% are the familial variety. In the Mayo Clinic experience, the median age of familial cases was 21 years and of sporadic cases was 51 years (Chong *et al.*, 1975). Familial MCT was more likely to be multifocal. Macroscopically, the tumours may appear well defined or locally infiltrating. Microscopically, the typical picture is of round or polygonal neoplastic C cells separated by dense, eosinophilic and amyloid-containing stroma. C cell hyperplasia may be found in the surrounding gland. The tumour is often slow growing, and the commonest sites for metastases are the cervical nodes and mediastinum.

Lymphoma

In many large pathological series of thyroid lymphomas it has been demonstrated that the overwhelming majority of these tumours are non-Hodgkin lymphomas arising on a basis of pre-existing Hashimoto's (autoimmune) thyroiditis (Compagno and Oertel, 1980). The disease tends to afflict elderly ladies, and the goitre which presents is often large and diffusely affects the gland. The majority are high grade diffuse lymphomas, (diffuse histiocytic histology by Rappaport classification and immunoblastic by Kiel classification) (Burke, Butler and Fuller, 1977). The possible transformation of lymphocytes in autoimmune disease such as Sjögren's syndrome and Hashimoto's disease, is of great theoretical interest. Regional lymph node spread is the earliest site of metastasis followed, often rapidly, by systemic dissemination.

Management

Although the management of the different types of thyroid cancer will be discussed individually below, the application of the follicular cell origin carcinoma management programme to all papillary carcinoma patients is controversial. This programme is based on the potential of recurrent carcinoma to concentrate radioiodine and the recognition that the avidity for iodine is very much less than normal thyroid tissue. All papillary tumours contain a follicular (colloid containing) element and so have the potential to concentrate radioiodine. However, the treatment scheme described below carries a morbidity, and many clinicians would not consider recommending more than conservative surgery for intrathyroidal papillary carcinoma or where microscopically the follicular element is small. It should also be stated categorically here that the correct management for a local recurrence of papillary carcinoma in the neck is re-operation — local removal, more radical resection or formal block dissection, as appropriate.

Follicular cell origin carcinoma

In patients with non-metastatic disease and also in many patients with metastatic disease, radical treatment intent requires a near-total thyroidectomy which only spares the parathyroid glands and recurrent laryngeal nerves. Locally extensive tumour is resected as far as possible and involved cervical and mediastinal nodes removed. A formal block dissection of neck nodes is not mandatory although it may become necessary.

Following surgery, the normal thyroid remnant is assessed in size by isotope scanning, although this is often clear from the operative report. A normal thyroid tissue ablation is then planned by radioiodine administration (*Figure 13.2*). This takes place when the surgical scar has healed, and before the patient has been started on replacement thyroid hormone. A small thyroid remnant is ablated by a single 80 mCi administration of iodine-131 (^{131}I); for patients with large thyroid remnants the ablation dose is split into first a 40 mCi ^{131}I administration and then 1 month later, if there is still functioning normal gland in the neck on a repeat isotope scan, a second 40 mCi ^{131}I dose. The patient takes liothyronine (T3) 20 μg orally three times daily, for the first 3 weeks of the 1 month gap.

There is an apparent paradox here in that a small remnant often requires a higher dose for ablation than a larger remnant; this is because the iodine transit time through the gland is less. Conversely, the first 40 mCi dose appears not infrequently to have ablated the normal thyroid tissue by the time that the 1 month scan is performed, and the second dose is not then given (although some normal thyroid activitiy may return much later and appear as a confusing site of concentration during the early screening programme). The protein bound radioiodine (PB^{131}I) load is high following thyroid ablation of a large remnant and, because of its greater biological half-

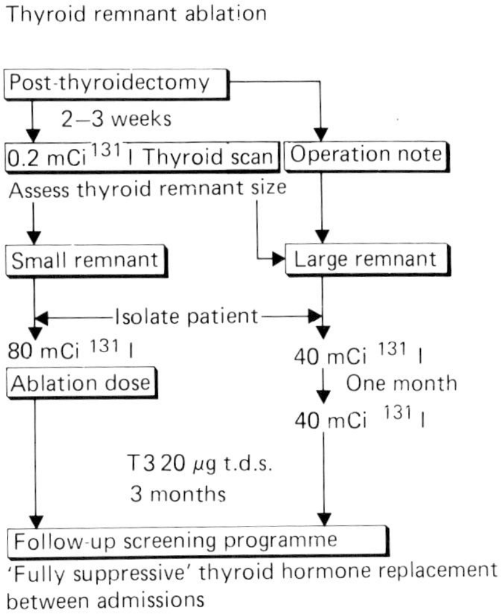

Figure 13.2 Algorithm of thyroid remnant ablation

life over that of the ionized salt, the whole body radiation dose is increased. Furthermore, this high circulating thyroglobulin level provides the reason for the several weeks gap between the two ablation doses. Another problem which may arise with ablation of large normal thyroid masses relates to early radiation thyroiditis with swelling (perhaps alarmingly so with compromise of the airway). This swelling occurs within the first few days after ^{131}I administration and can be reduced by cold compresses and systemic dexamethasone; tracheotomy is rarely needed. The risk of radiation thyroiditis is minimized by the split-dose ablation just described.

Following the ablation procedure, the patient is placed on replacement thyroxine in fully TSH suppressive doses for the rest of life (although the screening programme requires the use of the shorter half-life liothyronine near the times of screening). There is good evidence from the literature that patients who have had near-total thyroidectomy with thyroid remnant ablation and fully TSH suppressive thyroid hormone replacement have a better prognosis than others (Mazzaferri *et al.*, 1977).

Ablation of the normal thyroid tissue may take as long as 3 months, and the first screening point in the metastatic screening programme occurs 3 months after ablation. The frequency and details of the screening programme vary in different centres, only one scheme being exemplified here (*Figure 13.3*); the screening points are more heavily concentrated in the early follow-up years. Just before each screening point endogenous hypothyroidism is induced by removal of the liothyronine, and the TSH rises. Functioning metastases are more likely to declare themselves if the serum TSH is above 30 units/ℓ. If

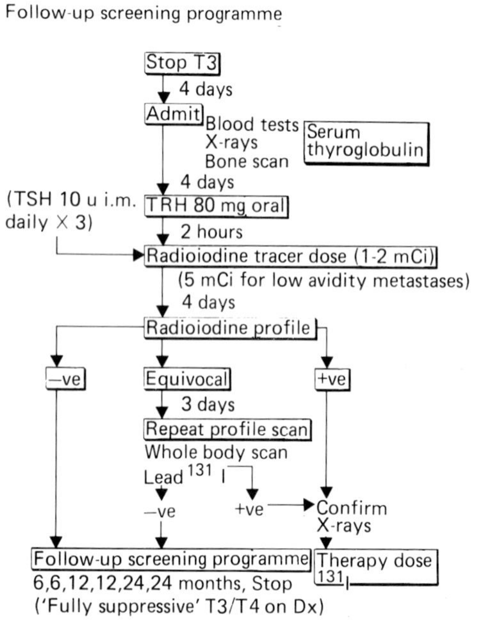

Figure 13.3 Algorithm of follicular cell origin carcinoma screening programme

liothyronine is stopped 8–10 days before the tracer radioiodine dose this TSH level is usually achieved; however, a dose of thyrotrophin releasing hormone (TRH) is sometimes given 2 hours before the tracer dose to augment the TSH level. In patients who have been on replacement thyroid hormone for some years the feed-back system may not lead to satisfactory rises in serum TSH on thyroid hormone withdrawal, and in these patients exogenous bovine TSH (which has the disadvantage of being potentially immunogenic) may have to be given intramuscularly prior to the tracer dose.

As functioning metastases of follicular cell origin carcinoma are of low avidity compared to normal thyroid tissue, so the tracer dose ^{131}I at the screening points is now 1–5 mCi, and a profile scan or whole body scan is performed 4 days later — the former being more sensitive, the latter more interpretable. Equivocal scan results can be for a variety of reasons and such a scan is repeated a few days later. One is then capitalizing on the fact that the turnover time of radioiodine in functioning tumour is 3–10 days, i.e. longer than the body pool. Thus functioning tumour metastases should still be retaining ^{131}I when the normal body pool (including compartmentalized amounts, e.g. salivary glands, stomach) has diminished towards background. Negative scan patients go back on thyroid replacement until the next screening point.

The profile scan should be sensitive enough to detect down to 0.02% of the dose at 4–5 days at any one focus. This scan should also be able crudely to assess turnover time of radioiodine in any tissue with uptake.

As a complementary investigation the PB^{131}I is determined after the tracer dose. In an athyreotic patient the circulating blood half-life of the ionized salt is approximately 12 hours and it should be undetectable by 1 week. Pochin (1967) observed that if, 6 days after a tracer dose of ^{131}I, the PB^{131}I was greater than 0.04%/ℓ then functioning (organifying) tumour tissue was present. Furthermore, this PB^{131}I measurement can crudely help in the assessment of body tumour burden.

A separate investigation which measures serum thyroglobulin levels has been heralded as a replacement screening test for the complex programme outlined above (Van Herle, and Uller, 1975; Black *et al.*, 1981). A feature of a follicular cell origin carcinoma with colloid containing follicles is thyroglobulin production, this usually going hand-in-hand with iodide trapping and binding. Patients on adequate doses of thyroid hormones have suppressed thyroglobulin production by normal thyroid tissue, and Black *et al.* reported that if the serum thyroglobulin level in these patients exceeded 5 μg/ℓ then there was 98% chance that metastatic disease was present. Black *et al.* proposed that this single serum analysis, which could be performed without withdrawal of thyroid hormone replacement, could replace the entire radioiodine screening programme. Thyroid ablation would still be necessary in relapsing patients prior to radioiodine therapy, but these would comprise the minority. This work is a potentially important contribution to the management of thyroid cancer, but the thyroglobulin assay, as used by other workers reporting their data to date, often has a lower sensitivity (although retaining a high specificity) than in the study just cited. These workers have extended this study to use radiolabelled antithyroglobulin to detect and localize thyroid metastases (Fairweather *et al.*, 1983); thus the possibility of therapy with antibody is now on the horizon. A minority of tumours are still able to concentrate radioiodine but do not produce thyroglobulin which is recognizable by the assay system (Grant *et al.*, 1984).

Pochin (1967) observed that under such conditions as described above, 80% of differentiated follicular cell origin carcinoma metastases concentrate radioiodine. A relapsed patient with a positive profile scan may expect to derive a useful response to a therapy dose of radioiodine if the tumour concentrates at least 0.05–0.10% of the dose/g, but one is hoping for a concentration nearer 0.50%/g. (A patient with an average tumour iodine turnover time who concentrates 0.1% of a 150 mCi dose/g of tumour receives 5000 cGy to the tumour, 0.5%/g gram delivers 25 000 cGy.)

The whole body dose received during radioiodine therapy is approximately 0.3 – 0.6 cGy/mCi.

The demonstration of such functioning metastases is an indication for therapy doses of radioiodine at 3-monthly intervals initially and then less frequently until such metastases have disappeared, six therapy doses have been given over a 2-year period, bone marrow tolerance has been reached or non-functioning tumour supervenes. White cell and platelet nadirs with a slow recovery (notably of the platelet count) to normal levels, or perhaps a plateau on the low side of normal, should all caution the clinicians that bone marrow tolerance has been approached. As shown in *Figure 13.4*, a standard therapy dose of 150 mCi ^{131}I is administered under conditions of high circulating blood TSH. Although there has been much published concerning the calculation of tumour dose, the philosophy of the present author is that if a minimum tumour iodine concentrating avidity has been exceeded, then a high fixed dose of radioiodine therapy (150 mCi) is given on each occasion.

Patients with miliary pulmonary metatases could suffer radiation pneumonitis and later pulmonary fibrosis from such high doses, and patients with spinal cord compression could suffer from early radiation oedema. Such patients should be treated with lower initial doses. Other complications of therapy are usually few, although early nausea and salivary gland swelling and/or pain, and bone marrow depression (especially after multiple therapy doses) are recognized. The gonadal dose may be sufficient to induce a radiation menopause, particularly in older premenopausal patients, or have a mutagenic effect in younger women. Pain in sites of metastases is said to be a good sign. The long-term major side-effect is the danger of inducing leukaemia (*see below*).

Although the thyroid ablation and screening programmes have made an impact on the survival figures for follicular cell origin carcinoma, and although good regression of functioning metastases has been demonstrated following ^{131}I therapy, it is difficult to quantify the impact of radioiodine therapy on the survival of patients in metastatic relapse (Pochin, 1967; Tubiana *et al.*, 1975; Mazzaferri *et al.*, 1977; Maheshwari *et al.*, 1981). In a review of patients with metastatic thyroid carcinoma outside the neck, Brown *et al.* (1984) reported that while pulmonary metastases could often be eradicated by ^{131}I therapy, metastases in bone responded less often.

The role of external beam radiotherapy in follicular cell origin carcinoma remains to be proven, but this treatment is recommended currently for locally invasive and incompletely resected tumours, unless the radioiodine uptake throughout the area of residual disease is high. Palliative radiotherapy to metastatic sites (particularly bone) is very useful in alleviating symptoms.

The chemotherapy data for follicular cell origin carcinoma of thyroid are scanty and unimpressive at present. That this group of athyreotic patients may have metastatic tumour which no longer concentrates

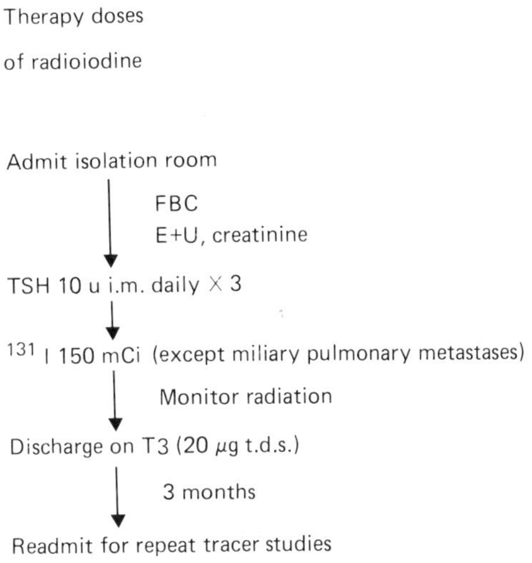

Figure 13.4 Algorithm of radioiodine therapy

radioiodine but yet may retain some unique tumour specific features such as cell membrane TSH receptors or some residual colloid formation, may allow monoclonal antibody attack in the future.

Anaplastic carcinoma

Anaplastic carcinoma of thyroid does not concentrate radioiodine, and locally extensive neck disease, particularly with airways or oesophageal involvement, should be treated by external beam radiotherapy. Some patients may be planned to high dose; others with widespread disease may be palliated through opposed portals (*see below*). Metastatic sites may demand external beam radiotherapy. There is no curative chemotherapy regimen known, and it is questionable whether the morbidity attending a partial response is worthwhile in this group of poor-prognosis patients.

Medullary carcinoma of thyroid

In the large Mayo Clinic experience reported by Chong *et al.* (1975), it seemed clear that surgery was the only potentially curative treatment modality. The present author follows the Mayo guidelines that aggressive surgery (which may include neck dissection and mediastinal exploration to clear involved lymph nodes), is the recommended approach. The multifocal nature of the familial MCT should demand a near total thyroidectomy in this group, although a more conservative thyroidectomy may be chosen in patients with sporadic forms of the disease. Thyroid hormone replacement is usually required.

The serum calcitonin level is an excellent tumour marker as it is fairly sensitive and specific for MCT (the levels being lower in familial MCT than sporadic MCT); the changes in serum levels correlate with changes in tumour burden, and it has a short half-life — less than 15 minutes. Although the calcitonin secreted by MCT is active in a bioassay, there is no metabolic syndrome associated with hypercalcitoninaemia. Serum calcitonin measurements should be performed pre- and postoperatively, and then serially to reflect the tumour burden remaining after treatment and the pace of any relapse. The patient followed in *Figure 13.5* demonstrates that apparently complete surgery had a minimal effect on the tumour burden as reflected by the serum calcitonin, and that the tumour continued to grow exponentially.

External beam radiotherapy can be useful palliatively (e.g. for locally extensive neck disease or for the unusual symptomatic bone metastases). No chemotherapy regimen is of proven value.

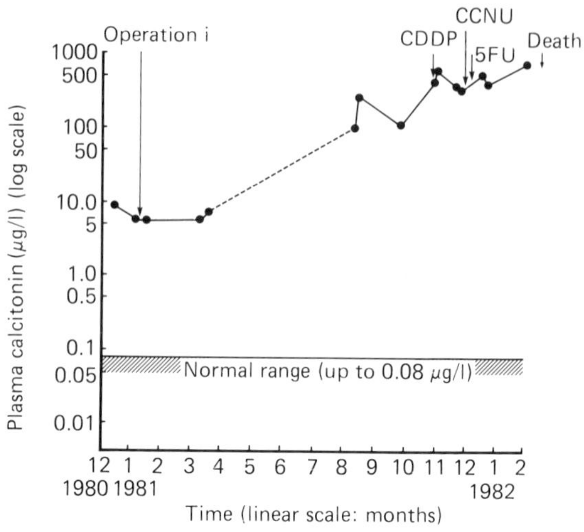

Figure 13.5 Serum calcitonin measurements in a patient with progressive MCT. The doubling time of this patient's tumour can be deduced from the slope of the graph. 5FU: 5-fluorouracil

Lymphoma

The management of malignant lymphoma of thyroid depends upon whether the disease appears localized or disseminated following clinical examination and certain staging procedures (*see* Chapter 8). If the disease appears localized to the thyroid (and regional nodes) the management is by radical external beam radiotherapy to these regions, followed by adjuvant chemotherapy (cyclophosphamide, vincristine, prednisone) with a real chance of cure. If the disease is disseminated then combination chemotherapy (usually with cyclophosphamide, hydroxydaunorubicin, vincristine, prednisone) gives excellent and worthwhile palliation in most cases.

Prognosis

The prognosis for patients with papillary carcinoma of thyroid is excellent and deaths should be unusual. In the large analysis by Mazzaferri *et al.* (1977), large or locally extensive papillary carcinomas were more likely to recur after therapy and the few deaths that did occur tended to be in this group. Papillary carcinoma was found to be more likely to recur locally in patients less than 30 years of age, but the death rate was higher in the older age groups. The conclusion from this apparently paradoxical observation is that regional (nodal) relapse in (young) patients is still highly compatible with cure following re-operation; this was confirmed by a separate analysis of cervical node status at presentation which did not influence survival. Relapses tended to occur slightly more frequently in the earlier follow-up years but a 2% annual rate for the first decade is a rough approximation. After 15 years follow-up, the cumulative recurrence rate was 23% but death rate was less than 4%, again emphasizing that the majority of patients with relapse are salvageable.

The outlook for follicular carcinoma is good but not so good as for papillary carcinoma. In the Mayo Clinic experience the follicular carcinomas which were non-invasive or microangioinvasive had an 86% 10-year survival, whereas those classified as angioinvasive had a 44% 10-year survival. It is noteworthy that just over two-thirds of all follicular carcinomas fell into the former group (Woolner *et al.*, 1961). The outlook for anaplastic carcinomas of thyroid is poor with the majority dying within 6 months of diagnosis.

Two large studies on the natural history of MCT have both found that with the aggressive surgical treatment policy outlined above, the 10-year survival in this slow-growing tumour type is 67% (Gordon, Huvos and Strong, 1973; Chong *et al.*, 1975). The former gloomy outlook for thyroid lymphoma may have improved in recent years. Compagno and Oertel (1980) found that just over half the thyroid lymphoma patients survived and that of those who died the majority had succumbed within 12 months of diagnosis. Patients with 'high grade histology' and more extensive disease at presentation fared worst.

Technical aspects of radiotherapy

Radioiodine — an unsealed source

There are many modes of decay of $^{131}_{53}I$ to the ground state of xenon ($^{131}_{54}Xe$). However, the majority of β-emissions are 0.61 MeV (with a range in tissue of approximately 2 mm) and the majority of γ-emissions are 0.36 MeV (with a *k* factor of 2.2, i.e. 2.2 R/h per mCi at 1 cm). The physical half-life of ^{131}I is 8.04 days.

It may be possible to calculate accurately the dose to a particular organ in which a radionuclide is concentrated. For the dose contribution from the β-emissions, it is necessary to know:

(1) the initial concentration of activity ($C = \mu$Ci/g of tissue
(2) the size of the organ
(3) the physical characteristics of the emission ($E\beta$ = mean β-energy (MeV) emitted per disintegration
(4) the effective half-life T_e which is related to the physical half-life (T_p) and the biological half-life T_b by the formula $1/T_e = 1/T_p + 1/T_b$. Knowing these, the total dose delivered is $73.8 \times C \times E\beta \times T_e$. The difficulty lies in the inability to know accurately the size and weight of the organ.

The γ-ray contribution to an organ is less than its contribution to a whole body because of the longer path length and sparsely ionizing characteristics of this emission. For a spherical organ, the dose contribution may be calculated from the initial concentration of activity of the radionuclide, the *K* factor and the radius of the sphere.

Using the ^{131}I ablation of the normal thyroid gland or remnant as an example, it may be stated that nearly 90% of the ablation dose is derived from the β-emissions. When whole body dose is considered, however, the γ-ray contribution is proportionately more. The whole body dose (which approximates the blood and bone marrow dose) can be calculated, but is best derived empirically from multiple blood sample measurements over several days after a ^{131}I administration. From such measurements, it may be stated that the whole body dose from ^{131}I given as therapy in thyroid carcinoma is usually in the range 0.3–0.6 cGy/mCi.

External beam radiotherapy

The treatment of thyroid malignancy by external beam radiotherapy provides an excellent object lesson in radiotherapy techniques. Several introductory statements are pertinent. The thyroid gland and its regional lymph nodes which extend into the mediastinum, are located just anterior to the critical normal tissue in this region: the spinal cord. The skin outline over the target volume changes enormously in both superoinferior and transverse sections (*Figure 13.6*). When considering a treatment scheme which avoids the spinal cord and yet treats the low neck, parallel opposed lateral portals are not possible because of the shoulders.

One can consider first the easiest example, the radical treatment of localized thyroid lymphoma. For this disease, a wide field is treated to include the whole neck and supraclavicular fossae and the upper mediastinal nodes down to the carina; the radical dose is less than that required for epithelial cancer. Parallel opposed anterior and posterior MV photon portals are employed in the first phase (*Figures 13.7a, b*). The patient lies in the mantle position and the upper field border is the same as for a mantle (i.e. the line between the chin dimple and the external auditory meatus — this line being vertical). The lower border is marked from the acromion diagonally 2 cm inferior to the clavicular border until it meets the mediastinal component of the field which extends down to the carina (found by simulation). Skin marks are usually employed rather than a template and both fields are permanently recorded by simulator films taken with solder wire outlining the portal for filming. The changing skin contour and body separation measurements from neck to mediastinum are nullified by bolus or compensation. As the dose for the first phase is not high, bolus is used around the neck and supraclavicular fossae. If compensation is

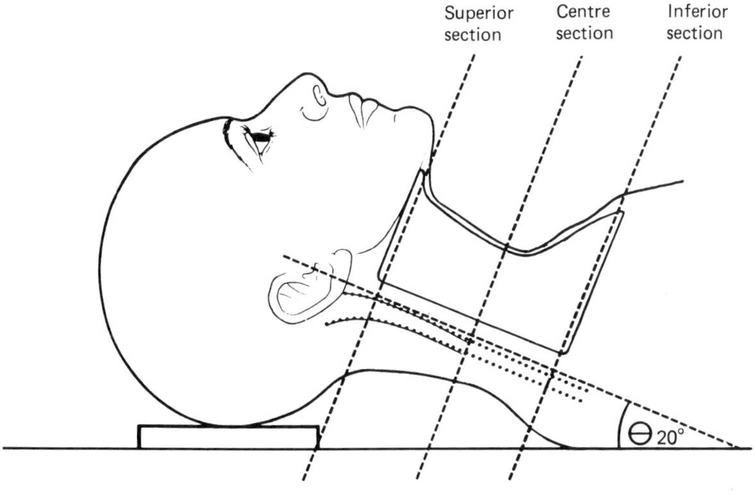

Figure 13.6 Neck sections through treatment volume

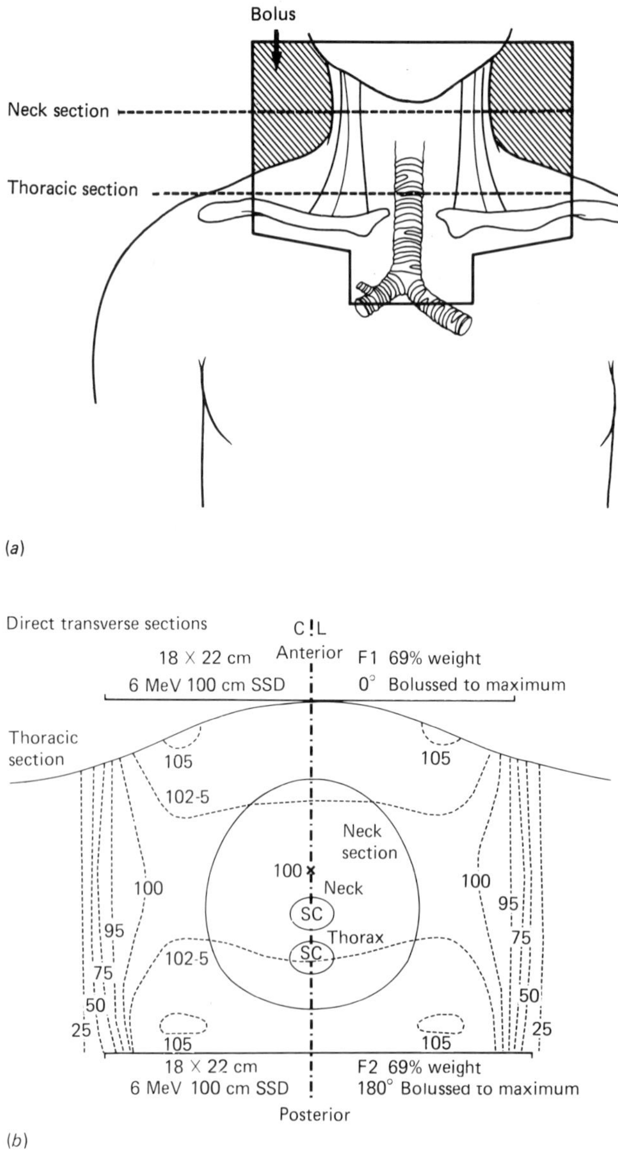

Figure 13.7 (*a*) Portal for treatment of localized thyroid lymphoma. (*b*) Dosimetry of fully bolussed, parallel opposed portal technique. SC: spinal cord; SSD: source skin distance

employed, only the surgical scar would require bolus. The prescribed dose is 3500 cGy midplane in 17–20 daily fractions; this does not exceed cord tolerance. The second phase of treatment is a 500–1000 cGy boost to the tumour bed and is usually administered through an anterior 14 MeV electron portal (*see below*). Where an electron beam of similar energy is not available, the parallel opposed MeV photon technique is continued for the boost, with lead protection to the spinal cord from the posterior portal.

For differentiated follicular cell origin carcinoma or MCT requiring external beam radiotherapy, the situation is more demanding as the spinal cord must not receive the full dose. The patient's treatment position is first found by simulation. The patient is supine with the head resting on an adjustable head block. The head elevation and flexion are adjusted until the cervical spine is straight (i.e. running parallel to the target volume and not bending into it) (*see Figure 13.6*). This position is reproducibly achieved each day by utilizing cardboard cut-out jigs or by an individual plastic facemask (shell), and the plan now continues parallel to the critical normal tissue throughout the length of the target volume. The target volume is defined from clinical examination, operative description and imaging. Although circumstances vary with individuals, the full length of the neck and upper mediastinum are usually included in the initial target volume but not the full width of the supraclavicular fossae. Two plans are usually the best alternatives. In the first (*Figure 13.8a*), MeV photons are employed from three fields: an open anterior and two wedged anterior oblique fields. The changing skin contours from upper neck to midfield to upper mediastinum make full tissue compensation absolutely essential to this type of plan. The spinal cord position is marked on the outlines taken through superior, midfield and inferior borders of the target volume and these three sections are superimposed in the composite plan. With full tissue compensation,

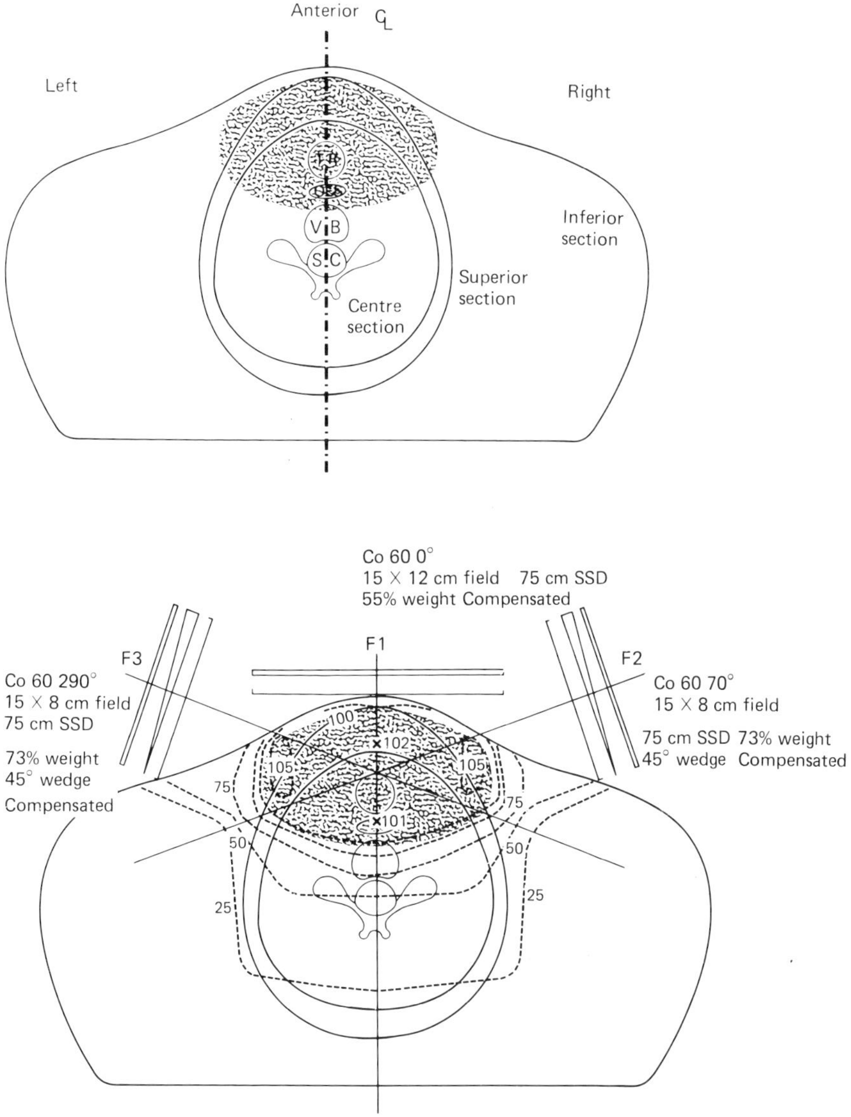

Figure 13.8 (*a*) Radical MeV photon plan for thyroid carcinoma. In the upper panel only the superimposed outlines (which are superior and inferior target volume sections in addition to the midline section) are shown. In the lower panel, the 3 field plan is added. ▨ Target volume; TR: trachea; OES: oesophagus; VB: vertebral body; SC: spinal cord; SSD: source skin distance

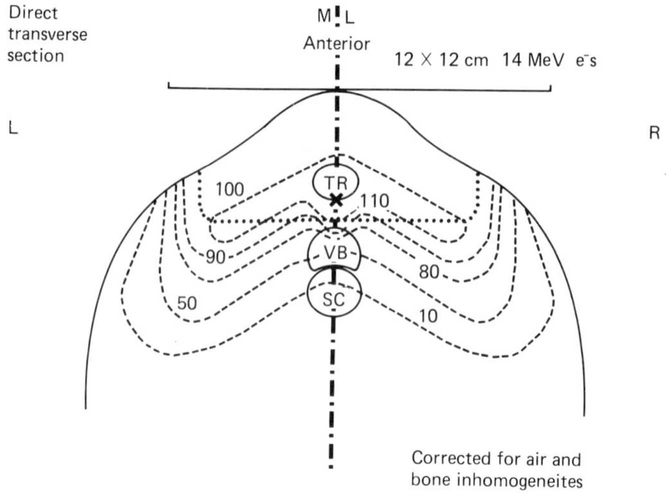

Figure 13.8 (*b*) Anterior MeV electron portal with the tracheal air gap compensated by an attenuation cap. Note that the sloping neck contour gives the ideal horse-shoe distribution in this 'idealized' neck. TR: air volume in trachea; VB: vertebral body; SC: spinal cord

these different outlines should not alter the optimal dose distribution unless the target volume or cord slopes in the third dimension. It would be unusual for the machine head to require twisting in the third plane in order to keep down the cord dose if the initial positioning procedure has been performed. The maximum spinal cord dose should be routinely documented on the treatment sheet.

The second type of plan (*Figure 13.8b*) is simpler. It comprises an open anterior 14 MeV electron portal beamed at the target volume with the patient in the supine position just described. The sloping neck contour allows the electron isodoses to 'bend' around the thyroid compartment of the neck and so homogenize the dose distribution within the target volume. The tracheal air gap could lead to forward projection of isodoses in the midline region and hence overdosage to the spinal cord (although the high density cervical vertebral bodies may compensate this). An attenuating wax midline block, overlying the trachea, is recommended to obviate this problem.

The prescribed dose, which in a good plan will be on the minimum tumour isodose, is 5000–5500 cGy in 25–30 daily fractions. It would be usual to reduce the length of the fields after 5000 cGy so that only the macroscopically involved regions are boosted to a higher dose. The skin reaction is obviously brisker with this electron technique.

A third external beam technique using a rotational bar and arc is described by Cunningham (1974). In this method, the horseshoe-shaped target volume (as seen in a transverse neck section) which partially surrounds the spinal cord, is treated by a 120° rotational technique using an anterior MeV photon source but with a screening bar placed in the central axis of the beam and moving synchronously with the rotation of the treatment unit. This screening bar will protect the spinal cord throughout the treatment.

Protection aspects of radioiodine therapy

The recommendations of the International Commission on Radiological Protection (ICRP) and the two Euratom Directives (1976, 1979), which lay down the safety standards for the European Community, bear directly on the therapeutic use of radioiodine. Every UK establishment using therapeutic radioiodine will shortly come into line, with the assistance of the UK Health and Safety Commission (HSC) and the National Radiological Protection Board (NRPB).

The unsealed source of radioiodine may only be 'manipulated' in designated and carefully equipped working areas (laboratories and specified hospital side wards with private lavatory and washing facilities), the drainage facilities leading directly to the main drainage effluent off the site. In these hospital side rooms, the floors, walls and ceiling must be covered with smooth, continuous, non-absorbant and easily cleansed surfaces (e.g. vinyl sheeting for floors and hard gloss paint for walls). Sinks and shower trays must be of stainless steel. The patient must use disposable eating utensils (e.g. paper plates, plastic cutlery). The area is designated by a radiation hazard warning notice which complies with the safety signs' regulations 1980 (i.e. they must comprise the radiation trefoil symbol inside a black triangle, with appropriate words). The notice gives details of the nature and activity of the isotope, the time and date of administration and any relevant nursing instructions. When large activities are administered, instructions regarding the time which staff and visitors may spend near the patient are outlined as well as the necessity for protective clothing. Pregnant women and children must be excluded from the area altogether. Local rules are outlined by the Radiological Protection Officer, who will supervise the wearing of monitoring 'badges' by the clinical staff. Radiation and contamination monitoring equipment must be available.

The patient who has received ablative or therapeutic doses of radioiodine will remain in such isolated conditions until (current UK practice) the maximum body iodine activity is 15 mCi or less, (if travelling home by public transport), or 30 mCi or less (if travelling home by private transport). Upon arrival home, the patient takes further precautions — avoiding playing with children or sharing a bed with a spouse until the whole body activity is deemed 3.5 mCi or less.

In the event of spillage of radioiodine solution, the spilled material should be treated with an excess of sodium thiosulphate solution to render it chemically stable prior to beginning the decontamination procedure. Contaminated clothing is immediately removed and prolonged washing/showering initiated without delay. Thyroid uptake of radioiodine can be blocked by the oral administration of an excess of stable iodine and 300 mg potassium iodide (KI) is administered orally to all persons potentially contaminated immediately after the incident and prior to thyroid and whole body serial monitoring. In those contaminated, the KI is continued (300 mg daily) for 10 days.

Thyrotoxicosis treatment by radioiodine

Radioiodine therapy is useful in some cases of thyrotoxicosis with diffuse thyroid hyperplasia. The radiation dose delivered to the hyperactive gland is usually sufficient to restore the euthyroid state. However, another important consideration has limited the indications for radioiodine administration for this benign disease: the whole body radiation dose received from such therapy has potential mutagenic and carcinogenic effects (leukaemogenic) — both these being stochastic effects of ionizing radiation. It may be stated here that the incidence of both these effects would appear to be extremely low (if detectable), and that consideration of these effects does not enter into management decisions during therapy of thyroid carcinoma (with the possible exception of intrathyroidal papillary carcinoma, *see above*). In the management of thyrotoxicosis, however, most British clinicians have limited the administration of radioiodine to older patients. Despite the recent conclusion of the UK Administration of Radioactive Substances Advisory Committee (ARSAC) that age restrictions should be removed (Williams and Halnan, 1983), the present author currently reserves radioiodine therapy in thyrotoxicosis to those past the reproductive years.

Radioiodine therapy is a reasonably certain way of treating thyrotoxicosis but takes at least several weeks to effect the reduction in the hyperthyroid state and carries a late risk of permanent hypothyroidism, which may not declare itself for up to 2 years after therapy. These factors influence management. A seriously thyrotoxic patient must be first controlled by more immediately effective therapy (e.g. carbimazole and propranolol) prior to definitive radioiodine therapy. As carbimazole and similar thiouracil drugs inhibit iodine organification and hence the concentration of radioiodine in the thyroid gland, it is then necessary to omit carbimazole for at least several days both before and after the radioiodine dose in order to achieve a therapeutic radiation dose to the gland. In the elderly, the severely toxic and those with cardiac complications, it is usually necessary to admit the patient to hospital over the period of therapy for observation. The adrenergic blocker may be continued during this period.

The philosophy on dose of radioiodine delivered differs in various centres. The present author prefers a single administration of 7–10 mCi (^{131}I). For larger (particularly multinodular) goitres or where one requires a more certain control of hyperthyroidism, a higher dose is recommended (10–15 mCi), even if the later risk of permanent hypothroidism is higher. All patients are carefuly followed-up; a minority will not be controlled and may require a second therapy dose 3 months later, while perhaps 10–20% of patients will eventually become hypothyroid requiring lifelong thyroxine replacement. Kendall-Taylor, Keir and Ross (1984) prefer to administer a higher (15 mCi) dose to all patients with its greater certainty of thyrotoxicosis control and early occurrence of iatrogenic hypothyroidism allowing early administration of thyroid hormone replacement. Not all workers would agree with this policy.

Adrenal tumours

The adrenal glands lie superomedial to the kidneys, paravertebrally in the retroperitoneal fat. The right gland is closely related to the liver, inferior vena cava and duodenum, while the left is separated from the stomach by the omental bursa and inferiorly is related to the superior border of the pancreas.

Tumours may arise in the cortex or medulla. Although benign cortical adenomas are not infrequently found at autopsy, most are non-functioning and of no clinical importance. The majority of functioning cortical tumours are found in female patients; those occurring in prepubertal patients tend to present with virilization while those in postpubertal patients present with Cushing's syndrome. An adrenal cortical adenoma producing aldosterone (Conn's syndrome) is a very rare cause of hypertension. Diagnostic tests include the endocrine demonstration of non-suppressable and excessive levels of circulating adrenal steroids and the relevant diagnostic imaging (e.g. intravenous urography (IVU), CT scan, angiography). Treatment is by surgical excision (adrenalectomy) — for both adenoma and carcinoma.

Adrenal carcinoma occurs in a younger age group than most epithelial cancers and in one study the average age of female patients was 37 years and of men 48 years (Nader *et al.*, 1983). Over one-half of the patients presented with abdominal symptoms such as fullness, indigestion, nausea, vomiting, abdominal swelling.

Histologically, adrenal cortical carcinoma may show features of differentiation or, more commonly, are anaplastic. In the differentiated type the cells are often polygonal and ultrastructural studies may show the features of steroid-forming cells (e.g. prominent endoplasmic reticulum and mitochondrial cristae). Some adrenal carcinoma cells may contain glycogen and appear as 'clear cells' on haematoxylin and eosin staining; they must then be distinguished from renal carcinoma.

Clinically, adrenal carcinoma behaves as an aggressive tumour with a propensity to early local infiltration and venous invasion; the most common sites of metastases are regional nodes (para-aortic, para-caval), peritoneal surfaces, liver and lungs; the proclivity for bone and brain differs in various reported series. Iodocholesterol scanning was based on the high metabolic rate of cholesterol in adrenal tissue but the technique has proved disappointing for the detection of metastases. For apparently localized tumour, radical surgical resection is recommended, and each patient is individually assessed for postoperative radiotherapy. The latter is recommended where there is incomplete surgical resection of an apparently localized adrenal carcinoma. Parallel opposed megavoltage photon portals are usually employed to deliver a dose in the region of 4000 cGy midplane in 20 fractions over 28 days. The adjacent position of the kidney to each adrenal and also of the liver on the right must always be considered and may provide constraints on radiation planning and dosage; overlying small bowel and the proximity of the spinal cord also require consideration in planning.

Adrenal carcinomas function endocrinologically in approximately one-third of cases and relatively more frequently in females. Cushing's syndrome due to adrenal carcinoma may be palliated by metyrapone therapy (250 mg – 1 g four times daily, commencing at the lower dose). Metyrapone inhibits 11 β-hydroxylase (the enzyme that converts the metabolically inactive 11-deoxycortisol to cortisol). When used as the only therapy, metyrapone may be so effective as to provoke ACTH hypersecretion and overwhelming of the enzyme inhibition. For these reasons, and to prevent a potential Addisonian episode, it is advisable to administer glucocorticoids in ACTH suppressive dosage (e.g. prednisolone 10 mg daily in divided dosage). Some patients experience pronounced gastrointestinal upset on metyrapone and occasional allergic reactions have been documented. Aminoglutethimide inhibits the conversion of cholesterol to pregnenolone (an early step in steroidogenesis). Given orally (250 mg two to four times daily) this drug also usefully palliates Cushing's syndrome, although gastrointestinal intolerance and the occasional violent morbilliform rash may limit its usefulness. Combination therapy with metyrapone and aminoglutethimide may be useful where escalation of the dosage of the individual drugs has led to side-effects. Such therapy is useful in the preparation for surgery of a patient with functioning and apparently operable adrenal carcinoma and in the longer term palliation of the advanced, functioning tumour. The possibility of Addisonian crisis must be remembered in all patients treated with these agents and glucocorticoid cover is usual.

Unlike the above mentioned drugs which provide a palliative metabolic blockade, O,p'DDD is a specific therapy; the drug causes necrosis and atrophy of normal adrenal tissue and also of differentiated adrenal carcinoma cells. Hutter and Kayhoe (1966) reported a steroid response rate of 72% and an objective regression of tumour bulk in 34%. Other workers have subsequently confirmed this drug's usefulness in adrenal carcinoma but responses may be slow (months) and there are associated gastrointestinal (vomiting and diarrhoea) and neuromuscular symptoms (lethargy and weakness) in many patients. The drug is not myelosuppressive, nor does it have hepatic or renal toxicity. Glucocorticoid cover is advisable.

Cytotoxic chemotherapy has no established place in adrenal cortical carcinoma management.

Adrenal medulla

The adrenal medulla belongs to the sympathetic nervous system, and the neuroblastoma of childhood (*see* Chapter 10) and phaeochromocytoma may both arise anywhere there is sympathetic nervous tissue.

Phaeochromocytomas are uncommon, occurring in approximately 1/10 000 of the population (UK), and in less than 1% of the hypertensive population. Phaeochromocytoma has been noted in a familial association with neurofibromatosis (von Recklinghausen's disease) or other endocrine tumours, in particular medullary carcinoma of thyroid and hyperparathyroidism (Sipple's syndrome, *see below*). Approximately 10% of phaeochromocytomas are malignant, invading local areas or giving rise to distant metastases; 90% of phaeochromocytomas arise in the adrenal glands. The tumour cells are polygonal and contain cytoplasmic 'granules' which contain the catecholamine stores.

Clinically, a phaeochromocytoma may present due to its release of pressor amines into the vasculature; this release may occur in spontaneous bursts or be provoked by emotion, exertion, posture, food or tumour handling. These episodes of catecholamine release may lead to the 'intermittent attacks' of classical phaeochromocytoma. During such attacks a patient feels apprehension and usually headache and pallor, sweating and palpitation; the blood pressure is usually very high during attacks which may last from a few minutes to several hours. Other patients suffer sustained hypertension and no episodic attacks.

The diagnosis is suspected in any patient with attacks such as described and is remembered as a rare (but usually curable) cause of hypertension. The diagnosis is made biochemically by the demonstration of increased catecholamine formation (vanillyl mandelic acid or metanephrines), quantified in the urine over a 24-hour period. Adrenal tumours are localized most commonly by CT scanning or ultrasound (usually preceded by IVU), but venous sampling at different levels in the vena cava allows confirmation of tumour site and detection of multiple growths. Unlike arteriography, venous cannulation is unlikely to provoke a hypertensive crisis.

Recently, (^{131}I) meta-iodobenzylguanidine (^{131}I MIBG) has been introduced as a commercially available radiopharmaceutical agent which is localized in adrenergic tissue. In recent years, accurate scintigraphic localization of phaeochromocytoma has been possible using this agent (Sisson *et al.*, 1981). Treatment of a single, localized phaeochromocytoma is by surgical resection.

^{131}I MIBG therapy is an interesting new approach to management, and capable of delivering meaningful radiotherapeutic doses to some tumours. External beam radiotherapy has little established place in primary management and limited application in palliation, but 3000 cGy in 10 fractions to bony metastases will produce good pain relief. In inoperable tumours, pressor amine production may be usefully inhibited by α-methyl tyrosine.

Apudomas and multiple endocrine adenomatosis

Pearse first recognized that throughout the body's different organs were a number of cell series with common cytochemical and ultrastructural properties. Cytochemically the most notable characteristic of these cells is their capacity for amine precursor uptake and decarboxylase (APUD) particularly of 3,4 dihydroxyphenylalanine (DOPA) and 5-hydroxytryptophan. The cells may also be identified by argyrophilia and ultrastructurally by the presence of specific endocrine storage granules. These storage granules contain any of up to 40 recently recognized peptide or amine hormones/transmitters. The term hormones/transmitters is used because many, perhaps most, of the peptides and amines stored and secreted by APUD cells are also found within the central nervous system as neurotransmitters. Gastrointestinal tract APUD cells often secrete their storage products to effect local responses on adjacent cells in a manner analogous to neurotransmitters (paracrine function). Indeed, the overlaps between the endocrine and nervous systems is such that Pearse regards the APUD cells as a 'third division of the nervous system' — a diffuse neuroendocrine system (Pearse, 1983).

This diffuse neuroendocrine system has a central division comprising the cells of the hypothalamo-pituitary axis and those of the pineal gland. The peripheral division's APUD cells are largely found within the gastrointestinal tract and pancreas, although the bronchial tree, urogenital tract, thyroid and parathyroid gland and adrenal medulla together with the autonomic nervous system also contain APUD cells.

APUD-omas are tumours of APUD cells which may be benign or malignant, and are often of importance because of the hypersecretion of APUD cells storage products. Apudomas are often described by the principal hormone secreted: e.g. insulinoma, glucagonoma, VIPoma, gastrinoma, prolactinoma etc. Other tumours retain their individual identities as parathyroid adenoma, medullary carcinoma of the thyroid, phaeochromocytoma, carcinoid. Highly malignant tumours such as malignant melanoma and small cell (oat cell) carcinoma of bronchus may also derive from APUD cells.

If one confines the discussion to gastrointestinal tract apudomas then treatment follows localization of the tumour by the imaging procedures, and surgery is often curative. Where there is malignant infiltration or diffuse hyperplasia/neoplasia of the APUD cells (e.g. some cases of Zollinger-Ellison syndrome), then surgery may be incomplete. In these instances, therapeutic procedures are often necessary to counteract the effects of the hypersecretion of the hormone/transmitter — either by drugs or other means, (e.g. total gastrectomy in Zollinger-Ellison syndrome). Cytotoxic chemotherapy has not made a major impact on the rare cases of malignancy arising from these tumours but dacarbazine (DTIC) and streptozotocin have both been described as active agents and may be useful in palliation.

Although many gastrointestinal tract carcinoid

tumours are also of neuroendocrine origin, the typical carcinoid syndrome which occurs when an advanced mid-gut carcinoid tumour has metastasized to the liver, is an important distinct entity. Attacks of facial flushing with loud borborygmi and diarrhoea occur in typical cases and the serotonin catabolite, 5-hydroxyindole acetic acid, is present in the urine in abnormal quantities. Serotonin antagonists (cyproheptadine, chlorpromazine, methysergide) may palliate these symptoms, as may phenoxybenzamine. Anecdotal literature reports of intra-arterial (hepatic artery) administration of 5-fluorouracil have suggested a role here for this cytotoxic agent, and other workers have claimed that systemic 5-fluorouracil, hydroxydaunorubicin and DTIC are active as single agents. Bronchial carcinoid adenomas are less likely to metastasize, the cells are less argyrophilic and the carcinoid syndrome is uncommon; the tumours may, nevertheless, be functional (e.g. causing 'ectopic ACTH' production). Surgery is usually curative.

The place of external beam radiotherapy in apudoma management is not well established, but the present author has had experience of patients with incomplete resection of a primary who have had long-term disease-free survival followng external beam radiotherapy, and he would therefore recommend postoperative radiotherapy in such cases. The technique for therapy would depend on the situation of the growth as would the dose prescription; most commonly, parallel opposed portals are employed and a dose of 4000–4500 cGy would be delivered in 20–25 daily fractions.

Multiple endocrine adenomatosis (MEA)

There is a tendency for several apudomas to occur together and for this pattern to be familial. In one syndrome (MEA I), parathyroid adenomas tend to be associated with pituitary adenomas and pancreatic islet adenomas. In MEA IIa there is a tendency for medullary carcinoma of thyroid to occur in association with phaeochromocytoma(s) and to a less extent parathyroid adenoma. In MEA IIb this triad occurs with a 'Marfanoid habitus' and mucosal neuromas. The clinical importance of these linkages is the need to screen for associated tumours upon discovery of one apudoma; also, following the diagnosis of MEA, there is a requirement to screen relatives as MEA has an autosomal dominant form of inheritance.

References

BLACK, E. G., CASSONI, A., GIMLETTE, T. M. B. *et al.* (1981) Serum thyroglobulin in thyroid cancer. *Lancet*, **2**, 443–445

BROWN, A. P., GREENING, W. P., McCREADY, V. R., SHAW, H.J. and HARMER, C. L. (1984) Radioiodine treatment of metastatic thyroid carcinoma: the Royal Marsden experience. *British Journal of Radiology*, **57**, 323–327

BURKE, J. S., BUTLER, J. J. and FULLER, L. M. (1977) Malignant lymphomas of the thyroid. *Cancer*, **39**, 1587–1602

CHONG, G. C., BEAHRS, O. H., SIZEMORE, G. W. and WOOLNER, L. B. (1975) Medullary carcinoma of the thyroid gland. *Cancer*, **35**, 695–704

COMPAGNO, J. and OERTEL, J. E. (1980) Malignant lymphoma and other lymphoproliferative disorders of the thyroid gland. *American Journal of Clinical Pathology*, **74**, 1–11

CUNNINGHAM, J. R. (1974) Physical aspects of external radiotherapy of the thyroid gland. In *Thyroid Cancer*, edited by J. O. Godden, pp. 81-88. Toronto: The Ontario Cancer Treatment and Research Foundation

FAIRWEATHER, D. S., BRADWELL, A. R., WATSON, J. S. F., DYKES, P. W., CHANDLER, S. and HOFFENBERGY, R. (1983) Detection of thyroid tumours using radiolabelled anti-thyroglobulin. *Clinical Endocrinology*, **18**, 563–570

GORDON, P. R., HUVOS, A. G. and STRONG, E. W. (1973) Medullary carcinoma of the thyroid gland. *Cancer*, **31**, 915–924

GRANT, S., LUTTRELL, B., REEVE, T. *et al.* (1984) Thyroglobulin may be undetectable in the serum of patients with metastatic disease secondary to differentiated thyroid cancer. *Cancer*, **54**, 1625–1628

HUTTER, A. M. and KAYHOE, D. E. (1966) Adrenal cortical carcinoma. Results of treatment with O,p'DDD in 138 patients. *American Journal of Medicine*, **41**, 581–586

KENDALL-TAYLOR, P., KEIR, M. J. and ROSS, W. M. (1984) Ablative radioiodine therapy for hyperthyroidism: long term follow up study. *British Medical Journal*, **289**, 361–363

McDOUGALL, I. R., COLEMAN, C. N., BURKE, J. S., SAUNDERS, W. and KAPLAN, H. S. (1980) Thyroid carcinoma after high dose external radiotherapy for Hodgkin's disease. *Cancer*, **45**, 2056–2060

MAHESHWARI, Y. K., HILL, C. S., HAYNIE, T. P., HICKEY, R. C. and SAMAAN, N. A. (1981) ^{131}I therapy in differentiated thyroid carcinoma. *Cancer*, **47**, 664–671

MAXON, H. R., THOMAS, S. R., SAENGER, E. L., BUNCHER, C. R. and KEREIAKES, J. G. (1977) Ionising radiation and the induction of clinically significant disease in the human thyroid gland. *American Journal of Medicine*, **63**, 967–978

MAZZAFERRI, E. L., YOUNG, R. L., OERTEL, J. E., KEMMERER, W. T. and PAGE, C. P. (1977) Papillary thyroid carcinoma: the impact of therapy in 576 patients. *Medicine US*, **56**, 171–196

MODAN, B., MARK, H., BAIDATZ, D., STEINITZ, R. and LEVIN, S. G. (1974) Radiation induced head and neck tumours. *Lancet*, **1**, 277–299

NADER, S., HICKEY, R. C., SELLIN, R. V. and SAMAAN, N. A. (1983) Adrenal cortical carcinoma: a study of 77 cases. *Cancer*, **52**, 707–711

PEARSE, A. G. E. (1983) The neuroendocrine division of the the nervous system. APUD cells as neurones or paraneurones. In *Dale's Principle and Communication Between Neurones*, edited by N. N. Osborne, pp. 37–47. Oxford: Pergamon Press

POCHIN, E. E. (1967) Prospects from the treatment of thyroid carcinoma with radioiodine. *Clinical Radiology*, **18**, 113–135

SAMPSON, R. J., WOOLNER, L. B., BAHN, R. C. and KURLAND, L. T. (1974) Occult carcinoma in Olmsted County, Minnesota: prevalence at autopsy compared with that in Hiroshima and Nagasaki, Japan. *Cancer*, **34**, 2072–2085

SISSON, J. C., FRAGER, M. S., VALK, T. W. *et al.* (1981) Scintigraphic localisation of pheochromocytoma. *New England Journal of Medicine*, **305**, 12–17

TUBIANA, M., LACOUR, J., MONNIER, J. P. *et al.* (1975) External radiotherapy and radioiodine in the treatment of 359 thyroid cancers. *British Journal of Radiology*, **48**, 894–907

VAN HERLE, J. and ULLER, R. P. (1975) Elevated serum thyroglobulin. A marker of metastases in differentiated thyroid carcinomas. *Journal of Clinical Investigation*, **56**, 272–277

WILLIAMS, E. S. and HALNAN K. E. (1983) Risks from radioiodine treatment for thyrotoxicosis. *British Medical Journal*, **287**, 1882

WOOLNER, L. B., BEAHRS, O. H., BLACK, B. M., McCONAHEY, W. M. and KEATING, F. R. (1961) Classification and prognosis of thyroid carcinoma. *American Journal of Surgery*, **102**, 354–388

14

Gastrointestinal carcinomas

T. J. Priestman

Introduction

For more than 50 years occasional reports have appeared in the medical literature indicating that irradiation might be of value in the treatment of various gastrointestinal cancers, but the evidence has never been sufficiently strong to gain wide acceptance and radiotherapy is still not considered part of the routine management of most gut tumours. In the last decade there has been renewed interest in the potential role of irradiation in the control of the common gastrointestinal adenocarcinomas, leading to a number of clinical trials which have been either recently reported or are currently in progress. The resulting data are often inconclusive or conflicting and allow few firm conclusions to be drawn. Against this background it is not reasonable to give authoritative recommendations on the indications for, and techniques of, therapeutic irradiation of gastrointestinal cancers. This chapter, therefore, sets out to summarize the natural history of the major gut tumours, identifying the causes of failure of current, primarily surgical, treatment and suggests possible areas where radiotherapy might be of value, describing those clinical studies which have set out to determine whether the addition of such treatment will improve response rates or survival.

The effects of irradiation on normal gastrointestinal tissues

The radiation tolerance of the gastrointestinal tract varies at different sites, with the duodenum and jejunum being the most sensitive regions. A summary of the effects of therapeutic irradiation on the gut is given in *Table 14.1*. The underlying histologic changes following radiotherapy are best documented for the small intestine where the acute reaction is represented by erosion of the epithelium, blunting of the villi and congestion of the submucosa, with capillary haemorrhages and reduction in lymphatic tissue in more severe cases. Chronic changes are characterized by progressive endarteritis which may result in ulceration, infarction or fibrosis and is accompanied by histological changes of atypical epithelial appearances with irregular crypt formation, thickening of the serosa, vascular sclerosis, submucosal thickening and fibrosis, lymphatic congestion and the condition of ileitis cystica profunda represented by the formation of submucosal cysts (Black *et al.*, 1980; Jensen *et al.*, 1983; Rubin, 1984). The risk of radiation damage may be minimized by keeping the treatment volume as small as possible, using the highest available beam energy — to ensure uniform distribution with the smallest integral dose — and reducing the daily fraction below 200 cGy when large fields are being treated (Roswit, Malsky and Reid, 1972). Care is especially necessary in those patients with a past history of inflammatory bowel disease or other conditions which might result in fixation of the normally mobile small bowel within the radiation field.

The radiosensitivity of the liver is now well established and doses of 3500 cGy to the whole organ, at 150–200 cGy/day, will result in radiation hepatitis in about 30% of patients, with the proportion rising to almost 50% when the dose is in excess of 4000 cGy (Ingold *et al.*, 1965). Clinically, the syndrome develops within 4–6 weeks of completing treatment and comprises anorexia, pain in the right hypochondrium, tender hepatomegaly, jaundice and ascites. The liver enzymes, particularly the alkaline phosphatases, are elevated. Usually these changes resolve spontaneously over 3–4 months but, especi-

Table 14.1 Summary of effects of irradiation on the normal gastrointestinal tract (based mainly on data from Roswit, Malksy and Reid, 1972 and Rubin, 1984)

Site	*Time of onset*	*Dose and incidence**		*Symptoms and signs*	*Underlying pathology*	*X-ray appearances*	*Management*
		5% risk	*50% risk*				
Stomach	Acute: 1–14 days			Anorexia, nausea, vomiting	Gastritis	Reduced motility and emptying ± spasm	Routine antiemetics
	Chronic: 1–24 months	4500 cGy	5000 cGy	Pain, haemorrhage, vomiting	Scarring, stenosis, ulceration and perforation	Reduced motility and ulceration, especially of posterior wall or antrum	Partial gastrectomy for intractible cases
Small intestine	Acute: 1–8 weeks			Pain, nausea, vomiting, bloody diarrhoea, abdominal distension	Denuding of the epithelium with blunting of the villi	Distended and distorted loops of bowel with air and fluid levels	Rest, i.v. hydration and electrolyte replacement Nil orally
	Chronic: 12 months –20 years, most cases occurring within 2 years of irradiation	4000 cGy	5000 cGy	Colic, anorexia, diarrhoea, fatigue, wasting, obstruction, ileus	Fibrosis, strictures, perforation, fistulae, abscesses, peritonitis	Matting, kinking, shortening and twisting of bowel with dilated loops and pooling of fluid	Resection, division of adhesions
Colon	Acute: 1–4 weeks	5000 cGy	6500 cGy	Diarrhoea and abdominal cramps	Oedema and non-specific inflammation		Low residue diet and routine antidiarrhoeal agents
	Chronic: 6 months – 2 years			Intractible colic	Fibrosis, ulceration	Narrowed, shortened, rigid bowel segment	Segmental resection
Rectum	Acute: 2–8 weeks	4000 cGy	5000 cGy	Watery diarrhoea, cramps, tenesmus	Oedema and non-specific inflammation with occasional haemorrhage		Low residue diet, routine antispasmodics and anti-diarrhoeal agents, steroid enemas
	Chronic: 6–12 months up to 10 years	5500 cGy	8000 cGy	Haemorrhage, constipation, pain	Ulceration, strictures, perforation, necrosis	Pipe-stem or hour-glass narrowing with fixity and rigidity	Colostomy and surgical repair

*For 100 cm^2 field treated at 200 cGy per day

ally with higher doses, there is a risk of progression to fatal liver failure. The underlying pathology appears to be damage to the central veins resulting in a form of veno-occlusive disease with hyperaemia and secondary damage to hepatocytes due to obstruction of the efferent veins (Ingold *et al.*, 1965; Reed and Cox, 1966). A further occasional consequence of hepatic irradiation, which may be seen with doses as low as 2000 cGy, is thrombocytopenia (Tefft, Traggis and Filler, 1969; Prasad, Lee and Hendrickson, 1977). This may result from small vessel damage leading to platelet sequestration (Kinsella, 1983). The changes described here occur after irradiation of the whole liver, but it is clear that, if 50% or more of the organ is adequately shielded, then doses of up to 5000 cGy may be given without serious consequences (Kraut and Earle, 1976).

Little is known of the radiation pathology of the pancreas and its sensitivity is not a dose-limiting factor in the irradiation of gastrointestinal lesions with the acinar and islet cells appearing resistant to normal therapeutic doses (Moss, Brand and Battifora, 1979).

Carcinoma of the stomach

One of the earliest reports of the use of therapeutic radiation described the control of gastric carcinoma (Despeignes, 1896). Subsequent megavoltage series have reported measurable regressions (Guttman, 1955) or relief of obstructive symptoms (Mantell, 1982; Childs, 1969) in patients with inoperable disease, and one study has reported a 5-year survival of 7% when radiotherapy was used as the sole method of treatment (Wieland and Hymmen, 1970). Despite these results, radiotherapy seldom forms part of the routine management of patients with stomach cancer, but dissatisfaction with the results of other treatments and results of a number of recent clinical trials of adjuvant therapy are bringing about a reconsideration of the potential role of irradiation in this condition.

Figures from two major British centres show that 66% of patients with gastric carcinoma are operable at the time of presentation, but only 28% will actually be suitable for resection and, although resection is considered potentially curative, the 5-year survival lies between 16 and 38% resulting in an overall figure of only 4% (Brookes, Waterhouse and Powell, 1965; Cassell and Robinson, 1976; Fielding *et al.*, 1980). For those patients who are not suitable for 'curative' resection the outlook is poor with median survivals averaging only 18 weeks (Kingston *et al.*, 1978).

Carcinoma of the stomach spreads by direct extension, lymphatic permeation, vascular and transperitoneal routes. These factors are taken into account in the current TNM staging of the International Union Against Cancer (UICC) (*Table 14.2*).

Table 14.2 TNM classification of carcinoma of the stomach

T	*Primary tumour*
Tis	Pre-invasive carcinoma (carcinoma *in situ*)
T0	No evidence of primary tumour
T1*	Tumour limited to the mucosa or mucosa and submucosa regardless of its extent or location
T2	Tumour with deep infiltration occupying not more than one-half of one region
T3	Tumour with deep infiltration occupying more than one-half but not more than one region
T4	Tumour with deep infiltration occupying more than one region or extending to neighbouring structures
TX	The minimum requirements to assess the primary tumour cannot be met
N	*Regional lymph nodes*
N0	No evidence of regional lymph node involvement
N1	Evidence of lymph node involvement within 3 cm of the primary tumour along the lesser or greater curvatures
N2	Evidence of lymph node involvement more than 3 cm from the primary tumour including those along the left gastric, splenic, coeliac, and common hepatic arteries
N3	Evidence of involvement of the para-aortic and hepatoduodenal lymph nodes and/or other intra-abdominal lymph nodes
NX	The minimum requirements to assess the regional lymph nodes cannot be met
M	*Distant metastases*
M0	No evidence of distant metastases
M1	Evidence of distant metastases
MX	The minimum requirements to assess the presence of distant metastases cannot be met

*The clinical evidence for T is the recognition of: (a) a malignant pedunculated polyp, (b) a malignant sessile polypoid lesion, (c) a cancerous erosion, or (d) an area of cancerous erosion on the margin of, or surrounding a peptic ulcer

The lymphatic drainage of the stomach is complex and *Figure 14.1* shows the principle local nodes which may be involved in tumour spread. Extent of spread clearly influences survival, and in a review of 3430 cases treated in the West Midlands, those with lesions confined to the mucosa had a 5-year survival of 65%, but when the growth reached the serosa the figure fell to 24%. Even for patients with node involvement, however, there was still a 6% 5-year survival, confirming the view that nodal infiltration *per se* is not necessarily a sign of incurability and that the number and distribution of involved nodes are more significant factors (Fielding and Alexander-Williams, 1985).

Past studies have shown that in patients coming to autopsy without resection 18% still have disease

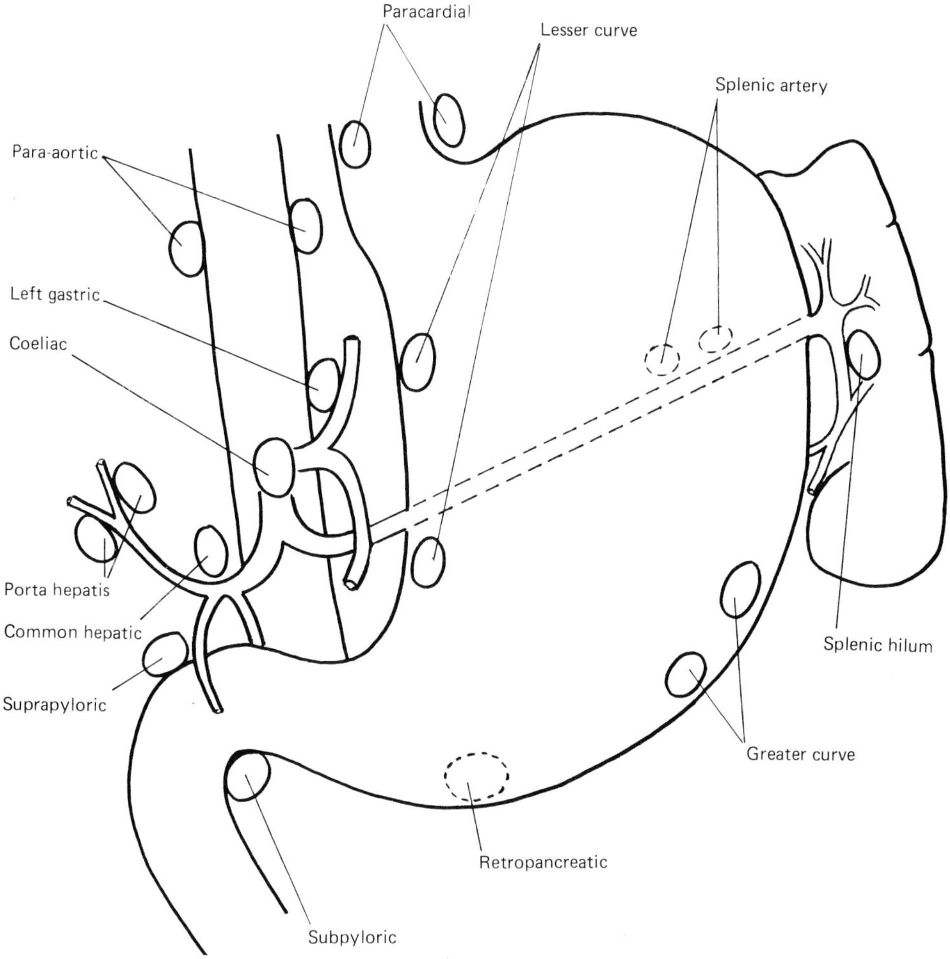

Figure 14.1 Principal local nodes which may be involved in carcinomas of the stomach

localized to the stomach and surrounding nodes (Stout, 1943; Horn, 1955), and a retrospective series looking at 107 patients who had second-look laparotomies after initially 'curative' surgery found evidence of tumour in 86 instances, and in 54% of these there was localized failure with no evidence of distant spread (Gunderson and Sosin, 1982). In all these cases the recurrent tumour could be encompassed within the radiation portals shown in *Figure 14.2a*.

In 1969 a prospectively randomized study in patients with unresectable tumour showed that the addition of 45 mg/kg body weight of fluorouracil in divided doses over the first 3 days of megavoltage irradiation (parallel pair with field size less than 400 cm^2 giving 3000–4000 cGy in 3–4 weeks) significantly improved survival (radiotherapy only 5.9 months, combined therapy 13.0 months, $P<0.01$) (Moertel *et al.*, 1969). It was subsequently noted that three of the 25 patients who received combined treatment survived more than 5 years and one, who died from other causes, had no evidence of gastric carcinoma at post-mortem (Holbrook, 1974). These findings were supported by a similar study from South Africa where objective improvement was noted in 55% of patients with advanced disease treated by a combination of fluorouracil and telecobalt irradiation (Falkson and Falkson, 1969). These results were largely ignored during the 1970s in favour of trials with adjuvant cytotoxic chemotherapy after gastrectomy. The results of these series have now been reported and prospectively randomized evaluations of fluorouracil and mitomycin (Fielding *et al.*, 1983), fluorouracil, cyclophosphamide, methotrexate and vincristine (Blake, Hardcastle and Wilson, 1981), fluorouracil and methyl-CCNU (Higgins *et al.*, 1983; Engstrom and Lavin, 1983), and fluorouracil, hydroxy-daunorubicin and mitomycin (Gagliano, McCracken and Chen, 1983) in combination with surgery have all failed to show any survival advantage compared with surgery alone.

The lack of success of these regimens together with

the realization that a significant proportion of deaths are due to local disease has led to a reappraisal of the possible place of radiotherapy as an adjuvant to surgery. Two series have looked at irradiation and 5-fluorouracil in combination with resection, and reported no survival advantage when compared with surgery alone or surgery plus chemotherapy, but in both instances the radiation doses were low, being 2000 cGy (Dent *et al.*, 1979) and 3000 cGy (Cohen and Zidan, 1981) respectively.

Evaluation of a higher radiation dose, 4500 cGy in 25 fractions over 5 weeks, is the object of a current British Stomach Cancer Group trial. In this study patients who undergo surgery and have a radical resection for lesions which have extended as far as the serosa or beyond and those who have a palliative resection for apparently localized disease are randomized to receive either no further therapy, radiotherapy to the tumour bed, or cyclical chemotherapy with 5-fluorouracil, hydroxydaunorubicin and mitomycin. The radiation is delivered through parallel opposed portals *(Figures 14.2a and b)*. To date over 200 patients have entered this study, but no results are available as yet.

In patients with locally unresectable tumour a recent study in the USA has re-explored the concept of combining radiation and cytotoxics. This Gastrointestinal Study Group trial, which compares 5000 cGy in a split course combined with fluorouracil followed by maintenance fluorouracil and methyl-CCNU with fluorouracil and methyl-CCNU alone, initially suggested that the chemotherapy arm was superior (Schein and Childs, 1978), but longer follow-up has revealed a significant survival advantage for those receiving combined treatment with 16% compared with 7% alive at 5 years ($P<0.05$) (Schein *et al.*, 1982). There is no doubt, however, that the combined therapy resulted in significantly more early morbidity and mortality and several authors have recently reported pilot studies combining high dose (≤4500 cGy) irradiation with intensive cytotoxic therapy in schedules which resulted in substantially less toxicity than was reported in the Gastrointestinal Study Group trial (Hass *et al.*, 1983; Gunderson *et al.*, 1983b; Schein *et al.*, 1983), and these schedules are likely to be incorporated in new randomized studies.

In all the series reported to date the radiation technique has employed megavoltage units and a parallel pair field arrangement. The treatment volume has usually been tailored to encompass known or suspected residual disease and this gener-

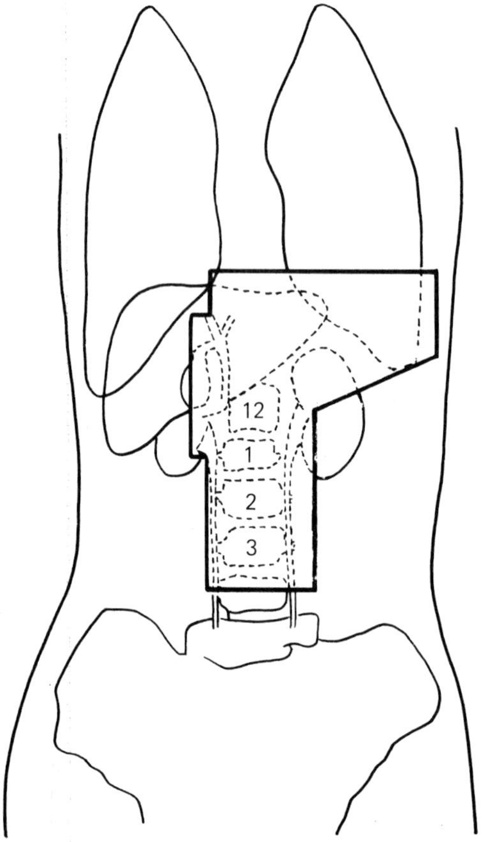

Figure 14.2 (*a*) Radiotherapy portals recommended in the British Stomach Cancer Group trials: the treatment volume includes the post-surgical gastric remnant, anastomoses, duodenal stump, gastric bed and the lymph nodes shown in *Figure 16.1*, including the porta hepatis and splenic hilum.

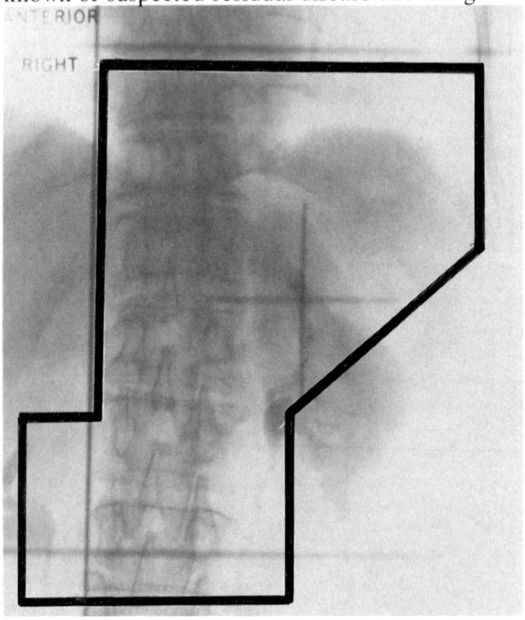

Figure 14.2 (*b*) With accurate treatment planning in conjunction with an IVP, one half to two-thirds of the left kidney may be spared and inclusion of the porta hepatis results in irradiation of only a small part of the right kidney

ally includes the porta hepatis and splenic hilum. The maximum field size is usually restricted to 400 cm^2 and supradiaphragmatic structures are shielded, particularly the heart in those patients for whom hydroxydaunorubicin therapy is planned. Tumour doses vary from 4500 to 6000 cGy, and side-effects appear to be reduced if the daily fractionation is kept below 200 cGy (Gunderson and Sosin, 1982). Inevitably, portions of both kidneys fall within the treatment volume but it appears that if at least two-thirds to three-quarters of one kidney are shielded then radiation nephritis is not a problem (Gunderson *et al.*, 1983b). This means that for proximal gastric lesions, where at least half the left kidney is usually in the field, the right kidney should be spared as much as possible, whereas for distal lesions adjacent to the duodenum it is the right kidney which bears the brunt of the radiation dose and the left may be appropriately shielded.

Alternatives to conventional megavoltage teletherapy are neutron beam irradiation and intraoperative therapy. In a series of 39 inoperable patients treated with fast neutron therapy at the Hammersmith Hospital, London, there were 19 with palpable epigastric masses of which 16 resolved; in addition, of 14 patients who came to autopsy, 10 had no macroscopic evidence of tumour (although all had microscopic disease). In this study, however, the stomach did not recover from the radiation damage and gastrectomy was recommended as a routine procedure 4–6 months after treatment (Catterall *et al.*, 1975). Another group reporting the results of combined neutron and conventional irradiation have claimed total tumour destruction in three out of seven patients with inoperable disease (Eichhorn, Lessel and Matschke, 1974).

Intraoperative radiotherapy is currently being practised in Japan and the technique allows a single high dose of radiation (2800–4000 cGy) to be given at the time of surgery. One recent series has reported on 50 patients with resectable gastric carcinoma treated with surgery and intraoperative irradiation, and claims improved survival compared with previous results from surgery alone (Abe *et al.*, 1980). For the present in Britain, however, facilities for neutron therapy and intraoperative irradiation are very restricted and these procedures must be considered as still largely experimental.

Carcinoma of the pancreas

Carcinoma of the pancreas accounts for some 5000 deaths in England and Wales each year. The overall 5-year survival is less than 5% (Tepper, Nardi and Suit, 1976; Borgelt, Dobelbower and Strubler, 1978). Radical resection is possible in about 20% of patients, but of these only 15–20% will survive 5 years (Tepper, Nardi and Suit, 1976) and in most series the operative mortality exceeds the 5-year survival rate (Baden and Sorenson, 1979). For patients who are deemed unresectable the median survival is only of the order of 3.5 months (Moertel, 1969), but in about one-third of cases extensive local disease, rather than distant metastases, is the criterion for inoperability (Tepper, Nardi and Suit, 1976) and for these patients the median survival is 6 months (Moertel, 1969).

The late presentation and aggressive nature of pancreatic adenocarcinoma are the main factors which account for the lack of success of surgery. When, in addition, the deep-seated location of the tumour and its proximity to radiosensitive structures, such as the kidney, are considered, it is not surprising that radiotherapy has been little used in this condition. Although pancreatic carcinoma has the reputation of being a radioresistant tumour, there have been a number of publications during the first 70 years of this century describing various techniques of irradiation and claiming significant palliation and, on occasions, possibly even improved survival. These reports have been described and evaluated in an excellent recent comprehensive review (Dobelbower, 1979).

Over the last 10 years a number of authors have presented retrospective series assessing the value of megavoltage irradiation with or without chemotherapy in localized unresectable pancreatic cancer and these results are summarized in *Table 14.3.* Following a retrospective survey from the Mayo Clinic showing that radiation doses of 3500–3750 cGy or less offered no survival advantage when compared with untreated patients (Childs, 1969), there has been a concensus that high radiation doses are necessary for pancreatic cancer and all these series have given 5000 cGy or more, seeking to reduce toxicity either by adopting split-course schedules, keeping daily dose to below 200 cGy or abandoning parallel pair techniques in favour of more precise treatment planning. Such planning relies on either marker clips placed at laparotomy or computerized tomography to define the tumour volume. By use of either the three field method, shown in *Figure 14.3a,* or a four field box technique, it is usually possible to encompass the tumour and a 1–2 cm margin within a treatment volume of less than 1 l. This means that the dose delivered to the kidneys, spinal cord and a large amount of small bowel is less than 50% of the tumour dose, whereas if parallel opposed fields are used these organs are included in the high-dose volume *(Figure 14.3b).* Using such localized radiation it has been possible to give tumour doses of up to 6700 cGy in 7–9 weeks without severe late complications (Borgelt, Dobelbower and Strubler, 1978). The series are retrospective and used a variety of treatment policies in a mixed patient population, but two points consistently emerge — overall survival is

Table 14.3 Radiotherapy ± chemotherapy for pancreatic carcinoma

Reference	*No. of patients*	*Radiotherapy schedule*	*Field size*	*Chemotherapy*	*Survival*				*Significant palliation (%)*	*Apparent local control (%)*	*Moderate or severe toxicity (%)*
					Median overall	*Median Rt only*	*Median Rt and Ct*	*% alive at 2 years*			
Haslam, Cavanaugh and Stroup, 1973	23	Three courses of 2000 cGy over 10 weeks. Parallel pair, ^{60}Co	11 x 13 cm on average	11 patients also had 5-fluorouracil	7.5 months	8 months	10 months	30	45	–	48
Borgelt, Dobelbower and Strubler, 1978	19	5900–6700 cGy in 7–9 weeks. Three or four fields on 45 MeV Betatron	Less than 1000 cm^2	7 patients also had 5-fluorouracil alone or in combination with other agents	12 months	8 months	17 months	26	–	–	9
Whittington *et al.*, 1981	48	5000 cGy in 5.5 weeks then 1500 cGy to a reduced volume. Four fields on 45 MeV Betatron	Not stated	15 patients had 5-fluorouracil alone or in combination	10 months	8 months	13 months	14	65	33	–
McCracken *et al.*, 1980	69	Three courses of 2000 cGy over 10 weeks. Parallel pair on ^{60}Co or 2–10 MeV accelerators	Less than 225 cm^2	All patients had 5-fluorouracil + MeCCNU. 30 patients also had testolactone	9.5 months	–	9.5 months	15	–	–	87
McCracken *et al.*, 1982	19	Two courses of 2500 cGy in 7 weeks. Parallel pair ^{60}Co or >2 MeV accelerators	Less than 225 cm^2	All patients had intra-arterial 5-fluorouracil	7 months	–	7 months	–	–	44	44
Nguyen Bugat and Combes, 1982	18	6000 cGy in 6 weeks Four fields on 25 MeV linear accelerator	15 x 10 cm or less	None	12 months	12 months	–	27	–	67	5

Rt: radiotherapy
Ct: chemotherapy

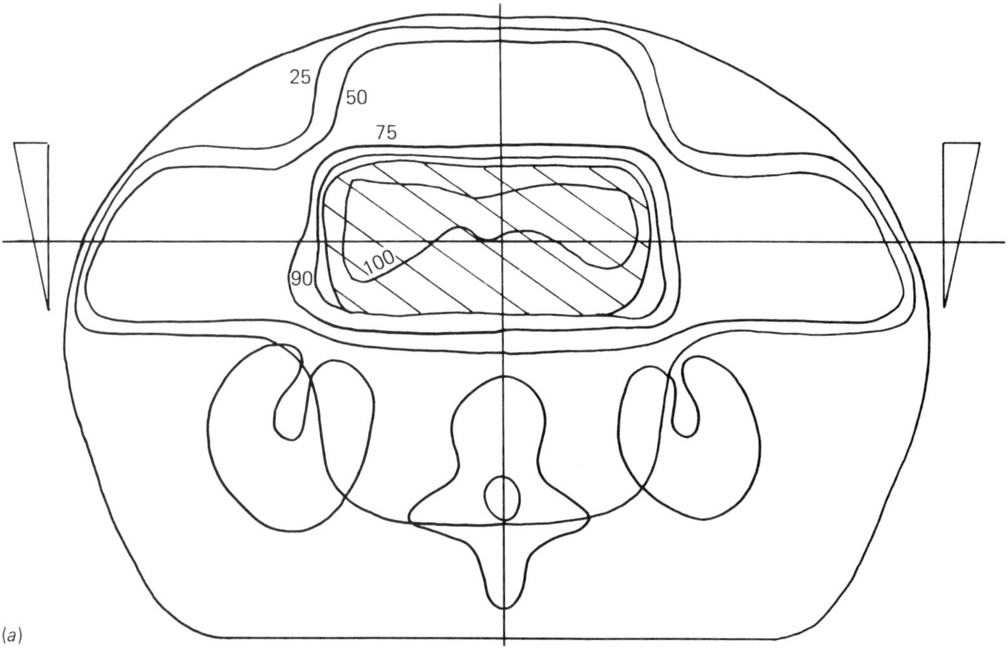

(*a*)

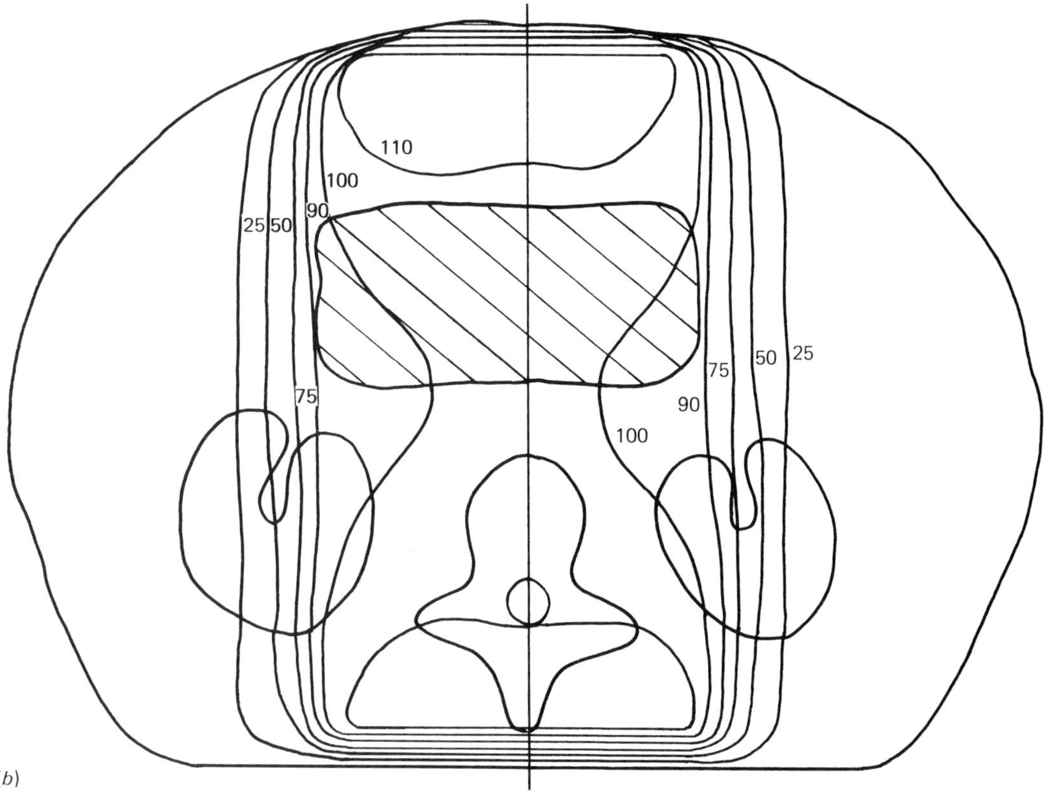

(*b*)

Figure 14.3 Differences in isodose distribution for irradiation of a pancreatic carcinoma using parallel opposed fields on a telecobalt machine (*a*) and an anterior and two lateral wedged fields on an 8 MeV linear accelerator (*b*)

improved when chemotherapy is combined with irradiation and treatment achieved local control in about one-third of patients. Toxicity has varied considerably in these reports, with moderate to severe reactions being encountered in 5–87%. Often these side-effects were due to simultaneous chemotherapy or were impossible to distinguish from symptoms due to progression of the underlying tumour. Problems directly attributable to irradiation appeared relatively uncommon, especially when precise beam direction, rather than parallel pair, techniques were employed (Borgelt, Dobelbower and Strubler, 1978; Nguyen, Bugat and Combes, 1982).

The value of retrospective series is always doubtful, but two recent randomized trials conducted by the Gastrointestinal Tumour Study Group have reinforced the view that combined therapy might offer a survival advantage. The first trial entered patients with locally unresectable disease and randomized them to one of three treatment arms: 6000 cGy alone, 4000 cGy plus 5-fluorouracil or 6000 cGy plus 5-fluorouracil. It was a prerequisite that all patients had disease which could be completely encompassed by parall pair radiation fields no greater than 400 cm^2, thereby excluding those with any evidence of distant metastases. The radio-therapy was given in two or three courses of 2000 cGy in 10 daily fractions with rest intervals of 14 days between each course and, in the chemotherapy arms, 5-fluorouracil at a dose of 500 mg/m^2 per day was given on the first 3 days of each treatment course. A total of 194 patients was evaluated and a clear survival advantage ($P<0.01$) was shown for both combined therapy arms as compared with radiation alone, but there was no difference between the two combined therapies. Overall the median times to progression were 12.6 weeks with radiation alone compared with 30.4 (4000 cGy + 5-fluorouracil) and 33 (6000 cGy + 5-fluorouracil) weeks, with 40% of patients from the combined regimens alive at 1 year compared with only 10% of those receiving radiotherapy alone. There was no difference between the groups in the number of treatment failures due to distant metastases, indicating that the beneficial effect of adding 5-fluorouracil was due to improved local disease control. There was no undue toxicity with any of the treatment regimens (Moertel *et al.*, 1981).

More recently, the same group have reported on the results of adjuvant therapy following potentially curative resection of pancreatic carcinoma (Kalser *et al.*, 1983). In this study, patients were randomized after surgery to no further treatment or to 4000 cGy plus 5-fluorouracil given by a similar schedule to that detailed above. Median survival for the controls was 11 months compared with 20 months in the treatment group (P=0.03), but 1 and 2-year survival was not recorded. These studies give weight to the contention that radiotherapy and chemotherapy can improve survival in pancreatic cancer, but the advantage is still small in real terms and is achieved only by a considerable period of treatment and the final conclusion must be that it is not justified to recommend these regimens as standard therapy at the present time.

Alternative radiotherapeutic approaches have been fast neutron therapy and iodine-125 implantation. Several authors have reported the results of fast neutron therapy either alone (Kaul *et al.*, 1981; Smith *et al.*, 1981) or in combination with photon beams (Al-Abdulla *et al.*, 1981). The results of neutron therapy alone are disappointing, with median survival times of 6–9 months and a clear inability to control local disease with doses of 1700–1950 cGy (neutron), and at these levels toxicity was marked and would seem to preclude dose escalation. In the combined photon–neutron series, 1-year survival was 40% compared with only 23% in those receiving photon irradiation alone, but the study was non-randomized and retrospective and the median survival time of 8.1 months for the mixed-beam group does not indicate any survival benefit compared with studies cited above using photons either alone or in combination with chemotherapy. This latter study also included a group treated by implantation of ^{198}Au seeds (Al-Abdulla *et al.*, 1981) intended to deliver 7000–10 000 cGy to tumour localized within the pancreas. Mortality was high with 24% of patients succumbing to peritonitis, cholangitis or septicaemia in the immediate post-operative period, but 32% (8/25) survived 1 year or more from the time of surgery. Implantation of ^{125}I has been used as an alternative method of boosting the dose of irradiation to the pancreas and giving an additional 10 000–15 000 cGy. When used for smaller unresectable tumours not involving the coeliac axis or superior mesenteric vessels this approach has resulted in median survivals of 12–14 months when combined with external beam doses of 3000–6000 cGy, with only a modest increase in toxicity (Whittington *et al.*, 1981; Shipley *et al.*, 1980; Syed, Puthwala and Neblett, 1983).

Two other approaches to pancreatic irradiation which have been considered are preoperative and intraoperative therapy. One series has claimed that preoperative irradiation of between 4400–4600 cGy in 5 weeks allowed radical resection in six of 11 patients previously considered of borderline resectability or frankly unresectable (Pilepich and Miller, 1980). Japanese reports of intraoperative therapy have been relatively discouraging with some palliation but no improvement in survival (Hiroaka, Nakagawa and Tashiro, 1975), but combining the technique with external beam therapy post-operatively has been claimed to lead to a median survival time in excess of 13 months in one recent series (Wood *et al.*, 1982).

Carcinomas of the extrahepatic biliary system

Carcinomas of the gall bladder and extrahepatic biliary tree account for only about 4% of all gastrointestinal tumours (*Table 14.4*). Tumours of the gall bladder are about twice as common as those of the ducts and occur three to four times more often in females than males. Cancers of the extrahepatic biliary system are seldom diagnosed preoperatively and are encountered during 0.2–0.5% of biliary tract operations (Treadwell and Hardin, 1976; Carmo *et al.*, 1978). Reported overall 5-year survival figures range from 0 to 12.5% (Waterhouse, 1974; Treadwell and Hardin, 1976; Kopelson *et al.*, 1977; Carmo *et al.*, 1978; Shieh, Dunn and Standard, 1981; Tompkins *et al.*, 1981). The likelihood of success is very dependent upon site and stage; about 20% of gall bladder cancers are localized to the wall of the organ and found only on pathological examination of cholecystectomy specimens. In these cases 5-year survival may exceed 60% (Shieh, Dunn and Standard, 1981). Another 20% of bile duct carcinomas occur in the lower third and may be treated by pancreaticoduodenectomy with reported overall survivals of more than 20% at 5 years (Inouye and Whelan, 1978; Tompkins *et al.*, 1981). For most biliary carcinomas, however, the prognosis is poor, and this is due to local extension, predominantly to the liver, rather than to distant metastases, which are an uncommon and late event (Carmo *et al.*, 1978).

Table 14.4 Relative incidence of gastrointestinal cancers (based on figures from Waterhouse, 1974)

	Male (%)	*Female (%)*	*Total (%)*
Stomach	14	8	22
Pancreas	5	4	9
Biliary system			
Gall bladder	0.5	2	2.5
Bile ducts	0.75	0.75	1.5
Large bowel			
Colon	13	19	32
Rectum	18	13	31
Anus	1	1	2
Total	52.25	47.75	100

The principal therapeutic approach to these tumours is surgical, but the value of radical procedures aimed at cure remains controversial. In most series less than 20% of patients have been candidates for radical surgery, the postoperative mortality has ranged from 18 to 50% and in those surviving surgery, local recurrences have occurred in some 30% (Treadwell and Hardin, 1976; Kopelson *et al.*, 1977). One recent British series looking specifically at carcinomas of the confluence of the hepatic ducts (Klatskin tumours) has suggested that recent developments in surgical technique and supportive therapy justify a more radical approach that might well result in improved survival (Blumgart *et al.*, 1984), but most authorities would argue that the surgeon's main role is in palliation aimed at relieving biliary obstruction (Bismuth and Malt, 1979; George, Brown and Foley, 1981). For those undergoing palliative procedures median survival times range from 2 to 5 months (Moertel, 1969; Bismuth and Malt, 1979).

In recent years a number of centres have reported the use of radiotherapy in the management of carcinoma of the extrahepatic biliary system. Because of the relative rarity of the condition all the series are small and none provides data from randomized studies. Taken overall the results are encouraging: jaundice due to obstruction was relieved in 15 of 18 patients, pruritus in 13 of 14, pain in seven of eight and shrinkage of tumour noted in six of seven (Green, Mikkelson and Kernen, 1973; Hudgins and Meoz, 1976; Kopelson *et al.*, 1977; Pilepich and Lambert, 1978). The radiation doses ranged from 1500–6000 cGy in 2–6 weeks, delivered through parallel opposed portals, and were well tolerated. Three patients treated by radiation alone have survived more than 3 years after treatment (Smoron, 1977; Pilepich and Lambert, 1978). It has been suggested that bile duct carcinoma is more responsive than gall bladder tumours (Smoron, 1977), but the overall results show no difference in radiosensitivity. Radiotherapy has also been given as an adjuvant following resection on a number of occasions. Once again none of the studies was randomized and differences in criteria of patient selection, treatment regimens and methods of reporting survival make accurate comparisons difficult, but all authors were agreed that the addition of radiotherapy did improve survival (Treadwell and Hardin, 1976; Kopelson *et al.*, 1977; Hanna and Rider, 1978; Pilepich and Lambert, 1978). In the largest series the results were compared with concurrent controls and showed that 49 patients receiving radiation doses averaging 4000 cGy in addition to surgery had a median survival of 11 months compared with 5 months for 19 patients receiving surgery alone ($P<0.02$) (Hanna and Rider, 1978).

These series have all used external beam therapy, but one recent report has indicated that high bile duct tumours may be suitable for internal radiotherapy with iridium-192 wire. Some 10–14 days after establishing biliary drainage by means of a U-tube or percutaneous transhepatic catheter, iridium-192 wire was inserted into the drainage tube to deliver a tumour dose of 4000–4800 cGy over 48 hours, after which time the wire was removed

(*Figure 14.4*). There were no complications attributable to irradiation and six of eight patients were still alive 11 months after treatment (Fletcher *et al.*, 1981).

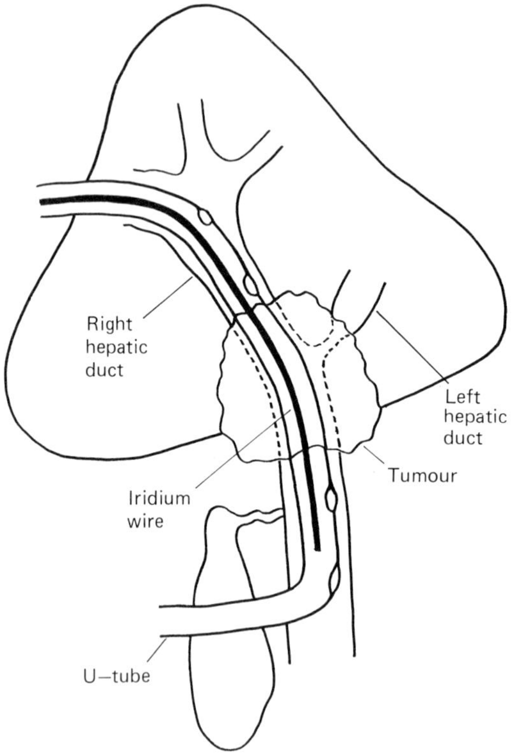

Figure 14.4 Technique for iridium wire irradiation of a carcinoma of the junction of the hepatic ducts

Because carcinomas of the extrahepatic biliary system are uncommon, it is difficult to organize randomized clinical trials to evaluate radiation therapy. The evidence available from the various pilot studies reported to date would suggest, however, that radiotherapy is of value in the palliation of inoperable disease and might well lead to improved survival in those who undergo resection.

Carcinoma of the rectum

Almost all the available data on the use of radiotherapy in large bowel cancer relate to the treatment of rectal carcinomas. Recently, however, there have been two reports of non-randomized studies which have claimed that giving doses of 4500–5500 cGy, by opposed fields, to the tumour bed following resection of B or C stage carcinomas of the caecum or colon has reduced the incidence of local recurrence and improved survival (Kopelson, 1983; Duttenhaver *et al.*, 1983). Despite the high doses, morbidity was said to be acceptable although Kopelson stressed the importance of treating patients in the lateral decubitus position to minimize the amount of small bowel included in the treatment volume. These series suggest that further exploration of adjuvant radiotherapy for locally advanced, but resectable, caecal and colonic cancers may be worthwhile.

In comparison with most other gastrointestinal carcinomas, the prognosis in rectal cancer is relatively good. Approximately 90% of patients have resectable tumours (Hughes, 1963; Roswit *et al.*, 1973; Phillips *et al.*, 1984) and the 5-year survival for those undergoing resection is just over 50% (Waterhouse, 1974). The major factor influencing prognosis is the degree of spread of the tumour and a variety of staging systems have been proposed to try to correlate clinicopathological findings with survival. The most widely used of these is Dukes' classification originally proposed in the 1930s. This has undergone a number of modifications by different workers and perhaps this is the major criticism of this system in that the stages mean different things to different people. It does, however, have the value of simplicity and is still widely used. *Table 14.5* shows the 1932 version of Dukes' classification (Dukes, 1932). *Table 14.6* summarizes the more recent, but more complex TNM system, which has still to gain wide acceptance.

Table 14.5 Dukes' 1932 classification of rectal carcinoma

Stage	*Definition*	*Incidence (%)*	*5-year survival (%)*
A	Carcinoma limited to wall of rectum with no extension into extrarectal tissues	18	70
B	Carcinoma has spread by direct continuity to extra-rectal tissues but not to nodes	35	50
C	Metastases present in regional lymph nodes	47	25

(Survival figures are based on those reported by the MRC Working Party, 1984)

Patients who relapse after excision have either blood-borne metastases or local pelvic recurrence. Clinical estimates of the incidence of pelvic recurrence vary from 10 to 50% (Medenhall, Million and Pfaff, 1983; Pilipshen *et al.*, 1984), but one series using second-look laparotomy put the figure at over 90% (Gunderson and Sosin, 1974). In some 50% of patients with local recurrence there is no evidence of distant metastases (Medenhall, Million and Pfaff, 1983; Pilipshen *et al.*, 1984). The principal factors

Table 14.6 TNM clinical classification of rectal carcinoma

T	*Primary tumour*
Tis	Pre-invasive carcinoma (carcinoma *in situ*)
T0	No evidence of primary tumour
T1	Tumour limited to the mucosa or mucosa and submucosa
T2	Tumour with extension to muscle or muscle and serosa
T3	Tumour with extension beyond colon to immediately continuous structure
	T3a Tumour without fistula formation
	T3b Tumour with fistula formation
T4	Tumour extending beyond the immediately adjacent organs or tissues
TX	The minimum requirements to assess the primary tumour cannot be met
N	*Regional and juxtaregional lymph nodes*
N0	No evidence of regional lymph node involvement
N1	Evidence of involvement of regional lymph nodes
	(note: the categories N2 and N3 are not applicable)
N4	Evidence of involvement of juxtaregional lymph nodes
NX	The minimum requirements to assess the regional and/or juxtaregional lymph nodes cannot be met
M	*Distant metastases*
M0	No evidence of distant metastases
M1	Evidence of distant metastases
MX	The minimum requirements to assess the presence of distant metastases cannot be met

predisposing to the development of local recurrence are the site, stage and degree of fixation of the tumour, with a significantly lower incidence of recurrence in Dukes' A lesions or those originating high (above 12 cm) in the rectum. The majority of pelvic recurrences become clinically apparent within 2 years of initial surgery (Medenhall, Million and Pfaff, 1983; Phillips *et al.*, 1984). For those with unresectable lesions the prognosis is poor, with a median survival of some 7 months (Williams, Shulman and Todd, 1957).

Although still frequently overlooked, the value of radiotherapy in the palliation of locally recurrent or inoperable rectal carcinoma is well documented. The earliest large series was reported from St Bartholomew's Hospital, London, (Williams, Shulman and Todd, 1957): complete symptomatic relief was achieved in 76% of patients with rectal bleeding, 48% with pain and 40% with mucous discharge. The majority of these patients received 6000 cGy in 6 weeks, but there is good evidence that lower doses give adequate palliation (*Figure 14.5*). Three series have claimed symptomatic relief in up to 80% of patients treated with 2000 cGy in 2 weeks or less (Wang and Schulz, 1962; Stearns and Leaming, 1975; James *et al.*, 1983). Doses of 3000 cGy or more are probably necessary to achieve actual tumour shrinkage in most instances (Wang and Schulz, 1962), although there is no indication that reduction in tumour size actually improves survival (James *et al.*, 1983).

When radiotherapy is used alone for control of pelvic recurrence it would, therefore, seem that a dose of 2000 cGy, given over eight to ten daily fractions with parallel opposed fields to the whole pelvis, is adequate to relieve symptoms in the majority of patients for 6–12 months and has the advantage that the course may be repeated, thereby affording further palliation (Stearns and Leaming, 1975). A survival advantage has been demonstrated in one randomized study in advanced disease when 5-fluorouracil was added to the treatment regimen (Moertel *et al.*, 1969). Patients with unresectable lesions who received radiotherapy and 5-fluorouracil had a median survival of 23 months compared with 17 months for those who had radiotherapy alone ($P<0.05$). Furthermore, three patients survived more than 5 years after treatment, two of them having no tumour when re-explored. Two subsequent retrospective surveys have also concluded that the addition of 5-fluorouracil enhances the palliative effect of radiation, although the influence on survival could not be clearly determined (Arnott, 1975; Vontgama *et al.*, 1975). These results would suggest that further investigation of combined therapy in advanced disease might be worthwhile.

While the value of radiotherapy in the palliation of advanced disease is clear, its role in primary treatment is less well defined. To some extent studies of adjuvant chemotherapy have diverted interest from irradiation in recent years but, despite a number of well controlled trials, there is no evidence that cytotoxic drugs improve survival and certainly they cannot be recommended for routine use after surgery (Carter, 1979). A retrospective study at the Memorial Hospital, New York, first raised the possibility that radiotherapy when combined with resection might reduce the incidence of local recurrence and improve survival. In this series, 727 patients received preoperative radiotherapy to a dose of 2000–2500 cGy in 2–3 weeks. The results were compared with 549 patients at the same hospital, treated over the same period, who received surgery alone. Overall survival at 5 years was 51% for those receiving combined treatment compared with 47.5% for patients having surgery alone. Analysis of the subgroups revealed a significant difference in patients with Dukes' C tumours: 37% of those who had been irradiated were alive at 5 years compared with only 23% of the controls. On the basis of these figures it was suggested that radiotherapy might improve survival particularly in patients with locally advanced but still resectable

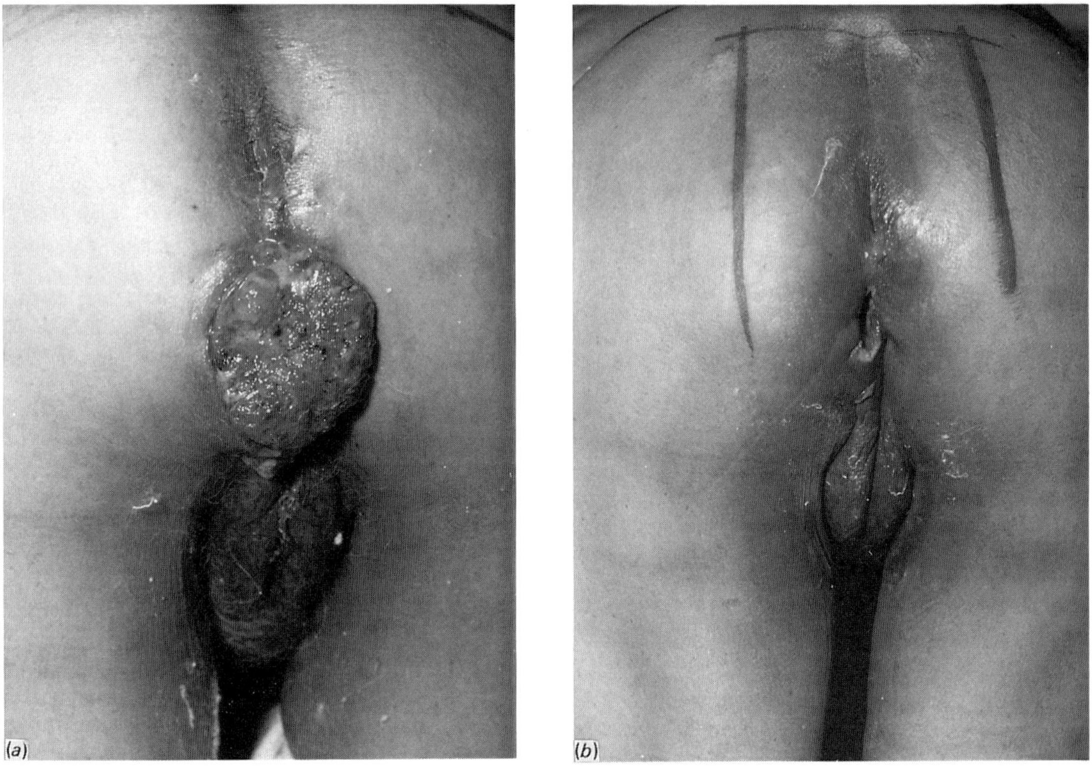

Figure 14.5 (*a*) and (*b*) Palliative irradiation in rectal carcinoma: resolution of fungating perineal recurrence following 4500 cGy midpoint dose in 15 treatments over 3 weeks from opposed anterior and posterior fields with an isocentric ^{60}Co unit

tumours (Stearns, Quan and Deddish, 1959). Since that time four randomized trials have reported the results of combining low dose preoperative radiotherapy with surgery. Only one (Rider *et al.*, 1977) has claimed a significant survival advantage compared with surgery alone and this trial had only a small number of patients (*Table 14.7*). The largest series has been coordinated by the British Medical Research Council. This failed to show any significant benefit from preoperative irradiation with doses of either 500 cGy as a single fraction or 2000 cGy given in 10 fractions over 2 weeks, although there was a trend towards longer survival in those patients with fixed tumours. This leaves two questions to be answered: are higher doses of radiotherapy likely to be more effective, and is there a role for irradiation to render inoperable tumours operable?

A number of non-randomized studies have explored the value of higher doses of radiation, 4000–5000 cGy in 4–5 weeks, given preoperatively. In three of these, a number of patients with previous biopsy-proven adenocarcinoma had no evidence of tumour when they came to resection after radiotherapy (Tepper *et al.*, 1968; Stevens, Allen and Fletcher, 1976; Friedman *et al.*, 1978) and a more recent, but again non-randomized, study showed a local recurrence rate of 20% in patients given 2000 cGy in five fractions with only 5% in those receiving 4500 cGy in 5 weeks (Walz *et al.*, 1983). None of these series reported an increase in operative mortality or subsequent morbidity as a result of radiotherapy, and a recent study of 4000–4500 cGy delivered preoperatively reported subsequent anastomotic failure in only one of 35 patients treated and a complete absence of local recurrence in 24 patients assessable for 10 months or more (Marks and Mohiuddin, 1983). A recent prospectively randomized study from the European Organization for Research and Treatment of Cancer has compared preoperative irradiation to a dose of 3400 cGy in 15 fractions over 18 days with the same regimen combined with 5-fluorouracil (Boulis-Wassif *et al.*, 1984). There was no significant survival difference between the two groups, but overall the incidence of local recurrence at 5 years was reduced to 10% and there was a feeling that survival was consequently improved by preoperative irradiation, although unfortunately, as there was no control arm with surgery alone, this was impossible to demonstrate conclusively. Concern over the possibility of radiotherapy increasing the difficulty of surgery, or of postoperative complications and anxiety over the accuracy of preoperative staging resulting from the

Table 14.7 Randomized trials evaluating preoperative radiotherapy for rectal carcinoma

Reference	*No. of patients*	*Technique*	*Results*
Stearns *et al.*, 1974	790 (but only 347 randomized)	18 × 16 cm parallel pair pelvic field, 2000 cGy at 250 cGy daily, surgery 2 days to 6 weeks postirradiation	No difference in overall survival or survival for different stages but those with Dukes' C lesions had fewer local recurrences
Roswit, Higgins and Keelin, 1975	700	Parallel pair to pelvis, 2000 cGy in 10 fractions over 2 weeks, booster dose of 500 cGy in 10 daily fractions to perineal field for low lying lesions. 60% orthovoltage therapy	Trend towards improved survival and reduced incidence of stage C tumours in irradiated group but results not statistically significant
Rider *et al.*, 1977	60	Single dose 500 cGy megavoltage 4 hours before surgery	Significant difference in survival, 40% for irradiated compared with 20% for controls
MRC Working Party, 1984	824	Either 500 cGy single treatment or 2000 cGy in 10 treatments over 2 weeks, megavoltage, parallel pair to pelvis	No significant difference in survival overall nor in any subgroup

view that adjuvant therapy is most likely to benefit only those with B and C lesions, has led to the suggestion of a sandwich approach to radiation: low dose preoperative therapy, resection and high dose postoperative irradiation. Two recent non-randomized trials have reported experience with this method, and both have claimed a reduction in expected local recurrence rates and suggested that survival is improved (Mohiuddin *et al.*, 1982; Gunderson *et al.*, 1983a).

Another approach is simply to give high dose radiotherapy postoperatively. This forms the basis of a large randomized European study in which patients with B and C lesions are randomized after resection to receive either no further treatment or 5000 cGy (delivered as 3000 cGy in 3 weeks, 2 weeks rest, then a further 2000 cGy in 2 weeks using one posterior and two lateral fields). So far only an interim report is available and this suggests a benefit for the Dukes' C patients and certainly confirms that the technique is reasonably safe with only three of 98 patients experiencing severe complications directly attributable to the radiation (Balslev *et al.*, 1982). The Gastrointestinal Study Group in the USA has also undertaken a study of high dose post-operative radiotherapy where patients receive 4600 cGy in 30–40 days. If this trial does show a benefit, it will confirm the results of a recent non-randomized series comparing 5000 cGy postoperatively with no further therapy for those with Dukes' C lesions. In this study, patients with low rectal lesions had a 70% disease-free survival after radiotherapy and surgery compared with only 22% after surgery alone (Localio *et al.*, 1983).

There is certainly good evidence from a number of series that preoperative irradiation may render non-resectable tumours resectable. Doses of 4000–5200 cGy in 4–6 weeks allowed complete resection in 27 of 44 patients previously considered inoperable in one series (Pilepich *et al.*, 1978) and 16 of 25 patients were similarly benefitted in another (Dosoretz *et al.*, 1983). This principle is being extended by the current Medical Research Council Study which is randomizing those with fixed tumours to receive either surgery alone or 4000 cGy in 4 weeks followed by surgery 1 month later.

These studies have used various different field sizes and placings for irradiation. *Table 14.8* lists the sites of local recurrence in a series of 41 patients with failure of local control after surgery alone. The majority of these would fall within the field of

Table 14.8 Distribution of local recurrence following surgery for rectal carcinoma (based on data from Medenhall, Million and Pfaff, 1983)

Site of failure	*Local recurrences (%)*
Presacral	36
Vagina	6
Bladder	6
Perineum	8
Pelvic side wall	8
Anastomosis	8
Other pelvic sites	12
Colostomy	2
Inguinal nodes	4
Peritoneal seedlings	8
Abdominal wall	2

approximately 15 × 15 cm parallel fields extending from, and including, the perineum inferiorly and the L5, S1 disc space superiorly with lateral margins 1 cm lateral to the bony pelvis; if there is residual disease present outside this volume then it is doubtful if cure could be achieved even with increased fields. Although three (one posterior direct and two post oblique wedge fields) and four field techniques have been used with the intention of reducing radiation-induced morbidity, there is no firm evidence that these approaches are superior to a simple parallel pair set-up.

Less conventional approaches to radiotherapy of rectal carcinomas include local irradiation, hyperbaric oxygen and fast neutron therapy. Local radiotherapy has been used with considerable success in selected primary rectal carcinomas. This endocavitary technique has been developed and refined in France by Papillon, who uses a special 50 kV contact superficial X-ray machine which may be introduced through a rectoscope giving a 3 cm diameter radiation field. The penetration of the radiation is limited, the depth dose being only 14% at 2 cm; this is a disadvantage in that only smaller lesions are suitable for treatment but an advantage in that very high doses may be given to the immediate tumour area (a typical course comprises 10 000–15 000 cGy in four treatments spaced over 6 weeks). To be suitable for treatment the tumour must be a polypoid, fairly well differentiated adenocarcinoma, not exceeding 3–5 cm diameter, within 12 cm of the anal margin. Failure to control the disease locally can be dealt with by an iridium-192 hairpin implant (*see* Chapter 16). Papillon has followed up 133 patients for 5 years, and 104 (78%) remain well and disease-free (Papillon, 1975). The reproducibility of Papillon's method and results has been demonstrated by similar studies in the USA (Sischy, Remington and Sobel, 1980).

Other specialized radiation techniques have been used in the management of recurrent or locally advanced rectal carcinoma. Eighteen of 22 patients treated with hyperbaric oxygen and radiotherapy achieved some symptomatic relief and eight of 15 patients with measurable disease had a complete response, no details of toxicity were given (Dische and Senanayake, 1972). Seven out of 13 patients had no evidence of tumour at intervals ranging from 9 to 18 months after fast neutron therapy. Again few details of treatment morbidity were recorded but, while it was noted that two patients developed intestinal obstruction during, and possibly due to, therapy, three others had no evidence of radiation damage at subsequent laparotomy (Catterall, 1972). Neither of these studies compared their results with conventional radiotherapy, but even if controlled studies were to demonstrate an advantage, the limited availability of such treatment facilities restricts their usefulness.

Anal carcinoma

The relative rarity of anal carcinomas means that few large series and randomized trials are available to guide management policies. The situation is further confused by disagreements on precise anatomical and histological classifications and the absence of a widely accepted staging system. Tumours are conventionally divided into those of the anal margin and those arising from the anal canal. The latter are some three times more common but have a slightly poorer prognosis (Morson and Pang, 1968; Beahrs and Wilson, 1976). The majority of cancers at this site are squamous cell carcinomas, but some 30% of lesions in the anal canal are basaloid tumours arising from the junctional zone above the dentate line. These are often also referred to as cloacogenic carcinomas. In terms of their natural history they are similar to the squamous cell carcinomas with a tendency to locoregional spread with blood-borne secondaries developing in less than 10% of patients. Lymphatic spread may be to either the inferior mesenteric, internal iliac or inguinal nodes.

A number of series have reported the results of external beam and interstitial radiotherapy for anal carcinomas either alone or in combination. Although 5-year survivals of up to 63% for anal margin tumours, treated by implant (Dalby and Pointon, 1961) and up to 80% for anal canal lesions, treated by teletherapy (Cantril *et al.*, 1983) have been reported, most patients have been managed surgically with survival figures at 5 years of 50–60% for lesions of the canal and 65–75% for the margin (Morson and Pang, 1968; Beahrs and Wilson, 1976).

The development of megavoltage irradiation has tended to limit the indications for interstitial isotope therapy to relatively early lesions situated low in the anal canal (*see* Chapter 16). It has been suggested the best results are obtained with superficial lesions, situated below the anorectal ring, less than half the circumference of the anal canal and less than 1 cm thick. Tumours meeting these requirements may be treated with a single plane implant giving 5500 cGy at 0.5 cm in 5–7 days with a good chance of cure and minimal risk of radiation fibrosis or necrosis (Bond, 1960). Iridium-192 using a template is ideal (*see* Chapter 16). Techniques for megavoltage external beam therapy have included single perineal fields, rotation, and three or four fixed fields to the pelvis, with or without a perineal boost. Doses have generally been in the range of 5000 cGy in 4 weeks to 7000 cGy in 7 weeks. At these levels necrosis or stricture formation requiring surgical correction occurs in about 10–20% of patients and 5-year survival averages about 40% overall for all stages. There is no evidence that any one treatment technique or dose schedule is clearly superior (Cummings, 1982) and within individual reported

Table 14.9 Mitomycin C and 5-fluorouracil combined with radiotherapy prior to resection for anal carcinoma

Reference	*No. of patients*	*Radiotherapy*	*Comment*
Nigro *et al.*, 1983	28	3000 cGy in 15 daily fractions, 15 × 15 cm parallel pair	20 patients had no microscopic evidence of tumour at resection and 22 were disease-free up to 8 years after resection
Quan *et al.*, 1978	10	3000 cGy in 15 daily fractions. No details of radiotherapy technique given	4 patients had no microscopic evidence of tumour and a further 5 no macroscopic cancer at resection. No survival data given
Sischy *et al.*, 1980	4	4000 cGy at 180 cGy daily 15 × 15 cm parallel pair to pelvis followed by 1000 cGy from direct perineal field in 10 daily treatments	No evidence of residual tumour in any patient at resection
Smith, Muff and Shetabi, 1982	4	3000 cGy in 15 daily fractions, four fields to whole pelvis	3 of the patients had no microscopic evidence of disease at surgery. No survival data
Michaelson *et al.*, 1982	37	3000 cGy in 15 daily fractions parallel pair to pelvis, field size increased to include inguinal nodes if necessary	17 patients had no microscopic evidence of tumour at resection and 78% were disease-free at 2 years

Table 14.10 Mitomycin C and 5-fluorouracil combined with radiotherapy as sole treatment for anal carcinoma

Reference	*No. of patients*	*Radiotherapy*	*Comment*
Bruckner *et al.*, 1979	3	3000–4500 cGy by external beam ± interstitial irradiation	Advanced cases unsuitable for surgery, all three gained complete response and disease-free at 1 year
Cummings *et al.*, 1982	13	5000 cGy in 10 fractions over 4 weeks, 3000 cGy by anterior and posterior opposed fields to whole pelvis in 12 daily fractions followed by 2000 cGy to primary and low pararectal nodes from lateral opposed fields in 8 daily fractions	All locally advanced though technically resectable, complete clinical regression in all patients and all disease-free at 12 months
Sischy *et al.*, 1982	15	4000–5000 cGy at 180 cGy daily by opposed fields to whole pelvis and inguinal nodes followed 3 weeks later by 1500–2000 cGy to primary from 10 × 8 cm perineal field ± further 1000–1500 cGy from iridium wire implant	Local control of disease in all patients although one died due to distant secondaries
Flam *et al.*, 1983	12	3000–4140 cGy given by a variety of techniques	Complete regression in all patients and post-treatment biopsies negative, 10 alive at 4–24 months with two deaths due to other causes (no evidence of tumour at post-mortem)

series there has been a tendency to tailor therapy to individual patients and their tumours rather than adopt a uniform approach, with the result that the optimum method for routine treatment remains to be defined.

Recently, a number of authors have reported the results of giving 3000–4000 cGy in 3–4 weeks preoperatively in combination with 5-fluorouracil and mitomycin C (*Table 14.9*). The various studies are not strictly comparable, but it does appear that, overall, at operation more than 75% of patients proved to be microscopically free of tumour as a result of the combined therapy, although the results were not so good when the chemotherapy and irradiation were given sequentially rather than synchronously (Michaelson *et al.*, 1982). In the light of these results workers have given radiotherapy combined with mitomycin C and 5-fluorouracil as the sole treatment for anal carcinoma. It is too soon to assess survival but the initial results are encouraging (*Table 14.10*), although in the one study where daily fractions exceeded 200 cGy quite severe toxicity was noted (Cummings, 1983). It is difficult to be certain of the significance of these results and at least one recent series has provided comparable results with radiation alone (Cantril *et al.*, 1983).

Almost 30% of patients with anal carcinomas will have involvement of the inguinal lymph nodes at the time of presentation (Woolfe and Bussey, 1968). Although instances of cure have been claimed following irradiation of groin nodes (Cummings, 1982), current British practice is usually to perform a block dissection unless the glands are fixed and inoperable (Goligher, 1984). The 5-year survival of patients with synchronous inguinal node metastases is about 16% whereas for those who subsequently develop gland involvement the outlook is considerably better with approximately 50% alive at 5 years (Sugarbaker, Gunderson and Macdonald, 1982), but again surgical removal is generally preferred to irradiation when metochranous nodes appear. Elective irradiation of clinically negative nodes has occasionally been advocated, but there is no clear evidence that this offers any survival advantage (Cummings, 1982) and the potential risk of lower limb lymphoedema argues against routine prophylactic irradiation.

References

ABE, M., TAKAHASHI, M., YABUMOTO, E., ADACHI, H., YOSHII, M. and MORI, K. (1980) Clinical experiences with intraoperative radiotherapy of locally advanced cancers. *Cancer,* **45**, 40–48

AL-ABDULLA, A. S., HUSSEY, D. H., OLSON, M. H. and WRIGHT, A. E. (1981) Experience with fast neutron therapy for unresectable carcinoma of the pancreas. *International Journal of Radiation Oncology, Biology and Physics,* **7**, 165–172

ARNOTT, S. J. (1975) The value of combined 5-fluorouracil and X-ray therapy in the palliation of locally recurrent and inoperable rectal carcinoma. *Clinical Radiology,* **26**, 177–181

BADEN, H. and SORENSON, T. I. (1979) The Whipple operation in 37 patients with periampullary carcinoma. *American Journal of Surgery,* **137**, 624–628

BALSLEV, I., PEDERSEN, M., TEGLBJAERG, P. S. *et al.* (1982) Post operation radiotherapy in rectosigmoid cancer Dukes' B and C. *British Journal of Cancer,* **46**, 551–556

BEAHRS, O. H. and WILSON, S. M. (1976) Carcinoma of the anus. *Annals of Surgery,* **184**, 422–428

BISMUTH, H. and MALT, R. A. (1979) Carcinoma of the biliary tract. *New England Journal of Medicine,* **301**, 704–706

BLACK, W. C., GOMEZ, J. F., YUHAS, J. M. and KLIGERMAN, M. M. (1980) Quantitation of the late effects of X-radiation on the large intestine. *Cancer,* **45**, 444–450

BLAKE, J. R. S., HARDCASTLE, J. D. and WILSON, R. G. (1981) Gastric cancer: a controlled clinical trial of adjuvant chemotherapy following gastrectomy. *Clinical Oncology,* **7**, 13–22

BLUMGART, L. H., HADJIS, N. S., BENJAMIN, I. S. and BEAZLEY, R. (1984) Surgical approaches to cholangiocarcinoma at confluence of hepatic ducts *Lancet,* **1**, 66–69

BOND, W. H. (1960) Discussion on squamous cell carcinoma of the anus and anal canal. *Proceedings of the Royal Society of Medicine,* **53**, 411–414

BORGELT, B. B., DOBELBOWER, R. R. and STRUBLER, K. A. (1978) Betatron therapy for unresectable pancreatic cancer. *American Journal of Surgery,* **135**, 76–80

BOULIS-WASSIF, S., GERARD, A., LOYGUE, J., CAMELOT, D., BUYSE, M. and DUEZ, N. (1984) Final results of a randomised trial on the treatment of rectal cancer with preoperative radiotherapy alone or in combination with 5-fluorouracil, followed by radical surgery. *Cancer,* **53**, 1811–1818

BROOKES, V. S., WATERHOUSE, J. A. H. and POWELL, D. J. (1965) Carcinoma of the stomach: a 10-year survey of results and of factors affecting prognosis. *British Medical Journal,* **1**, 1577–1583

BRUCKNER, H. D., SPIGELMAN, M. K., MANDEL, E. *et al.* (1979) Carcinoma of the anus treated with a combination of radiotherapy and chemotherapy. *Cancer Treatment Reports,* **59**, 395–399

CANTRIL, S. T., GREEN, J. P., SCHALL, G. L. and SCHAUPP, W. C. (1983) Primary radiation therapy in the treatment of anal carcinoma. *International Journal of Radiation Oncology, Biology and Physics,* **9**, 1271–1278

CARMO, M. D., PERPETUO, M. O., VALDIVIESO, M. *et al.* (1978) Natural history study of gall bladder cancer, **42**, 1422–1424

CARTER, S. K. (1979) 5-fluorouracil as adjuvant chemotherapy for large bowel cancer: is it appropriate for routine community use? *Cancer Chemotherapy and Pharmacology,* **2**, 81–84

CASSELL, P. and ROBINSON, J. O. (1976) Cancer of the stomach: a review of 854 patients. *British Journal of Surgery,* **63**, 603–606

CATTERALL, M. (1972) Clinical experience with fast neutrons. *Proceedings of the Royal Society of Medicine,* **65**, 839–843

CATTERALL, M., KINGSLEY, D., LAWRENCE, G., GRAINGER, J. and SPENCER, J. (1975) The effects of fast neutrons on inoperable carcinoma of the stomach. *Gut,* **16**, 150–156

CHILDS, D. S. (1969) Role of the radiation therapist in advanced management. In *Advanced Gastrointestinal Cancer* edited by C. G. Moertel and R. J. Reitemeier, pp. 58–62. New York: Harper and Row

COHEN, Y. and ZIDAN, J. (1981) Adjuvant therapy of stomach cancer by chemotherapy or radiochemotherapy. *Proceedings of the American Association for Cancer Research,* **22**, 459

CUMMINGS, B. J. (1982) The place of radiation therapy in the treatment of carcinoma of the anal canal. *Cancer Treatment Reviews*, **9**, 125–147

CUMMINGS, B. J. (1983) Carcinoma of the anal canal — radiation or radiation plus chemotherapy? *International Journal of Radiation Oncology, Biology and Physics*, **9**, 1417–1418

CUMMINGS, B. J., RIDER, W. D., HARWOOD, A. R. *et al.* (1982) Combined radical radiation therapy and chemotherapy for primary squamous cell carcinomas of the anal canal. *Cancer Treatment Reports*, **66**, 489–492

DALBY, J. E. and POINTON, R. S. (1961) The treatment of anal carcinoma by interstitial irradiation. *American Journal of Roentgenology*, **85**, 515–520

DENT, D. M., WERNER, I. D., NOVIS, B., CHEVERTON, P. and BRICE, P. (1979) Prospective randomized trial of combined oncological therapy for gastric carcinoma. *Cancer*, **44**, 385–391

DESPEIGNES, V. (1896) Observation concernant un cas du cancer de l'estemac traite par les rayons Roentgen. *Lyon Medical*, **82**, 428–430

DISCHE, S. and SENANAYAKE, F. (1972) Radiotherapy using hyperbaric oxygen in the palliation of carcinoma of the colon and rectum. *Clinical Radiology*, **23**, 512–518

DOBELBOWER, R. R. (1979) The radiotherapy of pancreatic cancer. *Seminars in Oncology*, **6**, 378–389

DOSORETZ, D. E., GUNDERSON, L., HEDBERG, S. *et al.* (1983) Preoperative irradiation for unresectable rectal and rectosigmoid carcinomas. *Cancer*, **52**, 814–818

DUKES, C. E. (1932) The classification of cancer of the rectum. *Journal of Pathology and Bacteriology*, **35**, 323–332

DUTTENHAVER, J., HOSKINS, B., GUNDERSON, L. and TEPPER, J. (1983) Adjuvant post operative radiation therapy in cancer of the large intestine. *Proceedings of the American Society of Clinical Oncology*, **2**, 120

EICHHORN, H.-J., LESSEL, A. and MATSCHKE, S. (1974) Comparison between neutron therapy and ^{60}Co gamma ray therapy of bronchial, gastric and oesophagus carcinomata. *European Journal of Cancer*, **10**, 361–364

ENGSTROM, P. and LAVIN, P. (1983) for the Eastern Cooperative Oncology Group. Post operative adjuvant therapy for gastric cancer patients. *Proceedings of the American Society of Clinical Oncology*, **2**, 114

FALKSON, G. and FALKSON, H. C. (1969) Fluorouracil and radiotherapy in gastrointestinal cancer. *Lancet*, **2**, 1252–1253

FIELDING, J. W. F. and ALEXANDER-WILLIAMS, J. (1985) Adenocarcinoma of the stomach. In *Surgery of the Stomach and Duodenum*, edited by C. Wastell and L. Nyhus. Boston: Little, Brown and Co. (In press)

FIELDING, J. W. L., ELLIS, D. J., JONES, B. G. *et al.* (1980) Natural history of early gastric cancer: results of a 10-year regional survey. *British Medical Journal*, **281**, 965–967

FIELDING, J. W. L., FAGG, S. L., JONES, B. G. *et al.* (1983) An interim report of a prospective randomized controlled study of adjuvant chemotherapy in operable gastric cancer. British Stomach Cancer Group. *World Journal of Surgery*, **7**, 390–399

FLAM, M. S., MADHU, J., LOVALVO, L. J. *et al.* (1983) Definitive non-surgical therapy of epithelial malignancies of the anal canal. *Cancer*, **51**, 1378–1387

FLETCHER, M. S., BRINKLEY, D., DAWSON, J. L., NUNNERLEY, H., WHEELER, P. G. and WILLIAMS, R. (1981) Treatment of high bile duct carcinomas by internal radiotherapy with iridium-192 wire. *Lancet*, **2**, 172–174

FRIEDMAN, P., PARK, W. C., AFONYA, I. *et al.* (1978) Adjuvant radiation therapy in colorectal carcinoma. *American Journal of Surgery*, **135**, 512–518

GAGLIANO, R., McCRACKEN, J. D. and CHEN, T. (1983) Adjuvant therapy with 5-fluorouracil, adriamycin and mitomycin (FAM) in gastric cancer — a SWOG study. *Proceedings of the American Society of Clinical Oncology*, **2**, 114

GEORGE, P. A., BROWN, C. and FOLEY, R. T. E. (1981) Carcinoma of the hepatic duct junction. *British Journal of Surgery*, **68**, 14–18

GOLIGHER, J. (1984) Carcinoma of the anal canal and anus. In *Surgery of the Anus, Rectum and Colon*, 5th edition, pp. 780–793. London: Baillière Tindall

GREEN, N., MIKKELSEN, W. P. and KERNEN, J. A. (1973) Cancer of the common hepatic bile ducts — palliative radiotherapy. *Radiology*, **109**, 687–689

GUNDERSON, L. L., DOSORETZ, D. E., HEDBERG, S. E. *et al.* (1983a) Low dose preoperative irradiation, surgery and elective post operative radiation therapy for resectable rectum and rectosigmoid carcinoma. *Cancer*, **52**, 446–451

GUNDERSON, L. L., HOSKINS, B., COHEN, A. C., KAUFMAN, S., WOOD, W. C. and CAREY, R. W. (1983b) Combined modality treatment of gastric cancer. *International Journal of Radiation Oncology, Biology and Physics*, **9**, 965–975

GUNDERSON, L. L. and SOSIN, H. (1974) Areas of failure found at operation (second or symptomatic look) following 'curative surgery' for adenocarcinoma of the rectum. *Cancer*, **34**, 1278–1292

GUNDERSON, L. L. and SOSIN, H. (1982) Adenocarcinoma of the stomach: areas of failure in a re-operation series (second or symptomatic look) clinicopathologic correlations and implications for adjuvant therapy. *International Journal of Radiation Oncology, Biology and Physics*, **8**, 1–11

GUTTMAN, R. T. (1955) Effects of 2 million volt roentgen therapy on various malignant lesions of the upper abdomen. *American Journal of Roentgenology*, **74**, 204–212

HAAS, C. D., MANSFIELD, C. M., LEICHMAN, L. P. and CONSIDINE, B. (1983) Combined non-simultaneous radiation therapy and chemotherapy with 5-FU, doxorubicin and mitomycin for residual localised gastric adenocarcinoma: a South West Oncology Group pilot study. *Cancer Treatment Reports*, **67**, 421–424

HANNA, S. S. and RIDER, W. D. (1978) Carcinoma of the gall bladder or extra hepatic bile ducts: the role of radiotherapy. *Canadian Medical Association Journal*, **118**, 59–61

HASLAM, J. B., CAVANAUGH, P. J. and STROUP, S. L. (1973) Radiation therapy in the treatment of irresectable adenocarcinoma of the pancreas. *Cancer*, **32**, 1341–1345

HIGGINS, G. A., AMADEO, J. H., SMITH, D. E., HUMPHREY, E. W. and KEEHN, R. J. (1983) Efficacy of prolonged intermittent therapy with combined 5-FU and methyl-CCNU following resection for gastric carcinoma: a Veterans Administration Surgical Oncology Group Report. *Cancer*, **52**, 1105–1112

HIROAKA, T., NAKAGAWA, I. and TASHIRO, S. (1975) Intraoperative irradiation therapy for unresectable pancreatic cancer. *Journal of the Japanese Society for Cancer Therapy*, **13**, 146

HOLBROOK, M. A. (1974) Gastric cancer: radiation therapy. *Journal of the American Medical Association,* **228**, 1289–1290

HORN, R. C. (1955) Carcinoma of the stomach: autopsy findings in untreated cases. *Gastro-enterology,* **29**, 515–525

HUDGINS, P. T. and MEOZ, R. T. (1976) Radiation therapy for obstructive jaundice secondary to tumour malignancy. *International Journal of Radiation Oncology, Biology and Physics,* **1**, 1195–1198

HUGHES, E. S. R. (1963) Results of treatment of carcinomas of colon and rectum. *British Medical Journal,* **2**, 9–13

INGOLD, J. A., REED, G. B., KAPLAN, H. S. and BAGSHAW, M. A. (1965) Radiation hepatitis. *American Journal of Roentgenology,* **93**, 200–208

INOUYE, A. A. and WHELAN, T. J. (1978) Carcinoma of the extrahepatic bile ducts: a ten-year experience in Hawaii. *American Journal of Surgery,* **136**, 90–95

JAMES, R. D., JOHNSON, R. J., EDDLESTON, B., ZHENG, G. L. and JONES, J. M. (1983) Prognostic factors in locally recurrent rectal carcinoma treated by radiotherapy. *British Journal of Surgery,* **70**, 469–472

JENSEN, M. H., SAVER, T., DEVIK, F. and NYGAARD, K. (1983) Late changes following single dose roentgen irradiation of rat small intestine. *Acta Radiologica Oncology,* **22**, 299–304

KALSER, M., ELLENBERG, S., LEVIN, B. *et al.* (1983) Pancreatic cancer: adjuvant combined radiation and chemotherapy following potentially curative resection. *Proceedings of the American Society of Clinical Oncology,* **2**, 122

KAUL, R., COHEN, L., HENDRICKSON, F., AWSCHALOM, M., HREJSA, A. F. and ROSENBERG, I. (1981) Pancreatic carcinoma: results with fast neutron therapy. *Internationl Journal of Radiation Oncology, Biology and Physics,* **7**, 173–178

KINGSTON, R. D., ELLIS, D. J., POWELL, J. *et al.* (1978) The West Midlands gastric carcinoma chemotherapy trial: planning and results. *Clinical Oncology,* **4**, 55–69

KINSELLA, T. J. (1983) The role of radiation therapy alone and combined with infusion chemotherapy for treating liver metastases. *Seminars in Oncology,* **10**, 215–222

KOPELSON, G. (1983) Adjuvant post operative radiation therapy for colorectal carcinoma above the peritoneal reflection II antimesenteric wall ascending and descending colon and cecum. *Cancer,* **52**, 633–636

KOPELSON, G., HARISIADIS, L., TRETTER, P. and CHANG, C. H. (1977) The role of radiation therapy in cancer of the extrahepatic biliary system. *International Journal of Radiation Oncology, Biology and Physics,* **2**, 883–894

KRAUT, J. W. and EARLE, J. D. (1976) Radiation therapy's role in the management of liver metastases. *International Journal of Radiation Oncology, Biology and Physics,* **1**, 977–979

LOCALIO, S. A., NEALAN, W., NEWALL, J. and VALENSI, Q. (1983) Adjuvant post operative radiation therapy for Dukes' C adenocarcinoma of the rectum. *Annals of Surgery,* **198**, 18–24

McCRACKEN, J. D., OLSON, M., CRUZ, A. B., LEICHMAN, L. and OISHI, N. (1982) Radiation therapy combined with intra-arterial 5-FU chemotherapy for treatment of localised adenocarcinoma of the pancreas: a South West Oncology Group Study. *Cancer Treatment Reports,* **65**, 549–551

McCRACKEN, J. D., RAY, P., HEILBRON, L. K. *et al.* (1980) 5-fluorouracil, methyl-CCNU and radiotherapy with or without testolactone for localised adenocarcinoma of the exorcrine pancreas. *Cancer,* **46**, 1518–1522

MANTELL, B. S. (1982) Radiotherapy for dysphagia due to gastric carcinoma. *British Journal of Surgery,* **69**, 69–70

MARKS, G. and MOHIUDDIN, M. (1983) Sphincter preservation for rectal cancer and the role of full dose preoperative radiation therapy. *International Journal of Radiation Oncology, Biology and Physics,* **9**, (suppl 1), 110–111

MEDENHALL, W. M., MILLION, R. R. and PFAFF, W. W. (1983) Patterns of recurrence in adenocarcinoma of the rectum and rectosigmoid treated with surgery alone: implications in treatment planning with adjuvant radiotherapy. *International Journal of Radiation Oncology, Biology and Physics,* **9**, 977–985

MICHAELSON, R. A., MAGILL, G. B., QUAN, S. H. Q., LEAMING, R. H., NIKRUI, M. and STEARNS, M. W. (1982) Preoperative chemotherapy and radiation therapy in the management of anal epidermoid carcinoma. *Cancer,* **51**, 390–395

MOERTEL, C. G. (1969) Natural history of gastro-intestinal cancer. In *Advanced Gastro-intestinal Cancer,* edited by C. G. Moertel and R. J. Reitemeier, pp. 3–14. New York: Harper and Row

MOERTEL, C. G., CHILDS, D. S., REITEMEIER, R. J., COLLOY, N. Y. and HOLBROOK, M. A. (1969) Combined 5-fluorouracil and supervoltage radiation therapy of locally unresectable gastrointestinal cancer. *Lancet,* **2**, 865–867

MOERTEL, C. G., FRYTAK, S., HAHN, R. G. *et al.* (1981) Therapy of locally unresectable pancreatic carcinoma: a randomised comparison of high dose (6000 rads) radiation alone, moderate dose radiation (4000 rads + 5-fluorouracil) and high dose radiation + 5-fluorouracil. *Cancer,* **48**, 1705–1710

MOHIUDDIN, M., KRAMER, S., MARKS, G. and DOBELBOWER, R. (1982) Combined pre and post operative radiation for carcinoma of the rectum. *International Journal of Radiation Oncology, Biology and Physics,* **8**, 133–136

MORSON, B. C. and PANG, L. S. C. (1968) Pathology of anal cancer. *Proceedings of the Royal Society of Medicine,* **61**, 623–624

MOSS, W. T., BRAND, W. N. and BATTIFORA, H. (1979) The gastrointestinal tract. In *Radiation Oncology*, pp. 332–365 St. Louis: C. V. Mosby

MRC WORKING PARTY (1984) The evaluation of low dose preoperative x-ray therapy in the management of operable rectal cancer: results of a randomly controlled trial. *British Journal of Surgery,* **71**, 21–25

NGUYEN, T. D., BUGAT, R. and COMBES, P. F. (1982) Post operative irradiation of carcinoma of the head of the pancreas area. *Cancer,* **50**, 53–56

NIGRO, N. D., SEYDEL, H. G., CONSIDINE, B., VAITKEVICIUS, V. K., LEICHAMN, L. and KINZIE, J. J. (1983) Combined preoperative radiation and chemotherapy for squamous cell carcinoma of the anal canal. *Cancer,* **51**, 1826–1829

PAPILLON, J. (1975) Intracavitary irradiation of early rectal cancer for cure: a series of 186 cases. *Cancer,* **36**, 696–701

PHILLIPS, R. K. S., HITTINGER, R., BLEOVSKY, L., FRY, J. S. and FIELDING, L. P. (1984) Local recurrence following 'curative' surgery for large bowel carcinoma. II The

rectum and rectosigmoid. *British Journal Surgery*, **71**, 17–20
PILEPICH, M. V. and LAMBERT, P. M. (1978) Radiotherapy of carcinomas of the extrahepatic biliary system. *Radiology*, **127**, 767–770
PILEPICH, M. V. and MILLER, H. H. (1980) Preoperative irradiation in carcinoma of the pancreas. *Cancer*, **46**, 1945–1949
PILEPICH, M. V., MONZENRIDER, J. E., TAK, W. K. and MILLER, H. H. (1978) Preoperative irradiation of primarily unresectable colorectal carcinoma. *Cancer*, **42**, 1077–1081
PILIPSHEN, S. J., HEILWEIL, M., QUAN, S. H., STERNBERG, S. S. and ENKER, W. E. (1984) Patterns of pelvic recurrence following definitive resections of rectal cancer. *Cancer*, **53**, 1354–1362
PRASAD, B., LEE, M. and HENDRICKSON, F. R. (1977) Irradiation of hepatic metastases. *International Journal of Radiation Oncology, Biology and Physics*, **2**, 129–132
QUAN, S. H., MAGILL, G. B., LEAMING, R. H. and HAJDU, S. (1978) Multidisciplinary preoperative approach to the management of epidermoid carcinoma of the anus and rectum. *Diseases of the Colon and Rectum*, **21**, 89–91
REED, G. B. and COX, A. J. (1966) The human liver after radiation injury. *American Journal of Pathology*, **46**, 597–611
RIDER, W. D., PALMER, J. A., MAHONEY, L. J. and ROBERTSON, C. T. (1977) Preoperative irradiation in operable cancer of the rectum: report of the Toronto trial. *Canadian Journal of Surgery*, **20**, 335–338
ROSWIT, B., HIGGINS, G. A., HUMPHREY, E. W. and ROBINETTE, C. D. (1973) Preoperative irradiation of operable adenocarcinoma of the rectum and rectosigmoid colon. *Radiology*, **108**, 389–395
ROSWIT, B., HIGGINS, G. A. and KEEHN, R. J. (1975) Preoperative irradiation for carcinoma of the rectum and rectosigmoid colon: report of a National Veterans Administration randomized study. *Cancer*, **35**, 1597–1602
ROSWIT, B., MALSKY, S. J. and REID, C. B. (1972) Severe radiation injuries of the stomach, small intestine, colon and rectum. *American Journal of Roentgenology*, **114**, 460–475
RUBIN, P. (1984) Late effects of chemotherapy and radiation therapy: a new hypothesis. *International Journal of Radiation Oncology, Biology and Physics*, **10**, 5–34
SCHEIN, P. S. and CHILDS, D. (1978) A controlled randomized evaluation of combined modality therapy (5000 rads, 5FU + MeCCNU) vs 5FU + MeCCNU alone for locally unresectable gastric cancer. *Proceedings of the American Association for Cancer Research*, **19**, 329
SCHEIN, P. S., SMITH, F. P., DRITSCHILLO, A., STABLEIN, D. M. and AHLGREN, J. D. (1983) Phase I–II trial of combined modality FAM (5-fluorouracil, adriamycin and mitomycin C) plus split course radiation (FAM-RT-FAM) for locally advanced gastric (LAG) and pancreatic (LAP) cancer: a mid-Atlantic Oncology Program study. *Proceedings of the American Society of Clinical Oncology*, **2**, 126
SCHEIN, P. S., SMITH, F. P., WOOLLEY, P. V. and AHLGREN, T. D. (1982) Current management of advanced and locally unresectable gastric carcinoma. *Cancer*, **50**, 2590–2596
SHIEH, C. J., DUNN, E. and STANDARD, J. E. (1981) Primary carcinoma of the gallbladder. *Cancer*, **47**, 996–1004
SHIPLEY, W. U., NARDI, G. I., COHEN, A. M. and LING, C. C. (1980) Iodine-125 implant and external beam irradiation in patients with localised pancreatic carcinoma. *Cancer*, **45**, 709–714
SISCHY, B., REMINGTON, J. H., HINSON, E. J., SOBEL, S. H. and WALL, J. E. (1982) Definitive treatment of anal carcinoma by means of radiation therapy and chemotherapy. *Diseases of the Colon and Rectum*, **25**, 685–688
SISCHY, B., REMINGTON, J. H. and SOBEL, S. H. (1980) Treatment of rectal adenocarcinomas by means of endocavitary irradiation: a progress report. *Cancer*, **46**, 1957–1961
SISCHY, B., REMINGTON, J. H., SOBEL, S. H. and SAVLOV, E. D. (1980) Treatment of carcinoma of the rectum and squamous carcinoma of the anus by combination chemotherapy, radiotherapy and operation. *Surgery, Gynecology and Obstetrics*, **151**, 369–371
SMITH, D. E., MUFF, N. S. and SHETABI, H. (1982) Preoperative radiation and chemotherapy for anal and rectal cancer. *American Journal of Surgery*, **143**, 595–598
SMITH, F. P., SCHEIN, P. S., MACDONALD, J. S., WOOLLEY, P. V., ORNITZ, R. and ROGERS, C. (1981) Fast neutron irradiation for locally advanced pancreatic cancer. *International Journal of Radiation Oncology, Biology and Physics*, **3**, 1527–1531
SMORON, G. L. (1977) Radiation therapy of carcinoma of the gall bladder and biliary tract. *Cancer*, **40**, 1422–1424
STEARNS, M. W., DEDDISH, M. R., QUAN, S. H. and LEAMING, R. H. (1974) Preoperative roentgen therapy for cancer of the rectum and rectosigmoid. *Surgery, Gynecology and Obstetrics*, **138**, 584–586
STEARNS, M. W. and LEAMING, R. H. (1975) Irradiation in inoperable cancer. *Journal of the American Medical Association*, **231**, 1388
STEARNS, M. W., QUAN, S. H. and DEDDISH, M. R. (1959) Preoperative roentgen therapy for cancer of the rectum. *Surgery, Gynecology and Obstetrics*, **109**, 225–229
STEVENS, K. R., ALLEN, C. V. and FLETCHER, W. S. (1976) Preoperative irradiation for adenocarcinoma of the rectosigmoid. *Cancer*, **37**, 2866–2874
STOUT, A. P. (1943) Pathology of carcinoma of the stomach. *Archives of Surgery*, **46**, 807–822
SUGARBAKER, P., GUNDERSON, L. L. and MACDONALD, J. S. (1982) Cancer of the anal region. In *Cancer: Principles and Practice of Oncology*, edited by V. T. DeVita, S. Hellman and S. A. Rosenburg, pp. 724–731. Philadelphia: Lippincott
SYED, N., PUTHWALA, A. A. and NEBLETT, D. L. (1983) Interstitial iodine-125 implant in the management of unresectable pancreatic carcinoma. *Cancer*, **52**, 808–813
TEFFT, M., TRAGGIS, D. and FILLER, R. M. (1969) Liver irradiation in children: acute changes with transient leukopenia and thrombocytopenia. *American Journal of Roentgenology*, **106**, 750–765
TEPPER, J., NARDI, G. and SUIT, H. (1976) Carcinoma of the pancreas: review of MGH experience 1963 to 1973. *Cancer*, **37**, 1519–1524
TEPPER, M., VIDONE, R. A., HAYES, M. A., LINDENMUTH, W. W. and KLIGERMAN, M. M. (1968) Preoperative irradiation in rectal cancer: initial comparison of clinical tolerance, surgical and pathologi-

cal findings. *American Journal of Roentgenology,* **102**, 587–595

TOMPKINS, R. K., THOMAS, D., WILE, A. and LONGMIRE, W. P. (1981) Prognostic factors in bile duct carcinoma. *Annals of Surgery,* **194**, 447–455

TREADWELL, T. A. and HARDIN, W. J. (1976) Primary carcinoma of the gall bladder: the role of adjunctive therapy in its treatment. *American Journal of Surgery,* **132**, 703–706

VONTGAMA, V., DOUGLASS, H. O., MOORE, R. H., HOLYOKE, E. D. and WEBSTER, J. H. (1975) End results of radiation therapy alone and combination with 5-fluorouracil in colorectal cancers. *Cancer,* **36**, 2020–2025

WALZ, B. J., KODNER, I. J., FRY, R., ROE, J., BREAUX, S. and HEDERMAN, M. (1983) Preoperative irradiation in two schedules for rectal cancer. *International Journal of Radiation Oncology, Biology and Physics,* **9**, (Suppl. I), 109–110

WANG, C. C. and SCHULZ, M. D. (1962) The role of radiation therapy in the management of carcinoma of the sigmoid, rectosigmoid and rectum. *Radiology,* **79**, 1–5

WATERHOUSE, J. A. H. (1974) *Cancer—Handbook of Epidemiology and Prognosis.* Edinburgh: Churchill Livingstone

WHITTINGTON, R., DOBELBOWER, R. R., MOHUIDDIN, M., ROSATO, F. E. and WEISS, S. M. (1981) Radiotherapy of unresectable pancreatic carcinoma: a six-year experience with 104 patients. *International Journal of Radiation Oncology, Biology and Physics,* **7**, 1639–1644

WIELAND, C. and HYMMEN, K. (1970) Megavoltherapie maligner neoplasien des magens. *Strahlentherapie,* **140**, 20–26

WILLIAMS, I. G., SHULMAN, I. M. and TODD, I. P. (1957) The treatment of recurrent carcinoma of the rectum by supervoltage X-ray therapy. *British Journal of Surgery,* **44**, 506–508

WOOD, W. C., SHIPLEY, W. U., GUNDERSON, L. L., COHEN, A. M. and NARDI, G. L. (1982) Intraoperative irradiation for unresectable pancreatic carcinoma. *Cancer,* **49**, 1272–1275

WOOLFE, H. R. I. and BUSSEY, H. J. R. (1968) Squamous cell carcinoma of the anus. *British Journal of Surgery,* **55**, 295–301

15

Malignant disease of the central nervous system

H. F. Hope-Stone

This chapter deals with tumours of the central nervous system (CNS) and spinal cord and the author will outline the role of radiotherapy — its appropriate technique together with the results of the treatment. Some of the children's tumours and those of the sympathetic nervous system are discussed in Chapter 10.

The primary intracranial tumours comprise about 1% of all deaths coming to autopsy. Metastatic tumours make up about 20% of the neoplasms. The gliomas account for 40%, meningiomas 12% and pituitary tumours 5%; the rest are made up of small groups of tumours. The classification of Russell and Rubenstein (1977) is still probably the most useful (*Table 15.1*).

Effects of irradiation on the CNS

No tissue of the human body is truly radioresistant. Given a sufficient dose, damage may be done to every organ, yet before 1940 the CNS was thought to be relatively free from the dangers of radiation damage. In 1941 Ahlbom first reported the possibility of spinal cord damage, but it was Boden (1948) who made all radiotherapists realize the potentially lethal effects of excessive radiation, both to the spinal cord and the brain stem. The pathogenesis is by no means certain, but most authors believe that it is due to vascular damage to the small arterioles leading to discrete damage to the glial cells. Demyelination will follow, but this has a latency period of 5 months to 5 years. At a later stage vascular occlusion with proliferation of fibrous connective tissue leads to arteriolar necrosis. The blood–brain barrier may be permanently altered and finally cell death takes place throughout the involved part of the nervous tissue.

The most sensitive parts of the CNS are the motor cortex, brain stem and spinal cord. The frontal and occipital lobes are less sensitive and the peripheral nerves relatively radioresistant, but even the latter may be damaged by devascularization secondary to radiation fibrosis, as seen in the effect on the brachial plexus (Stoll and Andrews, 1966).

The earliest clinical effects are seen in the spinal cord, and may be transient as seen in Lhermitte's sign when numbness and paraesthesiae follow neck flexion. This syndrome is most commonly seen in cervical spondylosis and multiple sclerosis, but true transient radiation myelitis is by no means uncommon and was well reviewed by Jones (1964). It occurs about 2 weeks to 7 months after irradiation (particularly of long sections of the spinal cord) as in the treatment of lymphoma. Doses as low as 2000 cGy in 4 weeks can produce this effect although it usually follows much higher levels (3000–4000 cGy). Fortunately it clears up rapidly, but it is important to recognize the phenomenon as it may be thought to be due to extradural neoplastic deposits. If treated with further irradiation this might have disastrous consequences.

More permanent radiation damage will only occur with higher doses, and in the spinal cord progressive radiation myelopathy will be seen when 4000 cGy in 15 treatments (or its radiobiological equivalent) is exceeded (Jones and Currie, 1982). The effect will be seen from a few months up to many years (usually within 3–4) after irradiation was given. Three types of lesion are seen:

(1) *Acute paraplegia or quadraplegia*. Boden (1950) described this phenomenon which is probably very rare. The paralysis is usually complete within a few hours and is invariably fatal.

(2) *Motor neurone disorder*. This usually affects the lower limbs and produces flaccid paralysis without sensory loss (Maier *et al.*, 1964).

(3) *Chronic progressive radiation myelopathy*. This commonly occurs after a latent period of 18 months. A progressive cord lesion is found and may lead to the Brown-Sequard syndrome and in turn to a spastic paralysis. Death follows in over 50% of cases, from ascending urinary tract infection or bronchopneumonia. Myelography may show an atrophic spinal cord segment, but in the future nuclear magnetic resonance imaging might outline the lesions more clearly.

Table 15.1 Classification of tumours of the central nervous system (modified from Russell and Rubenstein, 1977)

Glial
Astrocytoma
Grades 1 and 2 well differentiated
Grade 3 undifferentiated
Grade 4 glioblastoma multiforms
Oligodendroglioma
Ependymoma (includes ependymoblastoma, choroid plexus papillomas)
Pineal
Pinecytoma
Pineoblastoma
Teratoma (suprasellar germinoma)
Neuronal
Medulloblastoma
Sympathetic nervous system tumours
Neuroblastoma
Ganglioneuroma
Retinal
Retinoblastoma
Meningeal
Meningioma
Reticular
Microgliomatosis (non-Hodgkin's lymphoma, reticulum cell sarcoma)
Vascular
Angioma
Haemangioblastoma
Maldevelopment
Craniopharyngioma
Optic nerve and chiasm
Glioma
Pituitary
Eosinophil adenoma
Chromophobe adenoma
Basophil adenoma
Oncocytoma
Spinal cord tumours
Ependymoma
Astrocytoma
Glioma
Chordoma

Effects on the brain

Early transient effects will certainly occur but are not easily recognizable. Freeman, Johnstone and Voke (1972) described a somnolence syndrome occurring in some children receiving prophylactic CNS irradiation (1500–2000 cGy) for acute leukaemia. This was seen 6 weeks after irradiation and was associated with some EEG changes. The effect lasted for 3 weeks and then completely cleared up.

Early demyelination syndrome

This must be rare. Rider (1963) described only three cases in which demyelination, but not vascular changes, appeared to be important factors. Dose levels were high (5500 cGy in 16–27 fractions). Jones and Currie (1982) suggest this may have some relevance to the disastrous effect of neutron irradiation to the brain which was described in the MRC trial at Hammersmith (Catterall *et al.*, 1980).

Late brain necrosis

This also has a latent period of 3 months to 5 years. The clinical effects will depend on the part of the brain affected, but although not necessarily fatal, permanent damage may be produced in the motor or sensory areas. The optic pathways are usually only damaged by doses above the known clinical tolerance level of 4500 cGy in 4–5 weeks' treatment time. The hypothalamus may also be sensitive to these dose levels. Shalet *et al.* (1975) have reported reduction of pituitary growth hormone levels when this organ was in the high dose zone, although no other abnormality appeared to occur.

Radiological evidence of brain necrosis had not been easy to demonstrate until the advent of CT scanning, and even here interpretation may be difficult. *Figure 15.1* shows a scan of a patient (a boy aged 7 years) who was treated 2 years previously with a pair of parallel and opposed fields to a tumour dose of 4500 cGy in 20 daily treatments. The scan shows bitemporal brain damage but the child had no localizing symptoms. Nuclear magnetic resonance (NMR) might give us more information. *Figure 15.2* shows a white area in the left cerebellum (smaller than the actual field size used). The patient aged 60, who was completely asymptomatic from a neurological point of view, had a basal cell carcinoma of the skin of the left mastoid region treated 2 years previously with 10 MeV electron therapy. A dose of 5500 cGy in 4 weeks was given to the tumour — the cerebellum received a maximum of 2400 cGy. Perhaps other asymptomatic patients would show a similar effect if routine NMR scanning was performed after irradiation.

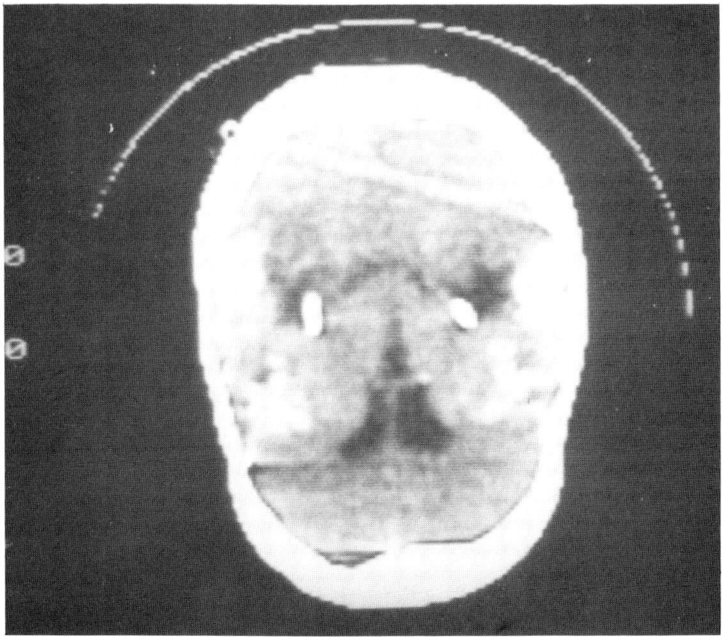

Figure 15.1 Bitemporal brain necrosis as seen on CT scan

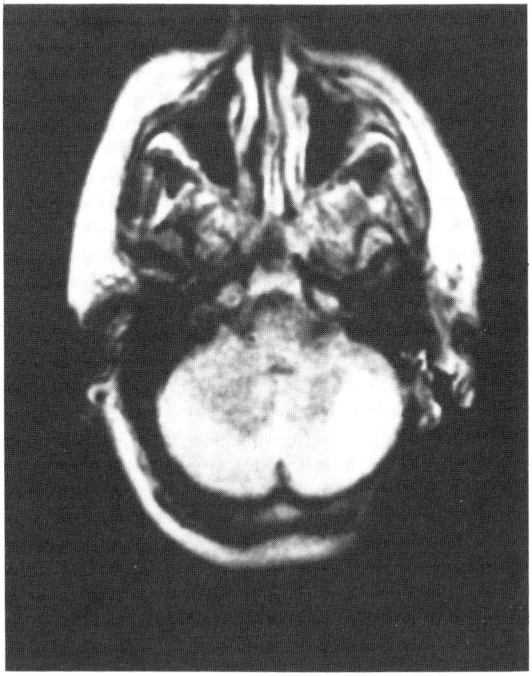

Figure 15.2 NMR scan showing possible irradiation effect on the (L) cerebellum — 2400 cGy from a 10 MeV electron field

Modification of brain tolerance

Hypertension is known to reduce the tolerance of the kidneys to irradiation in the experimental animal (Asscher, personal communication) and may affect spinal cord tolerance as well. Chemotherapy, and in particular methotrexate and CCNU, may have the same effect (Jones and Currie, 1982).

What are safe dose levels?

Spinal cord

In treating large lengths of the spinal cord Boden's original criterion of safety was 3500 Roentgens in 17 days. For small fields (<10 cm) 4500 would be safe, and using a Strandqvist's type of log plot, this would give a dose of 4200 cGy and 5000 cGy respectively over 42 days. Abbatucci *et al.* (1978) suggest the tolerance is higher – 5500 cGy in 27 fractions over 37 days. In the present author's opinion it would seem wise to err on the side of safety and it is suggested that 4500 cGy for short sections of the spinal cord (less than 10 cm) and 4000 cGy for longer sections (both in 20 daily fractions) is a reasonable compromise. Using 15 daily fractions the dose should be lowered to 3600 and 3200 cGy respectively. If the treatment time is prolonged and 25 fractions used, then 4500 cGy and 5000 cGy would be acceptable. The most important factor to remember is that reducing the number of fractions or treating on alternate days (a method to be deplored in the radical treatment of CNS tumours) requires an appropriate dosage reduction. Increasing the overall treatment time and the irradiation dose as well may not be as safe as it would appear, and there is little evidence that a better therapeutic response would be achieved.

Brain tolerance

The brain stem is a vital area where tolerance to irradiation is probably lower than elsewhere. A total of 4500 cGy in 20 daily fractions should not be exceeded. In the cerebral cortex, Lindgren (1958) found that the minimum dose which would produce necrosis was 4500–5000 cGy in 30 days. Kramer (1973) suggests that a dose below 7000 cGy is unlikely to produce changes (although he quotes five cases where damage did occur below this level). He advocates a maximum dose of 6500–7000 cGy over 6–8 weeks. The present author believes that 4500 cGy in 20 daily fractions or 5000 cGy in 25 fractions (or its radiobiological equivalent) should not be exceeded, as any possible benefit to be gained is far outweighed by the consequences which follow radiation damage to the brain. All fields should be treated daily, as treating only one field each day is more likely to lead to brain damage.

General policy

Not many of the brain tumours are particularly radiosensitive, and as a matter of policy it would seem unwise to use irradiation in patients who already have irreversible neurological damage, as they are unlikely ever to live a useful life. Palliation of symptoms in those patients with metastatic brain tumours might modify this approach.

Histological diagnosis is ideal and would seem essential, but at certain sites may be difficult or hazardous to obtain. Occasionally one will be forced to irradiate midbrain lesions (such as pontine glioma) without histological proof, but in the future, stereotactic biopsy techniques may help to overcome this problem.

When a large tumour mass is present and can safely be removed, this should certainly be encouraged as it will reduce the tumour burden which the radiotherapist is left to deal with (this is well shown in the results of treating medulloblastoma in the trial by the International Society for Paediatric Oncology (SIOP), (Bloom, 1983) – *see below*). A decompression alone may be all that is possible, and if carried out will improve the safety margin with regard to the production of irradiation oedema. This latter syndrome has always been regarded as a major problem for radiotherapists, but there is little clinical or experimental evidence that it really does occur. Providing the daily fraction of irradiation does not exceed 225 cGy and if dexamethasone (in a dosage of 16 mg daily) is used routinely, then the technique of a rising input of dose is not required.

Close cooperation between the neurosurgeon and radiotherapist is desirable, particularly if the patient has been transferred from another hospital, in which case the former's opinion should always be sought before starting irradiation.

Localization films, taken while the patient is fitted into a cobex skull cap, should be marked by the neurosurgeon who should outline the known site of the tumour. Generous margins around the marked area should be used particularly in the case of the gliomas, and it should be remembered that these can easily cross the corpus callosum to reach the opposite cerebral cortex. All patients, with the exception of the very fit or those with pituitary tumours, should remain in hospital for the first few days of treatment. If there are no side-effects from treatment they can initially go home for the weekends and then subsequently attend as outpatients (if living near enough), or stay in an adjacent hostel (if travelling times are too long).

Retreatment

Occasionally patients who have responded well to irradiation relapse, and the question of giving further treatment has to be considered if they are young and relatively fit. Even if the patients themselves have no views on the matter, relatives may well press for something to be done. The most important point to establish is whether there is definite recurrence or whether the problem could be one of irradiation damage, as in the latter case further treatment would be disastrous. If it is decided to treat again should one use irradiation or chemotherapy? The latter will only be palliative in nature and not without side-effects and, except in very radiosensitive tumours such as medulloblastoma or ependymoma, is not likely to be effective. In grade I and II astrocytoma which recur it might be worth retreating with irradiation providing at least 2 or 3 years have elapsed and the neurosurgeon and radiotherapist both appreciate that there will be a chance of necrosis occurring. In such a situation and with asymptomatic patients it would probably be best not to give any treatment: but if symptoms are present then the risk of necrosis should be accepted, as the alternative of death from tumour growth will be no worse. In this era some explanation of these problems will need to be given to the relatives and possibly to the patient as well. In the grade III and IV astrocytoma it is doubtful whether further irradiation should even be considered, but chemotherapy such as CCNU and vincristine parenterally, or methotrexate intrathecally or via a Omaya reservoir could be tried.

General management problems

As outlined above, cerebral oedema is rarely a

problem and normal fractionation can be used. However, in the patients receiving total CNS irradiation it would be wise to treat on a rising input basis reaching the maximum dose in 4–5 days. This method will help to increase bone marrow tolerance as well as to decrease the likelihood of irradiation sickness, particularly in children. Radiation sickness should not be a problem when only the brain is being treated, although occasionally patients do suffer from this, possibly for psychological reasons (as many patients expect to be sick while having irradiation). Oral or intramuscular antiemetics such as thiethylperazine (Torecan), metoclopramide (Maxalon) or domperidone (Motilium) can be used.

The main difficulty lies with those patients with cerebral irritability who cannot lie still, or those liable to attacks of epilepsy. In adults the former problem can be dealt with by mild sedation, but in young children some form of anaesthesia may be required (*see* Chapter 10). If epilepsy is likely, the patient will of course be receiving anticonvulsants but it would be wise to warn the radiographic staff (by appropriate distinctive wording on the radiation treatment sheet). A bite ring should be kept in the treatment room and if convulsions are occurring frequently the patient should be gently strapped to the treatment table (informing the patient why this is being done).

In all groups of patients some form of skull fixation is necessary. A plastic (cobex) skull cap or shell is required (*Figure 15.3*) and can be easily made in the mould room. After the localization films have been marked and the first set up checked by the radiotherapist, the plastic overlying the treatment area can be cut out of the cap (*Figure 15.4*), thus minimizing the skin reaction and improving the chance of good hair regrowth later. Megavoltage irradiation should always be used.

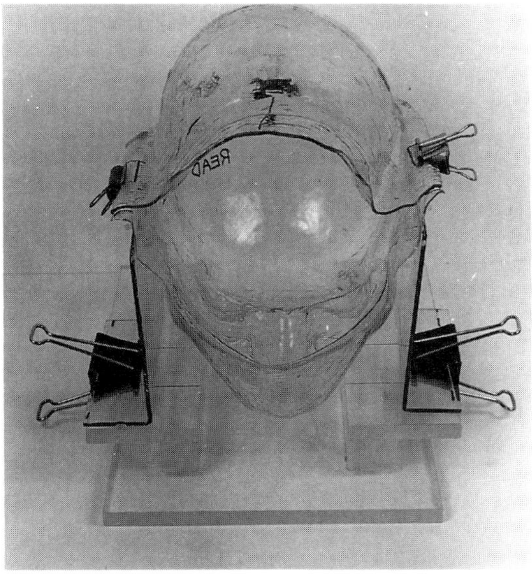

Figure 15.3 Plastic (cobex) skull cap (shell) for head immobilization

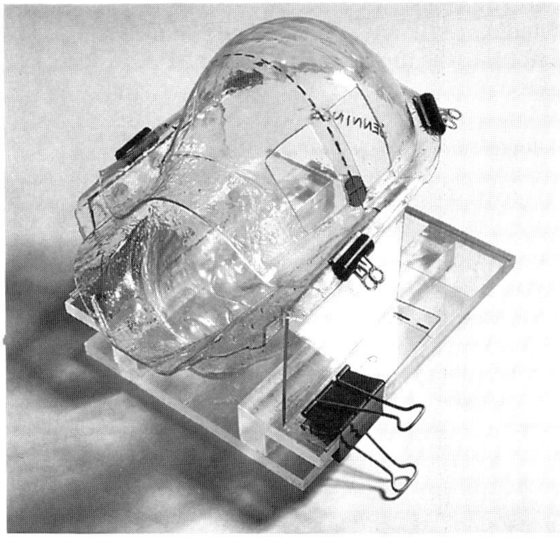

Figure 15.4 Shell with areas cut out to correspond to the irradiated fields

Since complete epilation will always follow irradiation, the patient (or parents if a child) will need to be warned of this side-effect. Most female patients will be pleased to wear a wig which should be ordered in good time. All patients should be reassured that some if not complete regrowth of hair will take place within 6–9 months (*Figure 15.5*).

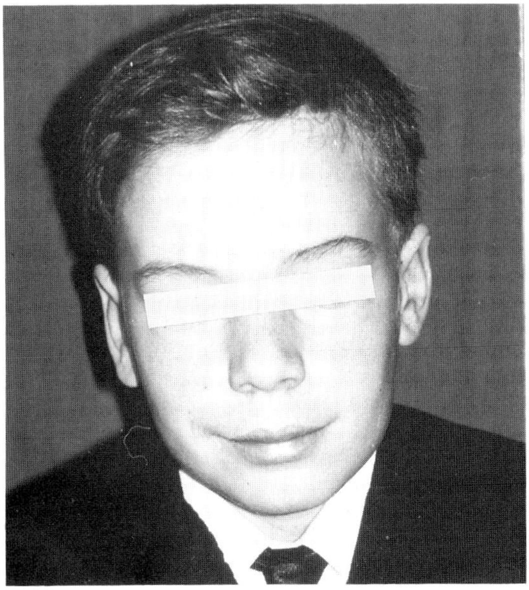

Figure 15.5 Good hair regrowth 3 years after whole brain irradiation for medulloblastoma

Skin changes of erythema and dry desquamation will occur, but can be reduced by cutting out parts of the cap which lie in the direct beam. Hydrocortisone Cream will relieve the irritation. Washing the hair during treatment should be avoided.

Long-term brain damage in adults should not occur if the dose levels outlined previously are adhered to. Residual brain damage from the tumour itself is the commonest cause of symptoms and may never completely disappear. In children one should not see mental retardation but growth hormone levels may be affected (*see below*).

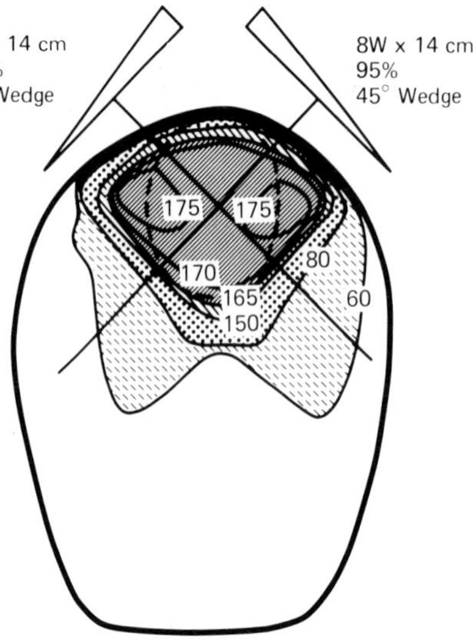

Figure 15.6 Isodose curves — pair of wedged fields to cerebellum, 5 MeV linear accelerator.
>165; 150–165; 80–150; 60–80; <60

Irradiation techniques and the results of treatment for individual tumours

Gliomas

Grades I and II differentiated astrocytoma

These slow growing tumours occur commonly in the posterior cranial fossa in young children, but also in the cerebral hemispheres in adults. They are best treated first by radical surgical excision. In children, at least, they can often be completely excised, and if this is done and the capsule is not ruptured then irradiation should not be required. If there is any doubt as to the completeness of the excision post-operative irradiation should be given. A tumour dose of 4000–4500 cGy (the lower dose being used if the child is less than 2 years old) is given using a pair of wedge fields with the patient lying in the prone position in a shell; 20 daily fractions are given over 4 weeks. The isodose curve is shown in *Figure 15.6.*

For larger tumours in adults a pair of parallel and opposed wedge fields may be preferred with the patient still in the prone position (*Figure 15.7a*). The dose of 4500 cGy will be reasonably homogeneous with this method (*Figure 15.7b*).

The results reported by Sheline (1977) suggest a 58% 5-year survival for grade I tumours treated with postoperative irradiation as compared with 25% without.

When the tumour occurs in the cerebral hemispheres it is rarely possible to remove it totally as it is relatively slow growing, the present author would advocate giving postoperative irradiation in patients who are quite fit. Two large wedge fields are usually sufficient (*Figure 15.8a and b*) but occasionally a three field technique will be required (*Figure 15.8c*). A total of 4500 cGy in 20 daily fractions is easily tolerated.

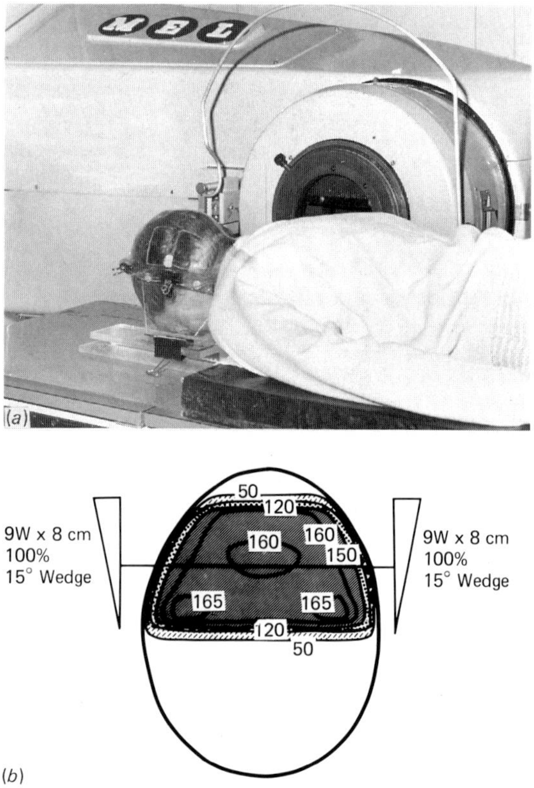

Figure 15.7 (*a*) Patient in prone position for opposed fields to the posterior fossa. (*b*) Isodose curves of this field arrangement, 5 MeV linear accelerator.
>150; 120–150; 50–120; <50

Grades III and IV malignant astrocytoma

These highly malignant tumours occurring in the

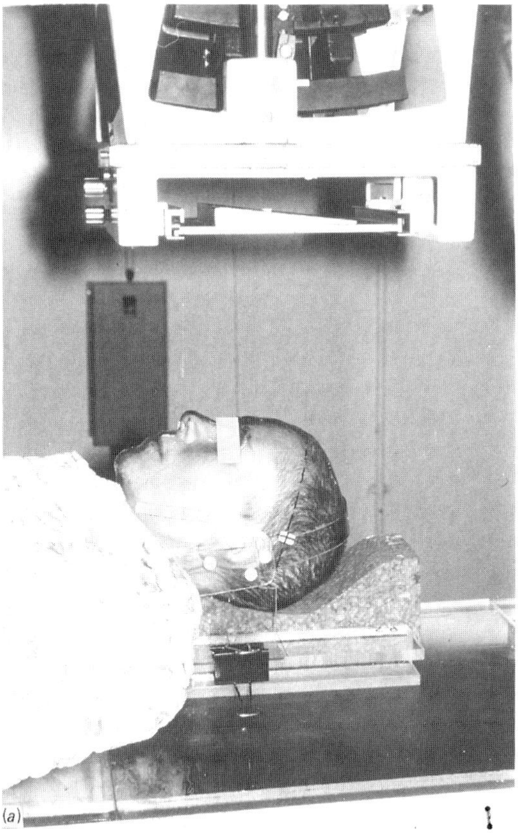

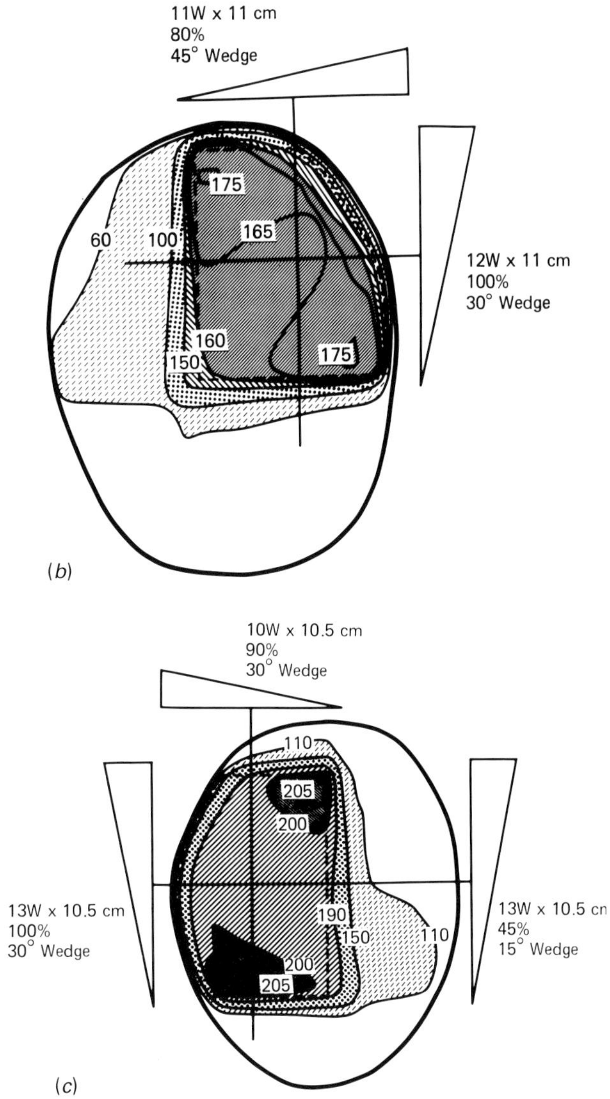

Figure 15.8 (*a*) Patient set up for 2 field technique. (*b*) 2 wedge field technique for grades I and II cerebral glioma 5 MeV. [hatched] >160; [dense hatched] 150–160; [dotted] 100–150; [light dotted] 60–100; [blank] <60. (*c*) 3 wedge field technique for grades I and II cerebral glioma 8 MeV. [hatched] >200; [dense hatched] 190–200; [dotted] 150–190; [light dotted] 110–150; [blank] <110

cerebral cortex have a very poor prognosis and it could be argued that any form of irradiation let alone surgery is a waste of time. Nevertheless, some patients do survive for 5 years or more — particularly grade III (Kramer, 1973). It would therefore seem reasonable to treat those fit patients who have had either a biopsy or incomplete excision. Large fields are required and it has been argued by Kramer (1973) that whole brain irradiation is always necessary. Certainly if both cerebral hemispheres are involved (*Figure 15.9a*) large parallel and opposed and possibly wedged fields will be needed (*Figure 15.9b*).

The present author feels that a maximum dose of 4500 cGy in 4 weeks is sufficient, but Jones and Currie (1982) suggest a minimum tumour dose of 5000 cGy in 27 fractions over 37 days, with an added boost to the tumour site of 500 cGy in three fractions (in selected young fit patients). Salazar, Rabin and McDonald (1976) suggest 5000–6000 cGy to the whole brain followed by a boost of 2000 cGy to the tumour itself. They claim a higher survival rate for this group of patients than those who received the lower dose.

In Kramer's series (1973) five out of 23 patients survived for 5 years. In a much larger series of cases, Sheline (1976) reported a 16% 5-year survival figure for grade III astrocytoma but no survivors for grade IV tumours. As the correct dose–time ratio is by no means certain, it is gratifying to know that the MRC in the UK have agreed to set up a multicentre trial to compare a conventional dose of 4500 cGy in 20 fractions to the whole tumour area using large fields, with the same dose and time to the same sized fields followed by a booster to the tumour area only of 2000 cGy in a further 10 fractions.

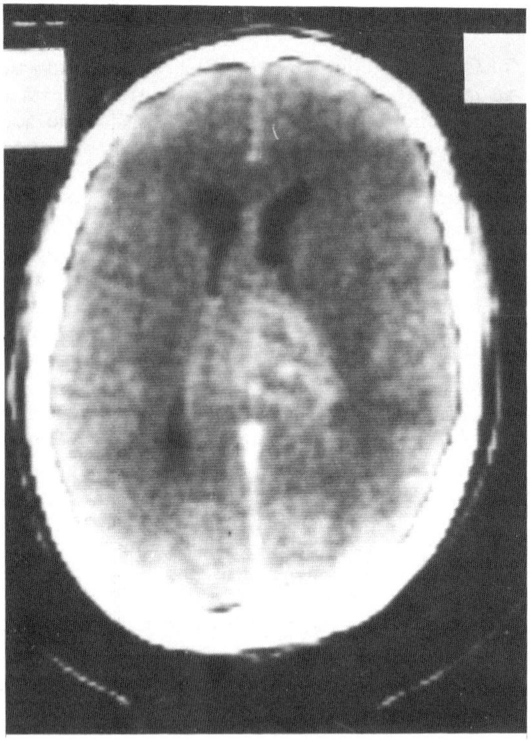

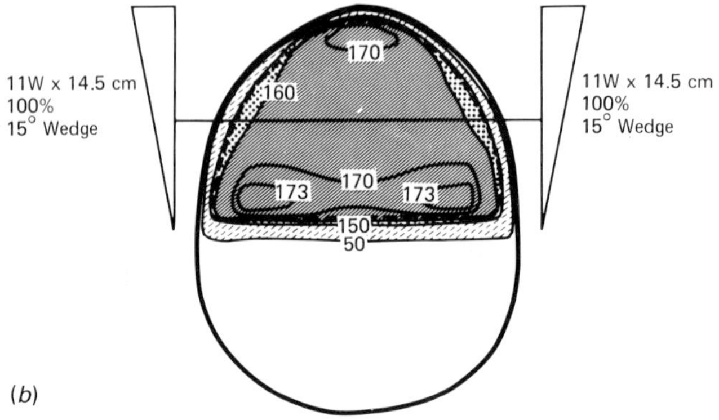

Figure 15.9 (*a*) CT scan showing glioma crossing midline (*b*) Isodose curves of large field technique for treating this patient, 8 MeV. [hatched] >160; [dotted] 150–160; [dashed] 50–150; [blank] <50

Oligodendroglioma

This is an uncommon tumour in man (5% of all CNS tumours) but apparently very common in dogs (Jones and Currie 1982)! They grow slowly, appearing in middle age and often present with epilepsy of unknown origin. The frontal lobe is a common site and somewhat less so is the occipital lobe. After an attempt at radical surgical excision, postoperative irradiation should be considered if the patient is reasonably well. It is difficult to judge how effective this may be, but Sheline (1977) reported a 10-year survival of 55% compared with 25% if surgery alone is used.

Ependymoma and choroid plexus papilloma

Although this is the second most common form of glioma, it nevertheless represents only 8% of all brain tumours. It is the most common of intramedullary spinal cord tumours and is found most often in children and young adults. Treatment policy has always been controversial, although radiation has the major part to play as they are difficult to remove surgically and fortunately they are very radiosensitive. The problem lies in their pattern of spread. Seedling metastases via the CSF are common, although this incidence depends on the grade of tumour and its site of origin. High grade tumours and infratentorial lesions are spread most commonly by this route. The spinal cord primary lesions and the supratentorial lesions do not often seed as they mostly have a low histological grade.

Treatment policy is therefore dictated by these two factors. It would seem logical to treat the supratentorial and spinal cord low-grade tumours with large fields to the local lesion only, giving a minimal tumour dose of 4500 cGy in 20 daily fractions (Garrett and Simpson, 1983). For all infratentorial lesions and with high grade tumours, total CNS irradiation is required using the same technique as described later for medulloblastoma. Jones and Currie (1982) suggest that if this treatment policy is followed an 80% 5-year survival figure can be achieved. A recent series reported by Garrett and Simpson (1983) gives a 78% 5-year survival in the low grade tumours but only 25–43% 5-year survival in those with high grade. The latter authors describe another prognostic factor: namely that if the functional status of the patient was poor before treatment then the outlook was adversely affected.

The use of adjuvant chemotherapy might be thought to offer some improvement in survival, but the SIOP trial (in which vincristine and CCNU were used) showed no improvement in survival as compared to the control group which only received postoperative irradiation: 54% surviving 3 years in the latter group against 38% in the former (Bloom, 1983).

Pineal and third ventricle tumours

These are rare tumours (0.5–1.0% of all intracranial neoplasms), but of interest because of their unusual presentation usually in the first and second decades of life. Russell (1944) described two groups: those arising in the pineal gland itself — the pineocytoma and pineoblastoma — and those arising elsewhere, the atypical teratoma now called suprasellar germinoma (Friedman, 1947).

The symptoms and signs are due to obstruction of the CSF pathways and pressure effects on the hypothalamus and pituitary, leading to abnormalities of sexual maturation, diabetes insipidus as well as visual field defects. Diagnosis in the past was often based on the clinical and radiological picture (*Figure 15.10a, b*) as obtaining histological proof was fraught with danger at this site. Today stereotactic biopsy techniques may overcome this.

Fortunately, these tumours are moderately radiosensitive, and surgery should be confined to obtaining histological proof of the diagnosis as well as to provide relief of the CSF obstruction. This was commonly performed in the past by a ventriculoatrial shunt, but if at all possible, this should be avoided as there is a theoretical danger that seedling metastases in the CSF would be spread into the rest of the body via the blood stream.

In view of the possibility of CSF spread total CNS irradiation would seem to be indicated, and is advocated by Sung, Harisiadis and Chang (1978),

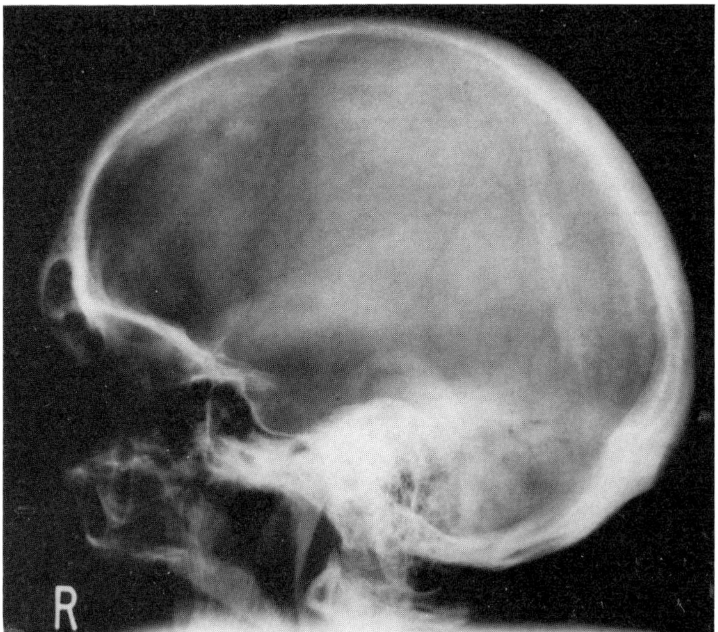

Figure 15.10 (*a*) Skull X-ray pineocytoma showing enlargement of pituitary fossa

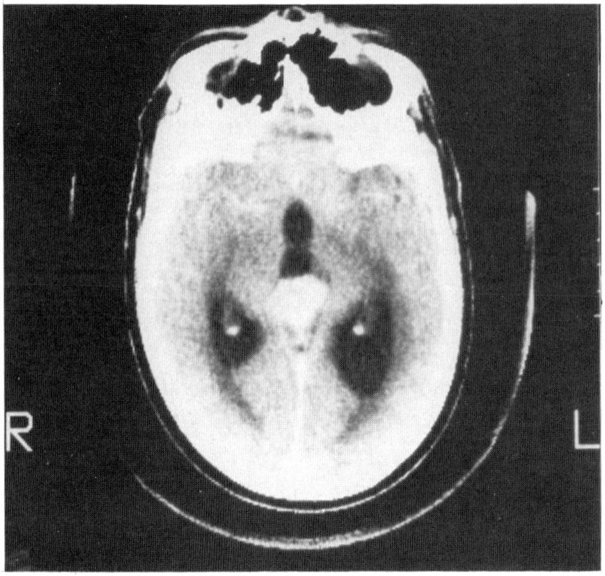

Figure 15.10 (*b*) CT scan of third ventricle tumour

followed by a booster to the tumour area only of 2000 cGy in a further 10 fractions.
although in their series of 73 cases only four patients (15%) were so treated. In this series, 10% of the true pineal tumours and 37% of the suprasellar germinomas metastasized via the subarachnoid space within 6 months to 5 years of diagnosis. Wara *et al.* (1979) reported on 113 cases but with only an 8% CSF metastatic rate.

The dose of irradiation may be more important as Sung *et al.* showed that 47% of patients who received a dose of less than 4500 cGy in 4–4.5 weeks developed local recurrence inside the irradiated volume, compared with only 10% who received 5000–5500 cGy in 5–6.5 weeks. It would seem therefore that the more undifferentiated tumours (pineoblastoma and suprasellar germinoma) are most likely to seed via the CSF and should therefore be treated with total CNS irradiation. A dose of 2500–3000 cGy to the spinal cord in 4–4.5 weeks, as advocated by Sung *et al.*, would seem reasonable. Using the same technique as in medulloblastoma (*see below*) this dose can easily be achieved, and the brain itself could be given 4500 cGy in 4 weeks (this dose is probably radiobiologically equivalent to the higher dose advocated by Sung *et al.*

For the well differentiated pinealoma (pineocytoma) two options are open. One is to irradiate the primary site only with a pair of parallel and opposed fields to a dose of 5000 cGy in 25 daily fractions. Alternatively, if there is any doubt about the exact histology, treatment should be given to the whole brain to include the entire subarachnoid space (anteriorly to include the cribriform plate and posteriorly the base of the skull), to 4000 cGy in 20 daily fractions and then the primary site boosted with a further 1000 cGy in five daily fractions. Any higher dose than this might well produce damage to the brain stem and hypothalamus and this could be just as dangerous as the possible risk of local recurrence.

Thalamus and brain stem

Until recently, tumours in this site have been inaccessible to histological diagnosis, but with the advent of stereotactic biopsy techniques the situation should change. In the past the diagnosis was usually not proven, and the reported results must therefore be viewed with suspicion. Cheek and Taveras (1966) described 11 cases of whom six survived more than 3 years. Sheline (1975) reported a 5-year survival of 41% in 27 patients. However, Allbright, Price and Guthkella (1983) have reported a 35% 5-year survival in 27 cases (all histologically proven) and without any operative morbidity. Up to now the only reasonable method of treatment has been to use a pair of parallel and opposed megavoltage fields to include a volume from the midbrain down to the foramen magnum and, as this area is particularly radiosensitive, a dose of 4500 cGy in 20 daily fractions should not be exceeded. Stereotactic implants of ^{125}I can now be considered, although dose levels need to be carefully considered (Gutin and Dormandy, 1982) (*see below*).

Medulloblastoma

This is the commonest brain tumour in children (*Figure 15.11*), and with an incidence of 10% of all children's malignant disease, one would expect to see about 80–90 cases per year in Great Britain. They also occur in young adults and make up about

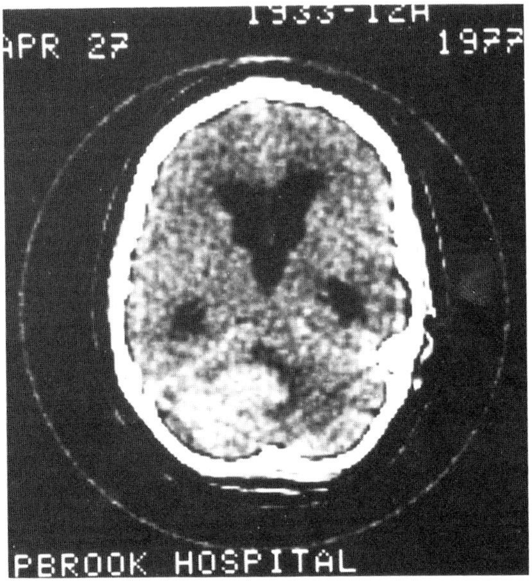

Figure 15.11 CT scan — medulloblastoma

7% of all brain tumours of neuroepithelial origin. Nevertheless because of rarity, no one department of radiotherapy will see many cases per year and there may be an argument for treating such patients in certain selected centres. Although these tumours are very radiosensitive, 5-year survival rates have varied tremendously both in the UK and the USA, ranging from as low as 5% to the 68% reported by Hope-Stone (1970).

The surgical approach in the past had often been only partial removal of the tumour to act as a decompression. This may not be in the best interests of the patient, as it has been shown in the SIOP trial (Bloom, 1983) that subtotal removal of the tumour is associated with a worse prognosis than complete excision. The temptation for the surgeon to carry out a bypass procedure, even with a millipore filter, should be strongly resisted as this will invariably increase the chance of seedling metastases reaching the blood stream and thus reduce any hope of curing the disease. The use of dexamethasone will so reduce cerebral oedema that there should be no need to carry out such a procedure. Irradiation to the whole cerebrospinal axis will be required and should be started as soon as possible after craniotomy. As treatment planning is very complicated the latter can usually be commenced even before the stitches are removed.

The aim of treatment is to give a homogeneous dose of irradiation to the whole of the central nervous system. This can be achieved in one of two ways, either by using the elegant London Hospital technique (Botrill, Rogers and Hope-Stone, 1965), with one large posterior spade-shaped orthovoltage field to treat the whole spinal cord and posterior brain, along with a single anterior megavoltage field; or alternatively, a series of matched megavoltage fields to treat the spinal cord and a pair of parallel opposed fields to treat the brain.

The theoretical advantage of the former method is that there is only the need to match two fields whereas with the latter more junctional points will be required which may lead to either under or overdosage at these sites. The use of an orthovoltage spinal field will also reduce the dose to the thyroid gland which, in children at least, may reduce the risk of producing an irradiation-induced carcinoma. The problem of differential bone absorption in the vertebrae when using orthovoltage can be overcome by the use of modern equipment such as the 300 kV (RT 305) which will give a half value layer of 2.7 mm Cu. The long treatment times associated with the older deep X-ray machines will also be markedly reduced with the RT 305 as at 90 cm focal skin distance a field length of 74 cm can be achieved with a dose rate of 30 cGy/minute. The overall time for 200 cGy will be only 15–20 minutes instead of the previous 45 minutes (Hope-Stone, 1980).

The children will still need to be sufficiently sedated (if under the age of 5 years) so that they will lie completely still for this length of time. This can always be achieved with a general anaesthetic but in most cases, it is not required. Under 2 years of age light sedation will usually suffice. Between 2 and 5 years, ketamine anaesthesia is preferred (*see* Chapter 10) as it will enable the child to wake up quickly without depression of the deep reflexes and thus take adequate daily nourishment. Over 5 years of age most children will cooperate even though the irradiation technique practised is one of the most complicated in use today. The biggest problem is one of cerebral irritation but even this can be overcome with the use of steroids and appropriate sedation.

The London Hospital technique

This was first described by Bottrill, Rogers and Hope-Stone (1965) and has been modified to take into account the possible danger of recurrence occurring in the subarachnoid space in the region of the cribriform plate. Three such cases were described by Hardy *et al.* (1978) and the method used to overcome this was reported by these authors.

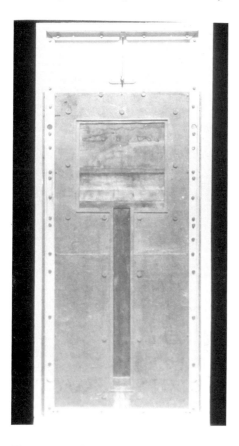

Figure 15.12 Differential copper filter embodied in lead shield (from Bottril, Rogers and Hope-Stone, 1965 by kind permission of the *British Journal of Radiology*)

The spinal cord is treated with a single posterior spade-shaped field down to the level of S2. As the spinal cord can never be at an equal distance from the radiation source the kneeling position as described by Bullimore and Mott (1982) is not used, and in any case, this is not easy to achieve in a fractious irritable child. Instead the patient is treated in the prone position which can easily be reproduced from day-to-day. The problem of the different distance from the radiation source to the patient's spinal cord is overcome by modifying the X-rays of a 300 kV machine using a differential copper filter which will compensate for these varying depths (*Figure 15.12*). The filter will also produce a dose reduction over the posterior portion of the brain; it is backed on the patient's side with aluminium (to absorb secondary irradiation). The whole filter is embodied in a lead shield which will completely protect the rest of the child's body.

The child lies prone in a specially constructed plaster cast (*Figures 15.13a and b*). Localization films are taken in the plaster cast with a single continuous lateral radiograph using a moving diagnostic X-ray field with a slit field (Hope-Stone, 1984). Lead markers are placed on the patient's skin at the same time so that an accurate position of the spinal cord can be obtained (*Figures 15.14a and b*).

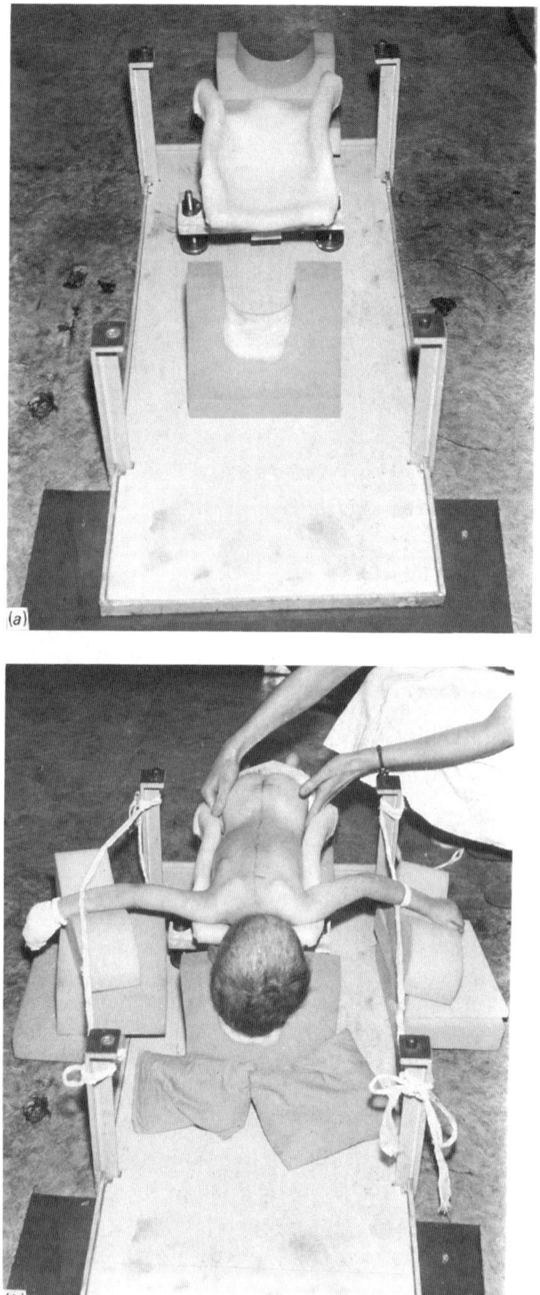

Figure 15.13 (*a*) Plaster immobilization cast. (*b*) Child lying prone in cast

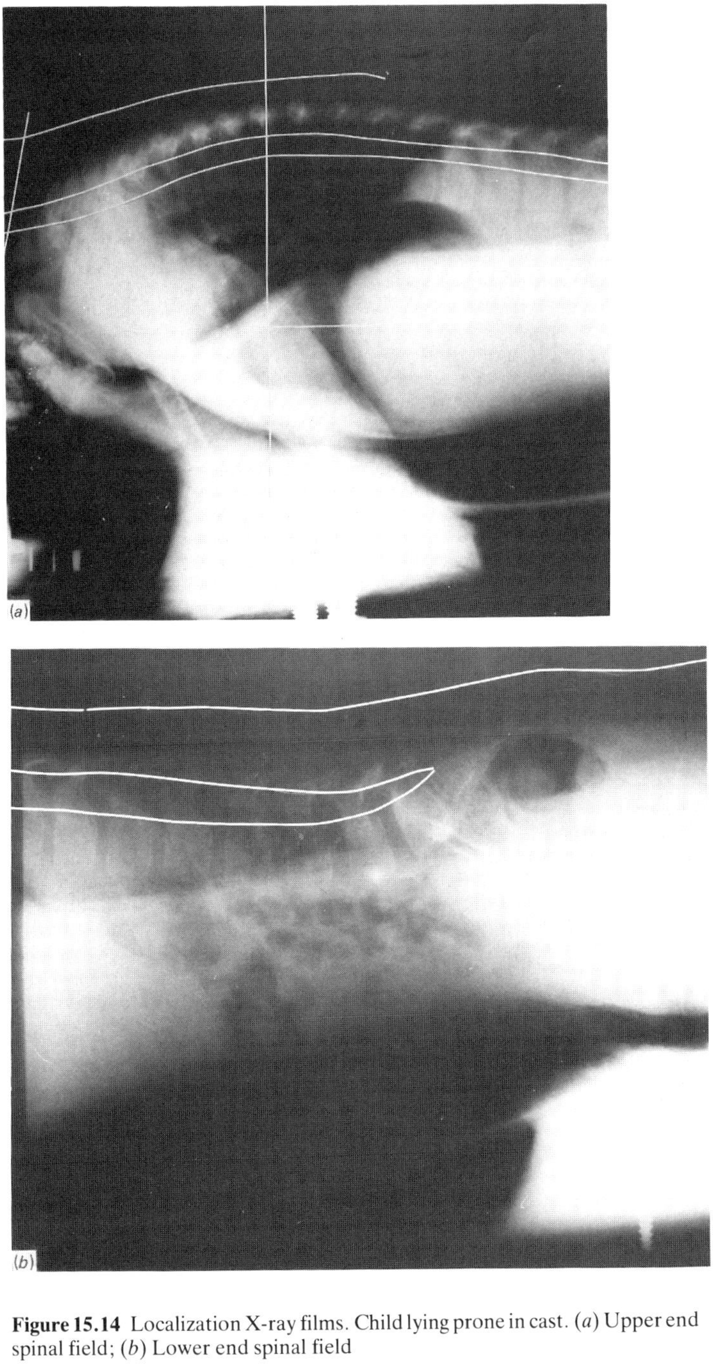

Figure 15.14 Localization X-ray films. Child lying prone in cast. (*a*) Upper end spinal field; (*b*) Lower end spinal field

When the child is lying prone in the cast, a plastic jig is used to set up the orthovoltage field (*Figure 15.15a*). Care must be taken to ensure that the child's spine is completely horizontal. The composite filter then replaces the plastic jig and bolus is used around the head (*Figure 15.15b*). A minimum dose of 3000 cGy to the spinal cord is given to children under 2 years of age rising to 3500 cGy for older children and adults. A width of 4.5–5 cm is used to cover the cord.

The brain is treated with a single direct anterior megavoltage field (^{60}Co or linear accelerator 5–8 MeV). A shell is made of cobex and the patient treated in the supine position with the shell being

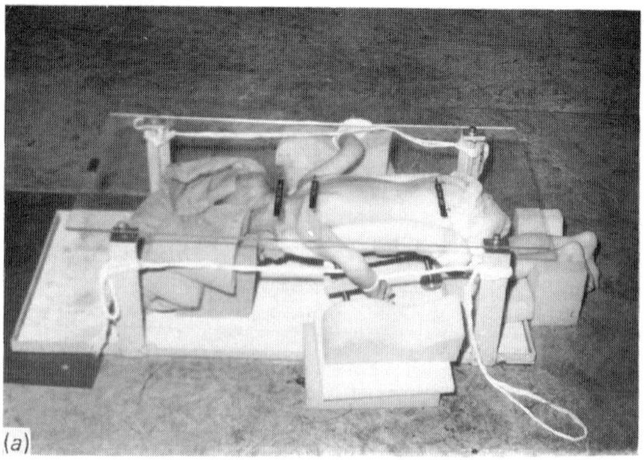

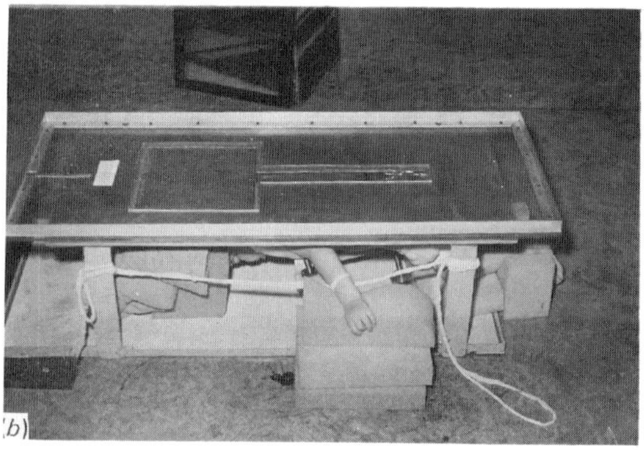

Figure 15.15 Child lying prone in plaster cast. (*a*) Plastic setting up jig in position — bolus bags around head. (*b*) Plastic jig replaced by copper filter (from Hope-Stone, 1970 by kind permission *Journal of Neurosurgery*, **32**, 83–88)

fixed to a base plate. The anterior field then covers the whole of the cribriform plate, the eyes being shielded indirectly with lead (*Figure 15.16*). An X-ray taken in this position shows the cribriform plate area to be treated (as seen between the parallel lines) (*Figure 15.17*). A lead compensator is used (*Figure 15.18*). A composite isodose curve is produced for the two sets of fields (*Figure 15.19*). The aim is to give a minimum dose of 4500 cGy to the posterior cranial fossa with a total maximum dose of 5000 cGy to the whole brain. The treatment time is usually 5 weeks. One important site to be watched carefully is the neck dip where the skin dose can be very high in some children. Ideally 4500 cGy should not be exceeded on the skin at any point but in the neck dip 5000 cGy may have to be accepted.

In older children whose spinal cord is longer than 74 cm and in all adults it is necessary to use a matching megavoltage technique (8 MeV) as the orthovoltage field will not be long enough. The anterior set up remains the same, but two long direct posterior spinal fields are used — the patient lying prone in a plaster cast. One moving junction point is used so that on each consecutive day the field is moved up or down 1 cm — the total distance to be moved will cover a length of 5 cm (*Figure 15.20*).

All patients are treated on a rising input basis starting at 50 cGy and working up by equal increments to 200 cGy. The anterior skull field can be

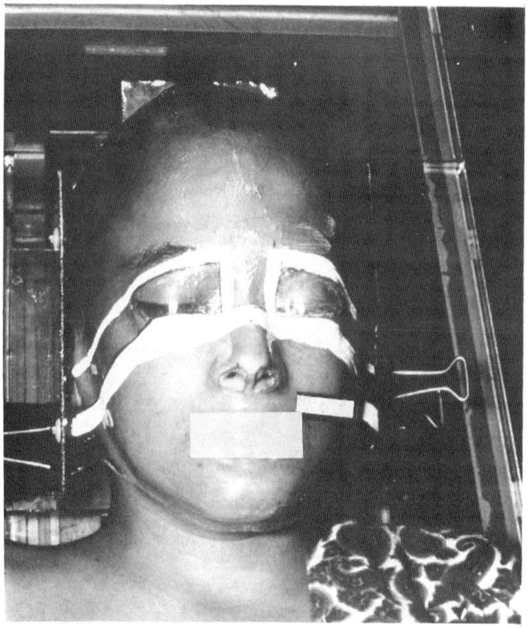

Figure 15.16 Anterior skull field. Eyes shielded indirectly with lead, cribriform fossa included in field

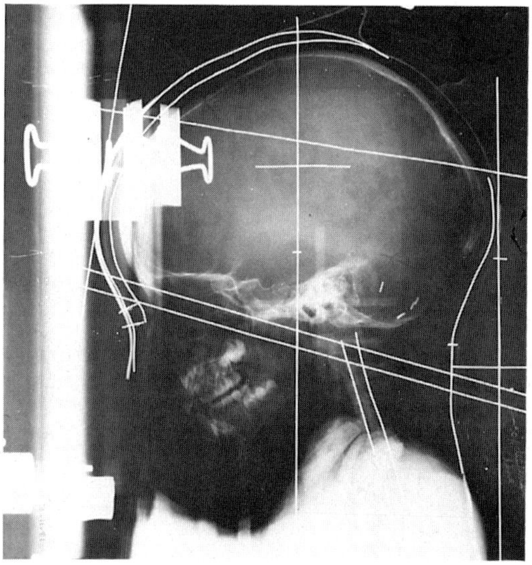

Figure 15.17 X-ray to show anterior skull fields. Cribriform fossa area lies between the parallel lines

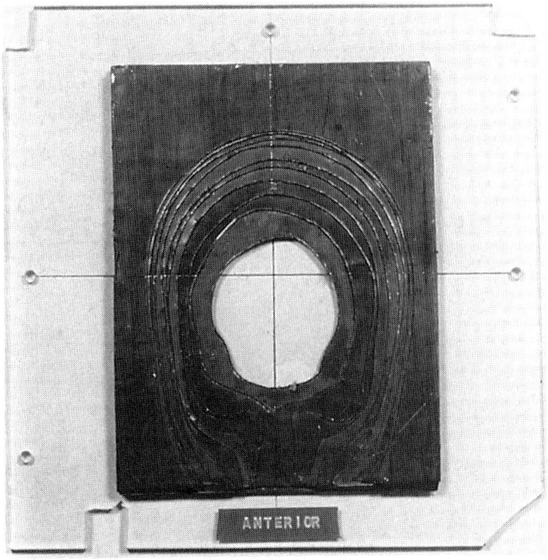

Figure 15.18 Lead compensator for anterior skull field

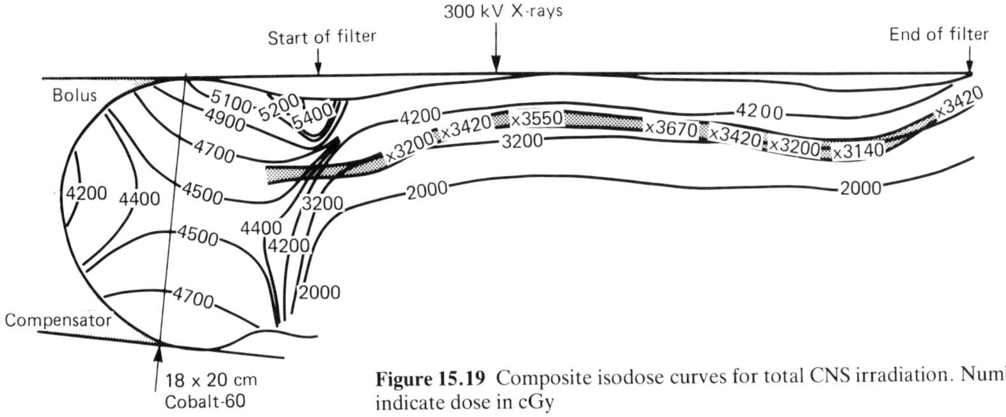

Figure 15.19 Composite isodose curves for total CNS irradiation. Numbers indicate dose in cGy

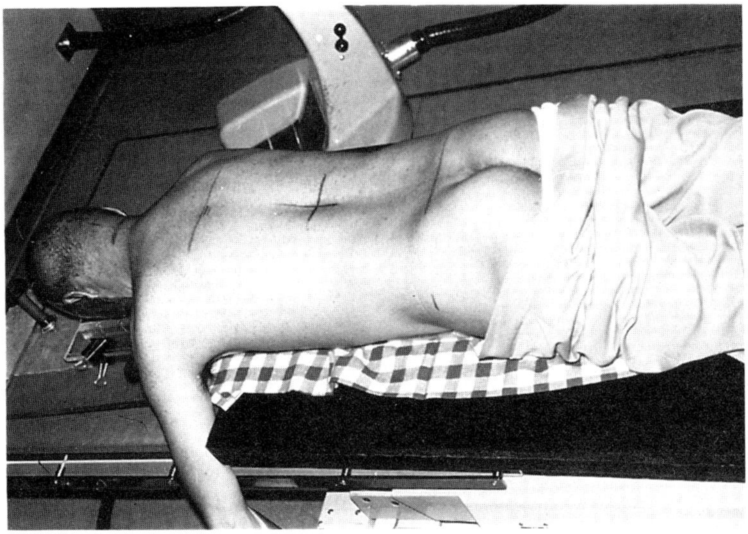

Figure 15.20 Spinal cord fields in total CNS irradiation of adult. Upper parallel lines show the position of the moving junction point

treated without the spinal cord field for the first 3 days as it is believed that treatment to the primary site should be started as soon as possible, particularly if only incomplete surgical excision has been carried out. In practice, this is often necessary as working out the details of the spinal cord filter may take an extra few days.

The use of a rising input technique is particularly important in these tumours as such a large volume of marrow producing bone is being irradiated and tolerance will be better achieved in this way. If the white cell count (WBC) falls below $3 \times 10^9\ell$ or the platelets below $100 \times 10^9\ell$ treatment should theoretically be stopped. In practice, reducing the daily input to 100 cGy will probably allow recovery, but if the WBC falls below $2 \times 10^9\ell$ then a few days rest will be required. When the platelets fall below $100 \times 10^9\ell$ the same approach may be used, stopping for a rest at $40 \times 10^9\ell$. The present author would, however, give an intramuscular injection of 50 mg of Deca-Durabolin as soon as the count falls below $100 \times 10^9\ell$ and this often will obviate the necessity of interrupting treatment.

Radiation sickness is rarely a problem. Skin reactions can be treated with 1% Hydrocortisone Cream. Epilation will always occur, and the parents must be warned accordingly and a wig provided as required.

Long-term side-effects have been described. Thyroid carcinoma was reported by Andrews and Kerr (1965) and kyphoscoliosis due to epiphyseal damage by Moss (1959). The latter has never been seen in the London Hospital series and this may be due to the more homogeneous dose given to the vertebrae (*Figure 15.21*). Convulsions due to fibrotic changes were described by Smith, Lampe and Kahn (1961). Overall growth may well be impaired due either to a direct effect on vertebral epiphyses or to a reduction of growth hormone level from irradiating the hypothalamic-pituitary axis (Shalet *et al.* 1981). The former can certainly occur but is not a major problem as the most likely outcome is that the children will be no taller when grown up than their parents. How commonly irradiation produces an overall reduction of growth hormone and therefore marked stunting in adult life remains open to conjecture. Shalet and Beardwell (1979) and Harrop *et al.* (1976) both describe a series of cases in

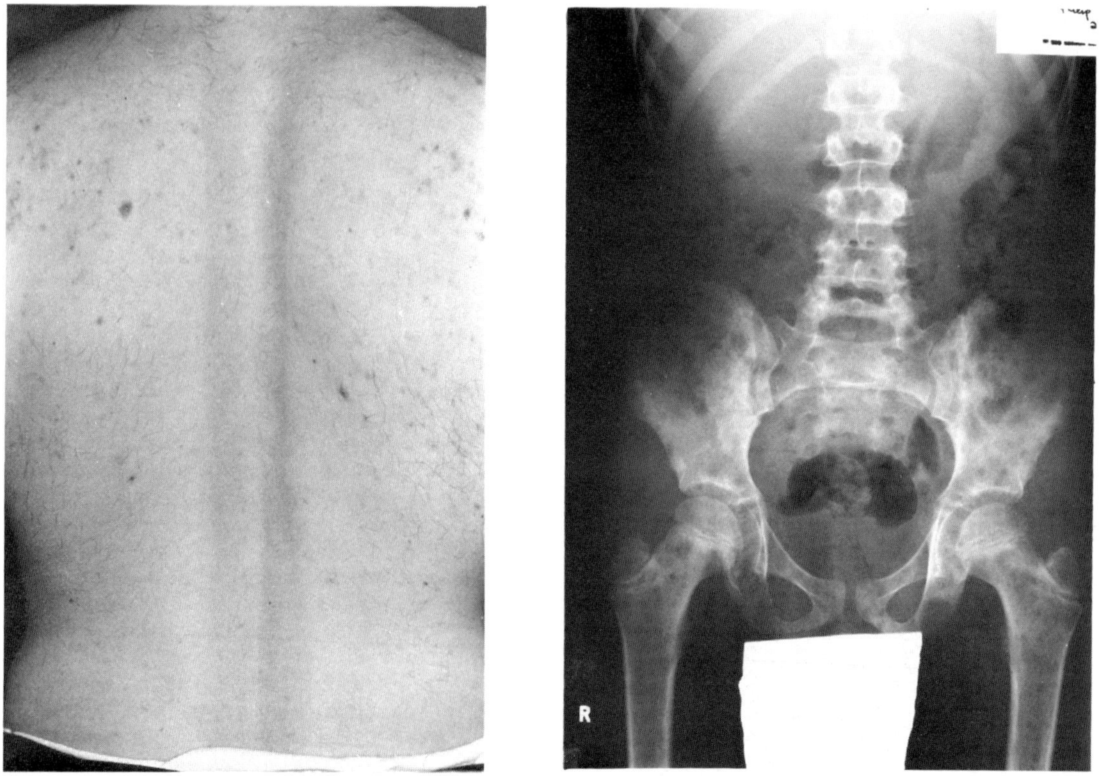

Figure 15.21 (*a*) Spine of 16-year-old boy treated 8 years previously for medulloblastoma

(*b*) Metastases to bone in medulloblastoma

which nearly one-half showed reduced growth hormone levels, but whether this was due entirely to the irradiation or to a combination of factors including the use of steroids, or even damage by the tumour is open to question.

Depression of thyroid function was also reported by Shalet (1982) who pointed out that if megavoltage was used, the exit dose from the spinal cord field would give significantly high doses to the thyroid gland. This could act as a carcinogenic agent to the growing thyroid in young children.

Results

In the first series reported from The London Hospital in a very small number of cases the 5-year survival figures were 77% (Hope-Stone, 1970). In a larger number of cases, 26 in all, reported from the same hospital a more realistic figure of 61% was found (Hardy *et al.*, 1978). The present author has updated those results and, in 41 cases, the 5-year survival is about the same, namely 50%. It should be noted that the 10-year figure is very similar which belies the notion that recurrence is common after 5 years.

Failure is usually due to local recurrence in the posterior cerebral fossa and occurs in 80% of such cases with or without spinal metastases (Bloom, 1983). As even the best results so far reported are not greater than 60% some form of adjuvant chemotherapy has been advocated. A multicentre trial to test this hypothesis was set up under the auspices of SIOP. All patients received total CNS irradiation with a maximum tumour dose of 5000–5500 cGy to the posterior fossa, 3500–4500 cGy to the rest of the brain and 3000–3500 cGy to the spinal cord — daily fractionation over 6–7 weeks being given. Slightly lower doses were used in children under 2 years of age. Half the patients received chemotherapy which consisted of weekly intravenous vincristine 1 mg/m^2 starting at the time of irradiation, and then after completion of treatment, monthly treatment was given using one dose of CCNU (100 mg/m^2) on day 1 with vincristine on days 1, 8 and 15. This was continued every 6 weeks for the next year. The most interesting result in the 144 children entered into the trial was that the actuarial 5-year survival using irradiation alone was about 42%, which does appear to prove that if all centres adhere to a rigid protocol of dose and technique then much better results can be achieved. The chemotherapy group (138 cases) did marginally better with a 51% actuarial survival figure, but the significance (P>0.56) is only nominal (Bloom, 1983). These results are similar to the last reported series from The London Hospital where chemotherapy was not used (*Table 15.2*).

However, a more interesting and important fact has emerged from the trial — namely that certain subsections did significantly better if given adjuvant chemotherapy. These were children less than 2 years of age (57% vs 31% in 26 cases) also, those children who had either subtotal surgical excision or who had brain stem involvement, did better. If these three high risk groups are put together there was a significantly improved survival (53% versus 25%). It would therefore appear wise to give all children in the high risk group adjuvant chemotherapy. A word of caution should be noted; namely that there may be a long-term danger of carcinogenesis from this combined method and it is therefore imperative that follow-up of these patients should be continued indefinitely.

Table 15.2 Results of radiotherapy and chemotherapy in medulloblastoma

	No. of cases	*5-year survival (%)*
Radiotherapy alone		
The London Hospital	41	51 (crude)
SIOP trial	144	42 (actuarial)
Radiotherapy + adjuvant chemotherapy		
SIOP trial	138	52 (acturial)
(Bloom, 1983)		

Metastatic or recurrent disease presents a problem. If bone involvement is widespread (*see Figure 15.21b*) symptomatic relief might best be obtained by chemotherapy as outlined above. If local or spinal cord recurrence occurs one can again consider chemotherapy providing previous drugs have not been given. There must, however, come a point where no such treatment at all should be considered, other than 'tender loving care' with appropriate sedation and analgesia.

Optic nerve glioma

These tumours, most commonly found in children, present with visual failure and proptosis, and eventually both eyes may be affected leading to complete blindness. The tumour grows slowly and insidiously and, if diagnosed early enough, may be amenable to surgical cure. Clintorian *et al.* (1964) reported 21 out of 24 patients alive at 24 years. If surgery is incomplete or impossible radical irradiation should be considered. A three field beam directed megavoltage technique can be used giving a tumour dose of 4500 cGy in 20 daily fractions (*Figure 15.22a*). Head fixation is imperative (*Figure 15.22b*).

Meningioma

Although accounting for about 15% of all primary intracranial tumours, the majority are benign and

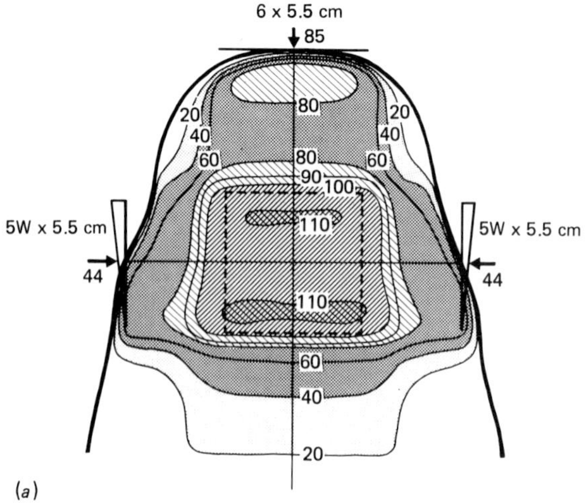

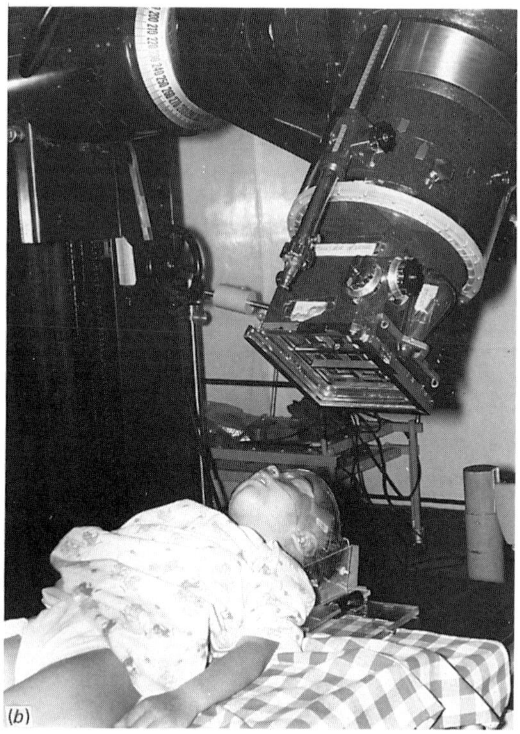

Figure 15.22 (*a*) 3 field technique for optic nerve glioma. >110; 100–110; 80–100; 40–80; 20–40; <20 (from Hope-Stone, 1976 In *Radiotherapy in Modern Clinical Practice* 1976, edited by H. F. Hope-Stone, p. 84 by kind permission of Granada Publishing Co. Ltd). (*b*) Head fixation for treating this patient

can be treated by surgery alone. Occasionally such a benign tumour may not be completely excised (these often being found in the region of the sphenoidal ridge) (*Figure 15.23*) and the question of irradiation to prevent subsequent local recurrence needs to be considered. This raises a difficult problem as no radiotherapist is anxious to give high dose irradiation to the brain for a benign condition. In a review of 213 cases, Wara *et al.* (1975) found that if post-operative irradiation was given (5000 cGy), the local recurrence rate was 22% compared with 74% if no such treatment was given. For a truly malignant meningioma where surgery is often incomplete postoperative irradiation should always be given. In all cases the present author sees no reason to risk irradiation damage to the brain, thus a tumour dose of 4500 cGy in 4 weeks, using relatively small fields, should not be exceeded.

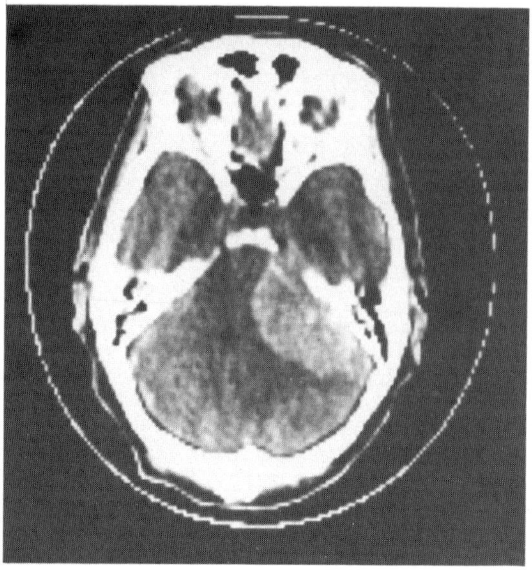

Figure 15.23 CT scan (R) petrous temporal meningioma

Primary non-Hodgkin's lymphoma (microgliomatosis — reticulum cell sarcoma)

This is a rare disease and the incidence appears to be 1.6% of all extranodular non-Hodgkin's lymphomas (Freeman, Berg and Cutler 1972). Even by 1983 there were less than 200 cases in the world literature (Gonzales and Shuster, 1983). Diagnosis can only be confirmed by excluding evidence of generalized lymphoma in the usual way (*see* Chapter 8). In theory, one would expect the same degree of radiosensitivity of these lymphomas as in other parts of the body, yet Gonzales and Shuster (1983), reporting on 15 cases, achieved less than a 20% survival. All patients received whole brain irradiation with doses ranging from 3000–6000 cGy in 3–6 weeks. Six cases showed evidence of CSF spread, but nine developed local recurrence. Gonzales looked at 70 cases in the literature and found a CSF seeding rate of 26%, but Sagerman, Collier and King (1983) showed no evidence of seeding at all in 15 cases. It would seem logical to treat the whole brain to 4500 cGy in 4 weeks as doses of 5000 cGy did not show any better results and the risk of irradiation damage would be greater (Gonzales and Shuster, 1983). In view of the latter author's 26% CSF seeding rate, it might also seem logical to treat the whole spinal cord to 3500 cGy using the medulloblastoma technique, but even with these two methods of treatment failure is still likely and the addition of chemotherapy may need to be considered.

Vascular tumours

Haemangioblastoma (*Figure 15.24*) should ideally be treated by surgery and this is usually successful (Northfield, 1973), but if they are very large and highly vascular, surgery even with prior embolization might be too dangerous. A moderate dose of irradiation in the region of 3500–4000 cGy given to the tumour site only will probably produce some shrinkage, although it is unlikely to eradicate the neoplasm completely. Nevertheless, symptoms will be improved and the danger of bleeding lessened, thus achieving long-term control in the same way as that of the glomus jugulare tumours (*see* Chapter 5).

Craniopharyngioma

Although relatively uncommon in Western Europe and the USA this tumour has a remarkably high incidence (5–7%) in Japan (Onoyama *et al.*, 1977). Occurring often before the age of 20, they grow slowly and present with visual failure, endocrine disorders (hypogonadism, diabetes insipidus and growth disorders) as well as signs of raised intracranial pressure. Surgery has always been the first line of treatment if only to make an accurate diagnosis. It is not usually possible to excise the tumour completely, particularly if there is suprasellar exten-

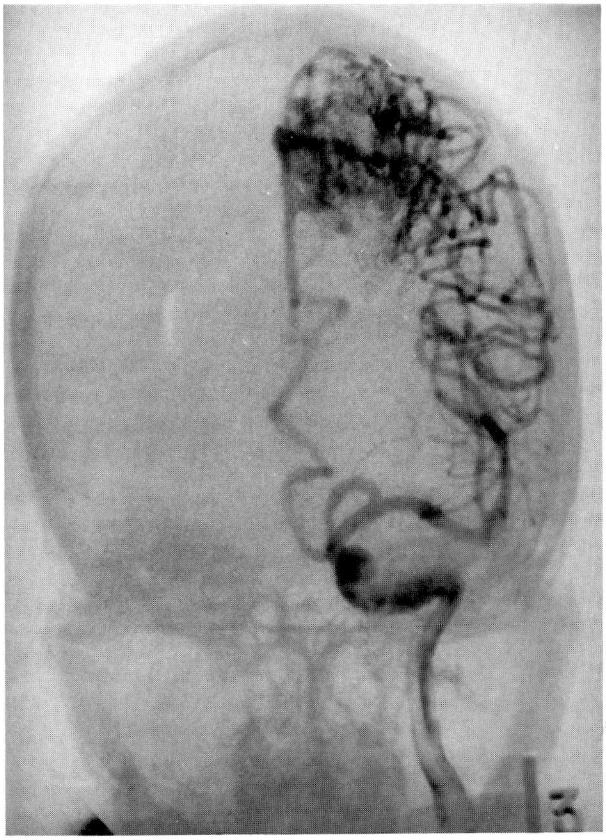

Figure 15.24 Haemangioblastoma of cerebral cortex

sion (*Figure 15.25a*) (many surgeons being content just to aspirate the cyst) (Sharman *et al.* 1974), thus postoperative irradiation is always required. Treatment can be given with a pair of parallel and opposed fields using a cobex shell. Beam direction is achieved with a back pointer (optical, mechanical or laser) (*Figure 15.25b*). Alternatively a 360° rotation technique can be used. Although 4500 cGy in 20 daily fractions would seem an adequate dose, Kramer, McKissock and Concannon (1961) advocated a minimum of 5500 cGy up to 7000 cGy in 6–7 weeks, and nine out of 10 patients survived for periods of 3 months to 7 years in this series. In Sharman's series, using 5000–5500 cGy in 20–22 fractions, 18 out of 22 patients survived from 2 to 7 years. Onoyama *et al.* (1977) showed that although a dose of less than 4999 rads (4999 cGy) produced a low survival rate, this was due to the poor postoperative condition of the patients which precluded a higher dose. Their highest survival rate occurred in the group receiving 5000–6000 cGy in 5–7 weeks (80% at 5 years and 73% at 10 years in 13 cases). Calvo *et al.* (1983) used a pair of parallel and opposed fields to give a dose of 5000–6000 cGy in 5–6 weeks in 18 patients and all were alive and well from 2–12 years. Vyramuthu and Benton (1983) reported a series of 15 cases treated in Edinburgh, again using a simple technique of parallel and opposed fields with dose levels of 4500 cGy in 28 days — 54% were free from recurrence at 5 years. None of the patients in the above reported series developed major side-effects except those treated by Kramer, Southard and Mansfield (1972) (to a dose

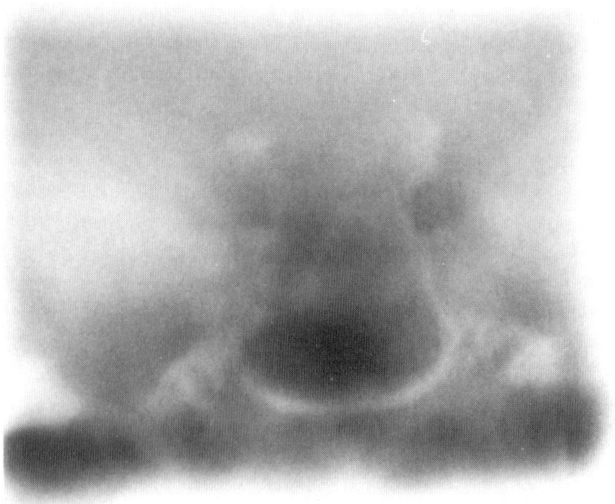

(*a*)

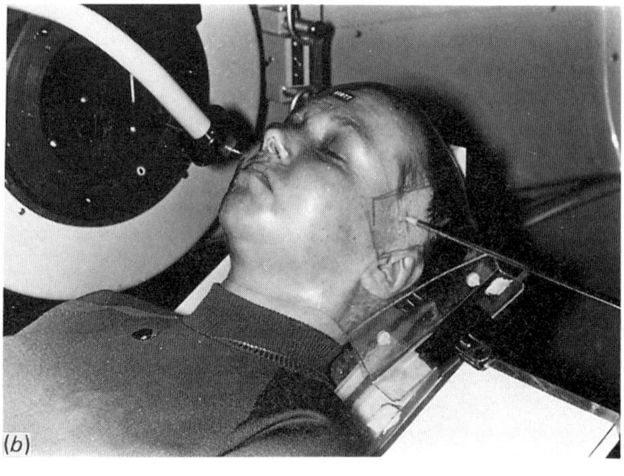

(*b*)

Figure 15.25 Craniopharyngioma. (*a*) Suprasellar extension as seen on tomography. (*b*) Mechanical back pointer set up for this patient

greater than 7000 cGy) in whom brain necrosis occurred.

In conclusion, the present author thinks that a simple radiation technique (after adequate surgery) to give a dose of 4500 cGy in 4 weeks would appear to be safe, and gives a reasonable chance of local control.

Pituitary tumours

Eosinophilic adenoma

This comprises about 37% of pituitary tumours, and presents with acromegaly in adults and giantism in children. Treatment is required if vision is likely to be affected, or if severe diabetes or hypertension occurs. Treatment to improve the facial features or general enlargement of the skeleton is not really necessary as most patients are hardly aware of the subtle changes that have taken place over the years. Surgery alone can be quite effective and, using the trans-sphenoidal approach, the temporary morbidity is relatively low, being less than 30% in 56 cases reported by Williams (1974) — although one case died from a postoperative embolus. Surgery has the great advantage of giving a definite histological diagnosis, and in the past was used to delineate any suprasellar extension, as suggested by the radiological picture (*Figure 15.26a*), but this can now be easily shown with a good CT scan (*Figure 15.26b*). In order to prevent recurrence postoperative irradiation is advisable in all cases. If a rapid response to treatment is not required then irradiation without surgery can be used providing one is sure of the diagnosis. Radiation alone will certainly arrest the growth of the tumour and make the control of hypertension and diabetes much easier, but it is unlikely to produce a marked reduction of growth hormone levels, thus the gross visual signs of acromegaly will not be improved. If the latter is required then bromocriptine should be given at the same time. Some authors would suggest that using the drug alone is all that is required, but unfortunately it is not particularly well tolerated by patients.

Radiation techniques

External megavoltage irradiation using a linear accelerator (5–8 MeV) is preferred to cobalt-60 on account of the sharp cut off of the margins of the beam, and it is possible to treat patients with a simple pair of parallel and opposed fields with an optical or laser back pointer (*Figure 15.27*). The fields should be as small as possible (3.5–5.5 cm) but should cover the known spread of the tumour (*Figure 15.28a*). A shell will immobilize the patient

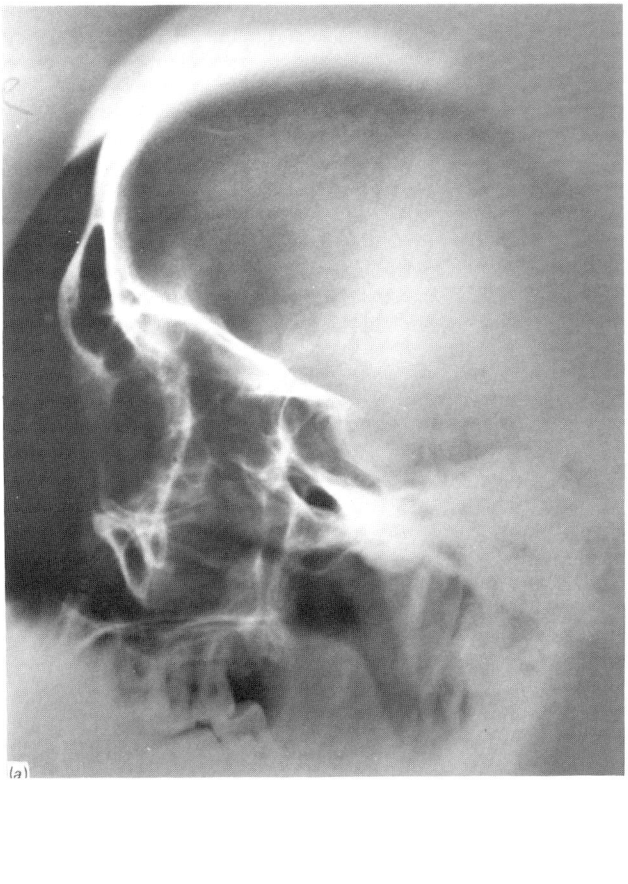

Figure 15.26 Pituitary tumour. (*a*) Skull X-ray to show enlargment of pituitary fossa

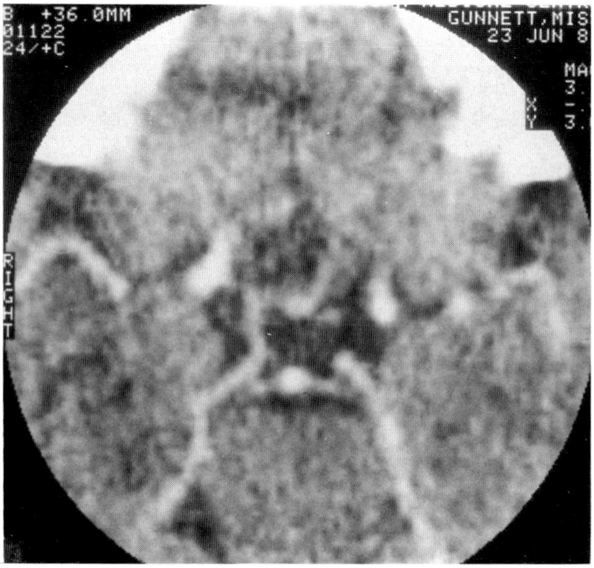

Figure 15.26 (*b*) Pituitary tumour. CT scan showing suprasellar extension

(*Figure 15.28b*) and localization films are taken on the simulator (*Figure 15.28c*); a verification film can be taken on the accelerator (*Figure 15.28d*). A dose of 4500 cGy in 20 daily fractions treating both fields daily can be given without fear of radiation damage. Indeed at The London Hospital since 1957, 280 patients have been treated in this way and there has not been a single case of brain necrosis, optic nerve injury nor obvious damage to the hypothalamus.

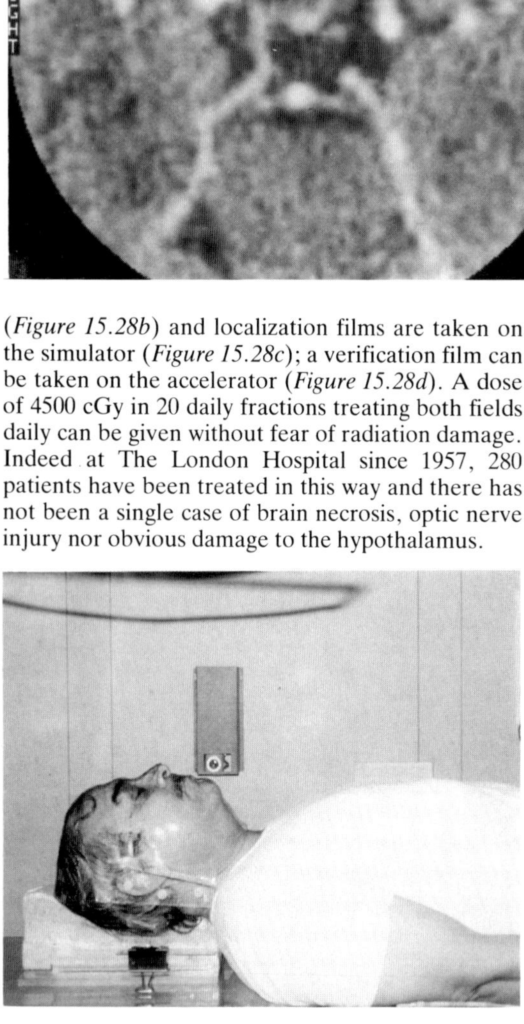

Figure 15.27 Laser back-pointer technique for treating pituitary fossa

A three field technique is preferred by some authors (Joffe, 1982), either using one direct anterior and two anterior wedged oblique fields, or changing the latter to oblique fields (*Figure 15.28e*); 280° rotation (sparing the eyes anteriorly) can also be tried. All three methods are designed to reduce the dose to the temporal lobe in particular but, as stated above, this is not a problem if appropriate dose levels are adhered to. The disadvantage of the more complicated technique is that the accuracy of the set-up will decrease with the number of fields used.

An alternative approach is to implant the pituitary, via the trans-sphenoidal approach with radioactive sources — yttrium–90 (^{90}Yt) is preferred to ^{198}Au as the latter gives a more diffuse irradiation and could damage the surrounding structures. Doses of up to 300 000 cGy can be given but the method is fraught with danger, particularly the production of irreversible optic nerve damage. Meningitis can occur, CSF rhinorrhoea can be a nuisance and hospital admission is required (Joplin, 1975). Unless the aim is to produce complete pituitary ablation, as in Cushing's and Nelson syndrome (*see below*), there seems little point in subjecting patients to a method of treatment with a relatively high complication rate, which will cause permanent panhypopituitarism in 50% of cases and require complicated replacement therapy for the rest of the patient's life. Using this technique for acromegalic patients will certainly produce dramatic regression of soft tissue and bony overgrowth. This may please the clinician but is hardly likely to impress the patient who is not aware of marked changes in his or her personal features.

Proton beam irradiation is a fascinating technique which requires a very expensive synchrocylotron or proton synchroton not usually available in most radiotherapy departments. Using the Bragg Peak phenomenon a very high dose of irradiation (6000 – 10 000 cGy) can be given to a very localized area theoretically without any danger to the surrounding structures. This method has been used at the

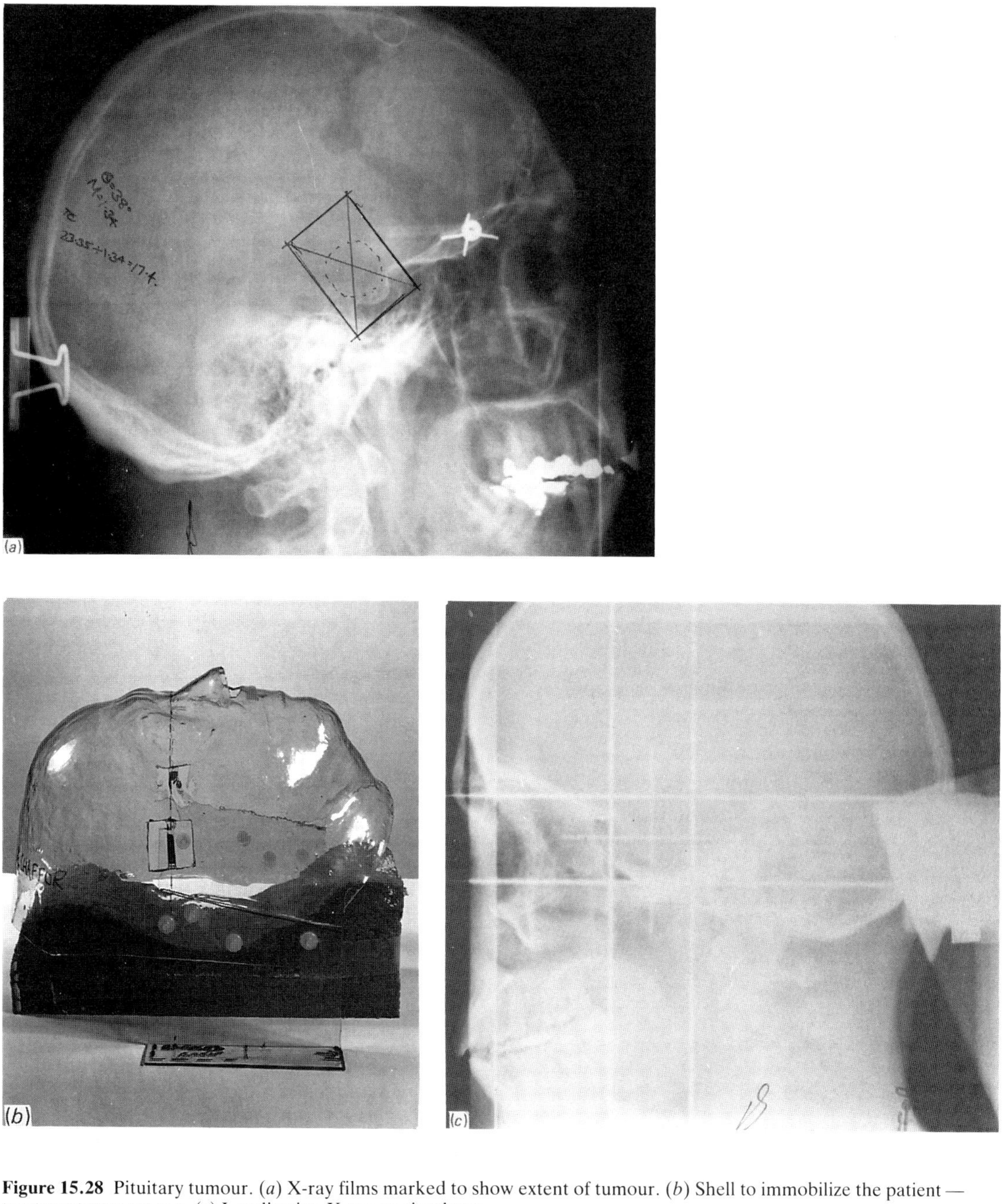

Figure 15.28 Pituitary tumour. (*a*) X-ray films marked to show extent of tumour. (*b*) Shell to immobilize the patient — treatment area cut out. (*c*) Localization X-ray on simulator

Massachusetts General Hospital by Kjellberg and Kliman (1974) with a 12 field technique — 7000 cGy was given to the pituitary tumour but sparing a thin shelf of the surrounding normal gland. Reported complications include temporary occulomotor palsies and minor seizures. This treatment has the advantage of being completed in 1.5–2 hours (and it only requires a 24-hour admission). On 254 cases of acromegaly the authors claim a 56% complete remission and an 85% partial remission, but the technique cannot be used for tumours showing suprasellar extension. The present author cannot see how such a complicated, expensive and potentially hazardous technique can be advocated for the routine treatment of acromegaly when simple treatment methods would suffice.

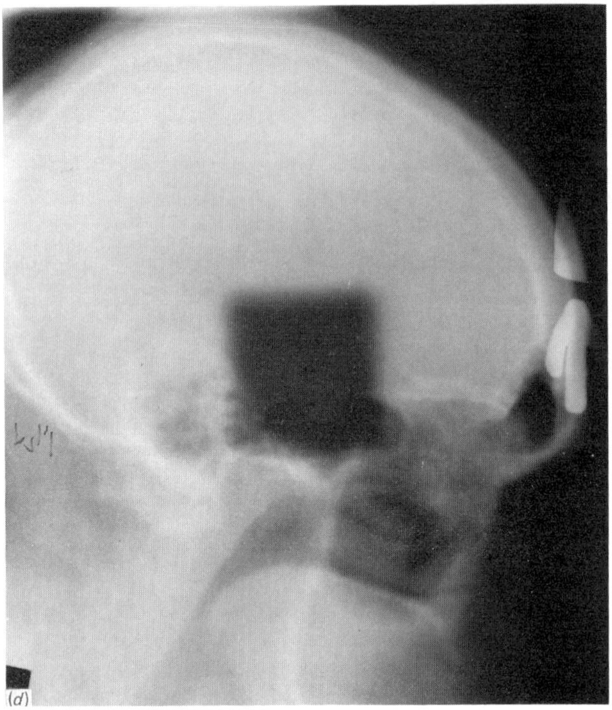

(d)

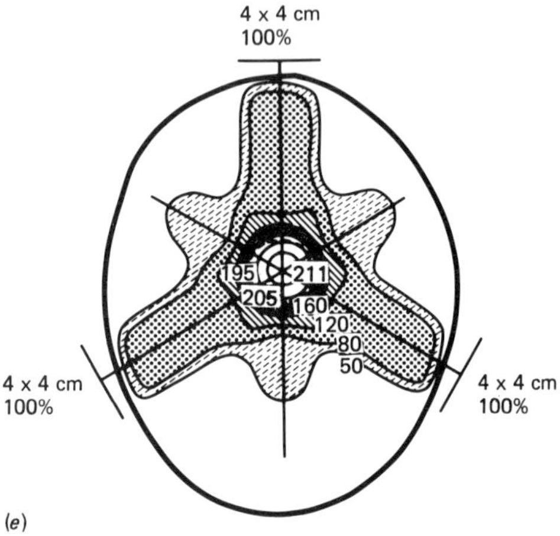

(e)

Figure 15.28 Pituitary tumour. (*d*) Confirmation film taken on 8 MeV linear accelerator. (*e*) Isodose curves of three field technique 8 MeV. ▭ > 195; ▨ 160–195; ▧ 120–160; ░ 80–120; ░ 50–80; ▭ <50

Chromophobe adenoma

This comprises about 50% of pituitary tumours, with bitemporal visual field defects being the commonest presenting symptom. Treatment is often with surgery in the first instance; by using an operating microscope with an ethmoidal or trans-sphenoidal approach, a histological diagnosis can be made and if there is rapidly failing vision this will give the quickest reduction of pressure on the chiasm. If there is no immediate urgency and the diagnosis is not in doubt, providing a CT scan is used to exclude suprasellar extension, radiation alone can be used as the tumours are relatively sensitive. The visual defects will rapidly respond to tumour doses of 4000–4500 cGy using the same simple technique as described above. Surgery might still be required if the vision does not improve within 6 weeks (Northfield, 1973), or if there is a subsequent rapid deterioration of vision. Chang and Pool (1967) reported visual improvement in 78% of cases receiving primary irradiation, but had an 11% tumour recurrence rate. If surgery is used initially then postoperative irradiation is certainly advisable, as complete excision is rare and recurrence very likely. The dose of irradiation would again be 4000–4500 cGy.

Prolactinoma

This tumour is commonly seen in young women who suffer from anovulatory infertility; prolactin-secreting pituitary tumours occur in one-third of hyperprolactinaemic patients presenting with amenorrhoea (Franks *et al.*, 1977). In a man the tumour may present with simple loss of libido. The diagnosis is usually made on clinical grounds and confirmed by finding raised levels of serum prolactin. There may be no gross radiological changes in the pituitary fossa, but a CT scan should be performed in order to be reasonably certain of the size of the tumour and the absence of suprasellar extension. The raised prolactin levels can usually be reduced by bromocriptine, and fertility improved, thus leading to pregnancy in due course, but unfortunately, owing to the stimulation by the high hormone levels in pregnancy, the tumour may start to enlarge again and produce pressure effects on the optic chiasm. For this reason, patients with this tumour who are taking bromocriptine should also receive pituitary irradiation (4000–4500 cGy in 20 daily fractions). If there are signs of suprasellar extension then surgery to remove the tumour should be performed in the first instance (Franks *et al.*, 1977).

Basophil adenoma

This comprises 10% of all pituitary tumours and may cause Cushing's syndrome, although this can also be due to primary adrenal adenomas. If the dexamethasone suppression test is positive then irradiation should be considered, even if the pituitary fossa is normal in size and the CT scan does not show definite tumour. This may be given by any of the methods previously described, or surgical hypophysectomy can be carried out. Richards, Thomas and Kilby (1974) reported an 80% response rate to 18 cases using the latter method, but the usual side-effects of transient CSF leaks, meningitis and diabetes insipidus were found. With external irradiation (4000–5000 cGy in 4–5 weeks), Orth and Liddle (1971) reported a 45% response rate in 51 cases. A recent report by Ahmed *et al.* (1984) suggests that the same good results can be achieved with a dose of 2000 cGy in 10 days if combined with metyrapone, thus reducing further any possible side-effects from irradiation.

Nelson syndrome

This occurs after bilateral adrenalectomy for Cushing's disease and is associated with an ACTH producing tumour of the pituitary gland. These lesions are usually aggressive, undergoing rapid expansion with compression and even invasion of supra- and parasellar structures. External irradiation can be used and would seem to be the treatment of choice, particularly if there is any spread of the tumour beyond the pituitary fossa, where the alternative method of a ^{90}Yt implant would not be feasible. The latter method, giving a tumour dose of 150 000 cGy to the whole of the gland, was described by Cassar *et al.* (1976) who claimed a 100% partial and 50% complete remission rate.

Malignant pituitary tumours

These are uncommon but are associated mainly with basophil adenomas and are only locally invasive. Occasionally even a chromophobe adenoma may show signs of malignancy with an increase of the mitochondrial elements and showing many cells with a large amount of mitoses — these have been called oncocytomas. Both types of tumours are probably best treated with radical surgery and postoperative irradiation, but if the former is not possible then irradiation alone, to a minimum dose of 4500 cGy in 4 weeks, should be given.

Spinal cord tumours

About 15% of all CNS tumours arise in the spinal cord and of the malignant tumours the gliomas are the most common.

Astrocytoma

This comprises about one-third of all the intraspinal tumours. The majority are well differentiated and therefore slow growing and are found more often in the upper rather than the lower end of the cord (*Figure 15.29*). Ideally, surgery is required both for diagnostic purposes and to remove as much of the tumour as possible. Irradiation will always be needed as complete surgical excision is rarely possible and some tumours are inoperable. Only the involved portion of the cord with a margin of 5 cm above and below needs to be treated. A wedge pair technique with the patient lying prone can be used (*Figure 15.30a*) to give a tumour dose of 4000 cGy in

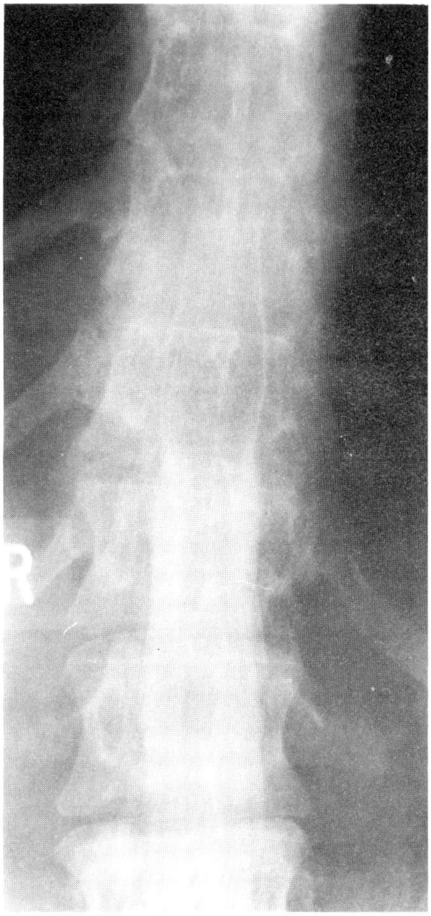

Figure 15.29 Myelogram astrocytoma spinal cord

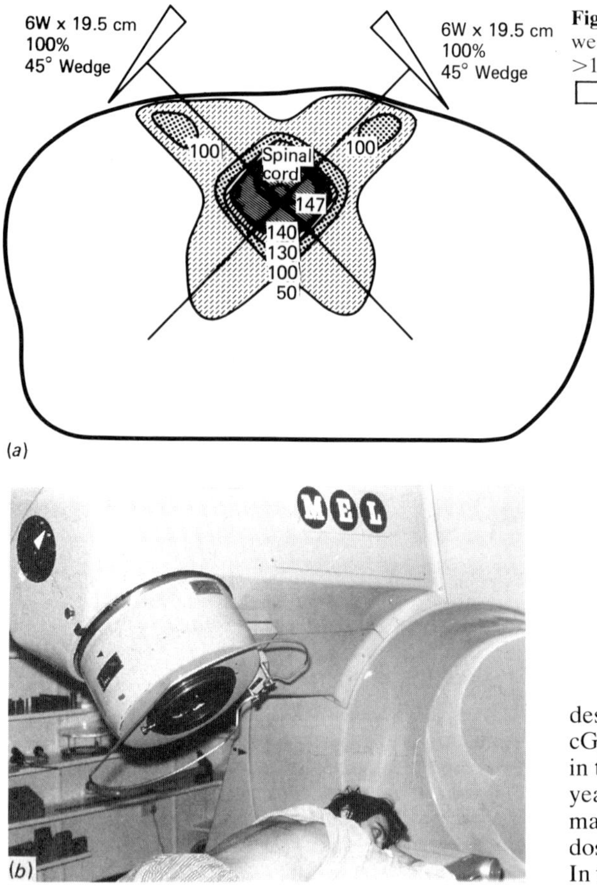

Figure 15.30 Astrocytoma. (*a*) Isodose curves to show field wedge technique for lower end of spinal cord 5 MeV. [hatched] >140; [hatched] 130–140; [stippled] 100–130; [stippled] 50–100; [blank] <50. (*b*) Patient lying prone in treatment position.

the cervical cord region and up to 4500 cGy lower down (*Figure 15.30b*). This is given in 20 daily fractions over 4 weeks. If tumour cells are spilt during the operation it may be necessary to consider treating the whole spinal cord as in ependymoma. Occasional multiple primary lesions occur (*Figure 15.31*) and the whole spinal cord will again need to be treated.

Ependymoma

This comprises about 60% of all spinal cord gliomas, the region of the cauda equina being the most commonly affected. Radical surgery is rarely possible as it would cause too much damage to the nerve roots leading to sphincter disturbance, impotence and paralysis of the lower limbs. Fortunately 90% of these tumours are well differentiated, and it would seem reasonable to treat only the known tumour volume with an adequate margin (at least 5 cm). A direct posterior megavoltage field is advocated by Peschel *et al.* (1983) unless the tumour is adjacent to the kidneys. These authors described eight patients who received 4500–5000 cGy in 4.5–5 weeks. There were no local recurrences in their series for periods ranging from 8 months to 8 years, and the acute and chronic morbidity was minimal. A wedge pair will give a more homogeneous dose and 4500 cGy in 4 weeks would seem adequate. In the rare malignant ependymoblastoma, consideration would need to be given to treating the whole CNS because of the danger of CSF seeding.

Chordoma

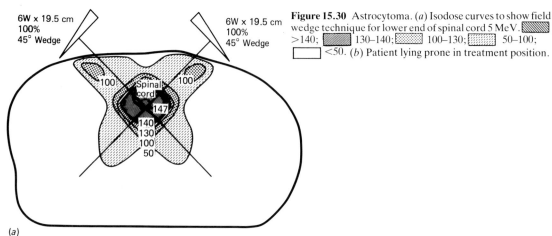

This is an uncommon malignant tumour occurring in middle-aged patients. It arises in notochordal tissues and is found most often in the base of the skull (clivus) in 33% of cases, the sacrococcygeal region in 50%, the rest being found in the remainder of the vertebral column. Ideally, radical surgical excision should be followed by irradiation as complete removal is rarely possible. Unfortunately, these tumours are not at all radiosensitive, but growth restraint may be obtained. Some authors recommend very high doses 6000–7000 cGy (Pearlman and Friedman, 1970). In 26 patients reviewed by Cummings, Hodson and Bush (1983) there was little evidence that doses greater than 5000 cGy produced any better local control than higher doses. However, four patients in their series were treated with hyperfractionation giving 100 cGy four times daily for 5 days and they all initially seemed to respond well. The present author would suggest that 4500 cGy in 20 daily fractions using one anterior and a pair of

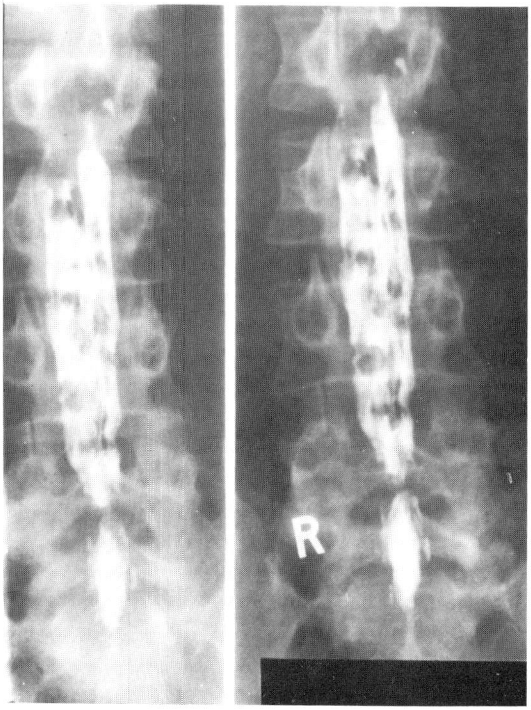

Figure 15.31 Myelogram to show multiple tumours in spinal cord astrocytoma

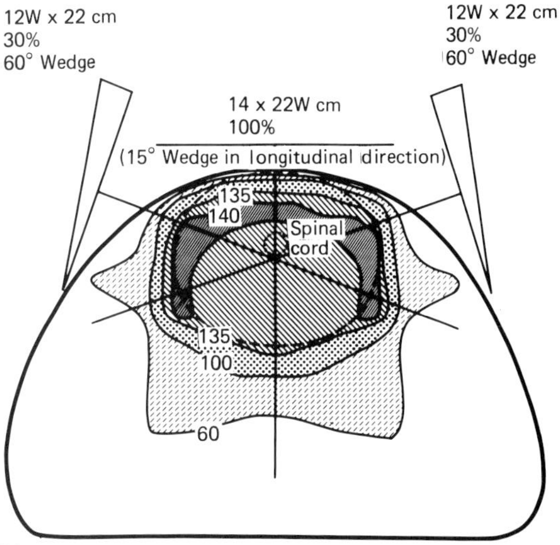

(*a*)

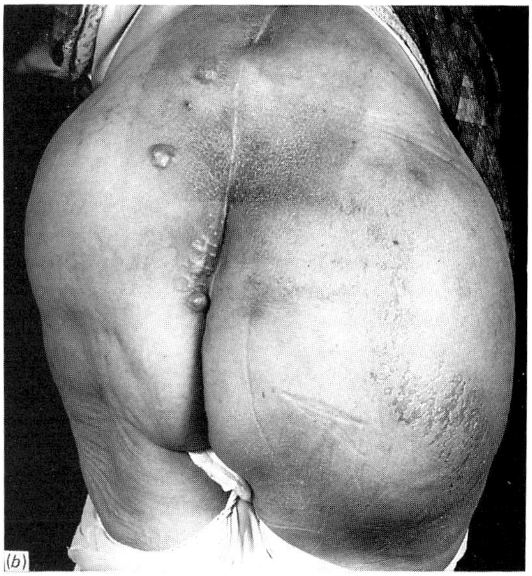

(*b*)

Figure 15.32 Chordoma. (*a*) Isodose curves of three field technique 8 MeV. [hatched] >140; [hatched] 135–140; [dotted] 100–135; [dotted] 60–100; [blank] <60. (*b*) Skin nodules after previous surgery and radiotherapy

oblique wedged fields (*Figure 15.32a*) would produce good growth restraint and a very low morbidity. Very high doses have been associated with quite marked pelvic soft tissue necrosis and bowel damage including fibrosis of the small bowel leading to intestinal obstruction (Saxton, 1981). Metastases may occur to bone or lymph nodes and, in one case at The London Hospital, occurred both in the cervical end of the spinal cord and in the skin of the buttock (*Figure 15.32b*); despite being a radioresistant tumour the skin lesions regressed at least temporarily with a dose of 3000 cGy in 2 weeks using a 300 kV orthovoltage machine.

Metastatic brain tumours

These make up 20% of all brain tumours (Russell and Rubenstein, 1977). The commonest primary site is the bronchus, closely followed by the breast and less often by the kidneys, colon, pancreas and melanoma. Metastasizing Hodgkin's disease is rare, being only 0.5% (of 2185 cases) in the Stanford series (Sapoznik and Kaplan, 1983). If the lesion can be shown to be solitary and there are no other metastases present, then surgical excision should be considered. Metastases from the kidney are the most likely to present in this way. If surgery is not contemplated then radical irradiation could be considered using a pair of wedged fields to give 4500 cGy in 4 weeks.

The majority of lesions are multiple, but in lung and breast primaries, even if apparently solitary, they should be considered to have other occult brain lesions and whole brain irradiation should be given. The easiest and often the quickest way to relieve symptoms is with corticosteroids. Dexamethasone 4 mg four times daily should be commenced immediately with concurrent alkalies or even cimetidine if there is any previous history of dyspepsia. In breast cancer the steroids may also act as part of normal hormone therapy and if there is a good response other methods of treatment may not be required; if there is no response whole brain irradiation should always be given as the prognosis from this primary site is better than most. A pair of parallel and opposed fields is used to treat the whole brain including the meninges (*Figure 15.33a*); if in doubt a simulator or verification film can be taken (*Figure 15.33b*). A cobex shell is not required. A total of 3000 cGy in 10 daily fractions gives as good a response as higher doses over a longer period of time (*see* Chapter 4).

The rare metastases from testicular tumours and the multiple metastases from the kidney can be treated in the same way. Metastases from Hodgkin's disease are probably worth treating to a higher dose. Sapoznik and Kaplan (1983) advocate 2000–3000 cGy to the whole brain with a boost to the site of the tumour of 2000–3000 cGy, the total time being 4–5 weeks. In five of their 12 reported cases survival was prolonged for 2–5 years.

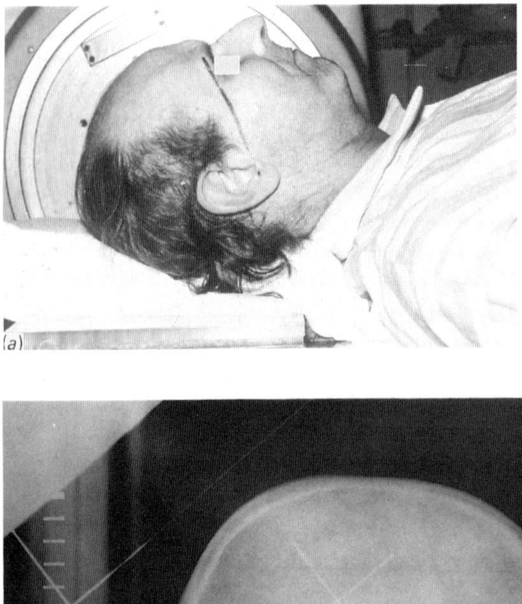

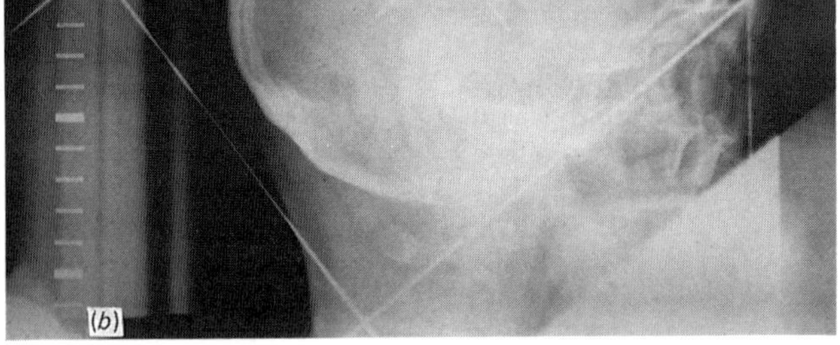

Figure 15.33 Whole brain irradiation. (*a*) Opposed fields; (*b*) Simulator verification field

Mestastases from other primary sites have an extremely poor prognosis and it is doubtful whether irradiation should be used at all. In carcinoma of the lung, Deeley and Edwards (1968) reported a 50% response rate but this lasted only 1 month. The only real indication for palliative irradiation in this group of patients is for relief of headache, nausea and vomiting not responding to steroids and symptomatic treatment. Such patients might be best treated with a single dose of 800 cGy using the same technique as above but continuing steroids and with appropriate antiemetics. The patient will not be upset by this treatment and can be discharged the next day if fit enough (Hope-Stone, 1976).

Spinal cord metastases

These most commonly occur as extradural tumours, from primary tumours in the breast, lung, kidney and prostate as well as from lymphomas and testicular neoplasms. Direct bone involvement will of course produce a similar neurological picture of spinal cord compression, as do soft tissue masses extending from the posterior thoracic or abdominal walls. Urgent treatment is required and any patient presenting with impending paraplegia should be accepted as an emergency. Admission to hospital with both neurosurgical and radiotherapy facilities is required as treatment must be started within 24 hours to prevent permanent paraplegia. A myelogram is obtained and laminectomy performed if a block is found at one level only. Surgery is also desirable to obtain a histological diagnosis if there is no known primary lesion. Occasionally the wrong clinical diagnosis is made, and instead of finding neoplasm, a tuberculous lesion may be discovered.

After laminectomy, as it is never possible to remove all the tumour (particularly from the anterior portion of the cord), postoperative irradiation must be given. A single direct posterior megavoltage field should be started the moment the stitches are removed and an incident dose of 3000 cGy (2500 tumour dose) is given in 10 daily fractions.

If the tumour is known to be radiosensitive, such as a small (oat) cell carcinoma of the lung, lymphoma or a testicular neoplasm, irradiation alone (to the same dose) may be used. This may also be used if the myelogram shows the presence of multiple lesions throughout the spinal cord (*see* Chapter 4).

Carcinomatosis meningitis

Leptomeningeal involvement is not uncommon from a primary tumour in the lung, stomach or breast. Diagnosis is made by identifying malignant cells in the CSF in a patient presenting with vague signs of headaches, cranial nerve palsies or changes in the mental state (with cerebral involvement), back pain, paraparesis and sphincter disturbances (with spinal involvement). Treatment should be considered as in 40% of cases this may be the only sign of spread of the tumour beyond the regional lymph nodes (Jones and Currie, 1982). Whole CNS irradiation using a simple technique with a series of matching direct megavoltage fields to the spinal cord and opposed lateral fields to the brain can be combined with intrathecal methotrexate (15 mg every 3–4 weeks). This drug must be used with care, leukoencephalopathy may occur and may be fatal.

New methods of treatment

Radiosensitizers

This is discussed in detail in Chapter 2. Hyperbaric oxygen combined with irradiation was tried in a pilot study by Chang (1977). There was no significant difference in survival between 38 patients so treated compared to 42 controls both receiving whole brain irradiation to doses between 3500 and 5000 cGy in 5 weeks.

Fast neutron irradiation was used in a control trial at the Hammersmith and the Royal Marsden Hospitals. A dose of 1560 cGy in 12 fractions over 26 days was compared with photon irradiation 5000–5500 cGy in 5–6 weeks. No survival improvement was shown. Demyelination took place in those brains treated with neutrons, so that although the tumour was destroyed, there was irreversible damage to the rest of the brain (Catterall *et al.*, 1980).

Chemical sensitizers

A hypoxic cell sensitizer would seem to be an excellent method to improve the radiosensitivity of brain tumours as it is easy to use in very ill patients and many of these tumours have a centrally necrotic area which must be poorly oxygenated. Unfortunately, the best available drug, mizonidazole, has not shown to be of any value in the recently reported trial in the UK (MRC, 1983). The most likely explanation is that because of the drug's toxicity which causes peripheral neuropathy, the dosage was markedly limited. New sensitizers will almost certainly be developed and may improve the response rate.

Combined chemotherapy and irradiation

Chemotherapy alone is a disappointing method of treating brain tumours (Hillebrand, 1979; Walker, Strike and Sheline, 1979), but adding chemotherapy to postoperative irradiation would seem worth trying. One controlled trial compared irradiation alone (5000 cGy in 5–6 weeks) with chemotherapy alone using CCNU (130 mg/m^2 repeated at 8-week intervals) and the third group received the combined treatment. Patients who received radiotherapy with or without chemotherapy had a significantly longer survival than those patients who had chemotherapy alone, but there was no difference in survival between the two irradiated groups (Reagan, Childs and Rhotan, 1976). In the UK, Garrett, Hughes and Ryall (1974) again showed no real improvement with CCNU and irradiation. The use of CCNU as an alternative again showed only a minimal improvement for the combined groups (Walker, Strike and Sheline, 1979).

One usefully effective combination is described by Athanussiou *et al.* (1983) in the management of CNS involved by chorion carcinoma. Systemic therapy and intrathecal methotrexate were combined with whole brain irradiation (3500–4500 cGy) and produced an 80% survival (1–20 years) in those patients primarily presenting with CNS involvement and a 25% survival in those who relapsed and had concurrent CNS involvement.

Radioactive implants

As the implantation of radioactive seeds has been shown to be a useful method of producing a very high localized dose of irradiation to the pituitary gland, it is not surprising that attempts have been made to use this technique at other sites. This had been technically impossible until the recent introduction of stereotactic methods to stimulate areas in the thalamus in Parkinson's disease, as well as to perform biopsies in hitherto inaccessible sites. It is now possible by a stereotactic afterloading technique to implant very small brain tumours with ^{125}I seeds. This isotope lends itself to this method as it has a relatively low energy (less than 35 kV X-rays) and low dose rate which means that it is not a serious radiation handling hazard for medical and nursing staff. Preliminary trials have been carried out (Gutin *et al.* 1981). Doses of the order of 3500–20 000 cGy were given either as permanent or removable implants. Other isotopes were used, particularly ^{192}Ir and ^{198}Au. The advantage of giving a very high dose is that there is some evidence that this will improve the overall survival but, in the past, the risk of giving such a dose has been the danger of producing brain necrosis (Walker, Strike and Sheline, 1979). A coaxial catheter system has now been devised to improve the accuracy of the implant (Gutin and Dormandy, 1982). At The London Hospital a modification of this method has been devised which will allow an afterloading technique to be used, but employing a reusable very highly active caesium source 3.5 mm long and 1.25 mm in diameter (Mantell, Klevenhagen and Afshar, 1986).

Conclusion

Except for the very radiosensitive neoplasms and pituitary lesions the treatment of brain tumours is not particularly rewarding. Nevertheless, it would seem to the present author that every case should be treated on its own merits. Hard and fast rules cannot be laid down for individual neoplasms, but the occasional excellent long-term results justify the great deal of time and effort required to treat most of these tumours.

References

ABBATUCCI, J. S., DELOZIER, T., QUINT, R., ROUSSEL, A. and BRUNE, D. (1978) Radiation myelopathy of the spinal cervical cord: time dose and volume factors. *International Journal of Radiation Oncology, Biology and Physics,* **4**, 234–248

AHLBOM, H. E. (1941) Results of radiotherapy of hypopharyngeal cancer at Radiumhemmet Stockholm 1930–1939. *Acta Radiology Stockholm* **22**, 155–171

AHMED, S. R., SHALET, S. M., BEARDWELL, C. G. and SUTTON, M. L. (1984) Treatment of Cushing's disease with low dose radiation therapy. *British Medical Journal,* **289**, 643–646

ALLBRIGHT, A., PRICE, R. and GUTHKELLA, A. (1983) Brain stem glioma of children. *Cancer,* **52**, 2313–2319

ANDREWS, D. S. and KERR, I. F. (1965) Carcinoma of the thyroid following irradiation for medulloblastoma. *Clinical Radiology,* **15**, 282–283

ATHANUSSIOU, A., REGENT, R. H., NEWLANDS, E. S., PARKER, D., RUSTIN, G. and BAGSHAWE, K. (1983) CNS metastases of chorion carcinoma. *Cancer,* **52**, 1728–1735

BLOOM, H. J. G. (1983) Results of SIOP trial in medulloblastoma. In *Proceedings of Vienna International Conference on Chemotherapy.* Annual Report

BODEN, G. (1948) Radiation myelitis of the cervical spinal cord. *British Journal of Radiology,* **21**, 464–469

BODEN, G. (1950) Radiation myelitis of the brain stem. *Journal of the Faculty of Radiologists,* **2**, 79–94

BOTTRILL, D. O., ROGERS, R. T. and HOPE-STONE, H. F. (1965) A composite filter technique and special patient jig for the treatment of the whole brain and spinal cord. *British Journal of Radiology,* **38**, 122–130

BULLIMORE, J. A. and MOTT, M. G. (1982) Paediatric Cancer. In *Treatment of Cancer*, edited by K. Halnan, pp. 743–768. London: Chapman and Hall

CALVO, F. A., HORNEDO, J., ABELLANO, R. *et al.* (1983) Radiation therapy in craniopharyngiomas. *International Journal of Radiation Oncology, Biology and Physics,* **9**, 493–496

CASSAR, J., DOYLE, F. H., LEWIS, P. D., MASHITER, K., VAN NOORDEN, S. and JOPLIN, G. F. (1976) Treatment of Nelson's syndrome by pituitary implantation of yttrium-90 or gold-198. *British Medical Journal,* **2**, 269–272

CATTERALL, M., BLOOM, H. J. G., ASH, D. V. *et al.* (1980) Fast neutrons compared with megavoltage X-rays in the treatment of patients with supratentorial glioma: a controlled pilot study. *International Journal of Radiation Oncology, Biology and Physics,* **6**, 261–266

CHANG, C. H. (1977) Hyperbaric oxygen and radiation therapy in the management of glioblastoma. In *Modern Concepts in Brain Tumour Therapy.* National Cancer Institute: Monograph no. 46

CHANG, C. H. and POOL, J. L. (1967) The radiotherapy of pituitary chromophobe adenomas. *Radiology,* **89**, 1005–1016

CHEEK, W. R. and TAVERAS, J. M. (1966) Thalamic tumours. *Journal of Neurosurgery,* **24**, 502–513

CLINTORIAN, A. M., SCHWARTZ, J. F., EVANS, R. A. and CASTOR, S. T. (1964) Optic gliomas in children. *Neurology,* **14**, 83–87

CUMMINGS, B. J., HODSON, B. M. and BUSH, R. (1983) Chordoma — the results of megavoltage radiation therapy. *International Journal of Radiation Oncology, Biology and Physics,* **9**, 633–642

DEELEY, J. and EDWARDS, R. (1968) Radiotherapy in the management of cerebral secondaries from bronchial carcinoma. *Lancet,* **1**, 1209–1212

FRANKS, S., JACOBS, H. S., HULL, M. G. R., STEELE, S. J. and NABARRO, J. D. (1977) Management of hyperprolactinaemia – amenorrhoea. *British Journal of Obstetrics and Gynaecology,* **84**, 241–253

FREEMAN, C., BERG, J. W. and CUTLER, S. J. (1972) Occurrence and prognosis of extra nodular lymphoma. *Cancer,* **29**, 252–260

FREEMAN, J. F., JOHNSTONE, P. G. B. and VOKE, J. M. (1972) Somnolence after prophylactic cranial irradiation in children with acute lymphoblastic leukaemia. *British Medical Journal,* **4**, 523–525

FRIEDMAN, N. B. (1947) Germinoma of the pineal — its identity with germinoma (seminoma) of the testes. *Cancer Results,* **7**, 363–368

GARRETT, M. J., HUGHES, H. J. and RYALL, R. D. N. (1974) CCNU in brain tumours. *Clinical Radiology,* **25**, 183–184

GONZALEZ, W. and SHUSTER, L. J. (1983) Primary non Hodgkins lymphoma of the CNS. *Cancer*, **51**, 2048–2052

GUTIN, P. and DORMANDY, R. (1982) A coaxial catheter system for after loading radioactive sources for the interstitial irradiation of brain tumours. *Journal of Neurosurgery*, **56**, 734–735

GUTIN, P., PHILIPS, T., HOSOBUCHI, Y. *et al.* (1981) Permanent and removeable implants for the brachytherapy of brain tumours. *International Journal of Radiation Oncology, Biology and Physics*, **7**, 1371–1381

HARDY, D. J., HOPE-STONE, H. F., McKENZIE, L. G. and SCHULTZ, C. (1978) Recurrence of medulloblastoma after homogeneous field radiotherapy. *Journal of Neurosurgery*, **49**, 434–440

HARROP, J. S., DAVIES, T. J., CAPRA, L. *et al.* (1976) Hypothalamic and pituitary function following successful treatment of intracranial tumours. *Clinical Endocrinology*, **5**, 313–321

HILLEBRAND, J. (1979) The results of the EORTC brain tumour group. In *Multidisciplinary Aspects of Brain Tumour Therapy*, edited by P. Paoletti, M. W. Walter, G. Butti and D. Knerick, pp. 235–243. Amsterdam: Elsevier/N. Holland

HOPE-STONE, H. F. (1970) Results of the treatment of medulloblastoma. *Journal of Neurosurgery*, **32**, 83–88

HOPE-STONE, H. F. (1976) Malignant disease of the nervous system. In *Radiotherapy in Modern Clinical Practice*, edited by H. F. Hope-Stone, pp. 71–107. London: Crosby, Lockwood and Staples

HOPE-STONE, H. F. (1980) Clinical application of the RT 305. *Medica Mundi*, **25**, 113–117

HOPE-STONE, H. F. (1984) Cobalt-60 teletherapy. *An International Compendium* compiled by M. Cohen and J. Mitchell. WHO and International Atomic Agency Vienna IAEA

JOFFE, S. N. (1982) Apudomas, pituitary and other endocrine tumours. In *Treatment of Cancer*, edited by K. Halnan, pp. 347–370. London: Chapman and Hall

JONES, A. (1964) Transient radiation myelopathy. *British Journal of Radiology*, **37**, 727–744

JONES, A. and CURRIE, J. (1982) Central nervous system. In *Treatment of Cancer*. edited by K. Halnan, pp. 223–248. London: Chapman and Hall

JOPLIN, G. F. (1975) The effect of ^{90}Yt implantation on endocrine functions and visual fields with functionless pituitary tumours with biopsy and radiological findings. *Clinical Endocrinology*, **4**, 139–163

KJELLBERG, R. and KLIMAN, B. (1974) Bragg Peak proton treatment for pituitary related conditions. *Proceedings of the Royal Society of Medicine*, **67**, 32–33

KRAMER, S. (1973) Radiation therapy in management of malignant gliomas. In *7th National Cancer Conference Proceedings*. pp. 823–826. Philadelphia: Lippincott

KRAMER, S., McKISSOCK, W. and CONCANNON, J. (1961) Craniopharyngioma treatment by combined surgery and radiation therapy. *Journal of Neurosurgery*, **18**, 217–226

KRAMER, S., SOUTHARD, M. and MANSFIELD, G. (1972) Radiation effects and tolerance of the central nervous system. In *Frontiers of Radiation Therapy and Oncology*, **6** pp. 332–343. Basel: Karger and Baltimore: University Park Press

LINDGREN, M. (1958) On tolerance of brain tissue and sensitivity of brain tumours to irradiation. *ACTA Radiology Supplement*, no. 170

MAIER, J. G., PENNY, R., SAYLON and SULAK, M. (1964) Radiation myelitis of the dorso-lumbar spinal cord. *Radiology*, **93**, 153–160

MANTELL, B. S., KLEVENHAGEN, S. C. and AFSHAR, F. (1986). An afterloaded applicator for the interstitial irradiation of brain tumours. *Clinical Radiology*, **37**, 35–36

MOSS, W. T., (1959) *Therapeutic Radiology — Rationale, Technique, Results*, 2nd edn., p. 402. St Louis: C.V. Mosby Co.

MRC (1983) A study of the effect of misonidazole in conjunction with radiotherapy for the treatment of grades 3 and 4 astrocytoma. *British Journal of Radiology*, **56**, 673–682

NORTHFIELD, D. W. C. (1973) *The Surgery of the Central Nervous System*. Oxford: Blackwell Scientific Publications

ONOYAMA, Y., ONO, K., YAMBUTU, F. and TAKEUCHI, J. (1977) Radiation therapy of craniopharyngioma. *Radiology*, **125**, 799–803

ORTH, D. R. and LIDDLE, G. U. (1971) Results of treatment in 108 patients with Cushing's syndrome. *New England Journal of Medicine*, **285**, 244–247

PEARLMAN, R. W. and FRIEDMAN, M. (1970) Radical radiation therapy of chordoma. *American Journal of Roentgenology*, **108**, 333–341

PESCHEL, R. E., KAPP, D. S., CARDINALE, F. and MANUELOIS, F. (1983) Ependymomas of the spinal cord. *International Journal of Radiation Oncology, Biology and Physics*, **9**, 1043–1046

REAGAN, J., CHILDS, D. S. and RHOTAN, A. L. (1976) Controlled study of CCNU and radioactive therapy in malignant astrocytoma. *Journal of Neurosurgery*, **44**, 186–190

RICHARDS, S., THOMAS, J. F. and KILBY, D. (1974) Transethmoidal hypophysectomy for pituitary tumour. *Proceedings of the Royal Society of Medicine*, **67**, 889–892

RIDER, W. D. (1963) Radioactive damage to the brain — a new syndrome. *Journal of the Canadian Association of Radiologists*, **14**, 67–69

RUSSELL, D. S. (1944) The pinealoma — its relationship to teratoma. *Journal of Pathology and Bacteriology*, **56**, 145–150

RUSSELL, D. S. and RUBENSTEIN, L. J. (1977) Pathology of tumours of the nervous system, 4th edn. p. 283. London: Edward Arnold

SAGERMAN, R., COLLIER, H. and KING, G. (1983) Radiation therapy of microglioma. *Radiology*, **149**, 567–570

SALALZAR, O. M., RABIN, P. and McDONALD, J. Y. (1976) High dose radiation therapy in the treatment of glioblastoma multiforms: a preliminary report. *International Journal of Radiation Oncology, Biology and Physics*, **1**, 717–727

SAXTON, J. P. (1981) Chordoma. *International Journal of Radiation Oncology, Biology and Physics*, **7**, 913–915

SHALET, S. M. (1982) Hormonal problems in patients treated for cancer. *Hospital Update*, April, 409–420

SHALET, S. M., and BEARDWELL, C. G. (1979) Hypothalamic pituitary function following cranial irradiation. In *CNS Complications of Malignant Disease*, edited by J. M. N. Whitehouse, H. E. M. Kay, pp. 202–217. London: McMillan Press Ltd

SHALET, S. M., BEARDWELL, C. G., MORRIS JONES, P. N. and PEARSONS, D. (1975) Pituitary function after treatment of intracranial tumours in children. *Lancet*, **2**, 104

SHALET, S. M., WHITEHEAD, E., CHAPMAN, A. J. and BEARDWELL, C. G. (1981) The effects of growth hormone therapy in children with radiation induced growth hormone deficiency. *Acta Paediatrica Scandinavica,* **70**, 81–86

SHARMAN, U., TANDOM, P. N., SAXENA, K., SINGHAL, N. M. and BARDAN, J. (1974) Craniopharyngioma treated by a combination of surgery and radiotherapy. *Clinical Radiology,* **25**, 13–17

SHELINE, G. E. (1975) Radiation therapy of tumours of the central nervous system in childhood. *Cancer,* **35**, 957–960

SHELINE, G. E. (1976) The importance of distinguishing tumour grades in malignant gliomas — treatment and prognosis. *International Journal of Radiation Oncology, Biology and Physics,* **1**, 781–786

SHELINE, G. E. (1977) Radiation therapy of brain tumours. *Cancer,* **39**, 873–881

SMITH, R. A., LAMPE, I. and KAHN, E. A. (1961) The prognosis of medulloblastoma in children. *Journal of Neurosurgery,* **18**, 91–97

STOLL, B. A. and ANDREWS, J. J. (1966) Radiation induced peripheral neuropathy. *British Medical Journal,* **1**, 834–837

SUNG, D. H., HARISIADIS, L. and CHANG, C. H. (1978) Midline pineal tumours and suprasella disgerminomas highly curable by irradiation. *Radiology,* **128**, 749

VYRAMUTHU, N. and BENTON, T. F. (1983) The management of craniopharyngiomas. *Clinical Radiology,* **34**, 624–633

WALKER, M. D., STRIKE, T. A. and SHELINE, G. E. (1979) An analysis of dose affecting relationship in the radiotherapy of malignant glioma. *International Journal of Radiation Oncology, Biology and Physics,* **5**, 1725–1730

WARA, W. M., JENKIN, D., EVANS, A. *et al.* (1979) Tumours of the pineal and suprasellar region — children's cancer study group — treatment results 1960–1975. *Cancer,* **43**, 698–701

WARA, W. M., SHELINE, G. E., NEWMAN, H., TOWNSEND, J. and BODDREY, E. (1975) Radiation therapy of meningiomas. *American Journal of Roentgenology,* **123**, 453–458

WILLIAMS, R. A. (1974) Hypophysectomy for pituitary tumours. *Proceedings of the Royal Society of Medicine,* **67**, 881–884

16

Interstitial therapy

D. Ash

Introduction

Soon after the discovery of radium by Marie Curie in 1898 it was recognized that it might have a role in cancer treatment by virtue of the fact that it could be implanted into the heart of a tumour. The first radium implant was reported in 1905, but it took several years before the development of safe and standardized radium needles allowed this treatment to become generally applicable. By the 1930s the Paterson/Parker rules of implantation and of dosimetry had been developed and allowed effective implants to be widely applied as they are to this day.

From the late 1950s onwards, however, the indications for radium implants fell as megavoltage machinery made it possible to deliver doses at depth more safely, and the need for radiation protection became more widely appreciated. Fortunately, at the same time the discovery and manufacture of artificial radioactive isotopes opened the way to the development of afterloading implant systems which can be used with minimal radiation exposure, and these are being increasingly adopted to preserve the unique advantages of interstitial therapy.

It must be admitted that no clinical trials have been performed to confirm the superiority of implantation over fractionated external beam radiation, although clinical experience over the last 50 years very strongly suggests it. The major practical and theoretical advantages are:

(1) Localized high dose with rapid fall-off
(2) Inhomogeneous dose with very high dose around each radiation source
(3) Low and continuous dose rate
(4) Short overall treatment time.

The first is probably the most important and often allows the tumour to receive a higher dose of radiation than would be tolerated by the larger volume of tissue which would have to be included in external beam radiation fields. The rapid fall-off of dose also allows relative sparing of adjacent critical normal tissue. Data on the value of low dose rate and short treatment times are derived from animal and *in vitro* experiments and have been difficult to confirm clinically.

General indications and contraindications

Specific indications for different tumour types and sites are discussed later but in general implants may be used in three main ways.

(1) Primary radical treatment

Small well localized tumours where the risk of adjacent lymph node spread is negligible may be treated to a radical dose with an implant which usually encompasses the tumour plus a 1 cm margin around it.

(2) Implant boost after previous external beam radiation

In cases where the tumour is fairly large and where there is a substantial risk of involvement of adjacent lymph node areas it is often best to give external beam radiation first and to deliver a dose which is sufficient to sterilize subclinical disease in nodes. The primary tumour can then be boosted by an implant which raises the dose to a curative level. Occasionally it may be necessary to perform the implant first and to follow it with external beam radiation, but in general, it is probably better to gain some regression with external beam radiation first.

(3) Perioperative implant

In a number of situations it is often helpful to combine local excision of a primary or recurrent tumour with a perioperative implant which positions the radioactive sources under direct vision at the site where recurrence is thought to be most likely.

Contraindications to implantation

Not all apparently localized tumours are suitable for implantation and it is sometimes best to rely on other treatment methods.

Target volume not identifiable

Because the dose falls off so rapidly around an implant there is a considerable risk of missing parts of the tumour unless the target volume can be accurately identified. If, therefore, the tumour margins are indistinct it may be better, at least initially, to treat with external beam radiation.

Tumour very extensive or with bone involvement

The amount of radioactivity which has to be implanted to encompass large tumours is often so great that, even though technically feasible, it is poorly tolerated by the patient and results in a high risk of necrosis.

Patients with bone involvement are not suitable for implantation both because the chances of cure are minimal and because the chances of producing bone necrosis are high.

Tumour access difficult

It is evident that unless the tumour is accessible an implant cannot be performed. If there are doubts about whether a geometrically satisfactory implant can be performed it may be better to rely on other means of treatment, as the risks of underdose or overdose within the implant volume are likely to be high.

Isotopes for implantation

The physical characteristics and protection requirements for different isotopes are summarized in *Table 16.1*.

Radium - 226

Radium has been in use for many years and has the advantage not only of long and proven usage, but also that the Manchester system is widely understood and readily applicable for most cases. The long half-life means that a stock of needles is always available and running costs are relatively low.

The main disadvantages are that implantation requires the handling of live sources and it requires 12 cm of lead to provide adequate protection. The limited range and rigidity of sources may sometimes require the implantation of a large number of needles and these can be uncomfortable for the patient.

Because the implant is performed with live sources speed is important, and unless the operator is very skilled it may not always be possible to achieve optimum geometry of source distribution.

Caesium - 137

In many radiotherapy departments caesium needles have replaced radium and have similar advantages and disadvantages. The half-life of caesium is only 30 years however, and as stocks of caesium needles come to the end of their useful life they are being increasingly replaced by afterloading systems which reduce radiation exposure to staff.

Gold - 198

Gold grains are still widely used and have the advantage of easy and rapid introduction through a specially designed gold-grain gun. They may be useful for small superficial lesions where a single plane can be implanted according to Paterson/Parker rules but more difficult to use for volume implants. Because the implant is not removable dosimetry cannot be modified after the seeds have been implanted, and radiation safety precautions are necessary for a few days after implantation. With a half-life of 2.7 days, however, radiation rapidly falls to a safe level.

Iodine - 125

Iodine can be made into seeds which can either be implanted singly in a similar way to gold grains or can be encapsulated in an absorbable suture which can be stitched into position in the tumour. In both cases the implant is not removable. A special applicator has been designed to aid source placement (Scott, 1972) and a system of dosimetry devised which takes into account the average dimension of the target volume

Table 16.1 Physical characteristics of isotopes used for interstitial therapy

Isotope	*Half-life*	*Energy range (MeV)*	*Tenth value layer (cm Pb)*
Radium-226	1620 years	0.19–2.43	12
Caesium-137	30 years	0.66	6
Iridium-192	74 days	0.30–0.61	2
Californium-252	2.65 years	2.3 (neutrons)	15 cm paraffin wax
Gold-198	2.7 days	0.41–1.09	0.25
Iodine-125	60 days	0.027–0.035	0.025

and, with the aid of a spacing nomogram, calculates the dose and the number of sources required (Anderson, 1976). Because of the low dose rate, ^{125}I may be especially suitable for slow growing tumours and has been used perioperatively to implant tumours of the lung, pancreas and prostate. There have been no studies comparing ^{125}I implants with other forms of local treatment, but excellent local tumour control rates have been reported (Kim and Hilaris, 1974). In spite of this, ^{125}I implants are not widely used.

Iridium - 192

Iridium is manufactured in the form of malleable wire (0.3–0.5 mm diameter) with a platinum sheath. It therefore has the advantage of flexibility and can be cut to any length. Because the mean gamma energy is only 412 kV, compared with 2 MeV for radium, only 2 cm of lead are required to provide adequate protection, and this combined with an afterloading technique substantially reduces radiation exposure to operating theatre and nursing staff.

Implants are performed with inactive source carriers in the first instance and because there is no exposure to radiation at this stage sufficient time can be taken to achieve optimum source geometry. This therefore allows a better distribution of dose. The dosimetry is usually performed according to the Paris system which was devised by Professor Pierquin and his co-workers (Pierquin *et al.*, 1977).

There has not been a controlled comparison of implants performed with radium or iridium, but a retrospective study by Pierquin showed a local recurrence rate of 3% for ^{192}Ir compared with 32% using radium (Pierquin *et al.*, 1970). A local tumour control rate of 95% has been reported for tumours less than 4 cm in diameter in the tongue and floor of the mouth implanted with ^{192}Ir (Pierquin *et al.*, 1971).

The disadvantage of ^{192}Ir wire is that the half-life is only 74 days and each batch of wire can only be used once or twice at most. It is therefore necessary either to have a regular order to maintain a stock or to order separately for each implant. In practice this is rarely a problem as delivery of the wire can usually be ensured within 3–4 days. It is, however, necessary to have a shielded instrument for cutting the ^{192}Ir wire and encapsulating it into the plastic tubes used for afterloading.

Californium - 252

Californium is an artificial isotope which is of interest because it emits neutrons. It therefore has the theoretical advantage not only of being implantable into the hypoxic centre of a tumour, but it also emits high linear energy transfer (LET) radiation. Clinical studies have been performed using afterloading implant techniques similar to those for ^{192}Ir, but unfortunately, the theoretical advantages promised were not observed clinically and this combined with formidable radiation protection problems has led to the abandonment of this isotope (Paine *et al.*, 1979).

Implant techniques for iridium - 192

The techniques used for radium needle and gold grain implantation have been fully described previously in standard text books and are not discussed further (Paterson, 1963), although they are relatively easy to use providing one has sufficient experience.

Before starting any implant a certain amount of pre-planning is necessary to identify the target volume and to decide the number and distribution of source lines to be used. It is usual to mark out the volume and the position of the sources on the skin or mucosa before inserting the source carrying tubes.

Plastic tube technique

The inactive source carrier is plastic tubing 1.6 mm diameter which is afterloaded with ^{192}Ir wire encapsulated into thinner plastic tubing 1.0 mm diameter. The outer plastic tube is positioned in the tumour by first inserting hollow stainless steel needles which are placed in parallel lines which follow the planned volume. Once in position, the stainless steel needles are replaced by plastic tubing. This is commonly done by the technique described in *Figure 16.1*. The stainless steel needle is replaced by a nylon cord over which the plastic tube is threaded and clamped and then pulled through to lie under the skin. A nylon ball is passed over the end of each tube to prevent undue pressure on the skin and the tube secured by lead discs. If X-rays are necessary to determine the separation of the plastic tubes within the tissue, an inactive fuse wire is passed down each tube so that it becomes clearly visible on X-ray. There is no exposure to radiation up to this point and radiation protection measures are unnecessary. The active phase of loading the implant can be performed behind a protective lead screen and takes a very short time. The ^{192}Ir wire, encapsulated in 1.0 mm plastic tubing, is passed down the implanted plastic tubing and clamped into position by crushing the lead disc at each end of the tube. Care should be taken to keep the entire length of active wire under the skin as there may otherwise be a hot spot at the point where the active wire passes through. The plastic tube technique is most commonly used for tumours on the skin and in the breast.

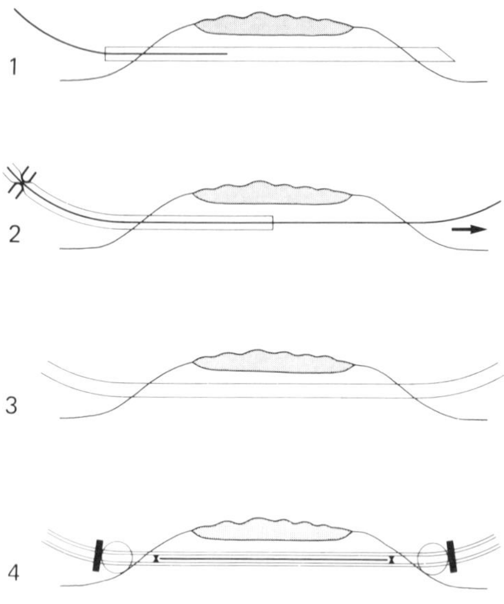

Figure 16.1 Steps in performing an afterloading plastic tube implant. (1) Stainless steel guide needle inserted and nylon cord passed down needle. (2) Guide needle removed and outer plastic tubing passed over nylon cord and clamped. (3) Plastic tube in position ready for afterloading. (4) Plastic tube afterloaded with ^{192}Ir wire encapsulated within inner tubing. Nylon ball and lead discs placed to fix implant in position

Plastic tube loop technique

For moderately large tumours of the tongue or floor of the mouth it is sometimes necessary to encompass the lesion by passing a series of loops of radioactive wire over it. The inactive phase consists of forming a loop of plastic tubing into which the active wire is afterloaded. A pair of stainless steel needles are first pushed up into the mouth from the skin below and are positioned to lie on each side of the lesion; a nylon cord is then passed up one needle and down the other to form a loop. The needles are withdrawn and plastic tubing threaded over the nylon cord and clamped at one end. The plastic tube is then pulled round into the mouth by the nylon cord to reform the loop. Three or four loops may be constructed in this way to cover the target volume (*Figure 16.2*).

Fuse wire is passed up each loop for the check radiograph and the active wire is then afterloaded into the tube and secured with nylon balls and lead discs.

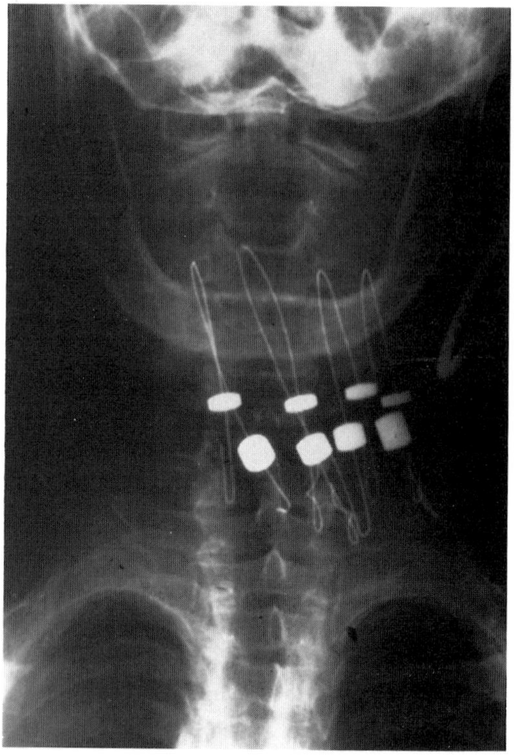

Figure 16.2 Plastic tube loop technique. Radiograph of loops in floor of mouth with fuse wire showing position of loops before loading

Hairpin technique

For smaller lesions in the mouth, ^{192}Ir wire is implanted in the form of hairpins made of 0.5 mm diameter wire rather than the thinner 0.3 mm wire used for the plastic tube technique. The inactive phase is accomplished by inserting stainless steel slotted hairpin guides (*Figure 16.3a*) which can be accurately positioned with the aid of an image intensifier or check X-rays. Once position and parallelism is assured a suture is passed under the cross piece of each guide. The implant is loaded by pushing the active hairpin (*Figure 16.3b*) down the guide and then withdrawing the guide needle while the bridge of the hairpin is held down. The suture is then tied over the bridge of the hairpin to secure the active wire in the mouth. On completion of the implant orthogonal check radiographs are taken for dosimetry (*see Figure 16.3*).

The hairpin technique can be used in the tongue, floor of the mouth and cheek, and may also have a place in the management of some rectal and gynaecological cancers. The volumes which can be implanted by this technique are restricted because of the fixed 1.2 cm separation of the limbs of the hairpins. For larger lesions the plastic tube technique may be preferable.

Template technique

It is sometimes difficult to maintain the parallelism of sources in an implant particularly where there is more than one plane. This problem may be overcome by using a rigid needle technique where the needles themselves act as the inactive source carriers and are maintained strictly in position by a plastic template. The needles are then afterloaded with the active iridium wire. Dose rate measurements have shown that the shielding effect of the stainless steel guide needles is negligible and accounts for a dose reduction of only 2–3%. Where the tissues will tolerate rigid needles a template technique will ensure accurate source geometry with consequent homogeneous irradiation. It also eases the dosimetry as source distances can be measured directly from the template. Templates are frequently used for cancers of the lip and breast (*Figures 16.4 and 16.5*).

Plastic tube miniature technique

For implants around the face, the implantation of 1.6 mm plastic tubes for afterloading may produce undue tissue trauma. For these sites a miniaturization of the technique has been developed. After measuring the target volume appropriate lengths of ^{192}Ir are encapsulated in 1.0 mm diameter thin plastic tubing. The active ends are kept in a shielded container leaving a long inactive end. A nylon or prolene suture is slipped into the inactive end of the plastic tubing for a distance of 8–10 cm and then clamped. The free end of the suture may then be threaded into a long straight needle which is used to pass the nylon thread into the tissue. Several parallel threads may be inserted before loading the implant by pulling the plastic tubing through under the skin and then positioning the active wire to lie within the target volume.

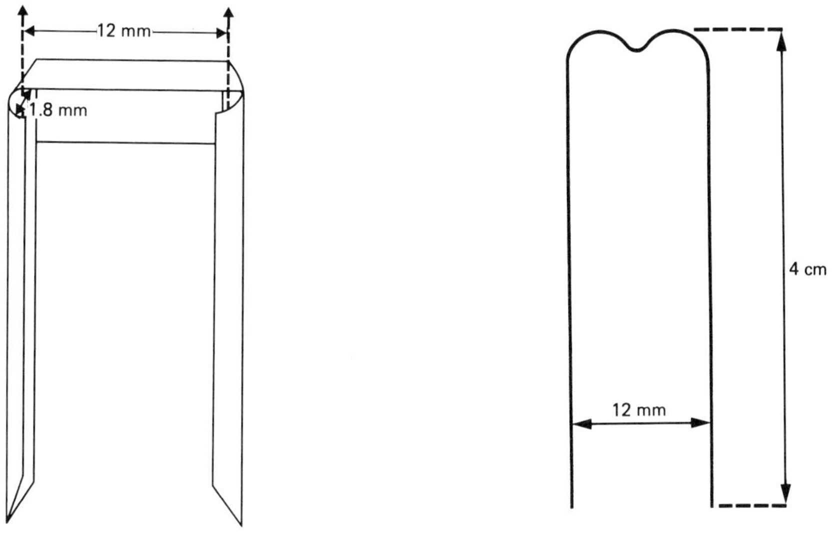

(*a*) (*b*)

Figure 16.3 (*a*) Stainless steel hairpin guide; (*b*) ^{192}Ir hairpin

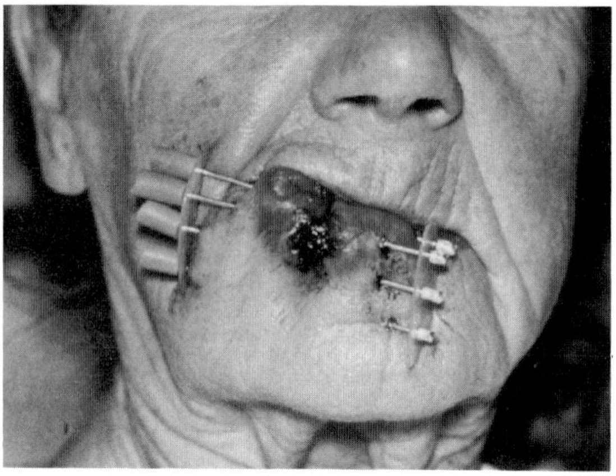

Figure 16.4 Lip implant with templates

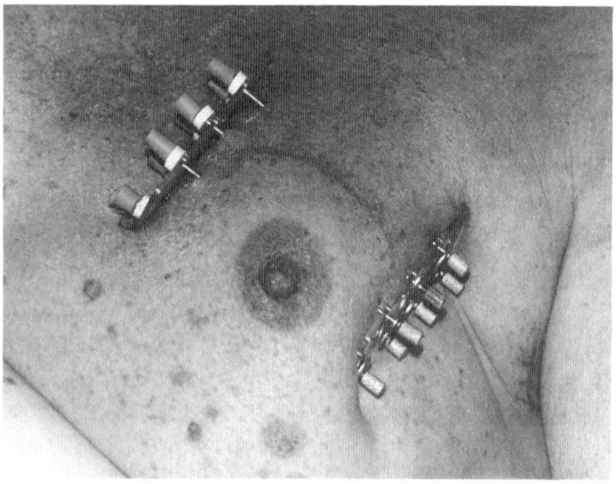

Figure 16.5 Breast implant with template

Moulds

Iridium - 192 can be used to load surface moulds in the same way as radium needles and gold grains have been used. These may be useful for lesions of the ear (*see* Chapter 12), scalp, dorsum of hand, or penis (*see* Chapter 3).

Dosimetry

The dosimetry of interstitial therapy is dominated by the inverse square law, and consequently lies in achieving a compromise between very high doses near each source which may result in necrosis and low doses at the margins of the target volume which may allow recurrence. All dosimetry systems therefore consists of two parts. First, the rules of implantation which ensure that radiation sources are distributed evenly throughout the target volume and second, a method for calculating the time for which the sources should remain in place to deliver the desired dose. In the Paterson/Parker system as originally described, the rules of implantation for radium needles were devised to ensure that a uniform dose with not more than ± 10% variation is received at a distance from the line of the sources which is usually specified as 0.5 cm. Once the form and radium content of the implant is known the time to deliver 1000 cGy can be looked up in a precalculated dose table and the time for the prescribed dose calculated. The methods and dosimetry are described in detail elsewhere (Meredith, 1967).

When long flexible lengths of ^{192}Ir became available for implant therapy it was evident that some implants could be performed more simply than dictated by the Paterson/Parker rules, and a new set of rules and dosimetry system was devised to take advantage of this. This has been called the Paris system (Pierquin *et al.*, 1978). The main departures from the Paterson/Parker system are that the dosimetry is based on the spatial distribution of sources actually achieved rather than an assumed ideal, and the dosimetry is calculated from the dose distribution in a plane in the centre of the implant rather than based on a plane outside the sources, which defines the treated volume. The distribution rules also differ, and unlike the Paterson/Parker rules the separation recommended for ^{192}Ir wires may vary with the length and number of sources implanted and it is not usual to cross the ends of the wires.

Distribution rules for iridium - 192 implants

(1) Active sources should be parallel and straight
(2) The lines should be equidistant
(3) The line or plane on which the midpoint of the sources lie (central plane) should be at right angles to the axis of the sources
(4) The linear activity of the lines should be uniform along the length of each line and identical for all lines
(5) The separation of sources may be varied from one implant to another. A minimum of 5 mm separation is acceptable for the smallest volumes rising to 20 mm for the largest
(6) For volume implants the distribution of sources in cross-section (central plane) should be either in equilateral triangles or squares
(7) Because it is not usual to cross the ends of the sources the overall length of active wire must be longer than the target volume by 25 – 30% depending on the number and separation of sources used.

It is necessary to define a number of terms used in the Paris system which will help to explain it.

Central plane

The plane at right angles to the axis of the midpoint of the sources. Dosimetry is based on the source geometry in this plane (*Figure 16.6*).

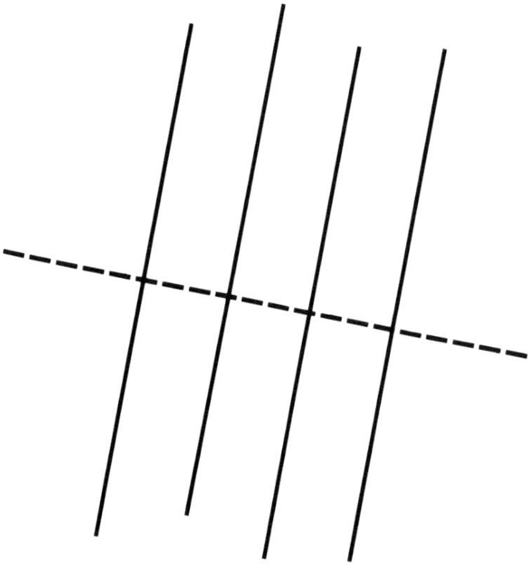

Figure 16.6 Central plane through an implant

Basal dose rate

The dose rate at a point in the middle of a pair or group of sources where the dose rate is lowest. In the case of a large implant there may be several pairs or groups of sources arranged in triangles or squares: for these a mean basal dose rate is taken for the implant as a whole (*see Figure 16.10*).

Reference dose rate

The reference dose rate is 85% of the basal dose rate. This serves to calculate the duration of the implant and the 85% isodose defines the treated volume.

Relation between source distribution and treated volume

Because the treated volume may vary with different source lengths and separations it is important to know the relationship between source distribution and volume so that adequate tumour coverage is ensured.

The length of the treated volume (l) is 70 – 80% of the length of the active sources (L) (*Figure 16.7*).

The thickness of the treated volume (t) is 50 – 60% of the separation between sources (T) (*Figure 16.8*).

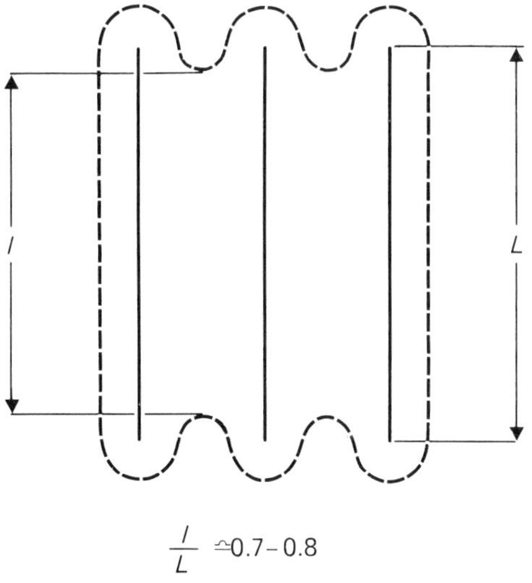

Figure 16.7 Relation between length of implanted sources (L) and length of treated volume (l)

The treatment margin around volume implants (m) is 30–40% of the separation between sources (M) (*Figure 16.9*).

Steps to be taken in dosimetry

Define the distribution of sources in the central plane

This may be done by direct measurement, by a tomogram taken through the central plane of the implant, or by geometric reconstruction of the central plane from orthogonal radiographs.

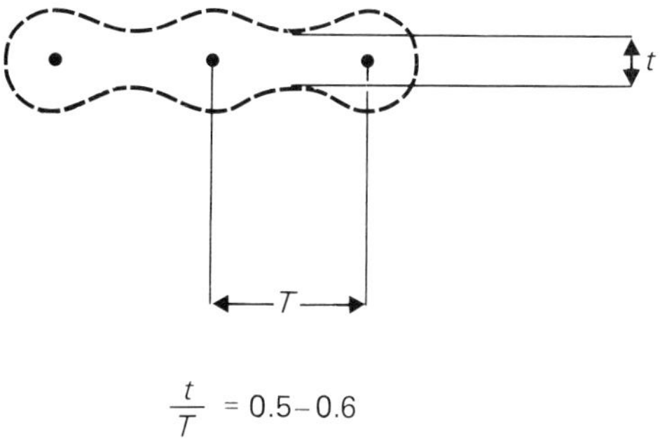

Figure 16.8 Relation between thickness of treated volume (t) and separation between sources (T)

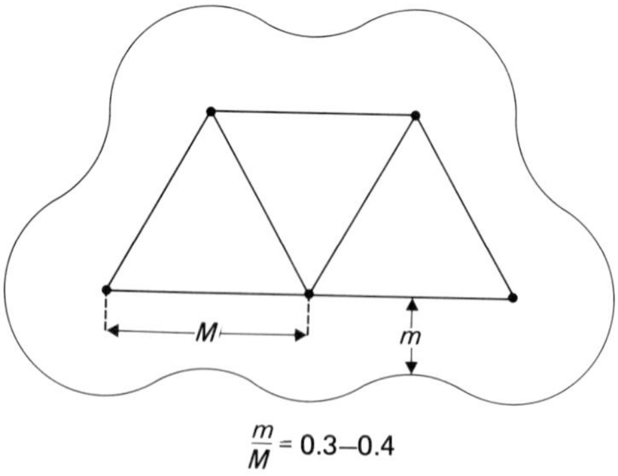

Figure 16.9 Relation between treatment margin (m) around volume implant and separation between sources (M)

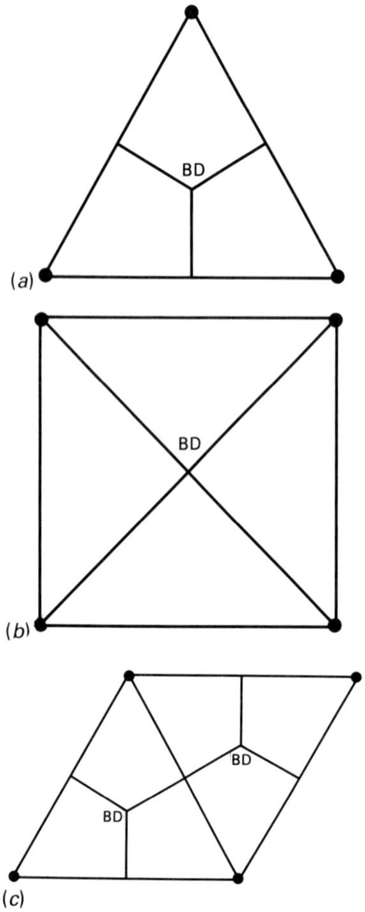

Figure 16.10 (a) Basal dose rate point for three wires with an equilateral triangle distribution in the central plane. (b) Basal dose rate point for an implant of four wires which form a square distribution in the central plane. (c) Basal dose rate points from the component triangles in the central plane of a volume implant

Define the points of basal dose rate

The points are geometrically defined as in *Figure 16.10*.

Calculate the dose rate at each basal dose point

This is done by using the dose/distance graphs of Hall, Oliver and Shepstone (1966) (*Figure 16.11*), from which the dose rate contribution of each source to the basal dose point can be measured depending on its distance from that point. If the sources have been properly inserted the variation between the component basal dose points within the implant should not be greater than ± 10%.

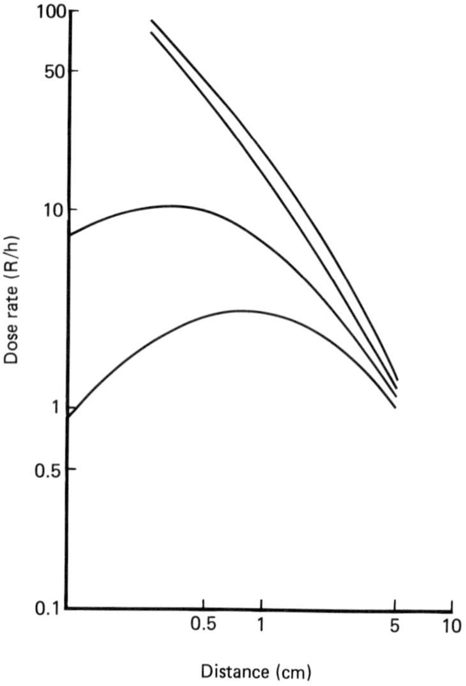

Figure 16.11 Graph of dose rate versus distance for ^{192}Ir wire

Calculate the reference dose rate for the implant

The reference dose rate is 85% of the basal dose rate. The dose rate graphs however give a dose rate for wire of unit activity i.e. 1 mg radium equivalent per centimetre. The activity of the wire actually used must be applied to get the true reference dose rate for the implant. In order to compensate for radioactive decay during the time of the implant it is usual to calculate the activity expected at the middle of the duration of the implant, rather than at the beginning.

Calculate the duration of the implant

This is done by dividing the prescribed dose (cGy) by the dose rate (cGy/hour). An example of how to calculate the dosimetry for an impant is given in *Figure 16.12*.

3 × 5 cm wires inserted.
Separation 12 mm with central plane distribution in the form of an equilateral triangle.

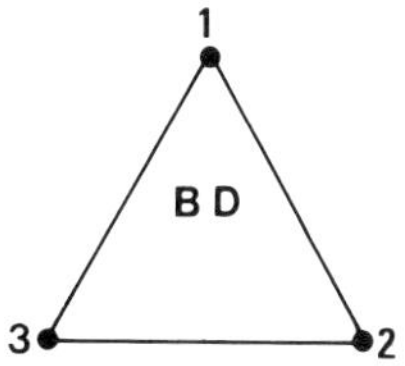

Wire	Dose rate at BD point	(Distance)
1	29.5	6.9 mm
2	29.5	6.9 mm
3	29.5	6.9 mm
	88.5	

Basal dose rate	= 88.5 cGy/h
Reference dose rate	= 88.5 × 0.85
	= 75.2 cGy/h
Activity of wire used	= 0.65 mg Eq Ra/cm
Therefore reference dose rate for the implant	= 75.2 × 0.65
	= 48.90 cGy/h
Dose prescribed	= 6500 cGy
Duration of implant	= 6500 ÷ 48.90
	= 132.9 h
	= 5 days 13 h

Figure 16.12 Example of dosimetry calculation for carcinoma of the lip template

Dose rate modification

It is usual with radium implants to aim at a dose rate of 40 – 50 cGy/hour, which delivers approximately 1000 cGy/day and a radical dose of 6000–7000 cGy in 6 or 7 days. It often happens however that the sources are a little closer together than planned, so that a higher dose rate is achieved and radical treatment may be completed in 4–5 days instead of 6 or 7. The question arises whether a reduction in overall dose should be made for a presumed increase in biological effectiveness of the higher dose rate. There remains considerable dispute over the effect of dose rate changes within the range encountered in interstitial therapy. In many centres correction to the overall time is made according to formulae and graphs derived from data collected during the early years of radium implant experience (Ellis, 1968).

Analysis of necrosis and recurrence rates in 263 patients treated by ^{192}Ir implants have shown no significant difference in the incidence of complications or recurrences at dose rates varying from 25 to 90 cGy/hour i.e. 6000 cGy in 3–11 days (Pierquin *et al.*, 1973). For the convenience of the patient the dose is therefore commonly delivered in approximately 5 days, and no dose rate correction is made.

Radiation protection requirements for iridium - 192 implants

The tenth value layer of lead to provide adequate protection from ^{192}Ir radiation is 2 cm and appropriate shielded containers are therefore used for transport of active wires.

The encapsulation of active ^{192}Ir wire into thin plastic inner-tubing is carried out using either a fully shielded instrument, or an unshielded instrument positioned behind lead blocks in a radiation source laboratory.

During the implantation procedure the active material is kept within its shielded container until ready for afterloading, which is performed using long handled forceps with the operator behind a mobile lead screen.

Protection for the nursing staff during the implant is provided either by nursing the patient in a single room with appropriately positioned mobile lead screens or with the screens alone, depending on the amount of radioactivity implanted.

The unloading procedure is done behind a lead screen and the used material transported back to the radiation source laboratory in its shielded container.

The radiation exposure encountered when using these measures is considerably less than for radium or caesium needle implants.

Indications and results of interstitial therapy

Cancer of the tongue

The tumours most suitable for implant therapy are those on the lateral border of the anterior two-thirds of the tongue. Those in the posterior third are better treated by external beam radiation and those at the tip of the tongue by surgery. For tumours less than 3 cm diameter the chances of subclinical involvement of the clinically negative neck are relatively low, especially if the tumour is well differentiated, and radical treatment with implant therapy alone (6000–7000 cGy) can be considered. If the tumour is larger or poorly differentiated it may be best to deliver a dose of fractionated external beam radiation (4500–5000 cGy) to the primary and adjacent node areas in the first instance and to boost the primary with an implant (2000–3000 cGy) 2–3 weeks after completion of external beam treatment.

The majority of implants can be performed using

the hairpin technique to produce a double plane encompassing the tumour (*Figure 16.13*).

The length of the hairpin limbs may be 2.5 – 5 cm depending on the size of the tumour. For superficial tumours it is sometimes tempting to use a single plane but this is associated with a high incidence of local recurrence, as the degree of infiltration of the tongue is often underestimated, and results in an inadequate dose to the deeper parts of the tumour.

The separation between the limbs of the hairpin is 1.2 cm, and if the tumour is thicker than this, further hairpin sources must be added or an extra single hairpin may be required. Alternatively, it may be better to use the plastic loop technique which allows larger separations to be used. Thanks to the excellent vascularity of the tongue the treatment is extremely well tolerated and the local control rates are high.

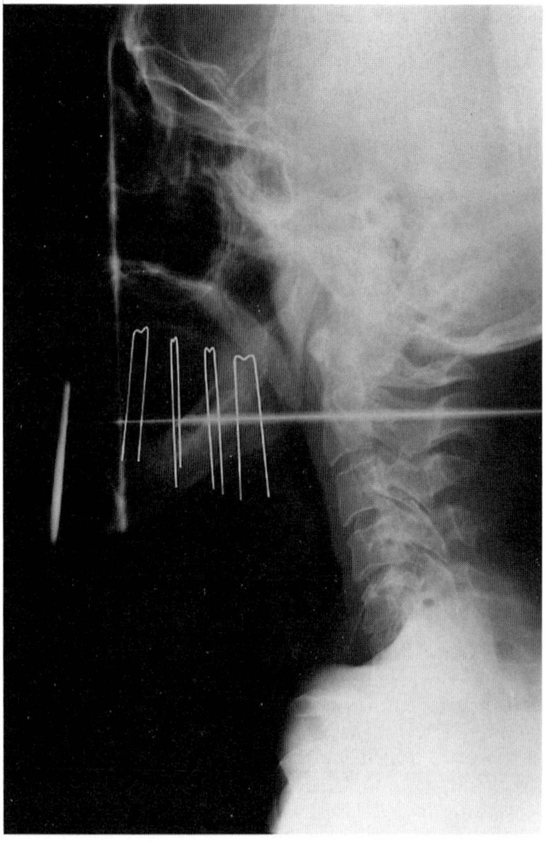

Figure 16.13 Radiograph of hairpin implant to the tongue

Cancer of the floor of the mouth

Similar considerations with regard to the combination of external beam radiation with implant therapy apply for floor of the mouth tumours as for tongue lesions, and implants may be performed using the same techniques. Because the mucosa of the floor of the mouth is considerably more fragile than that of the tongue, and because the mandible is much closer, morbidity may be greater at this site. If there is any suggestion of fixation of tumour to bone, implant therapy is contraindicated, as the risk of osteoradionecrosis of the mandible is considerable where the bone is included within the very high dose zone around each source.

Implant therapy is associated with a significant incidence of normal tissue damage and soft tissue necrosis may occur in up to 30% of cases. In the vast majority this heals spontaneously with conservative treatment. The incidence of necrosis is higher for floor of the mouth implants than for the tongue, and is clearly related to the volume of tissue implanted. A small number of patients may suffer bone necrosis.

The results of implant therapy for cancer of the tongue and floor of the mouth (Owen *et al.*, 1981) show that 92% of patients treated by implant alone achieve local tumour control, but for larger tumours where it is necessary to combine implant with external beam radiation this falls to 55%.

Cancer of the lip

Many small cancers of the lower lip can be treated by simple surgical excision with excellent results, but where the lesion occupies more than one-third of the lip more extensive plastic surgery with flap repair is required. For these patients radiotherapy provides a good alternative, and implant therapy in particular gives excellent functional and cosmetic results with a very low recurrence rate. The implant is usually performed using rigid afterloading needles maintained in place by a template.

Most lesions can be encompassed by three sources which form a triangle in the central plane, but more sources can be added for larger lesions (*see Figure 16.4*).

The teeth and gingiva can be protected by inserting a spacer between the inner surface of the lip and the teeth.

The results of treatment (Pigneux, Richaud and Lagarde, 1979) show that local control is achieved in 95.5% of cases. Nodal metastases are rare, and it is probably better to adopt a close follow-up policy with treatment on recurrence rather than give prophylactic treatment to clinically non-involved node areas.

Because of its very rich blood supply the lip tolerates radiation remarkably well and implant therapy has been used successfully to salvage recurrences after previous external beam radiation.

Cancer of the cheek

Tumours of the cheek are relatively uncommon but

can often be implanted with a single plane using the plastic tube technique. If the lesion is near the intermaxillary commisure a combination of an intra-oral loop plus a straight line source may be necessary to achieve adequate coverage at the posterior margin of the lesion.

Techniques have been described for implanting lesions of the palate and tonsillar fossa and for intracavitary treatment of tumours of the nasopharynx, but these are rarely used and well described elsewhere (Pierquin *et al.*, 1978).

Skin cancer

The majority of skin cancers can be adequately treated either by surgery or by fractionated external beam radiation. Implant therapy will produce a similar cure rate but the necessary admission to hospital is not justified for the majority of cases. There is a general impression that the cosmetic results of an implant given over 4–5 days are better than fractionated treatment given over a short period, so that where this is relevant or hospital admission is required for other reasons an implant may be indicated. Another useful indication is for lesions around the nose and ear where an implant or a mould (*see* Chapter 12) can be made to follow the changing contour of the skin and give a better dose distribution than can be achieved with external beam radiation.

Carcinoma of the anal canal and rectum

Squamous cancers of the anal canal are usually treated by abdominoperineal excision. They are, however, curable by radiation and anal function can be preserved in the majority. Unfortunately, the perineum tolerates radiation poorly and is a difficult site to implant satisfactorily. Excellent results have nevertheless been obtained by Papillon and his techniques and protocols are recommended (Papillon, 1982) (*see* Chapter 14).

Patients are initially treated by external beam radiation which is given to the primary tumour and to the posterior pelvis where nodal spread may occur. This is achieved by a combination of direct perineal field and sacral arc rotation, or by right angled wedged perineal and sacral fields.

After a dose of 3000–4000 cGy the tumour is implanted 6–8 weeks later using an afterloading needle technique with a template to maintain parallelism (*Figure 16.14*). The boost dose to the primary is 2000–3000 cGy.

The results of treatment reported by Papillon show a 5-year survival of 62% which is comparable with radical surgery, but 75% of patients retain normal anal function.

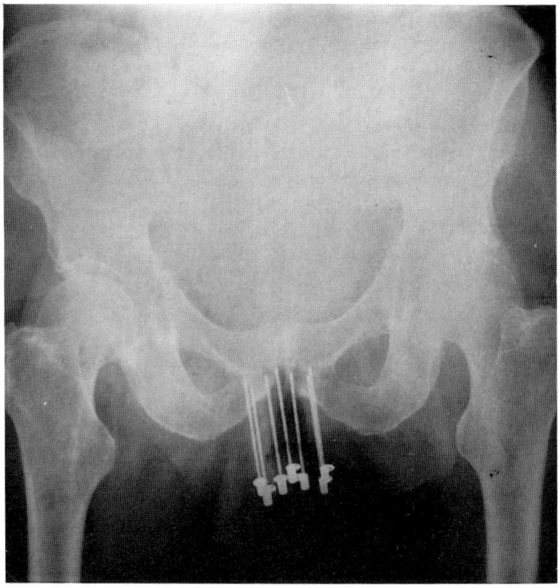

Figure 16.14 Radiograph of anal canal implant with template

Many low mobile exophytic cancers of the rectum can be cured by 50 kV contact radiation (Papillon, 1982), but in a few cases residual induration remains after three or four doses of 2000–3000 roentgens per treatment. For these cases a boost can be delivered by implanting a modified hairpin into the rectal mucosa, giving a further 2000 cGy.

In some elderly patients with more advanced rectal cancers where abdomino-perineal resection may not be feasible for medical reasons, an attempt at radical conservative treatment can be made by first giving 4000 cGy external beam radiation to the pelvis, and then implanting residual disease with the template technique used for anal cancer.

Carcinoma of the penis

Although amputation will readily cure most carcinomas of the penis, it is perhaps not surprising that many men would prefer conservation of their organ if possible. This can be achieved by radiation in one of three ways:

(1) External beam radiation
(2) Radioactive mould
(3) Interstitial implant.

External beam and mould radiation are discussed in Chapter 3 and both produce good results, although cosmetic and functional results of mould therapy are probably better than those of external beam radiation. One of the potential problems of mould therapy is that unless meticulous attention is paid to the construction and fitting of the mould there is a risk of the lesion and the sources parting from each other resulting in an underdosage which is impossible to calculate. This can be prevented by implanting the sources into the penis.

After adequate prior circumcision the patient is anaesthetized and catheterized and the implant performed with an afterloading needle technique with templates as in *Figure 16.15*. The usual dose delivered is 6000–6500 cGy.

During the period of the implant the penis is held in a foam block which keeps it away from the testicles and the inner thigh, thus reducing the risk of unnecessary radiation. Although it looks exceedingly uncomfortable the treatment is remarkably well tolerated. As with all techniques, however, there are 3–4 weeks of dysuria and local moist desquamation before healing takes place and meatal stenosis requiring dilatation may occur later in a few patients. Implants are contraindicated for lesions that infiltrate the corpora cavernosa or that are greater than 4 cm in any dimension.

The results of treatment by ^{192}Ir implant (Daley, Douchez and Combes, 1982) show a local control rate of 95% and the majority of sexually active patients retain their potency. The dose to the testes is 150–300 cGy and can be halved by the use of 2–3 mm lead shielding in those patients in whom fertility needs to be preserved.

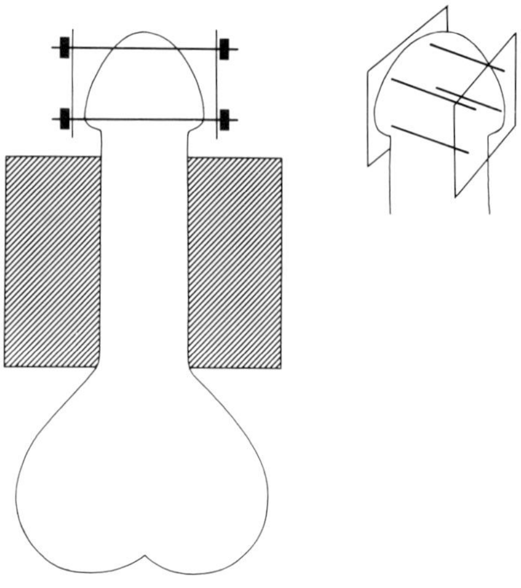

Figure 16.15 Diagram of implant technique used for carcinoma of the penis

Breast cancer

Implant therapy has a number of indications in the management of breast cancer.

(1) As a boost to the site of excision following lumpectomy and external beam radiation for primary breast conservation therapy
(2) As a boost to the tumour residue after external beam radiation for inoperable disease
(3) As salvage therapy for local recurrence.

Conservative treatment

After local excision of the primary tumour in the breast and biopsy of axillary nodes, a dose of 4000–5000 cGy is given to the breast and node areas by external beam radiation (*see* Chapter 4). An implant may then be performed to bring the dose at the site of excision up to 6000–7000 cGy.

This is performed either with a rigid template technique or with a plastic tube technique. The choice of technique may depend on the site in the breast. For deep and centrally sited lesions which may require more than one plane, the template technique would be most suitable, but for lesions at the periphery of the breast where a single plane is adequate, the plastic tube technique is usually preferable. Whichever method is used it is very important for the radiotherapist to know exactly where the tumour was before excision as the scar may not always be a sufficiently good guide and a geometric miss may easily occur. It is also important to avoid excessive irradiation of the skin either by allowing the active wire to protrude through the skin or to allow it to lie too near the surface. For tumours less then 2 cm in diameter, results show that at 10 years the local recurrence rate is 6 – 7%, and that nine out of 10 women have conserved their breasts with a good cosmetic appearance in more than 80% (Pierquin *et al.*, 1980).

For these small tumours, however, local recurrence rates are the same whether boost treatment is given with implant therapy or with external beam radiation (Calle *et al.*, 1978), and it is doubtful whether implants for all such patients can be justified. For larger tumours, on the other hand, the local recurrence rates with external beam radiation are higher and it is likely that an implant which can deliver a bigger local dose of radiation may improve results. The same is true for those cases where the tumour has not been excised.

Inoperable breast cancers are often associated with disseminated disease but it is, nevertheless, important to gain local control as the patient may live long enough to suffer distressing ulceration of their primary tumour. The dose required to maintain control of these large tumours is high, and after 4000–5000 cGy external beam radiation there is frequently a substantial residual mass. In such cases an implant can be delivered to the site of residual disease and a further 3500–4000 cGy can be given to bring the dose up to a total of 8000–9000 cGy. The cosmetic results are usually poor and are not only related to the dose of radiation used, but also to the fact that a large part of the breast was initially replaced by tumour and when this regresses little of the normal breast remains. The local control rates are however high, and the majority of patients die of metastases with their chest wall disease controlled (Bruckman *et al.*, 1979).

In spite of postoperative radiation chest wall recurrences still occur after mastectomy. As in the case of advanced primary tumours they are frequently associated with disseminated disease, but local control remains important. If the recurrence is localized and there are no obvious metastases, a single plane ^{192}Ir plastic tube implant can be performed and a dose of 5000–6000 cGy given. Even though the patient has already had external beam radiation the implant is usually well tolerated and local control regained in the vast majority of well selected patients. If there is diffuse dermal infiltration, however, marginal recurrence is common and other treatment methods should be tried.

Gynaecological cancer

The main role for radioactive isotopes in the management of gynaecological cancer is for intracavitary radiation of cancer of the cervix and body of uterus which is discussed in Chapter 9. There are a number of situations however where interstitial therapy may be valuable.

Cancer of the vagina

For limited superficial lesions radical implant therapy alone using the hairpin technique can be used or, in the case of larger superficial lesions, a vaginal mould can be prepared and plastic tubes fixed to the mould at the site of the lesion. For the more commonly presenting infiltrating tumours it is usual to give a course of external beam radiation to the primary and the pelvic nodes in the first instance and then to use implant therapy for a boost to the primary. If it has regressed sufficiently to fall within the range of a single plane implant performed with a hairpin or a mould then that may be used or a template technique similar to that used for cancer of the anal canal can be employed for more infiltrating lesions.

Tumours of the urethra

The most commonly occurring tumour at this site is a secondary deposit from endometrial carcinoma, but primary tumours of the urethra may also occur. Implant therapy either as primary treatment or as a boost after external beam radiation is performed under general anaesthesia. After inserting an indwelling catheter a circular plane of needles is implanted and subsequently afterloaded with active iridium wire. The ^{198}Au technique is described in Chapter 3.

Bladder cancer

Implant therapy for bladder cancer was practised extensively before megavoltage radiation, but with the availability of more penetrating radiation and the development of new endoscopic resection techniques, it has largely fallen out of use. In spite of these new developments, however, the local recurrence rates for infiltrating bladder cancer remain considerable, and the advantages of achieving a high localized dose of radiation are being re-evaluated. The results of 615 radium needle implants performed at the Rotterdam Radiotherapy Institute (Werf Messing, 1978) have shown unequalled local control rates but have not been repeated elsewhere (*see* Chapter 3).

Afterloading plastic tube techniques using ^{192}Ir wire have been developed to try to achieve similar results without the hazard of handling live sources.

Cystotomy is first required to expose the tumour and assess its suitability for implantation. The tumour should be less than 4 cm in diameter and not greater than 1 cm in thickness. The superficial part of the tumour is resected and plastic tubes are implanted into the base. The ends of the tubes are brought out through the skin and the desired site for the active wire is marked by metal clips in the bladder. The bladder and abdominal wound are then closed and the active wire is afterloaded into the prepositioned plastic tubes under fluoroscopic control which localizes the sources at the site marked by the metal clips. The implant which gives 2000–3000 cGy is usually combined with external beam radiation to the pelvis at a dose of 4500–5000 cGy. After delivery of the required interstitial therapy dose the active wire and the plastic tubes may be withdrawn without re-opening the bladder. To date there are too few patients with adequate follow-up to assess this approach fully.

Carcinoma of the prostate

Cancer of the prostate is usually a slow growing tumour with a long natural history and is relatively radioresistant. There is therefore a good theoretical basis for treating selected patients who have no metastases with a high localized dose of radiation given over a long time at low dose rate. This can be achieved by permanent implantation of ^{125}I seeds. The commonest technique is to expose the prostate surgically via a retropubic approach and, under direct vision, to implant the ^{125}I seeds with a specially designed applicator which distributes the sources equally throughout the gland. The number of seeds required depends on the tumour volume and the dose required. At the same operation a retroperitoneal lymph node resection may also be performed to deal with any regional spread.

For small well differentiated tumours with negative nodes, radical treatment by implant alone is given and a total dose of 12 000 – 15 000 cGy given. One-half of the dose is received in the first 2 months and the rest more slowly over the succeeding months.

For larger tumours and those which are poorly differentiated or with positive nodes, the implant is used in combination with external beam radiation to the primary and pelvic nodes. The results of treatment using these techniques (Guerriero, Carlton and Hudgins, 1980) have shown an overall 5-year survival of 90%.

Recent developments in endosonic ultrasound probes allow excellent visualization and screening of the prostate so that accurate implantation can now be performed percutaneously (Holm *et al.*, 1983).

Because of the long natural history of localized prostatic cancer the role of interstitial therapy remains unclear and it has not been adequately compared with external beam therapy techniques (*see* Chapter 3).

Implants for salvage therapy

When recurrences occur after previous radical external beam radiation, further radiation is often thought to be contraindicated because of the high risk of normal tissue damage. Perhaps because of the continuous low dose rate, re-treatment by interstitial therapy is better tolerated than external beam treatment and some patients can be salvaged in this way. It is first necessary to ensure that the lesion is suitable for implantation and that it is a true recurrence rather than a persistence of disease. It is tempting, because of the previous radiation, to give less than a radical dose with the salvage implant, but this is rarely rewarded with cure and a dose of at least 6000 cGy is required. There will inevitably be an enhanced risk of necrosis, particularly if large volumes are implanted, but some patients can be cured by salvage implant treatment even though they have recurred after previous irradiation.

Salvage implants may be attempted in the oral cavity and have been used to treat inoperable lymph node recurrences after radiation to the neck. For these cases a plastic tube technique is most commonly used. In a series of 124 cases of salvage implants for recurrent neck nodes reported by Pierquin *et al.* (1978), complete regression was achieved in 31 cases and substantial regression in a further 40. Salvage treatment of neck nodes in this way cannot be expected to result in cure, but useful palliation can be achieved with an acceptably small complication rate.

Conclusion

After a period of decline interstitial therapy is making a comeback. This is partly due to the development of new and safer afterloading techniques, but also the realization that local recurrence remains a considerable problem in many tumours and that the unique advantages of implant therapy have an important role in delivering the highest possible dose of radiation to the tumour without exceeding the tolerance of surrounding tissue.

References

ANDERSON, L. L. (1976) Spacing nomograph for interstitial implants of I-125 seeds. *Medical Physics,* **3**, 48–51

BRUCKMAN, J. E., HARRIS, J. R., LEVENE, M. B., CHAFFEY, J. T. and HELLMAN, S. (1979) Results of treating stage III carcinoma of the breast by primary radiation therapy. *Cancer,* **43**, 985–993

CALLE, R., PILLERON, J. P., SCHLIENGER, P. and VILCOQ, J. R. (1978) Conservative management of operable breast cancer — ten years experience at the Foundation Curie. *Cancer,* **42**, 2045–2053

DALY, N. J., DOUCHEZ, J. and COMBES, P. F. (1982) Treating carcinoma of the penis by iridium-192 wire implant. *International Journal of Radiation Oncology, Biology and Physics,* **8**, 1239–1243

ELLIS, F. (1968) Time fractionation and dose rate in radiotherapy. *Frontiers of Radiation Therapy and Oncology,* **3**, 131–140

GUERRIERO, W. G., CARLTON, C. E. and HUDGINS, P. T. (1980) Combined interstitial and external radiotherapy in the definitive management of carcinoma of the prostate. *Cancer,* **45**, 1922–1928

HALL, E. J., OLIVER, R. and SHEPSTONE, B. J. (1966) Routine dosimetry with tantalum-182 and iridium-192 wire. *Acta Radiologica,* **4**, 155

HOLM, H. H., JUUL, N., PEDERSON, J. F., HANSEN, H. and STROYER, I. (1983) Transperineal 125 iodine seed implantation in prostatic cancer guided by transrectal ultrasonography. *Journal of Urology,* **130**, 283–286

KIM, J. H. and HILARIS, B. (1974) Iodine 125 sources in interstitial tumour therapy. *American Journal of Roentgenology,* **123**, 163–169

MEREDITH, W. J. (ed) (1967) *Radium dosage — The Manchester System.* Edinburgh: E. & S. Livingstone

OWEN, J. R., MAYLIN, C., LE BOURGEOIS, J. P., BAILLET, F., SABATINI, B. and PIERQUIN, B. (1981) Iridium-192 implantation of tumours of the anterior two thirds of tongue and floor of mouth. *Journal of European Radiotherapy,* **2**, 93–102

PAINE, C. H., BERRY, R. J., WIERNICK, G., STEDEFORD, J. B. H., WEATHERBURN, H. and YOUNG, C. M. A. (1979) The use of brachytherapy with californium-252 in the treatment of human tumours (2 papers). Proceedings of a Seminar *Uses of 252 Cf.* Vienna: Karlsruhe IAEA

PAPILLON, J. (1982) *Rectal and Anal Cancer.* Berlin: Springer

PATERSON, R. (1963) *The Treatment of Malignant Disease by Radiotherapy*, 2nd edn. London: Edward Arnold

PIERQUIN, B., CHASSAGNE, D., BAILLET, F. and CASTRO, J. (1971) *Journal of the American Medical Association,* **215**, 961–963

PIERQUIN, B., CHASSAGNE, D., BAILLET, F. and PAINE, C.H. (1973) Clinical observations on the time factor in interstitial radiotherapy using iridium-192. *Clinical Radiology,* **24**, 506–509

PIERQUIN, B., CHASSAGNE, D., CACHIN, Y., BAILLET, F., FOURNELLE, C. and BUIS, F. (1970) *Acta Radiologica,* **9**, 465–480

PIERQUIN, B., CHASSAGNE, D., CHAHBAZIAN, C. M. and WILSON, J. F. (1977) *Brachytherapy*. St. Louis: Warren Green Inc.

PIERQUIN, B., DUTREIX, A., PAINE, C.H., CHASSAGNE, D., MARINELLO, G. and ASH, D. (1978) The Paris system in interstitial radiation therapy. *Acta Radiologica et Oncologica,* **17**, 33–48

PIERQUIN, B., OWEN, R., MAYLIN, C. *et al.* (1980) Radical radiation therapy of breast cancer. *International Journal of Radiation Oncology, Biology and Physics,* **6**, 17–24

PIGNEUX, J., RICHAUD, P. M. and LAGARDE, C. (1979) The place of interstitial therapy using iridium-192 in the management of cancer of the lip. *Cancer,* **43**, 1073–1077

SCOTT, W. P. (1972) Rapid injector for permanent radioactive implantation. *Radiology,* **105**, 454–455

WERF MESSING, B. VAN DER (1978) Cancer of the urinary bladder treated by interstitial radium implant. *International Journal of Radiation Oncology, Biology and Physics,* **4**, 373–378

17

The management of benign conditions

B. S. Mantell

The use of radiotherapy for the treatment of benign disease is regarded with disfavour today. Cannon, Randolph and Murray (1959) wrote of *Malignant irradiation for benign conditions*, while Glicksman and Toker (1976) considered that apart from a few 'die-hards' its use had virtually disappeared. However, the 'malignant' nature of radiation must be weighed against the potential side-effects of alternative agents such as corticosteroids and immunosuppressive drugs. Furthermore, conditions such as severe rheumatoid arthritis and relapsing polychondritis although 'benign' may, nevertheless, become potentially lethal. In considering radiotherapy for non-neoplastic disease, therefore, it is necessary to view the risks of radiation in the relatively small doses which are used in the light of the natural history of the condition or the distress it causes, and the dangers of its treatment by non-radiotherapeutic means.

The risks of radiotherapy

These may be regarded as genetic and carcinogenic. Alexander (1965) estimated that the dose of radiation required to double the mutation rate in man was between 15 and 100 cGy. The dose received at the level of the gonads can be measured at the first of a course of radiation exposures. Mantell (1978) used thermoluminescent dosimetry to measure the dose to the scrotum in a patient receiving a total of 1000 cGy to a foot for plantar fasciitis, and obtained a figure of 2.25 cGy. The risk of genetic damage in this case would seem to be insignificant. Due consideration must, of course, be given to the gonad dose in patients of reproductive age. It can be controlled by appropriate direction of beams, and by shielding if necessary. Suitable precautions to avoid irradiation of pregnant patients must be taken as in diagnostic radiology.

An increase in the incidence of leukaemia by a factor of 9.5 after radiotherapy for ankylosing spondylitis was reported by Court Brown and Doll (1965). This was, however, still extremley rare, as only 52 definite cases of leukaemia were found among over 14 000 patients who had been irradiated. An increase in cancer in 'heavily irradiated' sites was also noted, but this increase was by a factor of only 1.6. Smith and Doll (1982) studied the mortality of those patients in this series who had received only one course of radiotherapy. They demonstrated an excess of deaths from leukaemia of nearly fivefold, and a statistically significant 62% excess of deaths from cancers of the 'heavily irradiated' sites, that is those sites which would have been included in the radiation beams. It is of interest to note that in both the leukaemias and the other cancers the risk appeared to be much greater when irradiation was carried out above the age of 55 years than below the age of 25. The greatest risk of leukaemia occurred as soon as 3–5 years after treatment and had practically disappeared by 18 years, while that for the other cancers took more than 9 years to manifest and did not begin to fall until more than 20 years after radiotherapy.

In considering these figures, which may seem alarming at first sight, one must remember that some of these patients had been treated as long ago as 1935, often with very extensive fields involving much or all of the bone marrow. The actual number of patients who developed leukaemia is a far smaller proportion of those patients treated than is often believed.

Furthermore, in advising restriction of the use of phenylbutazone to the hospital treatment of ankylosing spondylitis the Committee on Safety of Medicines reported risks from this drug which seem even more disturbing than those associated with radiotherapy. In their study of 1963 reports of adverse reactions attributed to phenylbutazone, circulated to all UK doctors in their letter of 7 March 1984, the Committee noted no fewer than 445 deaths due to aplastic anaemia, white blood cell disorders, and thrombocytopenia.

Irradiation of the thyroid gland in childhood carries a risk of induction of malignancy which persists into adult life. Favus *et al.* (1976) reviewed the literature and reported a series of 1056 patients of whom 16.5% were found to have nodular thyroid disease. Sixty patients were shown at operation to have thyroid cancer, all of a low degree of malignancy.

Glicksman and Toker (1976) described a case of osteosarcoma which occurred 23 years after irradiation for bursitis. The dose of radiation administered was said to total 800 roentgens over a period of 3 months. This was, however, an 'air dose' using 200 kV X-rays with only 0.5 mm copper filtration, and the dose actually absorbed by the bone may well have been considerably greater than this figure would suggest. The 12 cases of osteosarcoma and fibrosarcoma occurring after radiotherapy collected by Steiner (1964) had all received doses (where recorded) of at least 3600 roentgens and sometimes much more. Kim *et al.* (1978), in a review of 47 cases diagnosed as radiation-induced sarcoma, were unable to find any case of bone sarcoma who had received less than 1100 ret, or of soft tissue sarcoma after less than 1400 ret (probably equivalent to approximately 3000 and 4000 cGy respectively fractionated over 4 weeks). Brady (1979) found no case of bone sarcoma in the literature attributable to a dose of less than 3000 cGy fractionated over 3 weeks.

It would seem, therefore, that while the risk of malignancy following low dose radiotherapy is a real one, it is extremely small and not the inevitable sequela it is sometimes thought to be. The small risk is certainly amply justified in a severe and potentially lethal condition such as advanced and active rheumatoid arthritis, and also seems acceptable in non-lethal disorders such as intractable plantar fasciitis, where the patient's life is seriously hindered by pain and impaired by mobility, or keloid where the cosmetic appearance may cause the patient much distress.

The rationale of radiotherapy in benign disease

In many cases this is clearly apparent, for example the powerful and prolonged immunosuppressive effect of total nodal irradiation (Fuks *et al.*, 1976) is utilized in the treatment of severe rheumatoid arthritis. Local postoperative radiotherapy is employed in the treatment of keloids to suppress fibroblastic proliferation. In other conditions, however, it must be admitted that treatment is essentially empirical. In capsulitis of the shoulder, for example, improvement may be ascribed to an anti-inflammatory effect, but the reason why many such patients whose pain and limited movement have not been helped by the conventional treatments, improve rapidly after a short course of low-dose radiotherapy is quite obscure.

Undoubtedly many of these cases are self-limiting, and may remit with or without treatment of any kind. The powerful effect of suggestion, especially when strange and impressive-looking equipment is applied to the patient, must also be remembered. In such conditions the true value of radiotherapy can only be established by controlled clinical trial. Such a trial would need to be double-blind and must inevitably involve the use of 'sham' radiation. This was in fact done by Rhys-Lewis (1965) in herpes zoster, and he was able to demonstrate that radiotherapy, previously regarded as useful in preventing and relieving the pain, was no more effective than placebo.

Discussion with the patient

It is now widely known by the general public that radiotherapy is given for cancer, and there is a possibility that the patient may fear that his condition is, in fact, malignant. It is therefore essential to make clear to the patient that while the treatment that is to be given is of the type often used for cancer, this is not the diagnosis in his case, and that the dose of radiation envisaged is much smaller than that used in the treatment of cancer.

The potential risks of the treatment must be described to the patient. In the case of a female of reproductive age a menstrual history must be obtained, and the necessity of avoiding pregnancy during irradiation explained. The present author believes it to be mandatory to tell the patient that there is a potential risk of the induction of cancer or leukaemia by the treatment, although the risk is very small indeed. Almost certainly it will be truthful to say that one does not know of a case where this has in fact occurred, as it is indeed such a rare complication. If the radiotherapist does not tell the patient of this remote possibility, someone else may do so, and very probably grossly overestimate the danger. Perhaps the only exceptions to the rule are elderly patients who might not expect to survive long enough in any case for radiation-induced malignancy to have time to develop, and those being treated for the life-threatening 'benign' diseases already referred to.

The likelihood of success must also be discussed with the patient. In the case of cosmetic treatment, as in keloid, the patient must have some reasonable ideas of the sort of appearance that can be expected. In locomotor conditions such as plantar fasciitis, where one is dealing with the hard core of patients who have failed with all the conventional treatments, one must be sure that it is understood that a trial of radiotherapy is being offered, and that there is a very real chance that no benefit will result. Radiotherapy should not be presented as a magical certain cure, even if this means denying the patient the full benefit of the power of suggestion!

Finally, the present author believes that the patient must be allowed to opt for radiotherapy himself, in the full knowledge that it may not do what is hoped. While he must realize that he is being exposed to the risks of radiation, he must have a sensible understanding of the minuteness of the hazard in the context of other therapies and of life itself. If the patient is hesitant about accepting treatment no pressure should be put on him. It is better to let him seek other advice, or if he prefers retain his symptoms, than to leave him with a nagging fear that he may have been done harm. The offer to treat him can be kept open to be taken up if and when he wishes.

The scope of radiotherapy for benign disorders

Radiotherapy has been tried, and benefit alleged, in an almost unlimited variety of conditions, from infertility to the mythical 'status thymicolymphaticus'. The disorders discussed in this chapter are ones of which the present author has direct experience and in which benefit seems to result from radiotherapy sufficiently frequently for him to feel justified in offering it when other measures have failed. For a fuller survey of the subject the reader is referred to Dewing (1965).

The management of thyrotoxicosis by radioiodine is a well-established practice, and is discussed in Chapter 13.

Ankylosing spondylitis

Treatment of this condition has probably done more than that of any other to earn for radiotherapy of benign disease its ill deserved evil reputation. Certainly Court Brown and Doll (1965) demonstrated a very significantly raised incidence of leukaemia in these patients, but this incidence, which was less than 0.5%, must be seen against the background of the severely disabling and even lethal nature of this 'benign' disease. The demand for radiotherapy here has been greatly reduced by the introduction of potent antirheumatic drugs, but a small number of patients are inadequately helped by these, or may be troubled by side-effects such as gastric irritation. Radiotherapy is often dramatically effective, giving some benefit in about 90% of cases and complete relief in 65–70% (Sharp and Easson, 1954; Morrison, 1955; Hart, 1961). In the present author's experience the patients are usually delighted and are apt to return demanding more radiotherapy when the disease relapses. It cannot be claimed that radiotherapy is a cure for ankylosing spondylitis, but as a palliative in those patients with relatively early disease whose joints are not yet ankylosed, but whose incapacitating pain is not controlled by the present conventional treatment, it is invaluable, and as discussed above may even be safer than phenylbutazone.

Patients should only be accepted from the rheumatologist, with whom the radiotherapist should work in close cooperation during treatment. It is important for physiotherapy including breathing exercises to be continued for maximum benefit.

Radiotherapy technique for ankylosing spondylitis

Scott (1939) used a wide field X-ray technique. He relates how his first case was treated with a diagnostic unit, in the absence of a radiotherapy machine! Other authors have described treatment of extensive areas of the spine and sacroiliac regions (Sharp and Easson, 1954; Morrison, 1955) because of the widespread nature of the disease. In the wake of Court Brown and Doll's report (1965) it now seems prudent to restrict the fields to the symptomatic areas. A blood count before treatment to exclude any blood dyscrasia which might later be attributed to radiotherapy is perhaps somewhat cynical but is none the less recommended.

The present author usually employs orthovoltage deep X-rays. This radiation may easily be applied for example to the spine, without the exit beam from a direct field causing nausea. It is perhaps more readily available than megavoltage which is heavily committed to malignant cases. The dose of radiation used is so low that skin reaction is non-existent. In contrast to the early workers the present author prefers to use the smallest fields that will include the symptomatic area. For example a field of 8×6 cm is adequate to treat a sacroiliac joint. An incident dose of 200 cGy given twice weekly to a total of 1000 cGy is usually sufficient to achieve rapid pain relief. Further areas may be treated as required, but it is preferable to avoid retreatment of an area if at all possible.

Rheumatoid arthritis

In contrast to ankylosing spondylitis, this common and incapacitating disease has in the past been affected but little by radiotherapy. The author has on occasions tried irradiation in the hope of relieving the symptoms from painful swollen joints which were not controlled by the usual treatments. Orthovoltage X-rays were used with pairs of parallel opposed fields to encompass the whole of the synovial tissue of a joint such as the knee. Doses of 1000 cGy at the midpoint in five fractions given twice weekly, or 2000 cGy in 10 fractions at the same rate were used. The results obtained can only be regarded as anecdotal, especially as rheumatoid arthritis is a condition well known for a fluctuant course of remissions and relapses and is therefore a favourite with purveyors of unproven and unorthodox remedies!

Accordingly, it is not surprising that some patients have benefitted by lessening of pain and reduction of effusion. The responses have in general been limited and transient, and in no way comparable with the dramatic improvement so commonly seen in ankylosing spondylitis. Steffen *et al.* (1982) were able to demonstrate inhibition of production of experimental arthritis in rabbits by a single dose of 600 cGy of 180 kV X-rays. They advocated the clinical investigation of radiotherapy in inflammatory forms of arthritis such as rheumatoid. It seems probable that the firmly established clinical condition is not entirely comparable with the laboratory model where radiation was used as prophylaxis before the arthritis was fully developed.

Ansell *et al.* (1963) described the intra-articular injection of colloidal radioactive gold in rheumatoid arthritis. They calculated the amount of isotope required to give an estimated 600–800 roentgens at the surface of the synovium. They reported a good response in 16 patients and some response in seven more out of a total of 30 treated. Gumpel, Williams and Glass (1973) used yttrium-90, thus avoiding the gamma ray hazard of gold-198. Gumpel and Roles (1975) in a controlled trial showed that injection of 5 mCi of yttrium-90 was comparable with synovectomy in efficacy, although it must be admitted that the value of synovectomy is not universally accepted.

Total lymphoid irradiation for rheumatoid arthritis

Cases of severe rheumatoid arthritis which have proved resistant to standard therapy may be treated with immunosuppressive agents. Cytotoxic drugs such as azathioprine, cyclophosphamide and methotrexate have been used, but have been associated with severe and sometimes fatal side-effects including the development of leukaemia (Cobrau, Sheon and Kirsner, 1973; Love and Sowa, 1975). Total lymphoid irradiation (Kaplan, 1980) has been shown to be apparently safe in this respect when used in the treatment of Hodgkin's disease. Baccarini, Bosi and Papa (1980) found no leukaemia or other second malignancy in 117 such patients treated by radiotherapy alone, while there were seven cases of acute non-lymphoid leukaemia in 496 patients who had received cytotoxic chemotherapy with or without radiotherapy; follow-up had been for a period of 2–10 years. Fuks *et al.* (1976) demonstrated a marked fall in the number of circulating T lymphocytes in these patients, which took several years to recover. There was reduction in the response of the lymphocytes to antigens, and a rise in the numbers of B and null lymphocytes with inversion of the ratio of T and B cells. They described a profound and sustained suppression of the absolute lymphocyte count and an increase in the ratio of suppressor to helper T cells. They concluded that total lymphoid irradiation may be a potent means of induction of long-term immunosuppression.

Kotzin *et al.* (1981) reported the use of total lymphoid irradiation as an immunosuppressive treatment for intractable rheumatoid arthritis, using a dose of 2000 cGy, half that used for Hodgkin's disease. Strober *et al.* (1983) reported a series of 11 patients so treated, of whom nine achieved a marked objective improvement in morning stiffness, swelling and tenderness of joints and general performance by 6 months. This improvement persisted without relapse for observation periods between 13 and 28 months from radiotherapy. Calin *et al.* (1983) reported a double-blind controlled trial of this treatment, in which 30 patients whose rheumatoid arthritis was uncontrolled by all the usual therapies, including cytotoxic drugs in 80%, were randomly allocated to total lymphoid irradiation using either 2000 or 200 cGy. Ten of 11 patients receiving the higher dose improved compared with one on the lower, while six of the latter suffered deterioration. These differences were highly significant.

Technique of total lymphoid irradiation

This is essentially the same as that used for Hodgkin's disease (Kaplan, 1980) except that the dose is reduced to half, and no interval is allowed between treatment of the upper and lower fields. The standard 'mantle' (*see* Chapter 8) is first treated; the present author gives a midpoint dose of 200 cGy daily for 10 days. Antiemetics are given routinely, and the haemoglobin, white cell count and platelets are checked twice weekly. During treatment of the mantle, planning of the 'inverted Y' for the lower half is proceeding, so that it can be started without a break as soon as the mantle is completed. An additional pair of parallel opposed fields to encompass the spleen is added to the inverted Y, and treatment proceeds at the same rate as did the mantle.

Relapsing polychondritis

The present author has treated a case of relapsing polychondritis by total lymphoid irradiation, with an immediate and dramatic response, as shown in the following case report.

Case report

A 43-year-old woman presented in December 1979

with a short history of malaise and anorexia associated with tingling discomfort in the pinnae, especially the left which exhibited a puffy inflammation. A diagnosis of relapsing polychondritis was confirmed by biopsy of the left pinna. She was treated with prednisolone in a dose of 20 mg daily as well as with azathioprine and chlorambucil, but the condition continued to progress. By 1983 the bridge of her nose had collapsed and she had developed cough and stridor due to chondritis of the trachea. Ultimately, faced with impending respiratory obstruction, total lymphoid irradiation was suggested. A mantle area was first treated to a dose of 2000 cGy in 10 daily exposures between 11 and 25 May, 1983. Irradiation of the abdominal and pelvic lymph nodes and spleen was begun on 1 June and a dose of 2000 cGy was completed on 23 June. The prolongation of this part of the course to 22 days was due to temporary stopping of irradiation because of a fall in the total white count to $1.1 \times 10^9 \ell$, attributable to radiation following previous cytotoxic therapy.

Almost immediately after the completion of radiotherapy the patient experienced a dramatic remission of her symptoms. The cough and stridor and the tingling of the ears ceased abruptly. There was transient recrudescence of the inflammation of the left ear as the prednisolone dosage was reduced but this resolved as the steroid was withdrawn more slowly. In November 1983 the patient was entirely asymptomatic on a prednisolone dosage of 7.5 mg/day, and this was slowly being withdrawn.

In December 1983 both ears, particularly the left, again developed puffiness and tingling. There was no recurrence of the tracheal symptoms and since the trachea had been irradiated directly in the mantle treatment but not the pinnae, it was decided to try the effect of irradiation of the left pinna. This was effected by means of 300 kV X-rays at a focus skin distance of 10 cm, in order to limit the depth dose. Lead shielding was used to confine the radiation to the pinna and to protect the parotid salivary gland. An incident dose of 2000 cGy was given in 10 daily fractions in January 1984. There was no immediate response, but 2 weeks after completion of radiotherapy the tingling ceased and the puffiness resolved. The right pinna was then treated in the same way. In July 1984 she was in complete clinical remission on prednisolone 2.5 mg/day. The prednisolone was withdrawn shortly afterwards. and there had been no relapse by November 1984.

Relapsing polychondritis is perhaps due to autoimmunity to collagen (Harisdangkul *et al.*, 1982), and the possibility of treatment by total lymphoid irradiation was suggested by its use in rheumatoid arthritis. The dramatic reversal of the severe and potentially lethal manifestations in this case was much more rapid than the response described in rheumatoid arthritis, and gave stable control of the disease when steroid and cytotoxic treatment had failed. The subsequent response of the the relapse in the ears to local irradiation suggests that a direct effect upon the autoimmune inflammatory process itself may also play a part in the control of this disease by radiotherapy.

Minor musculoskeletal disorders

Although neither lethal nor causing grave ill-health, conditions such as capsulitis of the shoulder and plantar fasciitis may give rise to a great deal of pain and may seriously impair the patient's ability to continue his normal life and occupation. In most cases the disorder can readily be relieved by simple and well-tried measures such as local injection of steroid or by physiotherapy. There always remains, however, a hard core of patients whose symptoms are resistant to all the usual treatments. In these one may reasonably consider radiotherapy which undoubtedly benfits some, but unfortunately not all, of these patients. The mechanism of response is quite obscure; it is tempting to ascribe it to an anti-inflammatory effect of radiation, but it must be admitted that a placebo effect has not been excluded, and that in many cases the disease is self-limiting. But such patients sometimes suffer many months or even years of discomfort, and if this can be curtailed or ameliorated by a small dose of radiation in some cases, a trial of radiotherapy is surely justified.

Painful heel syndrome

Pain and tenderness on the plantar aspect of the calcaneum (plantar fasciitis) or near the insertion of the tendo Achillis may cause considerable disability to patients who need to spend much of the day on their feet. The pain is presumably due to a local inflammatory reaction (Currey, 1975) and in most cases either subsides spontaneously or responds to steroid injection or other standard treatment. A few patients have persistent pain which is not so relieved, and many of these seem to be helped by radiotherapy.

Seventeen such patients were treated by irradiation to a dose of 1000 cGy in five fractions given two to three times a week (Mantell, 1978). Nine had bilateral symptoms, 13 had plantar calcaneal pain, eight tendo Achillis pain, and one had pain in the right plantar calcaneum and the left tendo Achillis. Their ages ranged from 19 to 70 years, two were female, and all had been referred by rheumatologists after the usual measures had failed. Parallel opposed fields of the order of 15 × 15 cm were centred on the painful area, in most cases using orthovoltage X-rays at 240–300 kV, but five patients were treated by telecobalt. Some of the patients with bilateral pain had both heels treated at the same time by tying the feet together. In all cases the dose was calculated at the

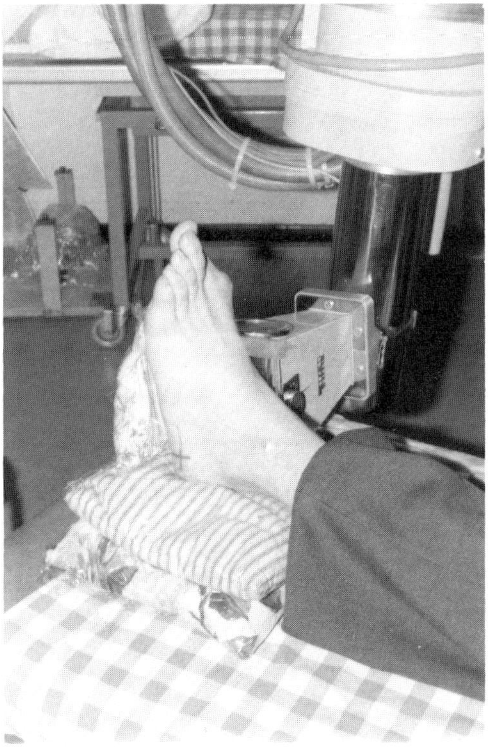

Figure 17.1 Radiotherapy for painful heel

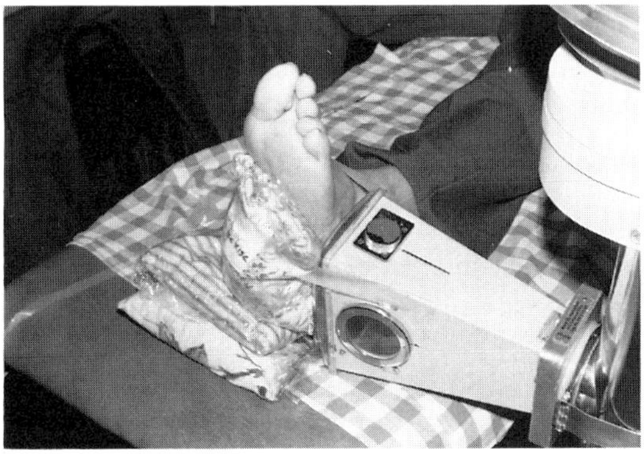

Figure 17.2 Painful heel; bolus applied

midplane, and bolus was used to make up for missing tissue (*Figures 17.1, 17.2 and 17.3*).

Of the 17 patients, nine reported complete relief of pain and two partial relief. Eight had improved by the end of the course of radiotherapy, and the others after 2 weeks, 2 months, and 3 months. Follow-up proved difficult and two patients were lost. The rest were followed-up for periods of between 2 and 43 months.

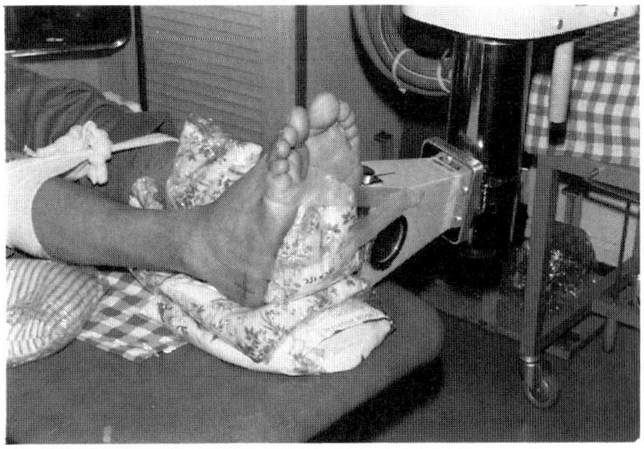

Figure 17.3 Painful heel; treating both heels together

Tennis and golfer's elbow

This measure of success with the painful heel syndrome encouraged the present author to try radiotherapy in these minor but potentially highly incapacitating conditions. Again, all the patients had persistent and refractory or repeatedly relapsing pain and had been referred by the rheumatologist after the usually effective remedies had failed. All were treated by orthovoltage X-rays using a single field, usually 8 × 6 cm, centred over the site of maximum tenderness. It was found that the easiest way to do this was to treat the patient prone in tennis elbow and supine in golfer's elbow. The arm was extended to a right-angle at the shoulder and supported on a second couch. An incident dose of 1000 cGy was given in five treatments twice per week, with bolus for air gaps (*Figures 17.4 and 17.5*).

Of 30 patients so treated 16 had no benefit, and two others obtained only transient improvement. Twelve, however, had lasting improvement, often complete and frequently very gratifying.

It cannot be claimed from these results that radiotherapy is of established value in these common conditions of heel and elbow. This work is in no sense a controlled trial and the possibility of placebo effect cannot be ruled out. Spontaneous remission is a possibility in some cases, but in others, for example a doctor whose painful heel had persisted for 20 years in spite of a variety of treatments but responded to radiotherapy, this seems unlikely. There is no doubt that the relief was very real to those patients whose condition improved after radiotherapy, whatever actually caused the improvement.

Capsulitis of the shoulder

This condition is characterized by a painful shoulder joint with severe limitation of mobility. Like the previously discussed disorders it is common, often self-limiting, but may respond to physiotherapy or steroid injection. The occasional patient with resis-

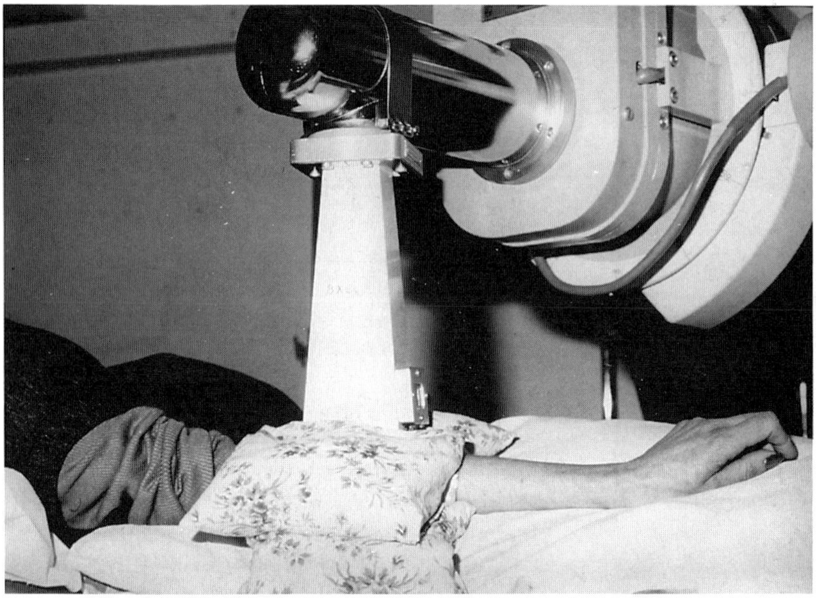

Figure 17.4 Radiotherapy for tennis elbow

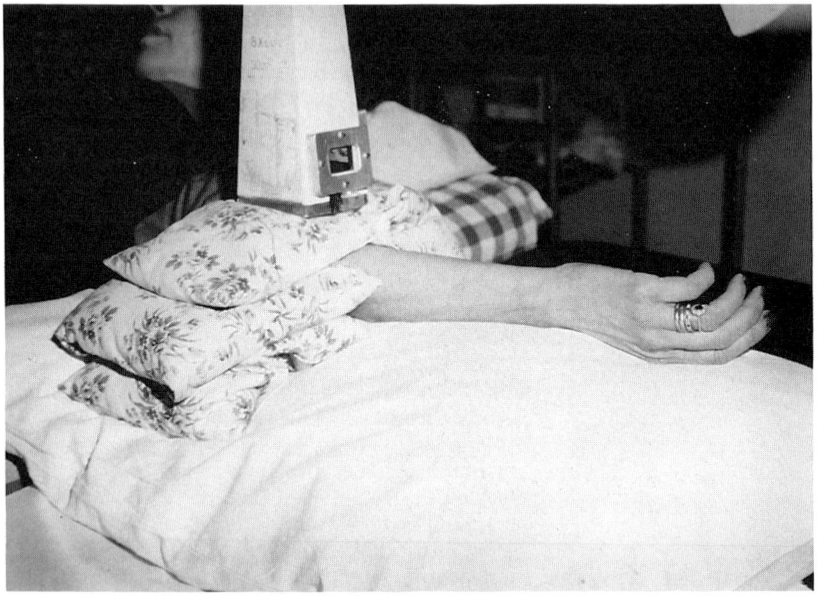

Figure 17.5 Radiotherapy for golfer's elbow

tant disease may remain incapacitated for months or years. Such patients are often helped by radiotherapy (Milone and Copeland, 1961), and the response can be particularly gratifying.

The present author usually treats these patients sitting, using orthovoltage X-rays. Anterior and posterior fields of the order of 15 × 10 cm are applied, approximately but not necessarily accurately parallel opposed, and a dose of 1000 cGy is given in five treatments twice weekly, to a volume including the whole shoulder joint (*Figures 17.6, 17.7 and 17.8*). Full bolus is used.

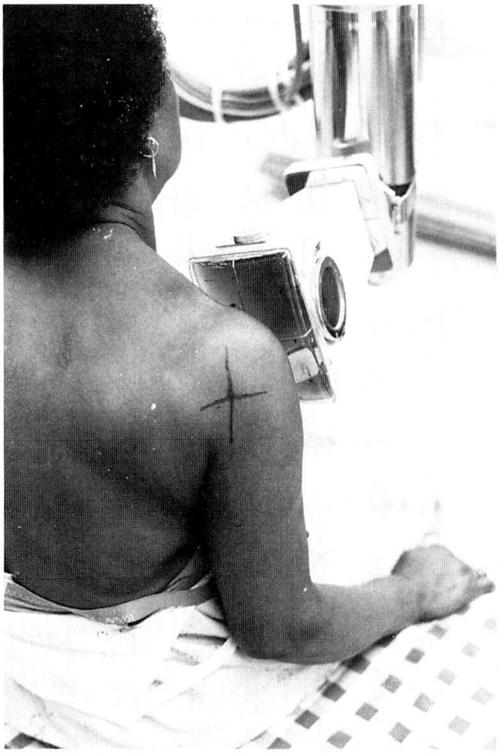

Figure 17.6 Radiotherapy for capsulitis of shoulder

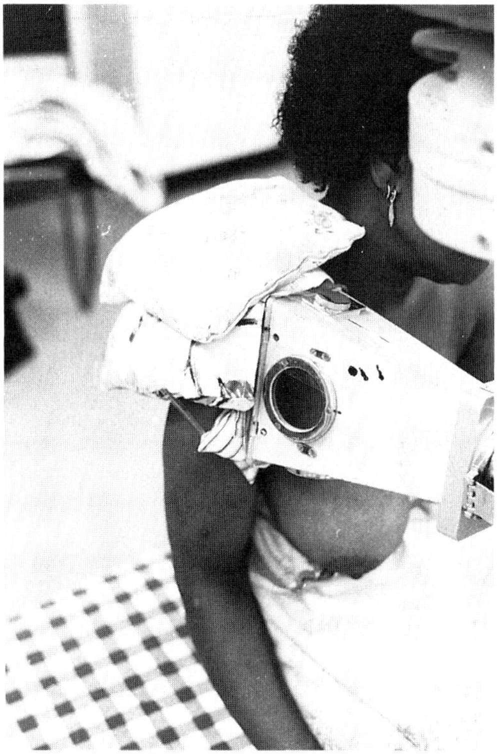

Figure 17.7 Capsulitis of shoulder; bolus for anterior field

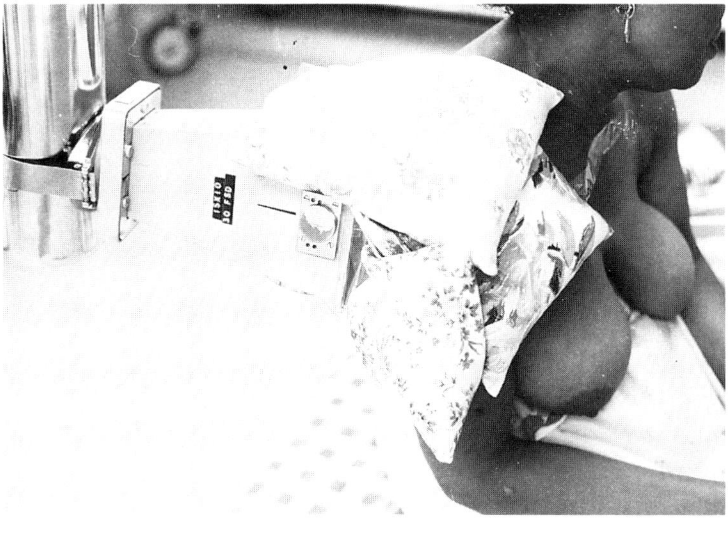

Figure 17.8 Capsulitis of shoulder; bolus for posterior field

In all these conditions as much rest as is reasonably possible should be given to the affected part during radiotherapy and until the pain has subsided. Activity may then gradually be increased.

Pigmented villonodular synovitis

This condition presents as a painful warm swelling of a joint, usually the knee. Aspiration of the joint may reveal a dark blood-stained fluid. The diagnosis is made by synovial biopsy, which shows the synovial membrane to be covered by masses of frond-like and nodular projections. Histologically these lesions are seen to be covered by synovial cells and to be full of dense cellular infiltration with haemosiderin pigment and areas of frank haemorrhage. The pathogenesis is obscure. Chung and Janes (1965) reviewed the literature with special reference to the hip joint, and added four cases of their own which were treated surgically. The condition may respond well to radiotherapy as described by Greenfield and Wallace (1950) who considered this to be the treatment of choice.

A radiation dose of the order of 3000 cGy in 15 fractions given daily over 3 weeks appears to be required, i.e. a considerably larger dose than is usually employed for benign conditions. A pair of parallel and opposed fields, either medial and lateral in the case of the knee, or anterior and posterior if preferred, is used. Orthovoltage radiation is adequate but may cause a skin erythema which can be avoided by the use of megavoltage which is also more easily applied, particularly with anterior and posterior fields to the knee.

Ectopic ossification

After hip-joint surgery ossification occasionally develops in the tissues around the joint, grossly impairing joint mobility. This may often be prevented by anti-inflammatory drugs, but in refractory cases, can also be prevented by irradiation used as soon as possible after surgery (Coventry and Scanlon, 1981). The hip joint and surrounding tissues are encompassed by anterior and posterior parallel opposed megavoltage fields measuring 10 × 10 cm. A dose of 2000 cGy in 10 daily treatments at midpoint seems to be adequate.

Coventry and Scanlon (1981) reported a series of 48 hips in 42 patients treated at the Mayo Clinic. They advised surgical removal of the ectopic bone followed almost immediately by radiotherapy; some of their patients began irradiation as soon as 2 days postoperatively, and all started within 10 days. They used the same dose and fractionation as given above but with larger fields, from 12 × 18 to 14 × 20 cm. They reported no complications of treatment and in particular no delay of wound healing. This is perhaps not surprising as a laterally placed incision will be carried out of the radiation fields even with their large dimensions. They insist on the need for *early* radiotherapy and feel that it is of doubtful value once ectopic bone has begun to re-appear as seen by X-ray. MacLennan *et al.* (1984) reported a series of 67 hips in 58 patients. Of the 67 hips only 11 achieved a less than perfect result. Four of the eleven had incomplete excision of ectopic bone, and five started radiotherapy more than 5 days after surgery. No reason for limited success was identified in the remaining two hips.

Total body irradiation for polymyositis

'The term *polymyositis* is used to describe a group of acquired, non-suppurative inflammatory muscle disorders in which diffuse voluntary muscle weakness is the cardinal feature' (Currey, 1980). There are many different clinical pictures, but it is the muscular weakness which they have in common. In a severe case, involvement of the pharyngeal and respiratory muscles may result in inhalation of secretions, respiratory failure and death.

Treatment is by high doses of prednisolone or, if necessary, with immunosuppressive therapy using azathioprine or methotrexate. Sometimes, however, these measures are inadequate to control the disease in a potentially life-threatening situation.

Engel, Lichter and Galdi (1981) described such a case in a 40-year old woman. When the patient's condition had deteriorated so gravely that mechanical ventilation and a nasogastric tube were required, they gave total body irradiation as twice weekly doses of 15 cGy to a total of 150 cGy over 5 weeks.

Improvement began during the second week of radiotherapy and progressed until muscular strength became normal. The patient remained in good health up to the time of writing, 13 months after radiotherapy. Hubbard *et al.* (1982) reported the case of a 44-year old man who relapsed twice after treatment with prednisolone and azathioprine and failed to respond a third time. He was treated with total body irradiation using the same regimen as that described above. He, too, began to improve during the second week of radiotherapy and returned to work after 3 months. He began to show signs of relapse, however, 6 months later. During this patient's treatment further objective evidence of response was obtained by serial measurement of muscle enzyme (creatinine kinase). This fell from an initial grossly raised level to almost normal by completion of radiotherapy. Muscle biopsy showed resolution of the characteristic inflammatory infiltration.

It is interesting to note that these patients have been treated by total body as distinct from total nodal irradiation. It might be expected that in polymyositis total body irradiation could be particularly advantageous in that a direct effect on the lymphocytes infiltrating the muscles might be obtained as well as a general anti-inflammatory action. Although it has been life-saving in some of the cases treated, it has secured only temporary remission rather than permanent cure. Further work will be required to determine whether more prolonged responses can be obtained by total nodal irradiation, or whether perhaps titration of total body irradiation to find a minimum dose which will induce remission would be the preferred approach. Such a minimum dose could perhaps be repeated many times.

Radiotherapy for menorrhagia

Menorrhagia due, for example, to fibroids is normally treated by hysterectomy. However, the occasional patient is found to be unfit for this operation. Obesity and cardiac or pulmonary insufficiency are the most frequent reasons. Low-dose irradiation to induce a menopause may be considered once malignant disease, which would require a different radiotherapeutic approach, has definitely been excluded.

The technique is essentially the same as that used for ovarian irradiation in breast carcinoma. Anterior and posterior parallel opposed megavoltage fields are used to cover the area in which the ovaries lie; measurements of 12 cm high by 15 cm wide, centred in the midline about a finger's breadth above the symphysis pubis are usually adequate. The position is confirmed by a simulator film; the fields should extend from about half way down the symphysis pubis to the lower part of the sacroiliac joint and out to the sides of the pelvic cavity. In very obese patients, whose skin may move considerably in relation to the bony pelvis, fields 2 or 3 cm more in both directions may be necessary to ensure the ovaries are covered. A maximum midline dose of 1200 cGy in three daily fractions is adequate.

Treatment of keloid

Luxuriant overgrowth of fibrous tissue in the healing of skin lesions is disfiguring. It may cause discomfort including troublesome itching and even pain, and may sometimes interfere with the movement of a joint. The condition of keloid formation particularly afflicts persons with pigmented skin, but may be found in all races. Simple excision is invariably followed by recurrence, the new keloid being larger than the first. Keloid formation may be inhibited to a considerable extent by pressure, and special garments and appliances are available for this purpose. Injection of a high potency steroid drug such as triamcinolone into a keloid may cause it to regress by atrophy of the fibrous tissue.

Keloids occur after a variety of injuries to the skin, including surgery, burns and even localized sepsis. Certain areas seem particularly at risk, including the pre-sternal skin, the lobes of the ears, and the skin around joints.

Irradiation of a keloid may produce appreciable regression, but only if the fibrous tissue is actively proliferating at the time of irradiation, that is within about 6 months of the precipitating injury. Once mature non-proliferating fibrous tissue has formed no response can be expected from irradiation, but it can be used to prevent regrowth of the keloid after excision. Even then, a fully satisfactory response cannot be guaranteed, and this must be made quite clear to the patient before treatment is embarked upon.

It is probably better to aim to reduce the bulk of keloid and to accept a less than perfect result than to attempt a total excision of all keloidal tissue and run the risk of producing a new keloid larger than the first. A satisfactory compromise can usually be obtained by subtotal excision leaving a narrow rim of keloid so that all the surgery is carried out within the originally involved area. Wound closure must be obtained without tension preferably using a subcuticular suture. A suitable pressure garment may be prepared and applied immediately after surgery.

Radiotherapy for keloid

The technique used is the same whether or not surgery has been performed. When a keloid has been excised the irradiation must start as soon as possible after surgery, once the wound has healed soundly enough to tolerate radiation without dehiscence. In practice this will be at about 7–10 days after operation, when the sutures are removed. Delay may result in the formation of new keloid tissue, and an impaired result. If, however, there is any threat of parting of the wound edge, radiotherapy must be delayed for a few days and the wound supported by adhesive strips. A pressure garment at this stage may be helpful in discouraging keloid formation while awaiting irradiation.

The present author normally uses superficial X-ray therapy at 140 kV. Smedal *et al.* (1962) used a closely shielded 2.5 MeV electron beam to give a dose of 1000–1200 cGy in a single exposure. Malaker, Ellis and Paine (1976) described an ingenious technique in which a nylon tube is implanted at the time of surgery, and afterloaded with a radioactive iridium wire when healing is adequate for irradiation. A dose of 2000 cGy is delivered at a point 2.5 mm from the axis of the wire opposite its midpoint. This method is only suitable for linear keloids.

The area to be irradiated is marked on the patient's skin. No margin should be used in order to limit the amount of tissue treated to the minimum necessary; the area is kept to the scar and residual keloid and will include any suture wounds. If a subcuticular suture has been used no suture wounds will be present. The marked out area is then traced onto transparent

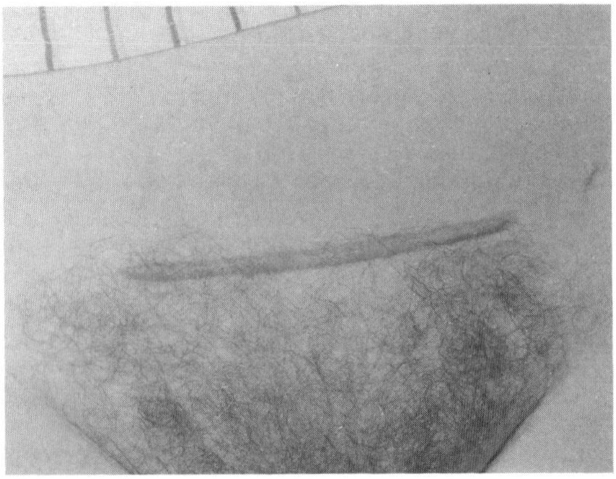

Figure 17.9 A keloidal Pfannenstiel scar

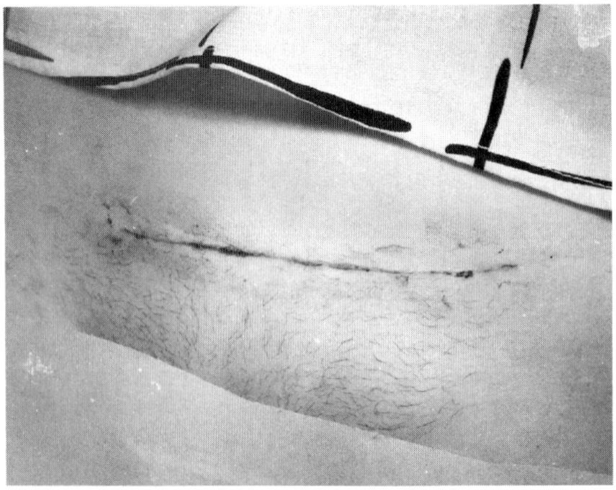

Figure 17.10 After excision of the keloid

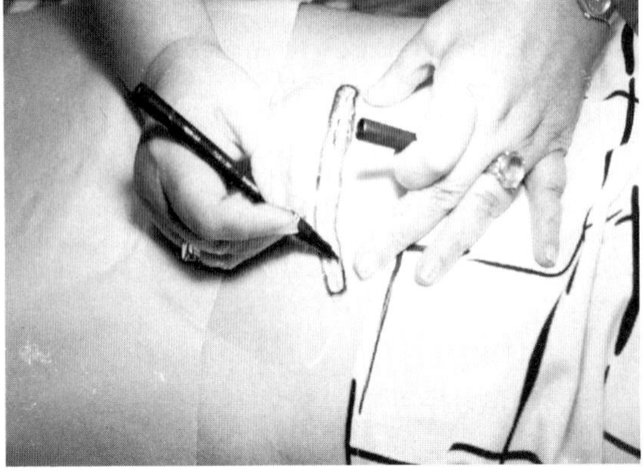

Figure 17.11 Tracing the skin marks onto cellophane

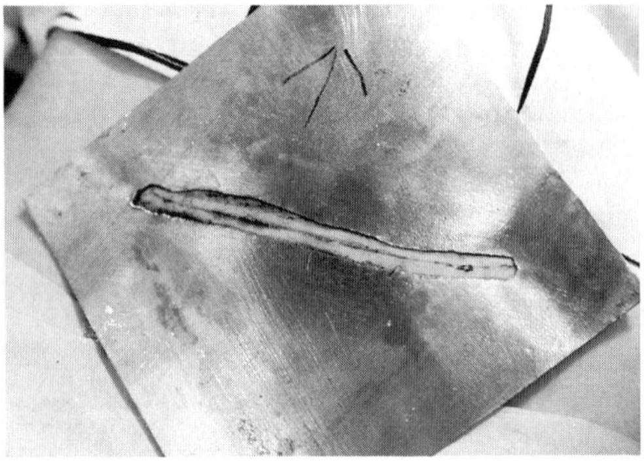

Figure 17.12 The lead cut-out in place

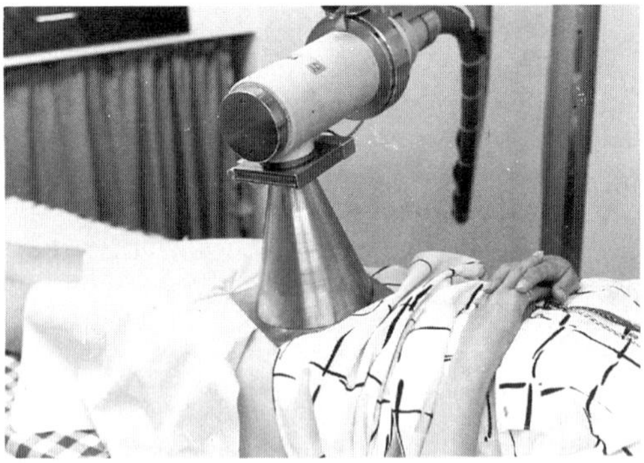

Figure 17.13 Superficial X-ray set-up for keloid

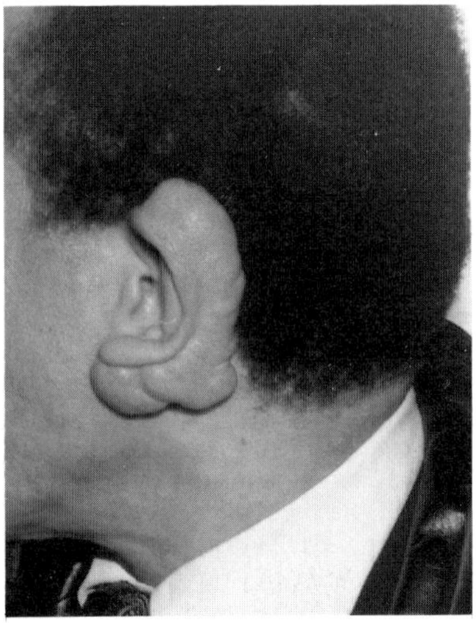

Figure 17.14 Keloid of pinna

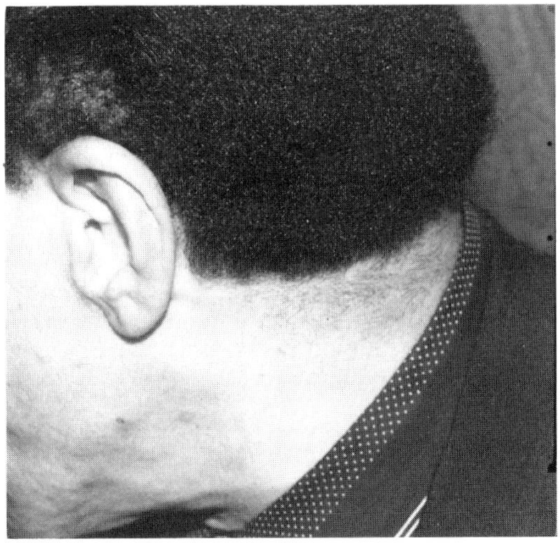

Figure 17.15 After excision and radiotherapy

material such as cellophane or scrubbed film and transferred onto thin (0.4 mm) lead; the area marked on the lead is then cut out providing a lead mask which should fit the marked skin area exactly (*Figures 17.9* to *17.15*).

Radiation dosage for keloid

The precise dose of radiation used is dependent upon individual preference, but is certainly much less than tolerance levels, and there is no need to use the sort of dose required for treatment of malignancy of the skin. Arnold and Grauer (1959) gave up to 3000 roentgens with 140 kV X-rays over about 4 weeks in up to six fractions of 500 roentgens each. The present author most frequently prescribes a dose of 2100 cGy at 140 kV in three fractions of 700 cGy at weekly intervals. It must be admitted, however, that this dose is not supported by specific experimental evidence, and may probably be varied with equal effectiveness. A single exposure of 1000 cGy seems to have been equally effective in the few cases in which it has been used.

If radiation is used in treatment of keloids in children, the possibility of induction of thyroid carcinoma, as described earlier, should be borne in mind with neck lesions. Inadvertent irradiation of epiphyses with possible distortion of growth must also be remembered when treating keloid at sites where this may occur.

Radiotherapy for plantar warts

Viral warts are common on any part of the skin, and in the vast majority of cases are readily treated by simple dermatological techniques. When they occur on the soles they may be particularly painful and are readily spread to other persons in circumstances where it is usual to walk with bare feet, as at swimming baths. In rare cases the normal treatments may fail to destroy a wart, and then it may be justfied to consider radiotherapy.

Several techniques for irradiation of plantar warts have been described, using low kV (superficial) X-rays. Grover (1965b) has reviewed these methods and has appended his own routine, which, he says 'seems to work very well'. The superficial keratin is first trimmed away, and a lead mask is prepared to treat the wart with a margin of 2 or 3 mm all round to allow for the tendency of warts to expand under the surface of the skin. A dose of 500 roentgens is recommended given once weekly to a total of four exposures. He states that the wart usually withers and disappears within 2 months of completion of radiotherapy.

It seemns worthwhile to remember the possibility of radiotherapy for the refractory plantar wart, although it is perhaps not entirely facetious to remark that during the many centuries that warts have been recognized, they have been cured by many extraordinary methods, including 'charming'!

It is of interest to note that one of the examples of results of 'malignant irradiation for benign conditions' quoted by Cannon, Randolph and Murray (1959) was an excruciatingly painful ulcer of the sole 2 years after a single X-ray treatment for a plantar wart, requiring excision and a pedicle flap repair. The X-ray treatment had apparently been given by an amateur radiotherapist!

Radiotherapy for benign conditions of the cornea

There are only two conditions of the cornea, apart from rare malignancies, in which irradiation is required with any frequency, pterygium and vascularization of a graft. It is important to avoid irradiation of the lens which might produce a cataract, and also to prevent any damage to the drainage of the aqueous which might give rise to glaucoma. At one time 50 kV contact X-rays with a special setting-up device were used to achieve the required dose to the cornea while sparing the underlying tissues, but the beta particles emitted by strontium-90 are a much more satisfactory alternative.

Strontium-90

This radionuclide decays to its daughter product yttrium-90 with a half-life of almost 20 years. Yttrium-90 itself decays with a half-life of 61 hours, and the two nuclides together form a long-lasting pure beta-particle emitter with a maximum energy of 2.2 MeV. Strontium-90 with a high specific activity and also a high degree of purity can be produced and from it an applicator suitable for use on the cornea can be constructed (*Figure 17.16*). This consists of a concave disc of a strontium-90 compound incorporated in rolled silver sheet formed to a spherical radius of 10 or 15 mm, mounted on a silver back and fitted with a handle. The surface dose-rate, measured with a scintillation probe, is provided with each applicator and must be adjusted yearly as the isotope decays. Full details of the applicators available may

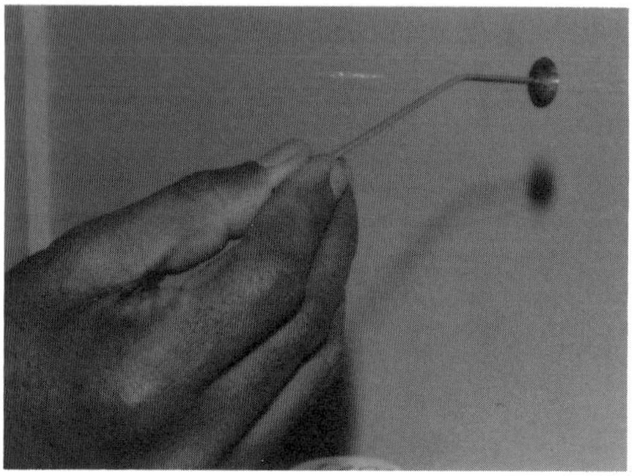

Figure 17.16 Strontium-90 ophthalmic applicator

be obtained from Amersham International (PLC) of Amersham, Buckinghamshire.

Strontium-90 produces a beta particle depth dose in tissue of 50% at about 1 mm, and 10% at about 3.3 mm, and since there is no gamma emission, protection is much simplified. The radiation is effectively absorbed in the clothing of the operator whose eyes are protected by a mask of clear perspex about 1 cm thick (*Figure 17.17*).

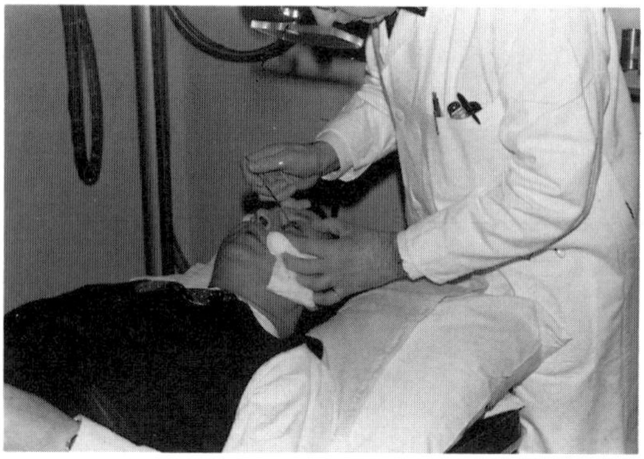

Figure 17.17 The strontium-90 applicator inserted; note the operator's eyeshield

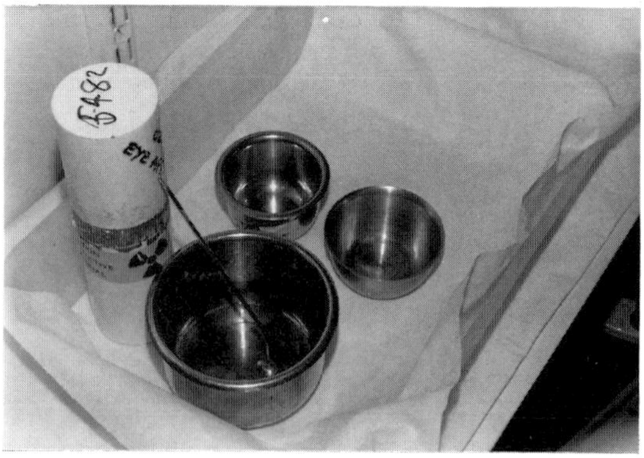

Figure 17.18 Sterilization of strontium-90 ophthalmic applicator; note lead storage case

The applicator is sterilized by immersion in a fluid such as cetrimide solution, and during sterilization the liquid itself and the walls of the containing vessel absorb the beta particles (*Figure 17.18*). The eye is anaesthetized by amethocaine or cocaine drops, the applicator is removed from the sterilizing fluid and washed in two changes of sterile saline. It is then applied to the affected area of the cornea, and held in place until the required dose of beta irradiation has been given. By means of this applicator a substantial dose of radiation can be given to the cornea, while the filtration angle lying at a depth of about 2 mm receives only about 25% of the dose at the surface of the cornea, and the sensitive posterior pole of the lens is almost unaffected.

As with keloid, the precise radiation dose to be given is a matter of personal inclination and experience. The present author uses the same dose for both pterygium and graft vascularization, that is 700 cGy at the surface of the cornea once weekly for three treatments. Lederman (1958) gave 600 roentgens once weekly for four exposures for pterygium, while Lentino *et al.* (1959) gave a dose of 2500 rep repeated after 2 weeks. In the treatment of corneal graft vascularization, Ainslie, Snelling and Ellis (1962) gave 400–500 rad repeated if necessry after a few days. They stressed the importance of irradiation as soon as vessels are noted, and observed that they regress very rapidly. It is the present author's practice to begin beta irradiation as soon as possible after excision of a pterygium, or in the case of graft vascularization as soon as the ophthalmologist has noted the appearance of vessels at the edge of the graft.

Radiotherapy for haemangioma

Congenital haemangiomas are common and may be unsightly. Naturally they cause far more distress to the parents of these infants than they do to the patients themselves. Low dose radiotherapy has been recommended in the past (Snelling and Greeves, 1955) but these lesions can confidently be expected to regress spontaneously. The present author would not advise irradiation in such cases. Large cutaneous haemangiomas of the port-wine type do not respond to radiotherapy.

Haemangiomas may occur in deep sites such as bone or central nervous system, and excision may be difficult or impossible. A tumour in the brain, spinal cord or meninges can act as a space-occupying lesion with the additional risk of bleeding. One in a vertebra may cause spinal cord compression. McWhirter and Dott (1955) emphasized that angiomas are true neoplasms of vascular tissue and as such are radiosensitive, while arteriovenous malformations consist of mature blood vessels and would not be expected to respond to radiation. These authors advise localized X-ray therapy over a period of at least 4 weeks to a total dose of 4500 roentgens or even more for a small lesion. The present author would advocate careful radiological localization of the tumour and irradiation of a volume large enough to include the whole lesion with a margin of about 1 cm all round to allow for any undetected local extension. A dose of 4500 cGy in 20 fractions over 4 weeks with megavoltage should be given. Gradual regression of the haemangioma over a period of several months may be expected (*see* Chapter 15).

Recently, a series of nine patients with vertebral haemangiomas treated by radiotherapy was reported by Faria, Schlupp and Chiminazzo (1985). All received 3000–4000 cGy by megavoltage at a rate of 200 cGy/day, 5 days/week. All had complained of pain which was completely relieved in five patients, and partially relieved in three. Only one patient failed to obtain any pain relief; the pain had been present for 12 years before treatment, and there was partial collapse of the involved vertebra.

Radiotherapy for epilation

Once employed for cosmetic purposes (Grover, 1965a), and as a common treatment for ringworm of the scalp, this is now virtually never used (but *see below*). A possible exception is for temporary removal of the hair from the skin surrounding a pilonidal sinus before excision in the hope that no further hairs will become entrapped before the wound has healed. A single exposure of 600 cGy using superficial (140 kV) X-rays is probably adequate.

Herpes zoster

Radiotherapy has often been used in the past in the hope of relieving the pain of acute zoster, or of preventing or relieving the extremely distressing post-herpetic neuralgia. Because of doubt as to whether irradiation was indeed effective in this condition, Rhys-Lewis (1965) undertook a randomized, double-blind trial. A total of 340 patients in the acute stage of herpes zoster, accumulated over a period of 10 years, was randomized to treatment or control groups. Radiotherapy was planned using orthovoltage X-rays to give an incident dose of 1000 roentgens, fractionated over 10 days, to the skin over the affected spinal segment. It was assumed that the site at which treatment was required was the ganglion, and it was estimated that the dose to the ganglion was of the order of 600 cGy. Both groups were planned and set up for treatment in exactly the same way, but in the control group the X-ray beam was not switched on. The cases were stratified according to whether symptoms were regarded as slight, moderate or severe, and in each case there was no difference in the proportion of patients improved whether or not radiation had actually been given.

Gynaecomastia

Patients with prostatic carcinoma on stilboestrol can have their painful breasts prevented with 500 cGy in three treatments (orthovoltage) given prophylactically.

Three anecdotes

Tuberculous lymph nodes

If non-caseous, such nodes consist largely of masses of lymphocytes. They may persist after adequate chemotherapy, and excision may then be considered. They may equally respond to a small dose of radiation, and the present author has seen such a patient with cervical nodes which disappeared after a dose of 500 cGy. The literature and the techniques and doses used in this condition are reviewed by Dewing (1965).

Salivary fistula

In the course of a disagreement with an acquaintance a young man received a stiletto wound to the side of the face which resulted in a salivary fistula. The constant pouring of saliva from the parotid gland was not only most unpleasant, but prevented surgical treatment of the fistula. A dose of 600 cGy over three treatments using a direct orthovoltage field succeeded in stopping the secretion of saliva for long enough to permit the fistula to be excised and the surgical wound to heal.

Hairy urethra

Another young man suffered a severe mutilation as the result of a road traffic accident, necessitating an attempt at reconstruction of his genitalia by the plastic surgeon. An excellent cosmetic if not entirely functional result was obtained, but unfortunately his new urethra became narrowed by calcareous deposits. Urethroscopy revealed that these were forming in the hairs which had grown in the skin from which the urethra had been fashioned and which had been taken from the thigh. Radiotherapy was requested in the hope of inducing epilation and thus preventing the reformation of the calcareous deposits.

After consideration of various external beam and intracavitary techniques it was felt that the only practicable method was to re-open the urethra surgically, irradiate it with superficial X-rays and then close it again. This was done; a dose of 4500 cGy in 10 daily fractions using 140 kV X-rays was given and an eminently satisfactory result was obtained. It was thought essential to use this large dose as less may have been followed by regrowth of the hairs. This case is perhaps an exception to the rule given by Dewing (1965), that there is *no* indication for permanent epilation in any benign skin disease!

References

AINSLIE, D., SNELLING, M. D. and ELLIS, R. E. (1962) Treatment of corneal vascularization by strontium-90 beta plaque. *Clinical Radiology*, **13**, 29

ALEXANDER, P. (1965) *Atomic Radiation and Life*, p. 180. Harmondsworth: Penguin

ANSELL, B. A., CROOK, A., MALLARD, J. R. and BYWATERS, E. G. L. (1963) Evaluation of colloidal gold-(Au) 198 in the treatment of persistent knee effusions. *Annals of the Rheumatic Diseases*, **22**, 435–439

ARNOLD, H. L. Jr and GRAUER, F. H. (1959) Keloids: etiology, and management by excision and intensive prophylactic radiation. *Archives of Dermatology*, **80**, 772–777

uBACCARINI, M., BOSI, A. and PAPA, G. (1980) Second malignancies in patients treated for Hodgkin's disease. *Cancer*, **46**, 1735–1739

BRADY, L. W. (1979) Radiation induced sarcomas of bone. *Skeletal Radiology*, **4**, 72–78

CALIN, A., CALIN, H. J., FIELD, E. *et al.* Double-blind controlled study of total lymphoid irradiation (TLI) in rheumatoid arthritis (RA). *Report of Heberden Society Annual General Meeting, 10/11 November 1983*, p.71

CANNON, B., RANDOLPH, J. G. and MURRAY, J. E. (1959) Malignant irradiation for benign conditions. *New England Journal of Medicine*, **260**, 197–202

CHUNG, S.M.K. and JANES, J. M. (1965) Diffuse pigmented villonodular synovitis of the hip joint. *Journal of Bone and Joint Surgery*, **47A**, 293–303

COBRAU, C. D., SHEON, R. P. and KIRSNER, A. B. (1973) Immunosuppressive drugs and acute leukemia. *Annals of Internal Medicine*, **79**, 131–132

COURT BROWN, W. M. and DOLL, R. (1965) Mortality from cancer and other causes after radiotherapy for ankylosing spondylitis. *British Medical Journal*, **2**, 1327–1332

COVENTRY, M. B. and SCANLON, P. W. (1981) The use of radiation to discourage ectopic bone. *Journal of Bone and Joint Surgery*, **63A**, 201–208

CURREY, H. L. F.(1975) Painful heel. In *An Introduction to Clinical Rheumatology*, edited by M. Mason, pp. 244–246. London: Pitman Medical

CURREY, H. L. F. (1980) Polymyositis and dermatomyositis. In *Mason and Currey's Clinical Rheumatology*, edited by H. L. F. Currey, pp. 170–180. Tunbridge Wells: Pitman Medical

DEWING, S. B. (ed) (1965) Tuberculosis. In *Radiotherapy of Benign Disease*, pp. 38–39. Springfield: Thomas

ENGEL, W. K., LICHTER, A. S. and GALDI, A. P. (1981) Polymyositis: remarkable response to total body irradiation (letter). *Lancet*, **1**, 568

FARIA, S. L., SCHLUPP, W. R. and CHIMINAZZO, H. (1985) Radiotherapy in the treatment of vertebral hemangiomas. *International Journal of Radiation Oncology, Biology and Physics*. **11**, 387–390

FAVUS, M. J., SCHNEIDER, A. B., STACHURA, M. E. *et al.* (1976) Thyroid cancer occurring as a late consequence of head-and-neck irradiation. *New England Journal of Medicine*, **294**,1019–1025

FUKS, Z., STROBER, S., BOBROVE, A. M., SASAZUKI, T., McMICHAEL, A. and KAPLAN, H. S. (1976) Long-term effects of radiation on T and B lymphocytes in peripheral blood of patients with Hodgkin's disease. *Journal of Clinical Investigation*, **58**, 803–814

GLICKSMAN, A. S. and TOKER, C. (1976) Osteogenic sarcoma following radiotherapy for bursitis. *The Mount Sinai Journal of Medicine*, **43**, 163–167

GREENFIELD, M. M. and WALLACE, K. M. (1950) Pigmented villonodular synovitis. *Radiology*, **54**, 350–356

GROVER, R. W. (1965a) Disease of the hair and scalp. In *Radiotherapy of Benign Disease* edited by S. B. Dewing. pp. 196–197. Springfield: Thomas

GROVER, R W. (1965b) Viral warts. *Ibid*, pp. 220–222

GUMPEL, J. M. and ROLES, N. C. A. (1975). A controlled trial of intra-articular radiocolloids versus synovectomy in persistent synovitis. *Lancet,* **1**, 488–489

GUMPEL, J. M., WILLIAMS, E. D. and GLASS, H. I. (1973) Use of yttrium-90 in persistent synovitis of the knee. *Annals of the Rheumatic Diseases*, **32**, 223–227

HARISDANGKUL, V., CHEN, C. J., LEWIS, R. E. and CRUSE, J. M. (1982) Relapsing polychondritis: immunohistochemical evidence suggestive of an autoimmune disease. *Internal Medicine*, **3**, 56–65

HART, F. D. (1961) A critical survey of the value of radiotherapy in the treatment of ankylosing spondylitis. *Clinical Radiology*, **12**, 130–131

HUBBARD, W. N., WALPORT, M. J., HALNAN, K. E., BEANEY, R. P. and HUGHES, G. R. V. (1982) Remission from polymyositis after total body irradiation. *British Medical Journal*, **284**, 1915–1916

KAPLAN, H. S. (1980) *Hodgkin's Disease*, 2nd edn, pp. 366–441. Cambridge, Massachusetts: Harvard University Press

KIM, J. H., CHU, F. C., WOODARD, H. Q., MELAMED, M. R., HUVOS, A. and CANTIN, J. (1978) Radiation-induced soft-tissue and bone sarcoma. *Radiology*, **129**, 501–508

KOTZIN, B. L., STROBER, S., ENGLEMAN, E. G. *et al.*

(1981) Treatment of intractable rheumatoid arthritis with total lymphoid irradiation. *New England Journal of Medicine*, **305**, 969-975

LEDERMAN, M. (1958) Radiotherapy of nonmalignant diseases of the eye. In *Progress in Radiation Therapy*, edited by F. Bushke, pp. 256–271. New York: Grune and Stratton

LENTINO, W., ZARET, M. M., ROSSIGNOL, B. and RUBENFELD, S. (1959) Treatment of pterygium by surgery followed by beta radiation. *American Journal of Roentgenology, Radium Therapy and Nuclear Medicine*, **81**, 93–98

LOVE, R. R. and SOWA, J. M. (1975) Myelomonocytic leukemia following cyclophosphamide therapy of rheumatoid arthritis. *Annals of Rheumatic Diseases,* **34**, 534–535

MacLENNAN, I., KEYS, H. M., EVARTS, C. M. and RUBIN, P. (1984) Usefulness of postoperative hip irradiation in the prevention of heterotopic bone formation in a high risk group of patients. *International Journal of Radiation Oncology, Biology and Physics*, **10**, 49–53

McWHIRTER, R. and DOTT, N. M. (1955) Tumours of the brain and spinal cord. In *British Practice in Radiotherapy*, edited by E. Rock Carling, B. W. Windeyer and D. W. Smithers, pp. 336–346. London: Butterworths

MALAKER, K., ELLIS, F. and PAINE, C. H. (1976) Keloid scars: a new method of treatment combining surgery with interstitial radiotherapy. *Clinical Radiology*, **27**, 179–183

MANTELL, B. S. (1978) Radiotherapy for painful heel syndrome. *British Medical Journal*, **2**, 90–91

MILONE, F. P. and COPELAND, M. M. (1961) Calcific tendinitis of the shoulder joint. *American Journal of Roentgenology, Radium Therapy and Nuclear Medicine*, **85**, 901–913

MORRISON, R. (1955) Chronic rheumatic diseases. In *British Practice in Radiotherapy*, edited by E. Rock Carling, B. W. Windeyer and D. W. Smithers, pp. 494–500. London: Butterworths

RHYS-LEWIS, R. D. S. (1965) Radiotherapy in herpes zoster. *Lancet*, **2**, 102–104

SCOTT, G. (1939) *Wide Field X-ray Treatment*, pp. 61–64. London: Newnes

SHARP, J. and EASSON, E. C. (1954) Deep X-ray therapy in spondylitis. *British Medical Journal*, **1**, 619–623

SMEDAL, M. I., JOHNSON, D. O., SALZMAN, F. A., TRUMP, J. G. and WRIGHT, K. A. (1962) Ten year experience with low megavolt electron therapy. *American Journal of Roentgenology, Radium Therapy and Nuclear Medicine*, **88**, 215–228

SMITH, P. G. and DOLL, R. (1982) Mortality among patients with ankylosing spondylitis after a single treatment course with x-rays. *British Medical Journal*, **284**, 449–460

SNELLING, M. D. and GREEVES, R. A. (1955) Diseases of the eye. In *British Practice in Radiotherapy*, edited by E. Rock Carling, B. W. Windeyer and D. W. Smithers, p. 355. London: Butterworths

STEFFEN, C., MULLER, Ch., STELLAMOR, K. and ZEITLHOFER, J. (1982) Influence of X-ray treatment on antigen-induced experimental arthritis. *Annals of the Rheumatic Diseases*, **41**, 532–537

STEINER, G. C. (1964) Postradiation sarcoma of bone. *Cancer*, **18**, 603–612

STROBER, S., FIELD, E. M., KOTZIN, B. L. *et al.* (1983) Treatment of intractable rheumatoid arthritis with total lymphoid irradiation (TLI): immunological and clinical changes. *Radiotherapy and Oncology*, **1**, 43–52

18

The management of patients: a radiographer's viewpoint

Pauline Curtis

The dictionary defines 'malignant' as 'virulent, dangerous to life, heinous, unpropitious, having extreme malevolence'; such indeed is malignant disease. While progress in oncology continues to pursue all the possibilities of overcoming the disease, with advances in some areas, it can still retain an unpredictable nature. Radiotherapy departments bring together all the expertise of the team of radiotherapists, radiographers, physioists, mould room and nursing staff to give patients with malignant disease the best, most effective treatment. Undeniably radiotherapy is teamwork, but is there an awareness that the team is incompolete without the patients themselves? The fight against their life-threatening condition muist not only *centre around* that person but also *involve* them as individuals. Any member of the team having person contact with patients must see them, not as tumours in patients but as people coping with an abnormality. What is their view of the methods that are to be used? How can they be helped towards a well-informed and positive attitude to the treatment?

It may help to think about individuals before they become patients and to consider the public image of radiotherapy in the mind of the community, of which they are part. That image has developed over decades of myths and misconception; however, it cannot be denied that radiotherapy is frequently used as a useful tool in the palliative treatment of terminal cancer and the gruelling nature of many radical courses of radiotherapy is well-known. People are therefore often abserved by the community to die following a course of radiotherapy or to undergo considerable discomfort during the period of the treatment. The benefits of radiotherapy are less well publicized; beyond the confines of the radiotherapy department there are few allies who will vouch for its efficacy, even amongst the rest of the medical fraternity. The team has a responsibility to help correct this view wherever suitable opportunities present; community health workers and staff from other parts of the hospital team should always be welcomed to the department as much patient anxiety can be dispelled at an early stage by educating those in contact with patients.

This chapter will follow an individual from the time when he or she is still merely a member of the community, through the treatment to the follow-up period, highlighting the difficulties experienced throughout this time and showing how the person may be helped to bear them.

For some people the most difficult part of all is to share the knowledge of an abnormal sign, especially if it is not causing physical distress. Another period of great stress comes during the staging of the disease, which may be protracted; the patient has no definite answers to his questions and will only be able to speculate. At this time there may be a re-shuffle within the family circle and as a result the patient may find himself either supported or perhaps smothered by his relatives.

It is well to remember that the patient has already been through much disquiet before he is referred to the radiotherapy department.

Talking and listening

When the 'work-up' period of staging of the disease is completed, it is possible for the overall treatment policy to be discussed with the patient.

Who should conduct the interview is somewhat of a dilemma. The consultant is the person who is able to give the most authoritative overall view, but registrars need to gain experience in this area. The patient may wish to include his spouse at this interview or another person who is close to him. This has the advantage that two people are absorbing the information and therefore more is likely to be taken in. Patients and their families then know as much as one another so that no suspicion exists about information withheld. Telling a patient the nature and extent of his illness before a large cast of people on a ward round must never be allowed to happen.

The best place for the talk is in a familiar environment to the patient, such as the peripheral clinic at the patient's local hospital, or in the ward of the hospital with which the patient has become very familiar during the time of pre-treatment surgery or investigations. This situation is not always possible and sometimes the interview has to be conducted within the radiotherapy department.

The patient will find it easier to believe that he is being told the full truth and that the doctor is truly caring about his reaction to it, if they are sitting down together and looking at one another. The scheme of treatment can then be outlined and the patient briefly acquainted with any problems which might occur as a result of that treatment. At this stage the patient may not be able wholly to digest the import of what he is being told. He may advance all kinds of reasons why it would be difficult for him to have such treatment; reasons which can be fairly easily surmounted after some discussion at home. If there are difficulties, such as totally dependent handicapped relatives, the social worker may need to be involved.

An appointment for the relevant planning session is given, although no starting date for the treatment course can usually be given at this stage, except in cases of extreme clinical emergency. The starting date is dependent on many factors and to make promises to the patient that cannot be kept because of existing workloads, will undermine his confidence in the team from the outset.

Communications

These play a vital part in winning the understanding and cooperation of the patient; some aspects are considered here.

Information given out does not necessarily equal information received; many factors, especially anxiety, may prevent assimilation. It is best to listen carefully and find out where the patient's knowledge has taken him before giving further information. It may even be necessary to disabuse before informing. It is advisable not to assume when talking to medical or paramedical personnel who have become patients, that they already possess the knowledge they need. Hindrances to communication, in addition to fear and anxiety, may include the following: the nature of the disease, such as cerebral metastases; the drug status, for example the patient who is taken off thyroid drugs prior to an ^{131}I dose; lack of English (if the patient has no interpreter, it may be possible to find one within the hospital; most hospitals keep a list of bilingual speakers, but where possible advance notice of the time of the patient's appointment should be given to the potential interpreter). Deafness or major visual defects such as bilateral cataracts may cause difficulty. Children raise a separate problem and communications must be simplified. Disbelief or distrust may be a bar to 'hearing'; in extreme cases it may be necessary to give patients their notes to read before they believe that nothing has been held back from them. Finally, a lower than average level of intelligence or standard of education may lead to problems.

It is necessary to be sure that the patient knows that channels of communication are always open. The inclusion in the team of a cancer counsellor (often a specially trained nurse) means that those patients who need further time spent with them may have a chance to air their anxieties fully. Some patients find it difficult to ask questions of those who are in control of their treatment, as to do so seems to them to be implying criticism. General practitioners need to be informed briefly at the beginning of a course what is happening to the patient and under whose care they are, so that problems arising at night or at the weekend can be met with some knowledge of what is happening or who to contact in an emergency.

Those who listen hear that the patient is worried and sometimes hear the deeper worries implied, but not expressed, in questions they ask. Some of those most frequently heard will now be considered.

How does radiation work?; perhaps this is really asking *Does it work? Why does it not affect the other tissue?* is another common query. It is easy to sympathize with the patient asking these questions since, if a surgical approach is taken, the patient feels disease has been eradicated, whereas the concept of radiotherapy is difficult to comprehend. Patients are usually satisfied with the answer that time and effort are spent to focus only on the area in question and that the treatment is given over a period of time in small doses so that healthy tissue recovers while malignant cells do not recover so completely and are eventually eradicated. This normally provides a lead-in to an explanation about why treatment cannot be given in a single fraction. There may be worry about radiation-induced malignancy implied in this last question. This is best answered by the clinician, who may be asked by the patient to give actual figures relating to this possibility, and will have to explain the risks of having and *not* having the recommended treatment.

Will I lose my hair? is another question. Others include, *Will I be sick? Will I be all right to travel (on my own)? Will I be all right to drive myself?* These are all questions reflecting information picked up by the patients from other people. It is here that some questioning of their 'treatment knowledge' and disabusing them of erroneous facts can help. It is a good opportunity for showing them that radiotherapy departments treat many types and sites of malignant disease, giving rise to differing side-effects.

Adjuvant chemotherapy treatments, which the patient may also undergo, should be considered before denying that hair loss will occur. Epilation doses from external beam therapy, including beards, moustaches and eyebrows, should be considered and also care taken to warn patients of depilation from exit doses. Patients receiving treatment to their anterior neck may become very alarmed when a 'short back and sides' hairline emerges. In some departments each patient may be asked to sign a consent form in any cases where hair loss is expected.

Will I be sick? Will I be all right to travel (on my own)? Often these questions reflect a worry about the indignity of vomiting or experiencing frequency or urgency of micturition or acute diarrhoea in a public place. On the subject of feeling sick it is important to explain the difference between the likelihood of feeling nauseated and actually vomiting. While reassuring most patients that they are unlikely to experience actual vomiting, they should be informed that if they do, then antiemetics taken regularly will nearly always control this; it seems to the present author foolish to promise patients that they will not feel nauseated, because experience shows that a great many do. Some patients with an acute fear of vomiting may best be given a prescription for antiemetics to be taken prophylactically in order to give them a sense of security. Those having large volumes irradiated or extensive abdominal fields should certainly be given a prescription in advance of the start of treatment.

It is perhaps comforting for the patient to know that, if frequency of micturition and diarrhoea are likely to occur, these symptoms are ones which will not come upon them suddenly and that they will be specially advised with regard to diet and how to treat specific symptoms when they occur.

Patients may be experiencing frequency of micturition or dysuria before the start of treatment because of large bladder tumours. It is only fair to point out that the good effect of the treatment will take a considerable period of time, and symptoms may get worse during that period with the combined effect of disease and reaction from treatment. Lack of sleep is also a factor when the patient experiences much frequency, and a combination of tiredness, depression and discomfort may suggest that this patient needs to be hospitalized for the duration of treatment. Most patients can tolerate this — especially with the thought of going home for the weekend if they feel sufficiently well. For those having the added discomfort of incontinence some practical appliance may need to be found.

Will I be all right to travel? can imply those fears already mentioned, but also perhaps the fear of feeling dizzy or faint. This can usually be dispelled as groundless, with due regard to the patient's medical history, e.g. fits. Some patients seem to welcome the idea of being accompanied on the *first* treatment visit to have moral support, although problems often arise regarding fares if two people are travelling regularly. Unfortunately, the ambulance service in the UK is too taxed to permit escorts except for those patients whose medical condition really demands it. For some people the answer that they will be fit to travel alone is a welcome relief, and may get them away from an over-protective family. Children under 14 should always have an escort. It is vital to remember what a problem financial considerations can be for the patient; it is often his paramount concern. Attempts should be made to arrange times to suit old age pensioners' (OAP) passes, to advise patients regarding season tickets, to fit in with off-peak travel where possible, and to refer to a social worker when money is a major problem. Patients in receipt of supplementary benefit may automatically reclaim fares merely by presenting attendance slips at the appropriate office. Prolonged treatment courses can impose a heavy financial burden on some patients' budgets; often a request for hospital transport arises solely out of these constraints.

Radiotherapy departments may be in areas many miles from the patient's home. If the catchment area is really wide, hostel accommodation can usually be provided. Some journeys are so far that ambulance/train/ambulance service is more practical and economical. It must be noted that referral patterns in some areas of the British Isles are very bizarre. While appreciating that general practitioners and referring consultants are trying to get the best treatment possible for their patients and wanting to use known and trusted colleagues, long-distance referrals often make little sense, except if the disease is rare and specialist expertise and/or equipment is required. Patients living in rural areas faced with the metropolis often fear lack of familiarity with their surroundings. Every effort should be made to send helpful travel information and maps when giving patients initial appointments at the department.

May I drive myself? When answering this query it is well to take into account the effect of any antiemetics and analgesia.

Should I rest? A counsellor seeing many patients undergoing radiotherapy notes that tiredness is a *very* common factor. With some, of course, there is the hassle of unaccustomed travel to be added to the effect of treatment, and elderly patients often talk of needing a nap to get over tiredness on their return home. Those planning to continue working during treatment should be advised not to overtax themselves in their out-of-work hours, especially if treatment follows a spell of hospitalization and surgery. It is important also to make it absolutely clear that tiredness does not mean that the disease is advancing. It may be best to have several treatments before returning to work, to assess the amount of energy the patient has to spare.

Physical reactions such as a low blood count contribute to the tiredness and any depression will increase this; postoperative depression following major surgery often coincides with the course of radiotherapy. Patients must be warned that their tiredness will not vanish immediately on finishing the treatment.

Can I have a drink? The answer in most cases would be continue as normal, except that neat spirits are not advisable, especially for those having treatment involving the upper alimentary and respiratory tracts. In some cases patients rely on a tot of something to get them off to sleep, which is to be encouraged, and others may benefit from starting to use an aperitif before meals to enhance their appetite. Those with a tendency to alcoholism do not usually ask the question!

May I wash? or more commonly *I know I musn't wash!* — spoken with varying degrees of gloom but usually with a complete willingness to comply. It is best to dispel the gloom and capitalize on the willingness, because the short answer to such a question is, 'yes you may certainly wash, bathe and shower or wash your hair, but with certain modifications which we will tell you about when more has been decided regarding the treatment you will receive.' Guidelines regarding these aspects will be discussed later.

What is this treatment? Is this radium treatment? Usually questions asked by older people stem from the time when internal treatments and external beam units were both carried out using radium which must have made a big public impact; since then the advance towards megavoltage equipment seems to have had much less of an impact on the public. The patient is best disabused of the 'radium' concept and told that facilities have improved enormously since it was first used. *What is this treatment?* implies that the patient is aware of the radioactive element in the treatment and is more familiar with the concept of radioactivity as potentially dangerous, which is quite natural, considering that the media often focus our attention on hazards associated with nuclear power stations and the horror of nuclear weapons. The present author finds it helpful to start from the patient's own experience of having had diagnostic radiographs taken (it is unusual to find anyone who has never had one), they are aware of the beneficial use of X-rays and will have noted the precautions taken, thus they can be introduced to the use of ionizing radiations for treatment by scaling up the expectation of size of machines, length of exposure time and more remote control of exposures by operating staff.

Some people will undoubtedly fear over-exposure to treatment, i.e. being given an incorrect dose. A quietly confident manner of approach by all members of the team should help to dispel this. Preparation of patients regarding expected side-effects is essential so that reactions are not attributed to over-treatment. Quite naturally patients can be worried by the idea of the machines delivering the dose incorrectly. Two pieces of information to minimize this fear are that the machine is never left unattended by the radiographer and that by law all machines must be fitted with double-dosimetry panels, which means that there are two fail–safe mechanisms.

Will I be radioactive? May I mix with other people? may suggest that the patient has come into contact with someone who has undergone therapy with ^{131}I or low dose rate intracavitary or interstitial treatments. It is normally quite a simple matter to assure those patients receiving external beam treatments that they will not be radioactive, but sometimes this worry persists. In one instance a family telephoned a department of radiotherapy some years after a patient had finished treatment to ask if his clothes could be safely given away.

Specific details are given to patients who are to have ^{131}I or intracavitary and/or interstitial treatments regarding visiting (*see* Chapters 9 and 16), but it is important to underline the enormous help it is for such patients to see the staff team confidently caring for them with due regard to safety rules but without fear. (Local rules for the care of such patients should always be available and should cover all eventualities.) It is important also to emphasize how alone a patient can feel in these circumstances and frequent visits, albeit short ones, by all staff who are involved with the care of that patient, to relieve their isolated state, are often welcomed, a two-way intercom system will help to relieve that isolation. Ward rounds all too frequently neglect such patients and confine their attention to the notes and not to the patients themselves who have been counting on a chance to discuss aspects of their treatment.

Is it cancer? This question has been left to the end of this section because it is usually left to the tailpiece of the conversation and is often asked by the patient of the most junior person, such as a student radiographer or nurse. Perhaps the reader wonders why this question has not already been dealt with in the initial interview. The fact is the patient asks this question when he or she feels ready for the answer and not before; alternatively, having been told that they have a malignancy, the patients may now be hoping for a denial. It may have been discussed at the onset, but in many cases the question will be asked somewhere during the progress through treatment and, in some cases, will never be asked at all. Let those who dread being asked the question take heart and rather find it an encouraging sign. First, the patient is progressing along his path and has reached the point where he feels able to face the answer which he probably strongly suspects is 'Yes, you do have a type of cancer', and second, the management of the patient when he is aware of his disease usually becomes easier, although some patients do subsequently set off on journeys of exploration in addition to conventional forms of treatment, to ensure a cure for themselves. These can be complementary to the conventional treatment or frankly detrimental to the patient and teams should be aware of such holistic approaches and be able to advise patients who seek supplementary or alternative forms of help.

If, as often happens, a radiographer or student radiographer is asked the direct question by a patient, that person needs to use the opening to bring the doctor and patient together as soon as possible, so that the opportunity does not evaporate. However, the temptation to disappear like a startled rabbit to look for the doctor concerned should be resisted at all costs! Gently turning the questioning to the patient to ask what he has learned so far is helpful, as it assists the patient to clarify the facts in his own mind. When passed on to the clinician it gives a starting point for revealing the fuller story.

It may be worth mentioning two difficulties here. The first is that malignant diseases are lumped together by the majority of the general public, so that patients need to understand that the spectrum of diseases and prognoses is very wide. The other is the distinction between contained primary disease and widespread disseminated disease; a patient may have gleaned many pieces of information from other people's experience, being party to only some of the story (as when someone hears only one side of a telephone conversation). But they will not be able to distinguish between radical and palliative courses and will interpret further courses of treatment as a failure of the first.

It is well to remember that the answer 'yes' to the question *Has it spread?* coming after a radical treatment has already been accomplished, can be more devastating for a patient than the original diagnosis. Often the anguish of this news is underestimated. Whether the treatment is radical or palliative, the patient and the radiotherapy team have goals which they are striving towards, be they cure or improved quality of life. Hope in both situations is an essential ingredient. Hope is part of the treatment.

Do you see many cases like this? Will I be cured? If the patient is not aware of his diagnosis these questions may reflect a groping towards a request for that knowledge. The opportunity for a quiet talk with the clinician may be what is required, i.e. the radiographer may ask if the patient would like to talk to the doctor again for a few minutes. However, *Do you see many cases like this?* taken at face value raises the dilemma — does it help the patient to continue to fall into that special category in which they may have been placed by their friends and family as a result of their illness, or will they feel strengthened by the knowledge that this situation has been met before and conquered. It is possible to reconcile these aspects when a patient sees that the treatment is individually tailored to him by taking time and trouble at the planning stage. It is usually possible to reassure the person that many cases of this type have been dealt with successfully. Patients may be referred to a national centre for treatments of some rarer types of tumour and the reason for this explained to them.

Will I be cured? or sometimes *How will they know if I'm cured?* Some patients need a mathematical probability of cure as an answer to this. For some, assurance that the treatment scheme is extremely effective in most cases, that progress will be monitored closely and further problems tackled if they do arise, is sufficient.

Having spent a good deal of time thinking about the best way of achieving the informed trust of the patient, consideration must be given as to how best the radiotherapy treatment can be given.

Planning

Ideally there should be a weekly session set aside by the consultant radiotherapist and the members of the team for the planning of the patient's treatment. There can be no substitute for a good interactive session with the patient, doctors and radiographers working out together many aspects both technical and practical; there will be much discussion between all three groups, consulting the physics department where necessary. It may also include the patient's family. It will certainly provide a good teaching forum for radiotherapists in training and student radiographers. The radiotherapists who saw the patient initially should try to be present at the planning stage to provide continuity and to introduce other members of the team. If the patient attends as an outpatient and is attending the radiotherapy centre for the first time, he may benefit from being sent helpful details concerning the locality, bus and train routes and parking facilities (some local car parks give special consideration to patients). If an inpatient, it is well to telephone the ward to liaise regarding a suitable time to dovetail with other items in the patient's programme and with his analgesia, if necessary; to check if all the information is available; to see how fit the patient is with due regard to height of couches and thus the most suitable mode of transport for him, and finally how long the patient will remain in the ward before discharge.

Guidelines for the planning session

All the staging data should be available; it can cause anxiety for the patient and extra work for all staff if decisions are made without the full information and changes are made later. Information regarding any previous treatment should also be to hand.

Decisions should be made on the following:

(1) Is it a radical or palliative treatment?
(2) Is the patient to be entered in a clinical trial; if so, are any extra tests required?
(3) Is external beam irradiation to be used alone or in combination with:
    (a) radiosensitizers, e.g. oxygen therapy, hypothermia, drugs
    (b) interstitial treatment, e.g. iridium wire implant to a residual breast mass
    (c) intracavitary treatment, e.g. gynaecological insertions
    (d) chemotherapy
    (e) surgery.

Consideration should be given to the following long-term effects, many of which will be irreversible and may need to be discussed with the patient:

(1) Induced menopause — does the patient understand that her periods will not cease immediately and that contraceptive precautions may therefore need to be continued?
(2) Sterility — is sperm banking required?
(3) Growth stunting, which will need to be discussed with the parents of the child
(4) Epilation — a wig may be ordered when the hair is still present
(5) The possible need for replacement hormones when a change in endocrine status occurs after treatment to endocrine glands.

The patient may need time to consider these effects, before giving verbal or written consent, depending on the policy of the department, particularly in relation to an induced menopause.

The type of radiation should be considered with due regard to:

(1) The tissue to be treated
(2) The depth of lesion within the patient, noting also whether there is any involvement of the skin or superficial areas
(3) The surrounding tissue and adjacent radiosensitive structures.

A choice between photons, neutrons and electrons needs to be made. Perhaps all these facilities may not be available at every centre and the patient may need to be referred elsewhere if there is a conviction that this treatment is proven to be effective in a particular disease. Finally, the total dose should be stated along with the fractionation to be used.

Technique

The position of the patient is extremely important, perhaps to ease an adjacent organ out of the way, e.g. tilting the chin when treating the parotid reduces the problems of eye dosage, using a bite block to position the tongue and lower jaw when treating the antrum, reduces soreness of the mouth.

Immobilization devices may be needed to hold the patient in the treatment position. There are many other ways of reproducing these positions and instructions for these should be recorded on the treatment sheet.

Localizing imaging techniques

There is a wide range now available, including simulators, CT facilities, real-time ultrasound scanners and xeroradiography; radiotherapists and therapy radiographers find it more useful than ever to interact with their diagnostic counterparts where there is access to these types of equipment. The urgency of starting treatment should take into account clinical need, the preparation necessary, and the existing machine workloads. An assessment of the patient's condition before treatment, the side-effects expected and therefore the best advice to patients regarding working, travelling and admission to hospital or a hostel (for all or some of the course) should also be considered. The relevant recommendations the patient needs, e.g. skin and dietary care, should be discussed.

This list has been arranged, as far as possible, in a chronological order. The number of items appears very lengthy but a glance will show that, if the first item is prepared well in advance for all patients expected at a session, many of the early items may be decided before the session begins, resulting in both the radiotherapist and the radiographer knowing the treatment policy. This will give patients a greater sense of security as they will know from the outset of their visit that thought has already been put into their treatment. Another advantage of this pre-planning is that it avoids alarming technical discussion taking place in the presence of the patient; it is of course impossible to eliminate this entirely and radiographers need to try to interpret for the patient any jargon that could be misconstrued, e.g. 'I think we'll do (CT) cuts here, here and here'! Pre-planning also means that other members of the team, mould room staff, physics department staff, nurses and treatment unit radiographers may be alerted and plan their programmes accordingly, which will maximize the amount achieved for the patient in one visit.

A good understanding by each section of the team regarding the work of the others is desirable to achieve smooth running of a department. While some departments maintain a static group of radiographers within the planning area, others prefer to rotate some or all of their staff through all the treatment units and the planning area, thus keeping everyone *au fait* with recent developments and ensuring that no impractical treatments are planned. Radiographers find it valuable to see the rationale behind the treatments which they are called on to carry out, whether it be by this method of staff rotation or in departmental meetings where non-routine cases are discussed.

Some thought with regard to mould room staffing is required. The work in this section demands a combination of talents and skills with regard to patient care, engineering ingenuity and inventiveness together with a background knowledge of radiotherapy. Staff are recruited to mould rooms from many different backgrounds. Radiographers who possess the necessary engineering skills or are willing to obtain them, may prove ideal. In some larger departments, radiographers make up part of the mould room team, possibly rotating through this area as well as to other areas of the department.

The patient in the mould room

It is often useful to make an individually moulded immobilization device for patients as definitive plastic head and neck shells in particular reduce the time needed to set-up the patient in the treatment position and removes the onus from the patient of remaining in that position unaided. It also negates the need for localizing marks or tattoos to be applied directly to the patient's skin. A careful explanation of these advantages should be given to the patient before he goes to the mould room (*see* Chapter 12).

It is particularly vital, if an impression is needed, that the patient understands fully what will happen in order to prevent panicking when impression material is used on the face. For non-English speakers an interpreter should be found or a written explanation given in the patient's own language. Centres treating many children often use a book with photographs of the process or videos to show to the patients and their families beforehand. Sometimes the children may watch the process happening to another child and be allowed to help with that. Children can have shells made for them, one for treatment and one which may be decorated by themselves and later taken home to 'show off'.

Naturally the fear uppermost in most patients' minds, when impression material is to be used on the face, is that of being unable to breathe during the process and those with a blocked nose may need a hollow bite-block to preserve a good airway.

During the impression-taking those having their eyes covered must be made aware that they have not been left alone.

When the immobilization device is fitted, it should be attached to a base plate which has a quick-release mechanism and the patient should be shown that it takes only seconds to remove them from the shell.

Often the patient appears to relax in the environment of the mould room where all is done for and to them. They have finished entering into the dialogue regarding the treatment programme and feel that things are under way. Many find the processes used there intriguing and may offer good advice regarding new gadgets and inventions drawn from their own work experience.

Special instructions

Recommendations to patients regarding any special care during treatment are best given in written form but should always be reinforced verbally by the radiographer and/or the radiotherapist, involving other family members in the discussion if this seems appropriate. The radiographer will explain:

(1) The reactions expected
(2) When they may be expected, i.e. delay of onset but continuing to reach their peak some time after cessation of treatment visits
(3) How they may be minimized.

General guidelines are offered here regarding advice to patients to help them to minimize skin, mouth and pelvic reactions, but most departments will have their own sets of instructions and new staff are advised to discover the policy of their new workplace.

Skin care

Advice should be given when the following information is available:

(1) Beam to be used, *either* superficial, orthovoltage X-rays, electrons or neutrons from low energy generators *or* megavoltage, neutrons from high energy generators
(2) Dose and fractionation
(3) Area to be treated
(4) Any previous treatment to this area, if so, what beam was used?
(5) If megavoltage is to be used, is any part of the area to have 'build-up' applied to counteract the skin sparing effect
(6) Type of skin. (Fair, or is the patient red-headed as both are prone to excessive reaction)
(7) Technique to be used so that exit areas may be known
(8) Use of sensitizers, if any.

Guidelines may be formulated under the following headings.

Area concerned

The patient may wash normally except in the area indicated to them by the radiographer, who will include the exit doses in that description, if thought necessary.

Cleansing

Cleansing of the area is desirable to keep it free of infection but with the following modifications:

(1) Warm water should be used, rather than hot
(2) No soap or shampoo should be used, apart from those suitable for babies
(3) The patients should endeavour not to eradicate any skin marks
(4) No talcum, antiperspirant, after shave or proprietary preparations, e.g. Savlon, Nivea. Many patients will have found these preparations panaceas in the past and will find it hard to desist from rushing to the bathroom cabinet for their old friend
(5) Lotions or ointments will be prescribed by the department staff if and when necessary.

Friction

Friction should be avoided in the following manner:

(1) Bathing gently with warm water and patting area dry with a soft towel
(2) No tight clothing should be worn in the treated region; stiff shirt collars and corsets are no longer worn but tight jeans can prove very abrasive and knickers with leg elastic should be discouraged where inguinal reactions might be expected. Patients having the breast treated should be encouraged to wear a soft brassière that is neither boned nor made of man-made fibres; better still, if the patient is comfortable without wearing one at all, is to leave this garment off altogether. It is not advisable to wear a breast prosthesis until treatment is finished and any reaction subsided. Many patients find it comfortable to wear a cotton tee-shirt next to the skin when having the breast treated as it provides the double function of an absorbent covering and protection for other clothing from skin marks
(3) Male patients receiving treatment to the face or neck should use an electric shaver, which can be made available in the radiotherapy department.

Heat and cold

(1) Concentrated heat should not be applied to the area, e.g. hot-water bottles and hair-dryers
(2) The area should be protected from harsh winds during the period of treatment
(3) Deliberate sunbathing of the area should be discouraged for at least 1 year after the treatment; for patients with skin carcinoma it is advisable to use a total ultraviolet blocking agent (such as a silicon barrier cream) when in strong sunlight to prevent further skin lesions and to protect previously treated areas.

It is important that the skin is examined on the last day of treatment and the patient given careful advice on how to proceed. One should remember that after a number of weeks of constant supervision, the period following the end of treatment often leaves the patient feeling slightly bereft. It may be advisable to organize occasional visits from the district nurse if the patient has to cope with moist desquamation; an aqueous solution of gentian violet remains the favourite remedy for this situation for many but increasing use is being made of soothing hydrogel wound dressings, e.g. Vigilon and Geliperm, as well as Flamazine ointment under melolin pads. An explanation of when special recommendations may be stopped is essential otherwise patients may be found still following them on the third follow-up visit!

Mouth care

There is no doubt that patients receiving treatment to all or part of the oral cavity will experience painful mucosal reactions, dryness or thickened saliva because of the salivary glands being irradiated, temporary loss of taste and risk of infection. It is often these patients who find it most difficult to complete their course of treatment. This situation is aggravated if the patient is a heavy smoker or addicted to spirit drinking. Habits of addiction are not easily changed but patients must be made aware at the outset of their own responsibilities to minimize the reaction as far as possible and given every encouragement in their efforts.

Guidelines for patients

Patients should be advised on the following:

(1) Pay particular attention to mouth hygiene by using chlorhexidine or similar gentle mouthwashes regularly and brushing their teeth with a soft toothbrush after all meals

(2) Take food and drink warm rather than hot or iced and reduce amounts of seasoning and spices, dilute spirits and avoid smoking
(3) The food content should be high in protein and taken in a form that is easily swallowed, e.g. scrambled eggs, milk puddings, yoghurt, soups, fish (smoked fish are often found more acceptable, having more taste). Liquidizers or food processors may be available on loan from the department
(4) If eating is painful, a mouthwash of soluble aspirin used before meals may be sufficient to provide analgesia.

A very close watch should be kept on patients having the mouth treated, especially those having chemotherapy and/or steroids, and if thrush develops, the radiotherapist should be informed.

The patient's weight should be monitored and, if rapid weight loss occurs, he may need to be admitted for hospital care.

Dental hygienists are often able to alleviate problems caused by a dry mouth, by providing an artificial saliva of the correct pH for the patient.

Pelvic treatments

While differences of opinion exist regarding the best way of minimizing bowel reactions, most people favour a low residue diet to rest the bowel as much as possible. A simple guide to foods recommended and discouraged should be made available, but in discussing these with the patient, it should be made clear that these are intended as a guide and not as a rule. It is well to remember that the patient's current diet may be designed to wrestle against chronic constipation, may be vegetarian, or may be dictated by the caterer of the local Meals-on-wheels. Where families can be involved in the discussion regarding diet, they should be encouraged to experiment to find meals tempting to the patients, which yet control the state of their bowels. This is an important aspect and can make the families feel involved in the treatment. Where dieticians or nutritionists are to be found on the hospital staff, they may be asked to keep a close watch on these patients, monitor their weight and advise where necessary; otherwise it is the radiographer who will monitor these reactions closely.

The word 'diet' is synonymous with 'reducing' in some people's minds and it may be necessary to point out to patients that this is contrary to our aim.

Guidelines for patients can be summarized as follows:

(1) Follow the diet recommendations given to you when you notice change to a more frequent bowel habit, or if diarrhoea occurs (which may not start until some way through the treatment)
(2) Report to the radiographer or doctor if diarrhoea persists, despite the change in diet, so that a prescription may be given
(3) Drink plenty of fluids if suffering from diarrhoea.

Gynaecological treatments

These may be carried out by a combination of external beam and intracavitary treatments, by intracavitary treatment alone or combined with surgery. If the intracavitary insertions are effected without a general anaesthetic it is important that one of the team is deputed to talk to the patient throughout the procedure. The indignity of the situation can otherwise be overwhelming. Many patients will want to know if sexual intercourse is advisable during the treatment and they should be warned that it may lead to increased internal soreness. However, post-treatment vaginal patency must be ensured where continued sexual activity is envisaged and patients may need counselling regarding use of lubricants and dilators following a course of pelvic irradiation. In general, resumption of normal sexual relations is not recommended during the first 6 weeks after completing treatment.

The treatment of children

Paediatric oncology poses many problems, both practical and emotional. It is undoubtedly easier to undertake in a centre where staff are more experienced in working with children and consequently more relaxed in their attitude, and the whole team is geared for this specialized form of therapy which demands very close team work. Children approaching treatment are greatly helped by being with others who are already experiencing it, parents likewise. Families of the child-patient come under much stress during the often prolonged period of treatment, marriages may suffer and siblings react against the excessive attention paid to their sick brother or sister. The whole family unit may need skilled care and financial help to assist with frequent hospital visiting. In the UK the Malcolm Sargent Cancer Fund for Children is active in both these areas, initially funding paediatric social workers in centres where there is a large paediatric practice and giving prompt financial help when it is genuinely needed.

When a child is referred for radiotherapy, they have usually already been subjected to a number of frightening and invasive investigations and may already be experiencing a course of chemotherapy. They are now faced with another area which may in their minds be fraught with painful procedures. It is for this reason that some radiotherapy teams do not wear a uniform when treating children.

Close teamwork is especially vital in the treatment of children. The paediatrician and the radiotherapist together must talk to the parents regarding the overall treatment policy and discuss thoroughly any long-term effects and gain parental consent before proceeding.

The following basic principles apply to treating children:

(1) Always tell the child what is going to happen with absolute honesty
(2) Set aside plenty of time when treating children — to neglect to do so is foolish
(3) Keep the number of staff to a minimum, especially at the planning stage. Too often droves of onlookers crowd to see 'an interesting case'. This must not be permitted
(4) Try to maintain the same group of radiographers throughout the treatment course — children value continuity even more than adults
(5) Build as much fun into the proceedings as possible
(6) Always attempt to win the child's cooperation before resorting to sedation, but if sedation does prove necessary, liaise carefully with the anaesthetist and ward staff or parents so as to minimize the disruption to the child's normal routine, otherwise they may miss meals or sleep patterns may become disturbed (*see* Chapter 10)
(7) Parents, understandingly, are often more apprehensive than the child; as their fear may communicate itself to the child, it is sometimes advisable to ask them not to be present during planning and treatment procedures, having explained what will be done in their absence.

Immobilization

If a child will not tolerate a conventional shell for treatment, it may be necessary to choose the most comfortable position possible and use one radiographer to maintain a close watch from the moment the child is left alone in the treatment room. For treatments of the trunk, it may prove helpful to make a plaster of Paris back or front shell to help maintain a supine or prone position easily; these can be lined with a soft material and provide a quick and easy method of positioning the child (*see* Chapter 15). It is worth remembering that children feel happier if they can maintain visual contact with the radiographer and therefore the position of the patient's head with respect to the viewing window should be considered, rooms with closed circuit TV systems being less suitable. Full use should be made of the intercommunication system, perhaps using it for a story to be read or told. Whether or not the child is sedated, a support must be provided to prevent them falling off the couch, possibly a modified seat belt arrangement or something more substantial for infants.

Body image

Children may be upset by changes in their body image; hair loss is particularly hard to bear for some. Children are often self-conscious about wearing wigs. One imaginative father shaved his own hair and maintained a bald pate until his son's hair regrew.

Steroid therapy causing facial puffiness will sometimes mean that a shell becomes too tight but the child may be loathe to admit that there has been any change.

It is easier for children to accept these changes where a group of them is sharing the experience.

The adult patient on treatment

The initial treatment

One of the radiographers from the unit makes sure the patient understands the following:

(1) They will be positioned as they were in the planning room, but will, on this occasion, be on their own for several minutes while the treatment is given
(2) During this time they are constantly being watched and an intercommunication system is in operation if they wish to call
(3) They will feel nothing unusual while the treatment is given
(4) The treatment can be interrupted if necessary
(5) That the special instructions given in planning have been understood
(6) Finally the patients should be asked if they have any further questions.

The doctor responsible for planning the treatment may wish to see the patient 'set-up' on the first occasion to satisfy himself that all is well and possibly to show where thermoluminescent dosimeters should be placed to obtain given doses at specific points. The link that this provides with a member of staff the patient already knows is an additional boost to the patient's confidence. If the set-up is unsatisfactory, discussion of the problem should either include the patient or take place out of his earshot. As the treatment course proceeds the patient is seen at regular intervals by the doctor, but on the intervening visits is carefully monitored by the radiographers who will report any worrying symptoms which may occur, e.g. stridor, or a rapid drop in the blood count, if necessary having the patient examined before proceeding to treat. Radiographers often encourage patients to write down questions they want answered by the doctor as otherwise when the moment comes the question is gone!

Staffing of treatment units follows, where possible, the guidelines laid down jointly by the Royal College of Radiologists and the College of Radiographers; (extracts from these recommendations are given in *Table 18.1*). Rotation of staff should always maintain some continuity on each unit.

Table 18.1 Radiographer staffing in radiotherapy departments. (An extract from recommendations laid down jointly by the Royal College of Radiologists and the College of the Radiographers for departments in the UK)

Recommended staff establishment
Superficial X-ray units
1 Radiographer
1 Senior radiographer II
(NB Where the unit is either (i) multifactorial or (ii) specialized (e.g. strontium), 1 Senior radiographer I is required instead of 1 Senior radiographer II)
Orthovoltage X-ray unit
1 Radiographer
1 Senior radiographer II
Caesium unit
1 Radiographer
1 Senior radiographer II
Telecobalt unit
2 Radiographers
1 Superintendent IV
Linear accelerator
2 Radiographers
1 Senior radiographer I
1 Superintendent radiographer III
(NB Extra staff may be required where the linear accelerator has an electron facility)
Simulator-treatment planning
1 Radiographer
1 Senior radiographer I
1 Superintendent radiographer III required when complex techniques involved

Follow-up clinics

The timing of the first follow-up visit is sometimes given to coincide with the climax of the treatment reaction, especially when this may be severe or the patient is likely to need support and encouragement, or it may deliberately be timed to wait until the treatment reactions have completely settled so as to assess the response.

As patients are often seen by the radiotherapist at the hospital whence they were referred, many are lost to view by the ward staff and radiographers at the radiotherapy centre who welcome news of the progress of old friends. If no encouraging good news is forthcoming a distorted picture of treatment success emerges, since patients are only seen again if requiring further treatment. Radiographers usually welcome chances to attend follow-up clinics held within their centre. It is ideal to hold follow-up clinics within the radiotherapy department itself, although this is often impossible through considerations of space.

A review of the progress of a patient through a course of radiotherapy reveals an overwhelming need for time to be spent *generously* with the patient. In most departments and for most members of the team, this is in increasingly short supply. If it can be avoided, the patient should not be aware that this is the case.

The aim of all departments should be to balance technical excellence with the equally important appreciation of the patient as an individual.

19

The role of the physicist in radiotherapy

S. C. Klevenhagen

Introduction

Radiation therapy has always been, from its early days and throughout its development, associated with physics. The discovery of X-rays, of natural radioactivity and of the effect of ionizing radiations on living tissue marked the beginning of use of radiation for the treatment of cancer. As a result of this close partnership, radiotherapy has always been able to assimilate quickly any developments in radiation or nuclear physics into clinical practice. The same applies to treatment equipment, which benefitted from the developments in high energy radiation physics, including various forms of particle accelerators. The physics capabilities for producing man-made isotopes, developed on a wider scale in the 1950s, have revolutionized brachytherapy, and in recent years the development of modern imaging techniques such as computed tomography (CT scanning), ultrasound, magnetic resonance (MR), together with computing technology, have contributed much to improvements in tumour diagnosis and localization, precision of treatment planning, as well as to the accuracy of radiation delivery to the tumour volume.

Most developed radiotherapy centres have physical scientists in their supporting teams. In very broad terms the role of physicists in radiotherapy is to provide the necessary scientific expertise and back-up service in all aspects of the usage of radiation beams in clinical practice. The radiotherapists, in prescribing the dosage in the management of patients, rely on the data provided by physicists. To ensure that the physics data are accurate and reliable is probably the most important responsibility associated with the physicist's work in this field.

Physicists are involved in a wide spectrum of radiotherapy activities encompassing external beam therapy, brachytherapy, treatment planning and computing, dosimetry and quality assurance, servicing of treatment machines and associated equipment, radiation protection, development and research, workshop activities, sealed sources laboratory, CT scanning, magnetic resonance and other imaging techniques, staff training and teaching, and liaison with medical, radiographic and technical staff (*Table 19.1*).

This list demonstrates that there is a large diversity of scientific disciplines which today form the radiotherapy physics support service. Physicists therefore, apart from their academic qualifications in pure physics, are required to enlarge and extend their expertise into allied fields, such as computing, electronics, equipment technology, imaging, radiation protection, etc. Often, however, physics departments, particularly those working with large radiotherapy centres, have on their staff a full complement of specialists, including computing scientists, electronics graduates and others with appropriate technical supporting staff to cover the whole spectrum of responsibilities.

Although physicists have been involved in the development of radiotherapy from the beginning, this association was, in the first instance, in the form of consultancies or part-time appointments. It is believed that the first full time appointment of a physicist to a hospital in the UK (The Middlesex Hospital, London) took place in 1910. During the formation of the Hospital Physicists' Association (HPA) in Britain in 1943 some 53 physicists were listed as active in hospital physics. The HPA survey on physics support facilities for radiotherapy carried out in 1980/1 revealed that in about 50 radiotherapy centres in the UK there were approximately 200 physicists engaged directly in radiotherapy work without taking technicians into account. This growth

Table 19.1 Overview of the physicist's involvement in radiotherapy

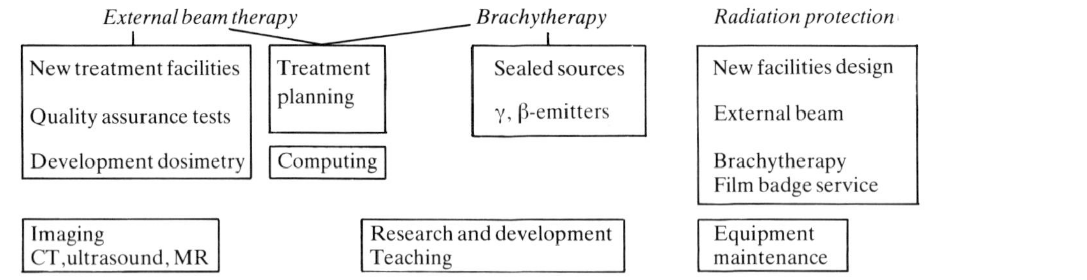

of physics support is a reflection of the growth of radiotherapy facilities and the complexity of the physics and technology involved.

In summary, the decision to provide a community with radiation therapy facilities not only involves a decision to secure the services of a radiation oncologist, to purchase and house the therapy equipment, and to arrange for its long-term maintenance, but also provides for the support of a suitably qualified and experienced physicist who has the appropriate equipment and facilities at his disposal.

The content and depth of the physics applied to radiotherapy can be quite involved. However, the aim of this chapter is not to describe the physical principles of any of the radiotherapy methods or techniques but to focus the reader's attention merely on the scope of the physicist's involvement in radiation therapy.

In the early days of radiotherapy almost all physicists were directly engaged in the everyday radiotherapy activities. This has changed to a large extent. Because of the increased complexity of the physics support a great deal of work is now being carried out in physics laboratories. The results of this work are often presented to radiotherapists only in a final, often simplified form. This 'invisible' physics contribution constitutes a significant part of the contemporary physics effort towards radiotherapy.

External beam therapy

The radiation beams produced by megavoltage machines such as cobalt-60 or linear accelerators are the most frequently used form of radiation in radiotherapy treatments. The physics and technology involved is much more sophisticated than that concerned with orthovoltage therapy, and consequently a large proportion of the physicist's time is devoted to this area of radiotherapy.

Among the tasks performed by physicists, the most important are:

(1) Acquisition of data concerning radiation beam physical characteristics
(2) Quality assurance tests of beam parameters and equipment performance
(3) Computing and treatment planning
(4) Contribution to development of treatment techniques
(5) Radiation protection.

The main function of physicists in dosimetry is to acquire, preferably by measurements, as much information as possible about the physical characteristics of the radiation beams employed in their radiotherapy centre. This knowledge is usually acquired immediately after a new therapy facility is brought into the centre. In the long term, physicists should institute a quality assurance programme designed to test the radiation beam parameters and equipment performance in the continuing use of these facilities. Further, physicists should outline a procedure to be used daily to determine that the therapy machine is operating under the conditions for which the data were obtained.

It is necessary for the physicist to have the appropriate equipment and instrumentation to perform the required dosimetry. It is also recommended that he has access, preferably direct, to computer facilities so that meaningful physical and mathematical evaluation of treatment plans agreed with the radiotherapist may be rapidly performed prior to the initiation of radiation therapy.

Dosimetric activities can conveniently be divided into three distinct groups:

(1) Dosimetry on new treatment facility and acceptance tests
(2) Long-term quality assurance tests
(3) Development dosimetry.

A new treatment facility

The involvement of physicists in the external beam therapy starts at the time of the decision by the hospital authority to purchase and install a radiation facility. This decision should be made with the advice of a physicist, whose responsibility in this task would be to help in the choosing of the equipment to suit the local requirement. The physicist's role is also to plan the installation from the radiation protection point of view and to survey the installation after completion so that it complies with the official radiation protection rules and law as well as meeting the general safety law. It is the physicist's function to certify that the therapy equipment is performing according to specification after it is installed. The decision to accept the machine is based on tests which are designed to confirm that the installed machine conforms to the specifications agreed between the radiotherapy centre and the manufacturer prior to the purchase.

A typical list of acceptance tests for a linear accelerator would have to include confirmation of beam energy, check of the radiation output level, check of dose measuring channels, determination of beam symmetry and flatness, spot checks on central axis dose distribution and beam penumbra, beam alignment checks with isocentre and light indicators, test of collimating system performance and verification of the radiation leakage level through the treatment head. A fuller list of checks is given in *Table 19.2*. They should be carried out roughly in the order indicated. There is, for instance, no point in undertaking extensive depth dose or tissue-maximum-ratios (TMR) measurements only to find afterwards that the collimator does not determine the field sizes properly. On the basis of such checks, the physicist would advise the radiotherapy department whether the machine is conforming to their requirements. Having accepted the equipment, the physics department would then continue measuring the beam's physical characteristics in the widest possible sense with emphasis on achieving high accuracy of the measured data. This second stage of dosimetry would deal with measurements which go far beyond the equipment acceptance tests and would be designed to look at the physical parameters of the radiation beam in greater detail (*Table 19.3*).

The first parameters which the physicist needs to determine are the beam quality or energy, and the radiation distribution pattern which the beam produces in the absorbing medium. These measurements are usually performed in water, which is considered to be a convenient and suitable substitute for soft tissue.

Beam energy (or quality) is an important parameter which needs to be determined at the outset of dosimetric work, as this information is required in many subsequent measurements. It is needed for a choice of various correction and calibration factors employed in radiation dosimetry. In clinical application, beam energy provides an indication about the tissue penetrating capabilities of the beam and the radiobiological effectiveness.

Important information about the beam properties in therapeutic application is the radiation distribution in the irradiated medium. These data are very carefully measured in terms of depth doses and often in the form of tissue–maximum dose ratios or tissue–air ratios. The latter form are convenient for use in isocentric treatment technique. Such measurements would be carried out for all field sizes, various beam energies and both photons and electrons if this modality is available. Similar measurements would need to be carried out on a neutron beam if a centre wanted to use such radiation. Centres which have neutron beam facilities, particularly those produced by a cyclotron, require strong scientific supporting teams to deal with the complexity of this treatment technique. A discussion of this aspect of the physicist's work lies beyond the scope of this chapter.

The programme of measurements on a new radiation beam would have to include studies of the build-up effect, electron contamination of a photon beam, photon contamination of an electron beam, neutron production in cases of photon beams above 15 MeV, careful output calibration and determination of its dependence on field size, measurements of parameters for irregular fields, determination of wedge factors and many others. Most of the measured data are normally prepared in a form suitable for use in a computerized treatment planning system or are fed directly into the computer.

Many of the parameters measured during the initial commissioning of a treatment machine are incorporated in the long-term quality assurance programme as a base line for comparison and checking of the radiation beam and the equipment performance. Each physics department should run an efficient quality assurance programme.

Quality assurance tests

Once detailed data on beam characteristics and equipment performance have been obtained during the initial dosimetry, it is necessary to monitor these parameters in the continuing use of the treatment machine. This is achieved by quality assurance.

The need for a quality assurance programme to ensure that cancer patients are treated adequately and with procedures and equipment which are safe and operate correctly, is undisputed. The result and effectiveness of treatments are affected by various uncertainties in the treatment procedures, which may include inaccuracy in tumour localization, errors in field placement, patient immobilization, beam calibration and other dosimetric errors, equipment malfunctioning and many others. It is obvious therefore that quality assurance in radiotherapy has to include checking and control of both clinical and physical parameters. It is very important that patients are carefully monitored during the treatment course and that unexpected reactions to the treatment are analysed with respect to possible clinical, physical or technical mistakes. This requires a carefully designed

Table 19.2 Typical linear accelerator acceptance tests

Radiation protection survey	*Dosimetry*	
Leakage through head		
Treatment room surroundings	Photons	Electrons
	beam quality	beam energy
Machine alignment and beam geometry	dose calibration	depth doses
Determination of isocentre	beam symmetry and flatness	beam symmetry and flatness
Stability of gantry rotation	dose monitoring electronics	dose calibration
Quality of collimating system		
Light field and radiation field agreement		
Distance indicators, lasers		
Scale readouts		
Mechanical and electrical safety checks		
All systems to be checked		

Table 19.3 Post-acceptance dosimetry

Photons	*Electrons*	*Preparation of data for clinical use*
Depth doses at all treatment conditions	Exact dose/monitor unit calibration	All data to be issued for use in form of graphs and tables
TMR at all treatment conditions		
Full beam distribution	Full dose distribution for various treatment conditions	
Exact dose/monitor unit calibration		Most data to be fed into the treatment planning computer
Output variation with field size		
Surface dose values	X-ray contamination	
Electron contamination		
Penumbra	Effect of stand-off and oblique incidence	
Data for wedges		
Irregular and blocked fields		
Data for treatments at unusual distances	Effect of cut-outs (field blocking)	

and documented quality assurance programme of radiotherapy procedures with the participation of all the professional groups involved. The need for accurate and reproducible delivery of radiation dose follows from the steepness of the dose–response curve, which suggests that the accuracy of the dose delivery to the target volume should be within 5% of the clinical prescription.

The physicist's role in the radiotherapy quality assurance programme is to ensure that the radiation beam parameters and equipment performance guarantee the delivery of a correct dose to the target volume. To achieve this a carefully designed programme of tests is performed. These are carried out periodically throughout the use of radiotherapy facilities. These tests cover a wide range of physical beam parameters and/or equipment performance and involve many of the parameters listed in *Tables 19.2* and *19.3*, which were measured at the time of equipment commissioning. The data collected then are the base line of assessment of the radiation beam and equipment performance later.

How many parameters are checked and how often, depends on the quality assurance programme agreed, but some parameters are relatively stable and need not be checked frequently. It is not, for instance, necessary to check the beam energy or depth doses every week, but it is necessary to calibrate the beam output with this frequency. The interested reader will find full specification of quality assurance tests in protocols prepared by the various physics departments which provide services in radiotherapy or in publications of the British Hospital Physicists Association or the American Association of Physicists in Medicine.

Development dosimetry

Dosimetry concerned with developments in

radiotherapy is an almost never-ending occupation for a physicist.

Although most treatment techniques for the specific type and siting of tumours are similar in most centres there are many individual differences in the details of techniques. The use of wedges, compensators, weighting of multiple fields, shielding blocks, and set-up aids, differs from centre to centre and these individual differences create a necessity for identifying the effect of these on the radiation distribution in the treated patient by dosimetry.

This is particularly evident in the approaches to the more complex treatment schemes such as total body irradiation with photons for leukaemia, large volume treatments with irregularly shaped fields (Hodgkin's disease), treatment of the whole central nervous system (medulloblastoma, ependymoma), treatment of the breast, total skin irradiation with electrons and electron arc therapy. Again, as with the simpler techniques the general principles for the complex techniques are widely accepted but individual differences concerning details of the techniques are considerable between the various radiotherapy centres. Physicists are required therefore to investigate by individual dosimetry any newly proposed technique so that the radiotherapist will feel confident in using it.

Furthermore, treatment techniques undergo a continuous evolution. Even a technique well documented and developed in one centre can rarely be adopted for use in another centre without having to carry out some dosimetry to account for differences for equipment, accessories, performance in setting-up method and treatment planning facilities. Some sophisticated treatment methods require the full time involvement of a physicist. The classic example of this is the computer-controlled tracking technique (Brace, Davy and Skeggs, 1981), known also as conformation therapy. Both terms are used to describe treatments in which the high dose volume is shaped to fit the target volume in three dimensions. Tracking techniques are particularly suitable and successful in the treatment of tumours of the oesophagus, thyroid, bronchus, chain of lymph nodes or medulloblastoma. The major obstacle to the routine use of this technique is the complex and expensive equipment which is required together with the large physics support needed. These examples, it is hoped, illustrate the physicist's activities in clinical dosimetry as an ongoing commitment in a radiotherapy department.

Brachytherapy

'Brachy' in Greek means 'short' — thus the term brachytherapy refers to treatments where the source of radiation is placed close to the tumour. In French-speaking countries a term 'Curietherapie' is used to describe this radiotherapy technique, in appreciation of the contribution of Pierre and Marie Curie to radiation physics. In general terms, brachytherapy can be defined as a method of radiotherapy in which an encapsulated source or an array of sources is employed to deliver gamma or beta radiation at a distance of up to a few centimetres, either by intracavitary, interstitial or surface applicator.

Brachytherapy presents physicists with problems very different from those encountered in external beam therapy. These arise from the fact that brachytherapy sources are usually small in size and that the radiation intensity around them varies rapidly with distance. For these reasons the dosimetry in brachytherapy is very difficult.

A serious problem in brachytherapy is radiation protection since, unlike a beam from a linear accelerator (linac) or a cobalt unit, the radiation beam from a nuclide cannot be switched off, and this presents a particularly serious environmental radiation hazard during handling of sources, clinical use and storage. A considerable amount of physicists' time is devoted to radiation protection.

Because of the problems with the size of the sources and fast dose fall-off, the radiation distribution calculation methods in brachytherapy have developed in a different way from the external beam physics. Instead of relying on detailed measurements, theoretical models for calculating dosage from first principles have been developed and introduced into clinical practice. The Swedish physicist Sievert (1921) was the first to propose an integration method to determine the dose delivered from a single brachytherapy source (radium). At the same time, however, practice showed that calculation of dosage or treatment time for an array of sources such as for a surface applicator (plaque) was a tedious procedure. Consequently, practical simplified dosage calculation systems have been developed, among which the Paterson-Parker system from Manchester (Meredith, 1967) has gained large popularity over the years.

In the early days of brachytherapy, when the principal sources employed were radium and radon, physicists were much involved in calculations of treatment data. Either the established dosage systems could be used for this purpose or individual calculations had to be done in unusual cases.

A vast amount of experience in the use of radium and its clinical effects has been accumulated in the 50 years since it has been used in radiotherapy. This experience, and the neatly working radium-based system, was shattered considerably when the capability of nuclear physics to produce man-made isotopes became available on a wider scale in the 1950s. Those which were considered suitable as radium substitutes are listed in *Table 19.4*. The main attractiveness of the new isotopes over radium was seen in their features which guaranteed better safety in use. Their γ-emission was in the medium energy range which

Table 19.4 Radioactive sources commonly available for brachytherapy as the substitute for radium

Radionuclide	*Average photon energy (MeV)*	*Half-life*	*Exposure rate constant* (R cm^2/h per mCi)
Gold-198	0.42	2.70 days	2.38
Chromium-51	0.32	27.7 days	0.184
Iodine-125	0.028	60.2 days	1.45
Iridium-192	0.29	74.2 days	4.64
Tantalum-182	0.70	115.0 days	6.87
Caesium-137	0.66	30.0 years	3.27
Cobalt-60	1.25	5.26 years	13.07

meant that thinner protection barriers were required for shielding and protection compared to radium. No gaseous disintegration products were generated by these isotopes and the active material was produced in an insoluble non-toxic form. In addition, these nuclides became available in high specific activity which offered the potential for reduction of the physical size of sources, an important improvement in clinical application.

The list in *Table 19.4* shows that the substitutes differ not only from radium in their physical characteristics but they also differ among themselves. Apart from this, the new sources appeared in different shapes, sizes and encapsulations, including rigid tubes, needles, small spheres, grains and flexible wires. This variety of forms and physical characteristics called for extensive investigations on the question of suitability and scope of clinical applications of these nuclides. A great deal of work has been done in physics over the last 15 years in this field.

The main issues requiring consideration were:

(1) How the new source could be fitted into the well established dosage calculation systems or was there a need for new calculation methods
(2) How the various physical characteristics of the new sources affected the dose distribution in tissue compared to that known from radium
(3) How the various encapsulations and shape of sources affected the dosage calculation
(4) What was the correlation between radiation absorption and scatter contribution at the energies of the various nuclides
(5) What were the exact values of the γ-emission factors (corresponding to radium K-factor).

The situation in brachytherapy physics was, in addition, further aggravated by the proposed changes in general dosimetry. Consequently, the new brachytherapy dosage systems had to assimilate also the switch-over from exposure (Roentgen) to the concept of the absorbed dose (rad and Gray and the new unit of activity–Becquerel). The reader can be assured that those physicists who were involved in brachytherapy in the last 15 years were not left idle!

These developments in brachytherapy, apart from problems of physical nature, have introduced radiobiological factors which require consideration. On changing from an existing radium technique to the use of new nuclides, radiobiological factors may become relevant either because a change of the energy of radiation is involved (*see Table 19.4*) or a change of source activity, hence dose–rate is involved.

The effects due to change in energy have fortunately been found not to be so serious. In the energy range involved, the radiobiological effectiveness was found to be within ± 4% of that for the γ-rays of radium (Kirk, Grey and Watson, 1972). This is regarded as being of no practical consequence.

The situation is not so simple with regard to change in dose–rate (*see below*).

As the result of this work, and the clinical experience collected with the substitutes, only a small number of the tried and investigated nuclides have established themselves firmly in brachytherapy. Caesium-137 is now widely used, particularly in intracavitary therapy, although some high dose–rate afterloading systems employ cobalt-60 or iridium-192 because of their high specific activity.

Iridium, in the form of a wire, is also used widely in interstitial afterloading techniques, but for permanent implantation gold-198 and iodine-125 are the most widely used nuclides.

It might be worth pointing out that in contrast to all other sources, iridium wire is not classified as a 'sealed source' and so is not subject to the leakage and other tests usually applied to these. The wire is activated by neutron irradiation in a nuclear reactor and the cladding material becomes radioactive. By choosing platinum as the cladding material this effect is minimized and it has been shown that the activity in platinum is negligible.

As soon as computers were introduced into medicine, physicists found them to be useful for solving problems in brachytherapy physics. One of the most tedious tasks in this field used to be the calculation of radiation distribution around the sources. Consequently, most dosage systems which were developed for radium therapy employed a simplified approach to dosimetry considering only a limited number of points in tissue. The gynaecological therapy dosage system (*see* the Manchester system, Chapter 9) is a classic example of this, where only two or three points within the treatment volume are considered in the determination of the treatment time and dose delivered. The computing technology has created an opportunity for calculating distributions in more detail and in many planes around the sources deposited in tissue. To facilitate this, mathematical calculation models have been proposed. The equation shown in *Figure 19.1* is an example of an algorithm suitable for use in a computer for working out a full distribution resulting from a large number

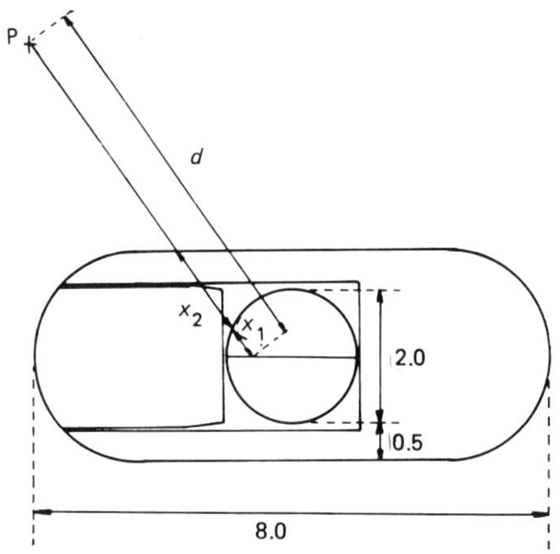

Method of calculation
The absorbed dose rate produced by the source at a point P in water can be determined from

$$D = Kf \frac{A_E}{2L_1} g \int_{-L_1}^{L_1} \exp(-\mu_1 x_1 - \mu_2 x_2) \frac{1}{d^2} T(d_1)\, dL$$

where

K is the exposure rate constant for caesium-137 ($K = 3{\cdot}3$ R cm^2/h per mCi)

f is the roentgen to cGy conversion factor (0.957) for soft tissue

A_E is the equivalent activity of the source

g is the correction factor to convert the equivalent activity of the source to true activity

$2L_1$ is the active length of the source

μ_1 is the energy absorption coefficient for the source material

x_1 is the path length of the radiation in the source material

μ_2 is the effective attenuation coefficient for stainless steel

x_2 is the path length of the radiation in the stainless steel capsule

Figure 19.1 Dose distribution calculation model for a caesium-137 source (adapted from Diffey and Klevenhagen, 1975)

of sources, such as those, for instance, used in the Curietron or Selecton afterloading systems.

A considerable problem in brachytherapy physics used to be the correlation between the sources' geometry and the anatomy of the patient. It is much easier now with the use of CT scanner images. There are now possibilities of displaying the brachytherapy distribution onto the CT images on the same treatment planning console. This is a very useful facility when consideration is given to the dose received by the critical organs in relation to the tumour as well as in the assessment of the effect of inhomogeneities on the radiation distribution.

Remote afterloading

Concern about radiation protection of the personnel involved in the use of sealed sources, particularly for the treatment of carcinoma of the cervix and the uterus where a large number of hospital staff was exposed to radiation, stimulated interest in the development of afterloading techniques. The concept of afterloading can be applied to any application of sealed sources in brachytherapy, either intracavitary, interstitial or at surface. Generally, the term afterloading describes a method whereby empty tubes, sleeves or applicators are first located in or on the patient and the radioactive sources are subsequently inserted into them after the applicator location has been confirmed as being correct.

The advantages of the afterloading technique are:

(1) Radiation exposure to staff is reduced or avoided completely
(2) It offers potential for increase in treatment capacity
(3) It provides an opportunity for improvements in treatment technique.

Afterloading can be performed manually or by a remote-controlled machine. In the former, the sources are introduced manually into the applicator previously placed in the patient. Remote afterloading utilizes some form of a remote-controlled machine for the insertion of sources, which also facilitates temporary withdrawal of them back to a safe when the patient requires attention by nursing staff. The better radiation protection which the remote afterloading offers is the most important aspect of this treatment technique.

The equipment for remote loading is far more complex and expensive than that used in the manual version. A machine for this purpose would comprise essentially a storage safe where the sources are kept when they are outside the treatment applicators. There are one or more delivery tubes connected to the safe, designed to mate at their distal end with treatment applicators fixed in or on to the patient. There is a mechanism for delivering the sources to the applicators for treatment or withdrawing them back to the safe as required. The machine must also have timers for each source to determine the treatment duration.

The concept of afterloading goes back to the early days of radiotherapy. Abbe (1906) described a treatment technique involving insertion, adjustment and attachment to the patient of empty tubes, into which radium could be inserted rapidly and easily. The main development effort, however, in afterloading physics and technology took place in the mid 1950s and early 1960s. In relation to gynaecological therapy, the pioneering work was done by Walstam (1962) who designed one of the first models of remote-controlled apparatus. This was followed by the appearance of several commercial systems which developed along two distinct applications: for low activity sources and for high activity sources.

The first group of these machines (e.g. Curietron or Selectron) was designed to simulate treatment conditions similar to those used in the old conventional radium therapy. The source is caesium-137 (tens of mCi activity; $10^3 \times$ MBq) resulting in treatment times of up to a few days. A typical dose rate to the Manchester point 'A', as a guidance for dosage in gynaecological therapy, would be of the order of 60 cGy/h; such a regimen of treatment is often referred to as low-dose rate regimen. Machines of this type are used in the ward where the patient is brought in from the theatre after the insertion of the applicator. No active material is handled in the theatres under such circumstances, therefore nobody involved in these procedures receives any exposure. Similarly, exposure to ward staff is reduced as nursing and other procedures are carried out only when the sources are retracted into the afterloading machine safe.

Ward design for use with the Curietrons is shown in *Figure 19.2*. The reduction of exposure to radiation experienced by staff involved in caesium insertions after the introduction of remote afterloading is illustrated in *Table 19.5*.

The second group of afterloading machines which utilize very high activity sources (e.g. Cathetron) cannot be used on a ward but must be installed in a separate, shielded room, of the type used for megavoltage therapy, and patients are treated in an analogous time regimen to that used in external beam therapy. The sources may be of a few Ci ($10^6 \times$ MBq) so that the treatment times are reduced to minutes.

The initially evident division on low and high activity systems is now losing its identity because many radiotherapy centres began changing their low intensity technique into what could be described as medium intensity (medium dose–rate) technique. This raises the dose rate at point 'A' to about 100–150 cGy/h, that is between two and three times higher compared to the conventional Manchester system. The benefit from the use of 'hotter' sources is the shortening of the treatment time. Fortunately, some afterloading machines such as the Curietron or Selectron have the internal safes designed with a sufficient safety margin and can accommodate caesium sources of either low or medium activity.

There are radiobiological factors to be considered in this change due to the dose–rate effect on the overall treatment time (or the total dose delivered to the tumour). The dose–rate effect is due to the fact that the effectiveness of the radiation on tissue varies with the dose–rate, particularly in the range 30–300 cGy/h which is exactly the region of concern in the afterloading technique. The question of how to allow for this correctly in the dosage or treatment time prescription has been given attention by many workers (for example Liversage, 1980). Although iso-effect formulae have been proposed to cope with this problem, it is thought that as yet there is not a sufficient volume of clinical evidence concerning treatment results to apply them indiscriminately in clinical practice. Clinical trials are being performed currently to find the answer to this problem (*see* Chapter 9).

Involvement in treatment planning

The successful treatment of cancer by radiation is a question of a skilful balance between the maximum probability of cure and the minimum probability of radiation-induced complications. Therefore, the radiotherapist must be in possession of precise knowledge of the radiation dose distributed throughout the irradiated volume of tissue in the patient prior to starting the treatment. This information should not only involve the dose to the tumour itself, but also the dose to normal surrounding tissue and organs, and most importantly the dose in the area of radiation-sensitive structures in the vicinity of the irradiated volume.

The activities in the radiotherapy department which involve tumour diagnosis, staging and localization, identification of the patient contour inhomogeneities and sensitive organs, followed by exploration of choices of treatment techniques and making decisions on technique of radiation application, determination of radiation distribution throughout the tissue volume involved and the final acceptance of the choice of treatment technique and radiation beam application, are referred to as treatment planning.

Treatment planning is a multidisciplinary activity involving staff from all the professions working in radiotherapy: medical, scientific, radiographic, technical, nursing and other related specialties. Successful planning of treatment depends on a unique contribution from each of these groups, and equally on effective communication and harmonious cooperation between them. The involvement of the medical staff in treatment planning is more precisely defined than that of physicists or radiographers. The current experience shows that the scope and demarcation of activities of the two latter groups may vary considerably from hospital to hospital depending on local requirements and concepts of responsibilities. The discussion in this chapter will be confined to the role which the physicist plays in the treatment planning procedures.

Radiotherapy planning is conducted through several distinct phases. The physicist may make a profound contribution to most and these include:

(1) Consultations with radiotherapists as to the general approach to the treatment planning for a given patient

(2) Collection of basic patient information
(3) Radiation field planning and isodose distribution charting
(4) Monitoring of settings, treatment time and other treatment data calculations
(5) Treatment implementation
(6) Verification dosimetry during treatments.

The physicist's familiarity with the radiation beam physical characteristics and their limitations, is often useful to the radiotherapist when he is considering a choice of approach to treating a given case. This applies to radiations of all types, whether generated by a machine or a sealed source. Consultations are particularly important in unconventional cases where

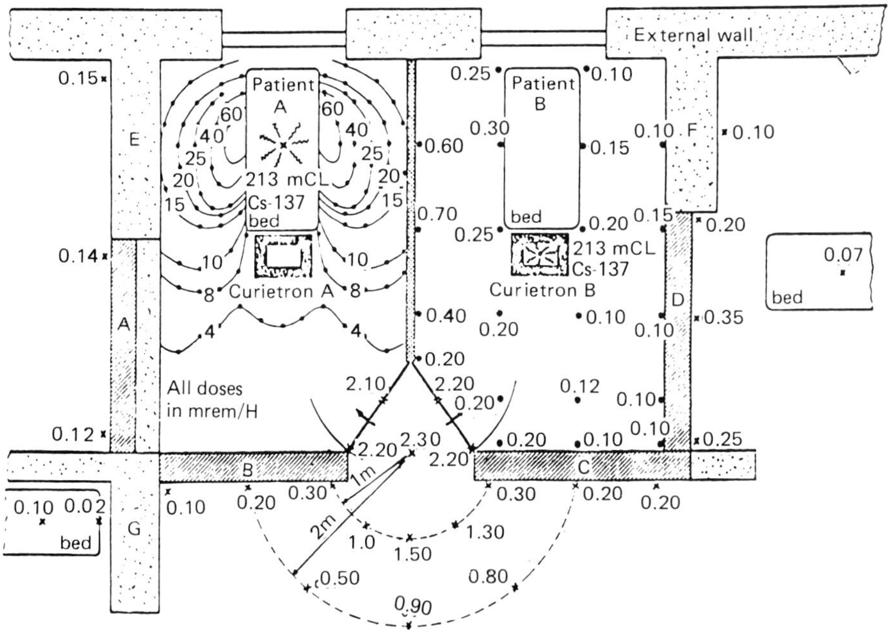

Figure 19.2 Protected room design for afterloading machines. The data show results of a radiation survey carried out for two treatment situations: dose rates marked with dots were measured with one set of sources *in situ* (patient A); dose rates marked with crosses indicate exposures as found outside the treatment room with both patients under treatment. (Adapted from Klevenhagen and Faulkner, 1981)

Table 19.5 A comparison of personnel doses recorded before and after the introduction of remote afterloading technique (Curietron)

All doses (mrems)		*Manual insertions only*		*Curietrons and manual insertions*	
		Yearly dose	*Monthly dose*	*Yearly dose*	*Monthly dose*
Consultant radiotherapist	1	308	26	180	15
	2	502	42	420	35
	3	380	32	182	15
Sealed sources custodian	1	615	51	360	30
	2	593	49	160	13
Average per custodian		604	50	260	22
Theatres	Sister	507	42	220	18
	Other staff	245	20	128	11
Curietron ward	Sister	426	36	120	10
	Other staff	332	28	98	8

the technique of usage of beams or sealed sources is not so obvious.

The important steps in treatment planning for any patient are the procedures aimed at the accurate localization and the determination of the full extent and position of the tumour relative to normal anatomical structures which may be very radiation sensitive. These steps also include determination of the patient's contour and their inhomogeneities. These procedures may involve several imaging techniques which are available to the radiotherapy centre. Conventional radiography with or without contrast media, isotopes, ultrasound, CT scanning and magnetic resonance, might all be employed at this stage. If megavoltage radiation beams are considered for the treatment, almost certainly the use of a treatment planning simulator would be necessary. The simulator will confirm that the selected beam arrangement leads to the traverse of the appropriate patient body section in the desired direction and that the beams are of the required dimensions. Radiographs taken with the therapy unit lack the desired diagnostic quality for this purpose. This is apart from the fact that time spent on a therapy machine for planning and field verification is wasted. Saving of treatment machine time is considered to be an important function of a simulator.

Most of the patient data collection and treatment simulation procedures are based on high technology imaging techniques, and physicists have the responsibility to ensure that the operational parameters of these methods are physically correct. This is important because the localization, simulation or scanning geometry must be perfectly matched to the distribution calculation geometry and to the geometry of the therapy unit on which the actual treatment will be carried out. Many of these problems are minimized if CT scanning images of the patient's appropriate cross-sections can be directly utilized during treatment planning. CT images give a precise description of the patient's cross-section and provide most useful information about internal structures provided the scanner is calibrated appropriately, and that the calibration is stable with time.

Scanners require constant testing to ensure this. The physical aspect of the CT scanning is discussed in more detail later (*see below*).

The magnetic resonance images are as yet little utilized directly in radiotherapy planning but the technology of MR is developing fast and already it promises to be useful in this field.

The currently used methods of collecting basic information either by imaging or contouring devices are being continously developed and improved. This is yet another area where physicists are active.

An important phase of radiotherapy planning is choosing the radiation beam arrangement, charting the combined isodose distribution and calculating the necessary treatment dosage parameters. In order to achieve a tumour dose considerably above the maximum normal tissue dose it is often necessary to use multiple beam-directed fields. Most radiotherapists would wish to have a complete isodose chart showing the resulting radiation distribution throughout the treated volume. In the past this was achieved by manual methods. This was time consuming and laborious. In addition, if this was carried out at only a few points in and around the tumour it would not now be considered adequate for determining the merits of a treatment plan.

The most convenient and accurate method of charting the distribution is by the use of a computer-assisted treatment planning system preferably linked with CT facilities. A computer treatment planning system does not necessarily need to be operated by physicists on an everyday basis. The degree of sophistication in design of the software allows it to be operated by staff who are less familiar with the physics principles involved in the calculations. More and more often, apart from the physicists and radiographers, the radiotherapists may wish to use the treatment planning computer. Involvement of medical staff in this phase of treatment planning may become more important with wider utilization of CT or MR images in planning computers. This will be encouraged by the necessity for accurate identification of the details of patients' anatomy and would speed up the procedures if repeated planning attempts have to be made with altered weighting or positions of fields before a satisfactory plan is obtained.

From this point of view, the role of physicists in this area of radiotherapy activities has changed considerably with the development of computers. Instead of concentrating on working out isodose distributions and doing dosage calculations, physicists take on overall responsibility for the scientific content of the radiation distribution calculation methods and isodose charting. A computer for this application is fundamentally a machine programmed to process physical information. This definition reveals the two main tasks which the physicists face: first, the treatment planning system must be designed for carrying out calculations in accord with the appropriate physical principles governing the radiation beams and their transition through body tissues; second, the information concerning the beams which the system is to handle and process must be correct and valid for the specific therapy, equipment and facilities in the given centre. Further, it is the task of the physicist to follow new developments in that area of physics which has application to treatment planning and to ensure that these are implemented in his own centre.

In practice, the routine treatment planning schemes as programmed on the computer cannot always be invoked, and special calculations or special treatment techniques must be developed. These may be simple or complex and often require considerable physics input. It is important that departures from the routine cases are recognized by medical or radiographic staff and the physicist consulted as appropriate. Treatment planning of intermediate complexity generally requires involvement of a physicist either directly or for checking. Routine plans produced by the radiographic and other staff should be overseen by physicists.

For solving individual cases, knowledge of the limitations and extent of the physical data and equipment is necessary. Quite often extra measurements on radiation beams may have to be undertaken to solve unusual problems, including preparation of these data for computer use, alterations in software or writing of new software. For all work in which calculations are done infrequently, the total responsibility for execution and checking of work is that of the physicist.

The purely computing aspect of the treatment planning process is discussed in more detail later (*see below*).

The implementation of the actual radiotherapy treatment is in the hands of the radiographers, and the physicist's role in this area is confined to devising techniques leading to reducing errors in setting-up and delivering the radiation. Among the approaches considered is the fully automated treatment technique (Brace, Davy and Skeggs, 1981), which is available in very few centres because of the cost of the equipment. More accessible are partially automated systems in the form of computer-controlled setting and recording of the various machine parameters (beam size, beam orientation, dose delivered). These systems are still a subject of practical assessment.

The physicist's involvement does not finish at the time of treatment implementation but extends to dose verification which may take place during actual treatment. Direct measurements on, in or through a patient's body may be desirable for several reasons, for example:

(1) Where important heterogeneities such as lung or bone are present in the treated volume and may affect the calculated dose distribution
(2) Where a sensitive organ such as the testis or the eye lies close to the main radiation beam
(3) Where there is a need to find by measurement a dose to the rectal wall during intracavitary treatment of the cervix uteri.

Among the methods available to physicists for dose verification on patients are ionization chamber, thermoluminescent dosimetry (TLD) and semiconductor detectors.

An ionization chamber is widely used in general dosimetry because of the reliability and precision of measurements it offers. For measurements on patients, however, it is not the most convenient of devices because it is relatively large with its stem and leads. It has the advantage of giving immediate reading of the dose provided its sensitivity is correctly chosen.

An interesting device is a semiconductor detector which fundamentally operates on the same principle as the solid-state diode or transistor employed so widely in electronic circuitry. The detector can be made of silicon which is about 2000 times denser than air. Together with the low energy deposition required in silicon to produce charges, this results in the semiconductor detector being about 20 000 times more sensitive than an ionization chamber of the same volume. These devices are, however, not free from problems. Their shortcomings include lack of repeatable operational characteristics, energy dependence, temperature sensitivity and radiation damage effect. These problems can be overcome to some extent in practical application. *Figure 19.3* shows a p–n junction semiconductor detector system which has been in use at The London Hospital for many years for measurements of rectal doses during caesium insertions in gynaecological therapy (Klevenhagen, 1976). By calibration of the detector in a suitable phantom and employment of appropriate circuitry, the energy and temperature dependence of the detector are minimized and the system is successful in clinical dosimetry.

The most popularity in recent years has been gained by TLD, except where an immediate reading of dose-rate is required. Thermoluminescence is a property of certain materials whereby the dose absorbed during measurement is stored until the material (dosemeter) is heated to about 200–400°C, when it is released in the form of visible light. The amount of light released is proportional to the dose absorbed. Dosemeters in form of lithium-fluoride microrods (6 mm × 1 mm in diameter) are particularly attractive for dosimetry *in vivo*, as they are small and rugged. They are very suitable for placing within the body in close proximity to the tissue or point of interest. The only probable disadvantage is the fact that the result of measurement is not immediately available since the dosemeter, whether in form of rods, chips or powder, must be taken to the read-out instrument for the assessment.

TLD is a convenient system in terms of its use on patients. It is, however, far more cumbersome when it comes to the physical aspect as TLD requires far more attention and care compared to, for example, ionization dosimetry. A full cycle of use of TLD consists of a combination of annealing, storage and handling, irradiation and readout and all these procedures require care and attention if the best performance is to be achieved.

Before making radiation measurements all dosemeters should be identically annealed when new to standardize their sensitivities and backgrounds. Annealing is a procedure which cancels any previous irradiation history of the dosemeters and makes them ready for use. The dosemeters can be repeatedly used

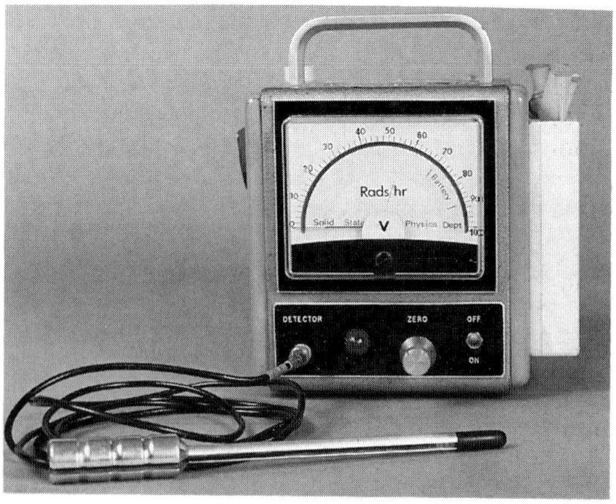

Figure 19.3 Semiconductor detector system for clinical dosimetry (Klevenhagen, 1976)

many times provided they are subject to annealing before making any new measurements.

One problem is sensitivity of the dosemeters which varies from batch to batch and needs to be determined when TLD are delivered and after every annealing. The sensitivity is energy dependent and several calibrations may have to be carried out, particularly if low energies or photon and electron applications are intended. Sensitivity depends also on their irradiation history and on the thermal treatment to which they are subjected in use. In addition, the calibration curve may exhibit supralinearity which means that the thermoluminescence output per unit dose is not constant for the dosemeter throughout the whole dose range. These factors illustrate the complexity of the TLD technique.

The storage and handling of dosemeters can affect TLD performance parameters such as sensitivity, stability, repeatability and threshold of detectable dose. Also important in the system is the TLD reader, into which the dosemeters are placed for heating and recording the light generated. The reader must be characterized by reliable and stable behaviour with time. Quality control of the reader performance is an important factor in running a good TLD service.

In all stages of TLD use there are possibilities for making mistakes. These can be minimized by employing careful experimental techniques. Despite the relative complexity of the procedures it is possible to attain reproducibility of TLD measurements within 5%, but this requires punctilious attention to details. It is sometimes found in clinical use that measurements on patients produce results of much larger spread. This can be attributed in most cases to the fact that the dosemeters are used in the area of the radiation beam where the dose with distance changes quite rapidly. A few millimetres difference in the dosemeter position may make a large difference to the dose recorded.

Computing in radiotherapy

It is difficult today to imagine modern radiotherapy and physics departments working without computing facilities. During the past decade the application of computers has increased considerably due to larger availability and lower cost of the hardware and widespread knowledge, particularly among physicists, of handling and using computers. Among the applications in radiotherapy the most important is that of computation of radiation distribution charts or so-called treatment plans. Other applications include treatment verification, acquisition of patient's anatomical data, record keeping and analysis of treatment results. Applications in treatment automation are developing slowly.

Computation of radiation distribution charts

Physicists take a deep interest in computing concerned with acquisition of radiation beam data and computation of radiation distribution in both external beam therapy and brachytherapy.

One of the most tedious tasks of the physicist in the past was to prepare by hand charts of isodose distributions resulting from combined radiation fields in external beam therapy. Two methods were popular. One was based on a summation of dose values over a large matrix of points. An alternative method was to use the superposition of isodose charts in pairs and obtain the resulting distribution by a direct interconnecting of points of equal dosage. Both of these were laborious and time consuming, particularly so if many alternative beam applications (plans) were to be considered. This work which sometimes took hours, can now be completed within minutes thanks to computers. Not only can the computer carry out calculations with greater speed, it also does them more accurately. It is easier therefore with computer planning to consider alternative ways of beam application or a change of any treatment parameters like wedges and field weighting, to optimize the distribution. Once the computer is supplied with the correct information on the radiation beams it uses in calculations, and it is programmed suitably, it can be operated by less specialized staff. As a consequence, treatment planning becomes more accessible to medical, technical and radiographic staff.

The advent of computer technology to radiotherapy made a large impact on the approach to the physics involved in treatment planning. In the conventional manual planning, in the past, the radiation beam was presented in the form of isodose lines charted separately for each of the applicable conditions. Each energy, field size and wedge required a separate chart. Other physical parameters relevant to the calculation of dosage, for instance the variation of beam output with field size, were also used in a convenient graphical form. Computers are, however, not very good at handling and performing calculations on data in this form. They prefer to operate on mathematical formulae. Because of this physicists were forced to think of alternative methods of beam presentation and thus, over the last few years, a new area of physics has gradually evolved concerned with radiation beam modelling and the development of computational algorithms.

Two aspects can be distinguished in this problem. One is the question of the model of an individual radiation beam which is suitable for computer use, and the second is the question of adding the individual beams to obtain the final multibeam distribution. The latter problem is simpler because in adding the various field contributions, the computation process can be easily programmed to mimic accurately the point summation manual method in that the contribution from each field in turn is added into each point of a dose matrix corresponding to the treatment region. More involved and complex is the problem of the form in which the individual beam is modelled and stored in the computer.

Ideally, one would like to have a mathematical formula (algorithm) to model the beam which would enable the distribution to be calculated. Many beam models have been developed by physicists with various degrees of success. In a photon beam difficulties have been experienced with beam modelling due to the influence of the treatment machine's individual design features affecting the calculation model and due to problems with unpredictability of scatter variation across the beam and with depth. In linear accelerators, the type of beam-flattening filter or electron scattering foil may make a given beam model inapplicable to a specific machine in the department unless suitable correction factors are employed.

One of the first and still successful calculation models for photons was proposed by Bentley and Milan (1977). In this model a single beam was represented in the form of a matrix of dose values corresponding to the dose distribution obtained from that particular radiation field. This model requires a relatively large quantity of data to be stored for each field. These have to be obtained by measurement of the central axis depth doses and beam profiles at five depths. This is an empirical approach to beam modelling. Although it involves a considerable measurement effort needed at the time of setting up the computer for planning, it has the advantage of depicting truly the individual beam features and thus is accurate.

A number of alternative methods of beam presentation have been proposed in which the main attention was focused on reducing the measurement of beam data to a minimum. Almost from the beginning, mathematical formulae were looked upon as a viable alternative. It was soon established, however, that measurement of data could not be dispensed with altogether, but rather that a combined empirical–mathematical model would keep to a minimum the amount of measured data required to characterize the individual therapy machine. This is, in fact, the stage of development which has been now reached. Most of the currently employed models use mathematical expressions to represent the beam, but a few measured data still have to be fed into the planning computer to customize the planning system to the user's own therapy beams.

Among the models developed for high energy photons is the Cunningham's model (Cunningham, Shrivastava and Wilkinson, 1972) which uses an approach based on the concept of separating the primary and scatter dose components. It is interesting to note that it incorporates a method of evaluating the scatter which was developed by Clarkson as long ago as 1941 when nobody anticipated how useful it would become in the computer age!

Other beam models are based on the observation that beam cross-plots (profiles) vary with some regularity with depth and field size. For instance, Van de Geijn's programmes are mathematical expressions based on this projective property of radiotherapy beams (Van de Geijn, 1965).

So far, however, it has not been possible to formulate a purely mathematical beam model which would produce a calculated beam distribution of sufficient accuracy to be acceptable. The calculation algorithms developed for fast electron beams have proved more successful in this respect. *Figure 19.4* shows an electron beam isodose chart calculated from the mathematical formula given in the *Equation 2*.

This shows a beam model which allows the isodose curves to be calculated in a unit density medium, for a beam of any shape with an allowance for the curvature of the entrance surface if applicable. This is an example of a physical approach in which the electron beam distribution is modelled by a mathematical formula derived from basic physical electron scattering and collision processes. The main representatives of this group are the age-diffusion model (Kawachi, 1975) and the multiple Coulomb scattering model (Hogstrom, Mills and Almond, 1981) described by Klevenhagen (1985). *Equation 2* is the result of the age-diffusion approach derived from the theory of diffussion of neutrons through media employed widely in nuclear reactors. This theory in turn is an extension of the Boltzmann equation concerned with molecular diffusion in gases. This is yet another example of how radiotherapy benefits from the direct assimilation of fundamental physics.

To be complete and satisfactory, a computerized planning system should be able to take into account all possible parameters which affect the calculated distribution. It should be able to deal with irregularities of the patient surface, with inhomo-

$$D_{(X,Y,Z)} = \frac{D_0}{2}\left\{\operatorname{erf}\left[\frac{X_0(Z)-X}{2(K\tau)^{1/2}}\right] + \operatorname{erf}\left[\frac{X_0(Z)+X}{2(K\tau)^{1/2}}\right]\right\} \quad \text{(Field width)}$$

$$\bullet \left\{\operatorname{erf}\left[\frac{Y_0(Z)-Y}{2(K\tau)^{1/2}}\right] + \operatorname{erf}\left[\frac{Y_0(Z)+Y}{2(K\tau)^{1/2}}\right]\right\} \quad \text{(Field length)}$$

$$\bullet \cos\left[G_1\left(\frac{Z}{R_p}\right)^2 + G_2\left(\frac{Z}{R_p}\right) + G_3\right] \quad \text{(Central axis depth dose)}$$

$$\bullet \exp\left\{-\left(\left[\frac{2\pi}{3R_p}\right] \bullet (K\tau)^{1/2}\right)^2\right\} \quad \text{(Central axis depth dose)}$$

$$\bullet \left[\frac{F}{(F+Z)}\right]^2 \quad \text{(Inverse square correction)}$$

Equation 2

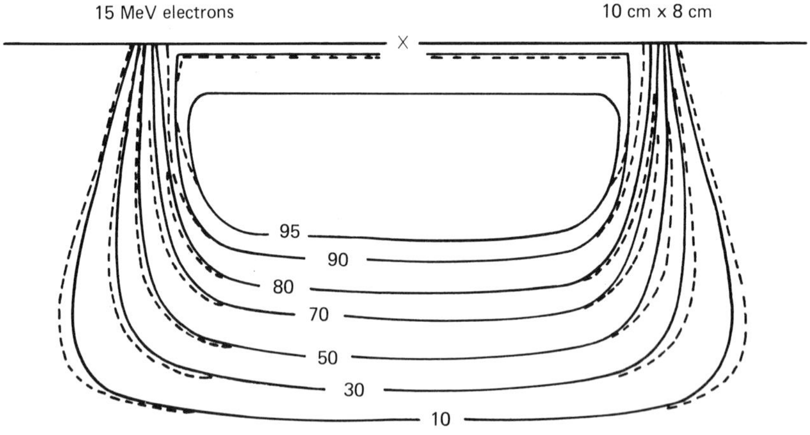

Figure 19.4 Isodose distribution for a 15 MeV beam generated by means of the age diffusion algorithm (continuous lines) compared with experimental curves (dashed lines)

geneities, wedges, various field weighting, fields of unusual shape or elongation, static or rotational beams. These features should be available for both photons and electrons. With the computer's ability to produce different plans very rapidly many existing systems have facilities to consider alternative treatment parameters and to produce an 'optimum plan'. The treatment planning system described by Redpath, Vickery and Duncan (1977) contains an optimization facility which, for a given combination of beam directions and sizes, finds the optimum weights and wedges for the beams, based on the criterion of uniformity of dose throughout the tumour volume.

The computer methods for treatment planning are now being taken one step further towards three-dimensional (3-D) treatment planning. This involves the computation of a dose distribution in 3-D, but obviously it requires a visualization of the body surface, the tumour and the relevant organs, throughout space. The availability of CT images has encouraged development in this area. The radiotherapist must be concerned about the extent of the tumour in a direction perpendicular to the plane of the beam axis, and be convinced that the radiation field in this direction adequately covers the tumour. Three-dimensional planning will offer him this information. However, such facilities are as yet only available in a few centres.

In the past 15 years physicists have put a considerable effort into the development of computational methods in treatment planning and this is still continuing.

Computed tomography in radiotherapy

The potential for utilization of CT scans in radiation therapy was immediately recognized when general purpose CT scanners became available. Optimal results in radiation therapy can only be achieved if accurate information is available about the tumour and the surrounding tissue. Computed tomography provides the radiotherapist with an imaging technique which gives this information. When scanning is carried out for radiotherapy purposes a series of contiguous transverse section images of the patient are made. These are used for diagnosis and staging as well as for the definition of the extent of the tumour, tissue inhomogeneities and the site of sensitive organs. CT also provides excellent information on the patient outline which is helpful in the selection of radiation portals.

Apart from being useful in tumour diagnosis, localization and staging, CT images are also successfully utilized directly in computer systems for calculating the exact radiation distribution in the patient, particularly in dealing with the problem of correcting for inhomogeneities.

The stages of the overall treatment planning process where CT finds application are shown schematically in *Figure 19.5*.

There are several practical problems associated with the use of a CT scanner for purposes of radiotherapy planning. The set up of the patient during the CT examination must match that of the proposed radiation treatment. To achieve this, the scanner's table top must be of a design (flat or curved) similar to that fitted on the treatment machine. Attention must be paid to the patient positioning during scanning, as it should be similar to that used during irradiation. An additional problem in 'matching' the CT examination and treatment situation, is the need to obtain images of the internal anatomical structures in locations corresponding to normal continuous breathing conditions such as exist when the patient is undergoing irradiation. The principle of motion–artefact-free diagnostic imaging observed widely in radiology does not necessarily apply to radiotherapy related CT scanning.

When the potential of CT in radiotherapy was realized, physicists started to work on the utilization of the CT images for the purpose of treatment planning. This led to the development of CT-linked treatment planning systems based on a computer. Such a system has a facility to use the CT-obtained data for displaying the images on the console of the treatment planning system and for calculating the radiation dose distribution taking into account the patient's outline and tissue inhomogeneities in the irradiated volume (*Figure 19.6*).

The significance of inhomogeneities in radiotherapy planning arises from the fact that the radiation distribution data related to the employed beams are usually measured in a medium of unit density with normal beam incidence on a flat surface. The practical problem with which the physicist is faced in treatment planning is the question of how to correct the idealized distribution to reflect the anatomy of a real patient. Both the inhomogeneities within the body and the irregularities of the entrance surface have a considerable modifying effect on the radiation beam distribution. Two factors contribute mainly to this effect: the different radiation energy absorption in the various tissues, and the alterations in the radiation scattering pattern caused by the inhomogeneities.

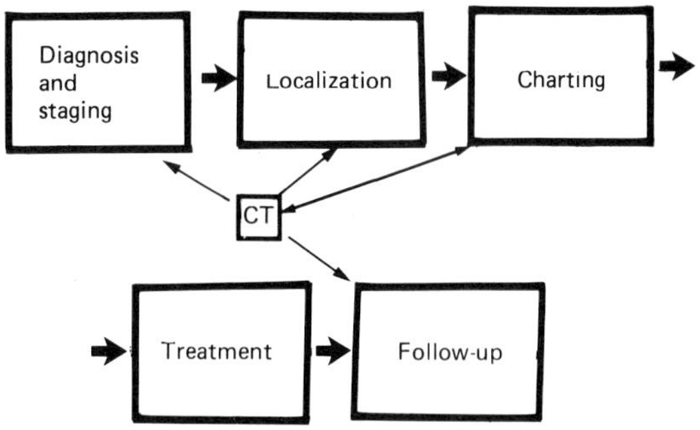

Figure 19.5 Applicability of CT scanning in the various stages of the treatment planning process. (Adapted from Parker and Hobday, 1981)

The inhomogeneities of importance in the body are the tissues and organs which differ from water (i.e. soft tissue) by density or atomic composition or both. Four inhomogeneities are important: lung and air cavities which differ from water only by density; bone, and of less importance fat, which are different from water in density and in composition. To allow properly for the effect of inhomogeneities on radiation distribution in a real patient, it is necessary to know their atomic numbers and physical densities as well as their dimensions, shape and exact position.

The external features of the patient's body, such as surface irregularities and obliquity also influence the beam distribution. CT scanners have proved to be superior imaging machines for the purpose of provision of all this information, useful in treatment planning in radiotherapy with both external beams and brachytherapy.

Two fundamental problems had to be resolved in developing CT-linked treatment planning systems. The first was to develop suitable software which would allow the results of the dose-distribution calculation algorithm describing the radiation beams to be superimposed on the CT images so that both match perfectly in terms of calculation geometry, patient outline, tumour position and other anatomical patient details. The second problem was to develop a technique for utilizing the CT number of CT image pixels for inhomogeneity correction.

Finding a solution to the latter problem was important as until the advent of the CT scanner only approximate corrections for the inhomogeneities were possible. The significance of CT to the development in this area is not yet fully appreciated by

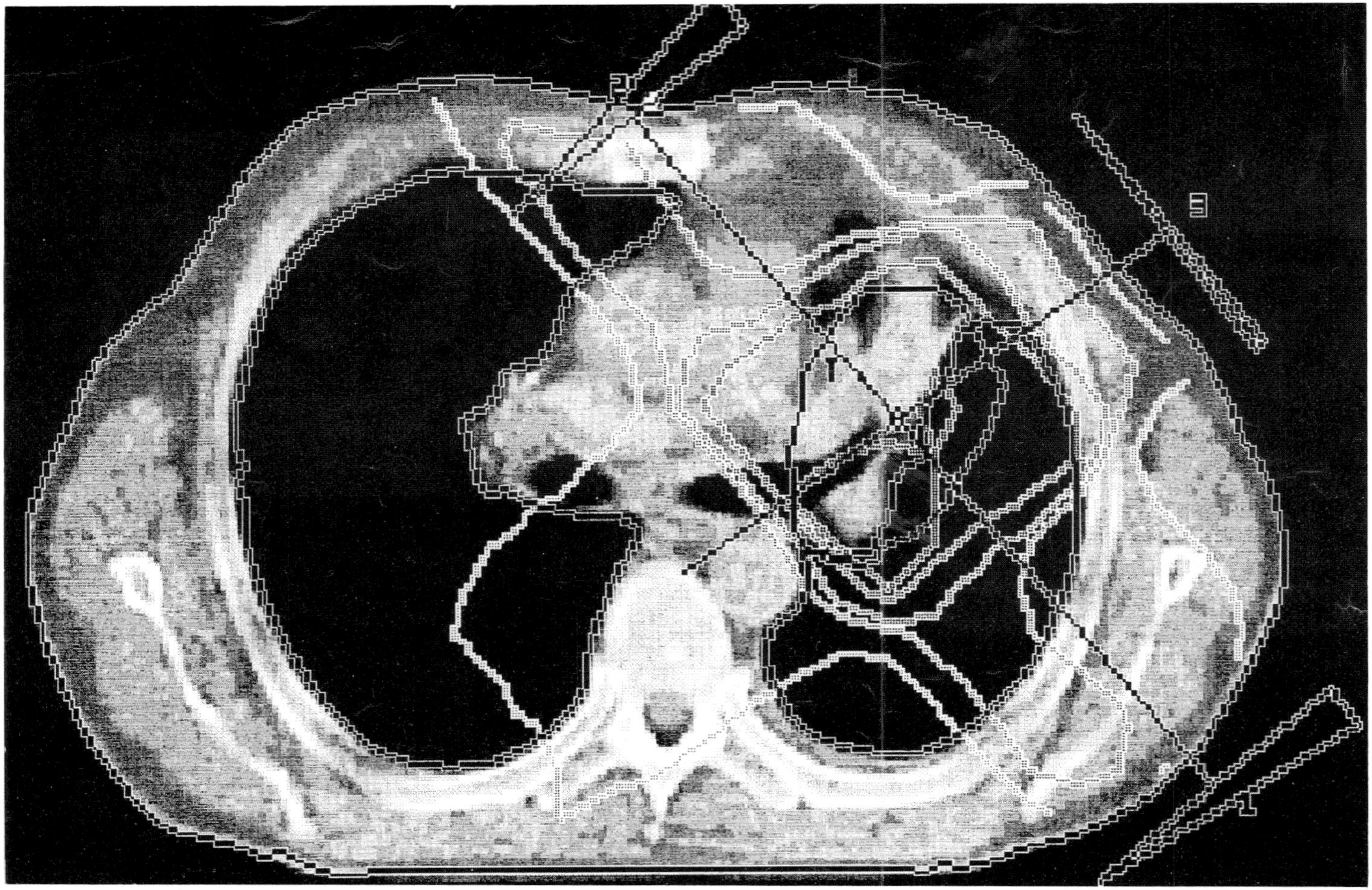

Figure 19.6 Superposition of radiation distribution calculated by a planning computer onto the CT patient image. (Courtesy of General Electric, USA)

radiotherapists. The correction technique is somewhat involved but will be briefly described in a simplified form.

The data of the CT images are viewed by projecting a picture onto a television screen, using fairly conventional techniques. The picture consists of elements of CT information — pixels. Usually a system would use a 256 × 256 pixel matrix to fill the television screen with a CT image or in high resolution systems a 512 × 512 pixel matrix. Each pixel of the CT picture has a value which represents the physical density, or more precisely, the radiation absorption value of a small volume in the body. In order to refer to absorption values it is necessary to assign a scale which is expressed either in terms of Hounsfield numbers or CT numbers. Effectively therefore, each pixel has its own CT or Hounsfield number assigned to it depending on its absorption value. It is this information on the various absorption values of the body cross-section that is utilized in the calculation of the radiotherapy beam distribution including inhomogeneity corrections. These possibilities were first realized in application to high energy photon therapy (Geise and McCullough, 1977; Parker, Hobday and Cassell, 1979; Cassell, Hobday and Parker, 1981).

When attempting to use the information provided by the scanner in the radiation distribution calculations the physicist has to overcome the problem of having tissue attenuation data (CT numbers) measured at the beam energy used by the scanner which are to be employed by the megavoltage therapy beam energy. Parker, Hobday and Cassell (1979) solved this problem by a direct determination of the relationship between the CT numbers and the relative electron concentration in the various tissues. The interest is focused on the electron concentration (electrons/cm^3) since this is the quantity which matters in the Compton type of interactions between radiation and tissue in the megavoltage energy region. Thus the image matrix of the patient body made up of CT numbers becomes an electron concentration matrix where the anatomy with the inhomogeneities is accurately localized and which lends itself to correction procedures.

The method of direct utilization of CT data has been developed further in application to electrons by Hogstrom, Mills and Almond (1981). The approach to an electron beam, however, is different since the relevant quantities in interaction processes between tissue and electrons are the collision stopping power and scattering power. The CT numbers which describe the patient anatomy therefore have to be related to these two parameters. This is done by calculating the CT numbers for various types of tissue using the attenuation coefficients for the average scanner X-ray energy obtainable from the appropriate physics tables. The linear collision stopping powers and the linear scattering powers may also be computed for the same tissues by employing a similar approach. Having obtained these data, the correlation between the CT numbers and the stopping and scattering powers may be established by plotting them together as illustrated in *Figure 19.7.*

By employing this procedure the CT image which, when it is taken on the scanner consists of CT numbers, is now converted into an image representing either electron concentration in each pixel or in the case of electron beam application, the stopping power and scattering power of each fragment (pixel) of tissue. At this stage the computer planning system has two CT images at its disposal. One is the conventional CT image and the second is one in which the pixels have been converted into parameters relevant to the interaction processes between the radiation traversing the body and the various tissue along the radiation path. The conventional image is used for marking the target volume, extent of inhomogeneities, sensitive organs and for the choice of radiation beams for treatment. The converted matrix of pixels is used for calculating the radiation distribution including correction for inhomogeneities.

A great deal of physics work has been put into developing methods of correcting for density in radiotherapy calculations. The advent of whole-body CT has generated an increased interest in this problem. There are several methods currently available of various degrees of complexity; among them the so-called 'effective TAR method' (Sontag and Cunningham, 1978) is, from the practical point of view, the most advanced, but it requires powerful computing facilities and a relatively long computation time. It should be noted that this method, if applied to energies above cobalt-60, requires replacement of TAR (tissue air ratios) by TMR (tissue maximum ratios).

The Sontag–Cunningham method of dose distribution calculation accounts for the effect of inhomogeneities on both the primary and scattered radiation components of the total dose at each point in the patient and considers individual tissue elements in three-dimensions.

For photons the corrections are most important in the thorax, where differences in midpoint tumour dose between corrected and uncorrected distribution plans may be as high as 25% (Parker and Hobday, 1981). The corrected plan gives much more accurate information about the distribution of radiation within the lung and around the lung boundary.

Inhomogeneity corrections are even more important for high energy electron therapy, where the changes in the range of electrons in tissues can result in very large changes to the estimated dose.

When the CT-aided treatment planning computer completes its calculations a more accurate dose distribution chart is produced in which the dose to the tumour and to the surrounding normal tissue (for example the spinal cord) is predicted with a higher degree of accuracy compared to other methods. This

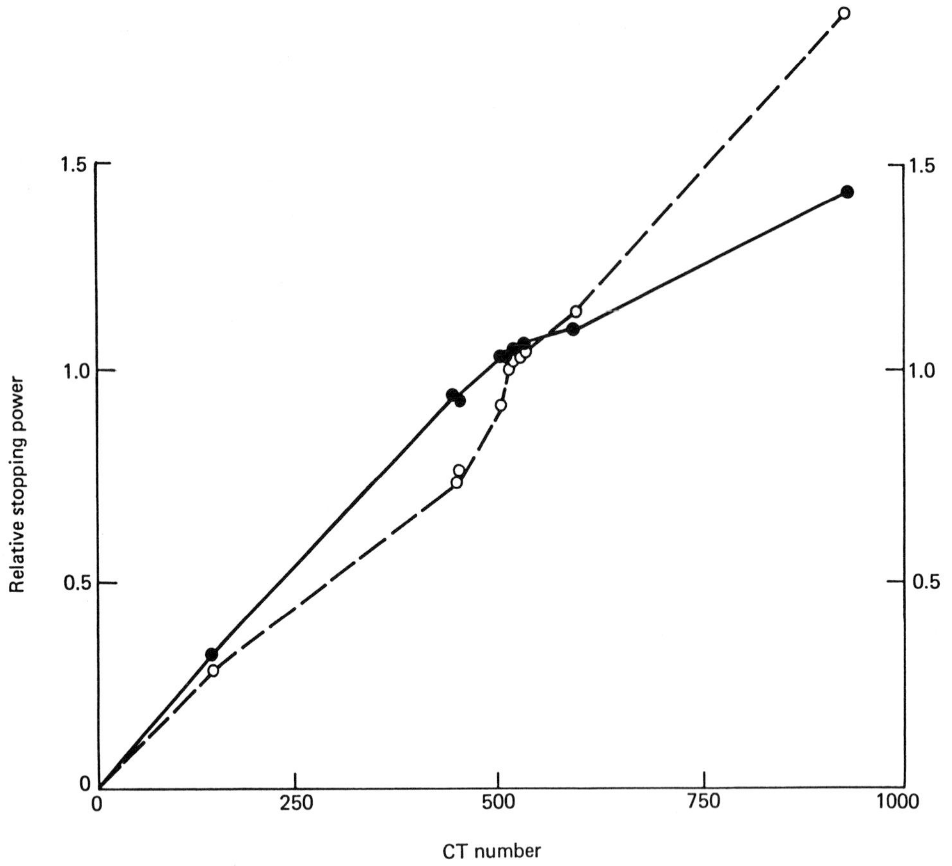

Figure 19.7 Relationship between CT numbers and stopping and scattering powers of electrons. ● Measured stopping power ratios; ○ measured scattering power ratios (from Hogstrom, Mills and Almond, 1981)

technique therefore makes a significant contribution towards minimization of failures in radiotherapy resulting from underdosage at the tumour volume and complications because of overdosage of normal tissue.

Further advantages of CT-aided planning lie in the fact that calculations in almost true 3-D geometry can be carried out. Radiotherapy planning usually considers a transverse plane through the centre of the treatment volume. It is important that the radiotherapist is aware of the isodose distribution in other planes. Coronal and sagittal distributions or many transverse sections throughout the target volume can be calculated and displayed.

The whole-body scanner provides opportunities for evaluation of alternative treatment techniques of a wider scope than were previously possible. CT scans may be easily obtained with patients in different treatment positions and an evaluation of alternative plans can be made. This can include comparison of integral dose, dose to critical organs, uniformity through the target volume, effect of inhomogeneity corrections, etc.

The final application in the whole procedure of treatment planning of the CT scanner is in monitoring the effectiveness of the radiation treatment and by serial scanning on follow-up.

Radiation protection

Each Authority in the UK Health Service must be served by an appropriately qualified and experienced physicist to act as radiological protection adviser (RPA). His duty is to visit regularly the facilities where radiation is used, to review in consultation with the radiotherapists the protection measures laid down. The clinicians are under obligation to inform the RPA when any change of equipment, usage, or environment occurs which may affect the radiological safety of the department. The physicist who is the RPA, is responsible for advice on all aspects of radiation protection, from planning new facilities to modifications of the existing ones. He must ensure that the environment is regularly surveyed and that the staff exposed to radiation from external sources is systematically monitored, preferably on an individual basis. If the radiation survey indicates that persons may, under normal working conditions, receive doses in excess of the level reasonable in the circumstances for the particular type of work, the RPA must indicate the measures to be adopted to rectify the situation. The RPA's responsibilities involve all areas of radiotherapy activities.

Radiation protection, in general, has two aspects; advisory and dosimetric, and physicists play an active role in both. The first involves provision of advice either through the appropriate committees or directly to radiotherapists, radiographers, technicians and administrators. Radiation protection dosimetry is the practical aspect of controlling the hazard arising from exposure to radiation and this is an important responsibility of the physicist.

Protection in external beam therapy

The physicist's task in external beam therapy is probably the simplest of all the tasks which he performs. The focal issue in this area of radiotherapy is the proper design of treatment room facilities at the time of equipment installation. Once the room for a treatment machine is suitably designed most of the problems of staff protection are solved. This is, however, not simple especially in the case of megavoltage installations. Room design for a linear accelerator has for example to be based on calculations which give consideration to all possible therapy beam orientations, scatter generated in the patient, in walls, floor and ceilings and to the leakage of radiation through the shielding around the radiation target (treatment head). At energies above 15 MeV, neutron production may become significant in magnitude and needs to be considered. The crucial areas in the design are the maze entrance and the machine control panel room which are heavily occupied by staff, particularly radiographers. A good practice in the design of these areas would be to aim to achieve radiation levels not in excess of one tenth of the permitted exposure. A large amount of expense is involved in the construction of suitably protected megavoltage treatment facilities, which are vital for the safety of all the staff. The physics calculations and advice therefore carry a considerable degree of responsibility.

The success of the design must be checked by a thorough survey of radiation levels in the whole of the environment of the newly installed machine. Proper documentation of this work must be made and held for future reference and inspections by the authorities who control the implementation of the radiation protection measures.

Once the treatment machine is in use and the survey is satisfactory, the routine protection work is confined to monitoring the staff exposure. This is conveniently achieved by using film dosemeters (film badges). Periodically, however, a survey of the treatment room environment needs to be repeated to confirm that no changes have occurred since construction of the room.

If the radiotherapy centre is equipped with a cobalt-60 or caesium-137 external beam machine, there will be a need to exchange the sources for new ones every few years when their activity is low. This work must be carried out by an experienced company and under a strict radiation protection survey. A great deal of thought must be given to such an operation prior to the source exchange.

Protection in brachytherapy

In contrast to the external therapy facilities where the radiation protection requirements must be already resolved at the time of building an appropriately designed room to house the equipment, radiation protection in brachytherapy is concentrated on the minimization of unwanted exposure during the usage of the sealed sources. Brachytherapy thus requires attention from this point of view all the time.

There are two fundamental rules concerning safe work with sealed sources. One is that the exposure to all personnel involved in the treatment procedure, apart from the patient, should be as small as possible. All activities related to storage, movement and handling of sources should be designed to achieve this. The second rule is that all sources which are on the hospital premises should be accountable for at any time and under any circumstances. There is no such thing to the physicist as a lost radioactive source. Should the unthinkable happen, and the source be 'lost', it must be retrieved.

The central area for brachytherapy activities is the radioactive sealed sources laboratory which has to be appropriately designed to provide the storage, cleaning, handling facilities and sources inventory. This may involve not only the conventional γ-ray emitters such as tubes and needles or facilities for afterloading sources, but also β-ray or neutron emitting sources. Afterloading equipment for gynaecological therapy or iridium wire preparation may also have to be included in a well developed sealed sources laboratory. It is a duty of the physicist to design such facilities to the highest possible safety standards.

The maintenance of the sealed sources during their useful life is usually simpler than the maintenance of equipment producing external therapy beams, although with the arrival of afterloading machines the situation has somewhat changed. Sealed sources such as tubes, needles, β-emitters or source trains of the Curietron type require only periodic checking for possible mechanical damage which, in fact, rarely occurs. The afterloading equipment itself, however, requires far more attention to keep it in serviceable condition. Once a year, radiation leakage and wipe tests on sources should be carried out to see that they conform to a generally accepted norm. When the sources are used for treatment on a patient, it is necessary to ensure that other patients not involved in a treatment with radiation are not exposed unnecessarily. Nursing and other staff must have adequate protection facilities. Ideally there should be a special ward designated for brachytherapy, surrounded by protective walls and equipped for afterloading facilities.

When using brachytherapy a great deal of the success with radiation protection is dependent on how well the staff involved is trained to do this work and whether they have written operational instructions, safety rules and emergency procedures at their disposal. Staff training should be carried out periodically to review the safety measures, discuss possible problems and maintain the awareness in radiation protection. The preparation of written instructions, and rules may appear a tedious task but is very necessary. The custodian of sealed sources, nurses, theatre staff, radiographers and all personnel who come into contact with the sources must all know the rules and regulations and what must be the correct procedures for problems and in emergencies. For legal reasons these rules must be in a written form to avoid any ambiguity and to secure the safety of all concerned. Physicists must be conversant with the code of practice and other regulations or any other legal requirements concerning the use of radioactive sources.

Research and development (R and D), teaching

As in any other field of medicine or science, radiotherapy would not make any progress unless an appropriate effort is put into research and development. Similarly, the physics underlying radiotherapy must be developing in parallel. There are several aspects of the R and D activities in which physicists are involved:

(1) Research on various aspects of ionizing radiation characteristics, on dosimetry, on interaction processes of radiation with matter and the effect of ionizing radiation on tissue and cells
(2) Development and/or assimilation of new improved treatment methods and techniques for clinical use
(3) Assimilation of research and development results which are produced in other radiotherapy and physics centres
(4) Assimilation of national or international recommendations currently concerning the best practice in physics and radiation dosimetry
(5) Interchange of information of research and development results through meetings and publications.

In teaching, the physicist's involvement covers various levels of academic standard both of undergraduate and postgraduate standard, including PhD level. This extends to practical training of which in-post training is a popular form.

References

ABBE, R. (1906) Radium in surgery. *Journal of American Medical Association*, **47**, 183–185

BENTLEY, R. E. and MILAN, J. (1971) An interactive digital computer system for radiotherapy treatment planning. *British Journal of Radiology*, **44**, 826–833

BRACE, J. A., DAVY, T. J. and SKEGGS, D. (1981) Computer-controlled cobalt unit for radiotherapy. *Medical and Biological Engineering and Computing*, **19**, 612–616

CASSELL, K. J., HOBDAY, P. A. and PARKER, R. P. (1981) The implementation of a generalized Batho inhomogeneity correction for radiotherapy planning with direct use of CT numbers. *Physics in Medicine and Biology*, **26**, 825–833

CLARKSON, J. R. (1941) A note of depth dose in field of irregular shape. *British Journal of Radiology*, **14**, 265–268

CUNNINGHAM, J. R., SHRIVASTAVA, P. N. and WILKINSON, J. M. (1972) Program IRREG — calculation of dose from irregularly shaped radiation beams. *Computer Programs in Biomedicine*, **2**, 192–199

DIFFEY, B. L. and KLEVENHAGEN, S. C. (1975) An experimental study and calculated dose distribution in water around caesium sources. *Physics in Medicine and Biology*, **20**, 446–454

GEISE, R. A. and McCULLOUGH, E. C. (1977) The use of scanners in megavoltage photon beam therapy planning. *Radiology*, **124**, 133–150

HOGSTROM, K. R., MILLS, M. D. and ALMOND, P. R. (1981) Electron beam dose calculations. *Physics in Medicine and Biology*, **26**, 445–459

KAWACHI, K. (1975) Calculation of electron dose distribution for radiotherapy treatment planning. *Physics in Medicine and Biology*, **20**, 571–577

KIRK, J., GREY, W. M. and WATSON, E. R. (1972) Cumulative radiation effect. *Clinical Radiology*, **23**, 93–105

KLEVENHAGEN, S. C. (1976) A theoretical and experimental study of p-n junction silicon radiation detectors operated in d-c mode. *PhD Thesis*, London University, London, UK

KLEVENHAGEN, S. C. (1985) *Physics of Electron Beam Therapy*. Bristol: Adam Hilger

KLEVENHAGEN, S. C. and FAULKNER, K. (1981) Radiation protection aspects of the Curietron. *AMPI Medical Physics Bulletin*, **6**, 145–150

LIVERSAGE, W. (1980) A comparison of the predictions of the CRE, TDF and Liversage formulae with clinical experience. *British Journal of Radiology*, Special report no. 17

MEREDITH, W. J. (1967) *Radium dosage, Manchester System*. Edinburgh: E. and S. Livingstone

PARKER, R. P. and HOBDAY, P. A. (1981) CT scanning in radiotherapy treatment planning: its strength and weaknesses. In *Computer Axial Tomography in Oncology*, edited by J. E. Husband and P. A. Hobday, pp. 90–109. London: Churchill Livingstone

PARKER, R. P., HOBDAY, P. A. and CASSELL, K. J. (1979) The direct use of CT numbers in radiotherapy dosage calculations for inhomogeneous media. *Physics in Medicine and Biology*, **24**, 802–809

REDPATH, A. T., VICKERY, B. A. and DUNCAN W. (1977) A comprehensive radiotherapy planning system implemented in Fortran on a small interactive computer. *British Journal of Radiology*, **50**, 51–57

puter. *British Journal of Radiology*, **50**, 51–57

SIEVERT, R. M. (1921) Die gamma-strahlungs-intensitäte in der umgebung von Radium-Nadeln. *Acta Radiologica*, **1**, 89–128

SONTAG, M. R. and CUNNINGHAM, J. R. (1978) The equivalent tissue-air ratio method for making absorbed dose calculations in a heterogeneous medium. *Radiology*, **129**, 787–794

VAN DE GEIJN, J. (1965) The computation of two- and three-dimensional dose distribution in cobalt-60 teletherapy. *British Journal of Radiology*, **38**, 369–377

WALSTAM, R. (1962) Remotely-controlled afterloading radiotherapy apparatus. *Physics in Medicine and Biology*, **1**, 225–232

20

Medical and radiotherapeutic oncology: the interaction

R. T. D. Oliver

Introduction

The two principal non-lymphoid adult tumours, in which more than 50% of patients with advanced disease are cured by combination chemotherapy — germ cell tumours of testis and gestational choriocarcinoma — share the characteristic that a proportion are curable by each of the single agents in the combination (Berkowitz *et al.*, 1980; Begent and Bagshawe, 1982; for review *see* Oliver, 1985). For the majority of other types of adult cancer the lack of cure by single agent chemotherapy and failure of combination chemotherapy, is almost the universal rule. Radiotherapy, in contrast, does produce a cure rate in a substantial number of adult tumours as a single agent, and must therefore be the front runner for any study of combination treatment. One possible factor in the lack of successful exploration of cytotoxic drug–radiation interaction is that the two modalities cannot be administered completely synchronously as has been possible for the combinations of drugs used in the two chemocurable tumours. This is because the principles governing scheduling of radiation and cytotoxic drugs are completely different. It is the intention of this chapter to consider the principles of combination chemotherapy, to review past experience of drug–radiation interaction and justification for the specific scheduling of drugs and radiation, and to develop a theme for a new generation of drug–radiation studies ending with a reappraisal of the place for medical oncology in the context of current structure of medical and radiotherapeutic oncology departments.

Cure of cancer with cytotoxic drugs

Cytotoxic vs cytostatic drugs

Antibiotics can be subdivided into cytostatic and cytotoxic types on the basis of whether the damage done to the bacterium was reversible, as in the former group, or irreversible as in the latter group. Cytotoxic chemotherapy as used in cancer practice, although designated cytotoxic because of the effects of the drugs *in vitro* can, in fact, also be subdivided on the basis of whether it produces cytotoxic effects *in vivo*, i.e. cure, as seen in leukaemia, lymphomas, testicular germ cell tumours or childhood solid cancer, or alternatively cytostatic effects, i.e. delay in tumour regrowth, which has been the only effect demonstrable in most trials of cytotoxic drugs in adult solid cancers. This is most clearly demonstrated by the adjuvant trials in breast and poor prognosis bladder cancer where there is clear evidence of delay to first recurrence (Bonadonna *et al.*, 1977; Glashan, Houghton and Robinson, 1977; Howells *et al.*, 1984; Herr, unpublished data), but equivocal benefit in terms of overall survival (Bonadonna *et al.*, 1984; Howells *et al.*, 1984).

Criteria for measuring response to cytotoxic drugs

Most of the justification for using the concepts of complete and partial response (Simon, 1982) to assess the benefits of cytotoxic chemotherapy, rather than those of growth delay as used in most experimental radiotherapy research (Fowler, Hill and Sheldon, 1980), or even the ultimate measure i.e. durable survival, was that they provided a more rapid way of assessing whether there was any drug activity. There have been three major disadvantages to this approach. First, the response criterion lacked any clinical parameter based on symptomatology, which although much more subjective was the reason why the patient was seeking treatment. The development of various performance status indexes such as the Karnofsky index or WHO/UICC performance status index (*Table 20.1*) was an attempt to compensate for this lack of objectivity of symptoms. Unfortunately, the results from using this type of index have not been totally reliable as they do not distinguish the effects of drug toxicity from symptoms of the tumour. The second disadvantage of using measurable metastases to assess response was that it cannot be an accurate assessment of the effect of the drugs on stem cells if the measurable metastasis consists of a large proportion of differentiated cells or host stromal cells and tissue as in patients with germ cell tumour who have a mature teratoma.

Table 20.1 Definition of performance status categories

UICC/WHO	*Karnofsky*	*Definitions*
0	100	Asymptomatic
1	80–90	Symptomatic, fully ambulatory
2	60–70	Symptomatic, in bed less than 50% of the day
3	40–50	Symptomatic, in bed more than 50% of the day, but not bedridden
4	20–30	Bedridden

The third disadvantage is the large number of patients with cancer who have failed conventional treatment, who do not have measurable disease, and who cannot therefore be assessed. More than 50% of bladder cancer cases (Oliver, 1980) and 80% of prostate cancer patients (Yagoda *et al.*, 1979) do not have measurable metastases terminally. As it is increasingly accepted that in the adult solid tumours cytotoxic drugs are not curative, although some do have a palliative effect, measurement of response in terms of improvement in performance status and not just in terms of producing shrinkage of totally asymptomatic measurable lesions will be increasingly important.

Response rate to single agent chemotherapy

The chemocurable tumours are set apart from other neoplasms by the high initial complete response rate and durable disease control rate seen with single agent therapy (*Table 20.2*). This is in contrast to most of the other adult tumours where rapid regrowth occurs when the drugs are stopped, even in those rare cases with small volume metastases who apparently achieve a complete response to single agent chemotherapy. There are two exceptions to this, i.e. oat cell carcinoma of the lung and ovarian carcinoma (Young, Knapp and Perez, 1982; Morstyn *et al.*, 1984), although few of the single agent studies in these tumours give enough long-term follow-up information to establish the cure rate at 10 years. In addition, in ovarian tumours where, on average, 7% achieve long-term disease-free cure with single agent chemotherapy (Young, Knapp and Perez, 1982), the possibility that the patients achieving long-term cures with single agent chemotherapy are atypical germ cell tumour, has not been absolutely excluded. This hypothesis is partly supported by the high incidence of placental alkaline phosphatase production by ovarian tumour tissue (Haije *et al.*, 1979) and the fact that more than 90% of testicular germinomas (i.e. seminomas) also produce placental alkaline phosphatase (Tucker *et al.*, 1985).

Subclassification of drugs and the principles of combination therapy

Cytotoxic chemotherapeutic drugs can be subclassified on the basis of their chemical and biological effects in terms of the phase of cell cycle at which they act (*Table 20.3*). All of the active anticancer cytotoxic drugs have action on DNA synthesis (*Figure 20.1*). However, there are factors other than the specificity of their chemical reaction which determine their arrival at the specific target, such as cell membrane

Table 20.2 Drug-induced complete response rates (%) in chemotherapeutically curable malignancies

	Single agents				*Combination*
Childhood acute lymphatic leukaemia	Vincristine 57	Prednisolone 47			92
Hodgkin's disease	Mustine 13	Vincristine 36	Procarbazine 38	Prednisolone 0	61
Testicular teratoma	Bleomycin 3	Vinblastine 16	Cisplatin 22		73
Choriocarcinoma	Methotrexate 47	Actinomycin 57	Chlorambucil NA		85

Table 20.3 Classification of cytotoxic drugs

	Alkylating agents	*Antimetabolites*	*Antitumour antibiotics*	*Others*
Phase/cycle specific		Methotrexate Procarbazine Hydroxyurea 6-mercaptopurine Cytosine arabinoside		Vincristine VM 26 VP16-213
Non-phase specific	Chlorambucil Cyclophosphamide Melphalan BCNU/UNU Cisplatin	5-Fluorouracil	Hydroxydaunorubicin Bleomycin Mitomycin Mithramycin Mitoxanthrone	

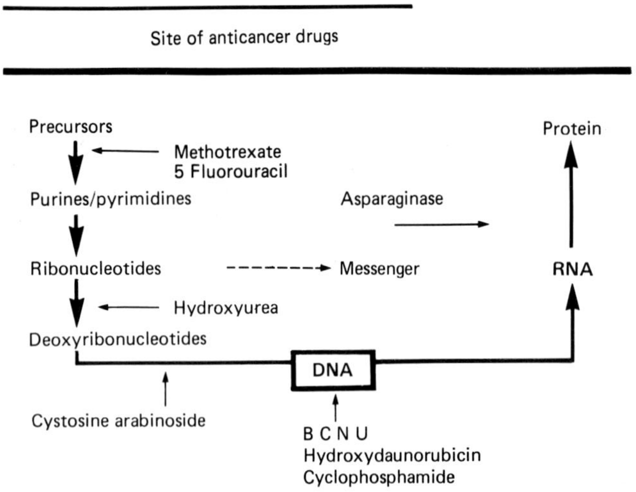

Figure 20.1 Sites of action of anticancer drugs in the cycle of DNA synthesis

transport, drug pharmacology and excretion (for review *see* Chabner and Myers, 1982).

The majority of the cytotoxic drugs are not specific for any phase in the cell cycle and are known as non-phase specific. With repeated use these drugs generate cumulative effects on normal stem cells. The remaining drugs are specific for the synthetic phase of actual DNA synthesis because they either inhibit enzymes invovled in DNA synthesis or are synthetic analogues of normal DNA bases. In general, these types of drugs always leave the non-cycling proportion of normal cells undamaged and so are safe for repeated use (Bruce, Meeker and Valeriote, 1966).

Over the last 30 years the methodology for assessment of new drugs and combinations has been formalized (Simon, 1982). It is now the convention that all new drugs are assessed initially for toxicity with dose escalation to the limit of tolerance in so called phase 1 studies on terminal patients for whom there is no conventional treatment or who have escaped from control by such treatment. Although evidence of anticancer activity is not demanded of any drug which progresses from phase 1 to phase 2 studies, few of the really successful drugs introduced over the last 15 years have not given some evidence of activity in phase 1 studies. In phase 2 studies selected groups of 20–40 patients with specific tumours are appraised when they first develop measurable lesions in order to obtain information on response rates. This enables drugs to be selected for combination studies which are then piloted in a phase 2 trial and, if more active than the single agent, go forward to a phase 3 randomized trial against conventional treatment in an adjuvant or adjunctive setting in combination with surgery or radiotherapy.

The guiding principle in selecting drugs for combination therapy has been to attempt to select drugs with differing side-effects (*Table 20.4*), although the selection of drugs used in the really successful combination treatments has often been based on the order

Table 20.4 Toxicity of anticancer drugs

Haematological	Most except bleomycin
Mucous membranes	Most with high doses, but especially methotrexate and bleomycin
Vomiting and nausea	Especially with platinum, nitrogen mustard and hydroxydaunorubicin
Alopecia	Hydroxydaunorubicin, etoposide, high dose vincas
Subcutaneous burns	Hydroxydaunorubicin, nitrogen mustard, DTIC
Cardiotoxicity	Hydroxydaunorubicin
Neurotoxicity	Vinca alkaloids, cisplatin
Second malignancies	Principally alkylating agents and radiotherapy especially if combined
Infertility	Alkylating agents

in which the drugs were tested first as single agents. In most of the curative combinations, the drugs are given synchronously or in close sequence with a gap for recovery between each cycle. The principal reason for intermittent as opposed to continuous use of drugs was the demonstration, particularly with the non-phase specific drugs, that damage to stem cells was cumulative with continuous treatment, leading to immunosuppression and bone marrow failure. In addition, the incidence of second malignancies, particularly leukaemia, was more frequent when the drugs were given in low doses for long continuous periods (Reimer *et al.*, 1977).

Although it is usual in clinical practice to give all the drugs within a combination in close succession, there is some evidence from *in vitro* studies that drugs scheduled with short periods of 1–24 hours in between each individual drug give an enhanced response, as has been demonstrated for methotrexate and 5-fluorouracil. When using this combination the optimum time interval has been shown to be 24 hours, with the methotrexate being given first. To date there has been no evidence in clinical trials of improved therapeutic indexes from sequencing of the two drugs in randomized trials (Browman *et al.*, 1983; Coates *et al.*, 1984) although part of this might be that quantitation of side-effects is not as easily measurable as regression of metastases.

Similar problems made it difficult to evaluate whether there was a therapeutic advantage for the more complex scheme of scheduling developed by Price and Hill (1981) on the basis of the principles developed by Bruce, Meeker and Valeriote (1966). These schedules undoubtedly reduce the risks of serious lethal bone marrow and gut toxicity and have been adopted widely to provide less toxic chemotherapy combination for use in the common adult cancers. Although this approach provided safe methods for giving multiple drugs together with relatively few side-effects, the lack of really active drugs for these tumours meant that the only advantage of these schedules was that they encouraged widespread use in a 'service setting' of multiple drugs without very critical appraisal.

The chemocurable tumours

Childhood tumours

The previous section has emphasized the problems of using conventional measurable response criteria to quantify cytotoxic drug activity in the relative chemoinsensitive adult solid neoplasms. Although measurable response criteria are still valid for chemosensitive childhood tumours, there are today other problems with regard to assessing their responses. These are: how to determine resistance to standard drugs in order to evaluate new drugs in patients resistant to conventional treatment; and when is it safe to stop treatment in responding patients, i.e. is maintenance necessary? Childhood leukaemia is the first model of a chemocurable malignancy (for review *see* Pinkel *et al.*, 1971) and was the disease in which many of the concepts which have dominated the use of cytotoxic drugs in malignancy were first developed. Although more than 90% of patients could be put into remission with vincristine and prednisone, the majority relapsed, and as half of them were in sanctuary sites i.e. the CNS, two adjunctive treatments were added. The first was maintenance chemotherapy which was continued for 3 years. When this was found not to prevent CNS relapses cranial irradiation and intrathecal chemotherapy were added. When compared to the initial impact of these procedures, the improvement in results in the last decade has been less impressive, the main gain being in trials looking at the value of adding other newer drugs in subsets of patients shown by multivariate analysis of earlier trials to be at risk of failing standard treatment (Simone, 1979). Equally, as multivariate analysis has identified the patients most at risk from treatment failure the question as to whether a full 3 years' maintenance therapy is required for the good prognosis patient now needs evaluation.

The chemotherapy of childhood solid tumours developed from the basis of the principles used for the treatment of leukaemia. Some of these, such as neuroblastoma in older children, proved more resistant than leukaemia (Simone, 1984). However, for most tumours, after an intensive induction phase, most frequently using vincristine, actinomycin (or hydroxydaunorubicin) and cyclophosphamide, and including where possible surgical excision of the primary and irradiation, maintenance was given for up to 2 years. Today in the most curable of these neoplasms (Wilms' tumour) the principal controversy centres on whether radiotherapy is necessary and how long maintenance chemotherapy is required (Lemerle *et al.*, 1983).

Hodgkin's disease

When combination cytoxic chemotherapy was first used to treat advanced Hodgkin's disease, the principles learnt from the treatment of childhood leukaemia were applied, and treatment was usually continued for 3 years after an initial induction phase lasting 9 months with courses of treatment at less frequent intervals being used as maintenance (De Vita and Serpick, 1970; Nicholson *et al.*, 1970). When trials were eventually undertaken it emerged that, although the longer treatment regimen did delay relapse, the overall outcome in terms of survival was identical (Sutcliffe *et al.*, 1978), and today treatment is usually stopped somewhat arbitrarily after six courses of treatment (or three courses from disappearance of all known disease), although the evidence that this is the minimum requirement is not very strong.

In Hodgkin's disease, data on the best second line chemotherapy are somewhat unclear. Some groups have reported salvage of failed mustine, vincristine (oncovin), procarbazine and prednisone (MOPP) treated patients, with hydroxydaunorubicin, bleomycin, DTIC and vinblastine (ABVD) (Santoro and Bonadonna, 1979), although others have not, or have been discouraged by toxicity problems. DTIC is very damaging to peripheral veins, and bleomycin produces increased pulmonary toxicity in patients who have had previous irradiation to the chest. However, there are reports of a lower incidence of second malignancy (Vallagussa *et al.*, 1982) and less damage to spermatogenesis with ABVD than with MOPP and a higher incidence of continuous disease-free survival when the two combinations (ABVD and MOPP) are used in sequence (Bonadonna *et al.*, 1984).

Recently, the evidence that etoposide has activity as a single agent has led to developments of combinations using this drug (McElwain and Selby, 1984; Santoro *et al.*, 1984). The prolonged period of primary chemotherapy (6–9 months) necessary before being able to determine that a patient has drug resistant disease is one of the factors which is slowing progress in this area. For the future, there is a need to define patients with poor prognosis and early indicators of poor response in good risk patients and to use second line treatment at an early stage in these patients.

Adult myeloid leukaemia

When curative chemotherapy first appeared (Clarkson, 1972; Crowther *et al.*, 1973) the principles learnt from treating the childhood leukaemias were applied in adult acute myeloid leukaemia and an initial intensive induction phase was followed by a maintenance phase of chemotherapy. In addition, some of the earlier studies also used immunotherapy with BCG and leukaemia cells inactivated by irradiation (Powles *et al.*, 1977). Although there was some benefit from the immunological treatment in several of the studies, this was ultimately thought not to be due to immunological mechanisms but due to the bone marrow of such patients being better able to tolerate chemotherapy when they relapsed (for review *see* Oliver, 1977). None of these studies showed any real benefit from maintenance chemotherapy, and the most successful regimens today use the maximum amount of treatment possible in the initial induction phase and give no maintenance therapy (Bell *et al.*, 1982; Lister *et al.*, 1980).

Germ cell tumours

Following the discovery that cisplatin was an active agent in treatment of metastatic teratoma (Higby *et al.*, 1974) there have been two principal approaches to the design of combination regimens. The first successful regimen was that of Einhorn and Donohue (1977) who simply added platinum as a third drug to the bleomycin and vinblastine regimen developed by Samuels *et al.* (1976) with an improvement of long-term cure rate from 35 to 58%. Those centres with long experience of developing combination regimens in malignant teratoma and other malignancies during the pre-platinum era simply added it as an additional drug to their already complicated regimens. As a consequence their initial combinations consisted of multiple drugs (up to 10 drugs) in alternating combination regimens given initially for 12–24 months (Newlands *et al.*, 1980; Vugrin *et al.*, 1981).

The initial results from these more complicated regimens were in some instances a little better than the bleomycin, vinblastine, cisplatin (BVP) regimens. With maturation of the results, however, little difference can be demonstrated between the two approaches after making allowance for the era when the patients were treated (MRC Testicular Tumour Working Party, 1985) (*Table 20.5*) although two constant findings have emerged. All studies using maintenance treatment after initial induction have shown no added benefit (Einhorn and Williams, 1980), and all of those using multiple alternating combinations have been able to reduce the dosage of the drugs other than cisplatin, and simplify their regimens, thus reducing treatment times down to 6 months or less without loss of effect (Vugrin, Whitmore and Golbey, 1983; Newlands *et al.*, 1983).

Those studies using only the three drugs (BVP), although initially starting with 9 weeks' treatment, ultimately achieved better results in patients with advanced disease when 12 weeks' treatment was given, and this has become the standard method. Although some centres using BVP without a tradition of retroperitoneal lymph node surgery gave more than 3 months' treatment, this was at the expense of increased morbidity. The significant factor in demonstrating that more than 3 months' chemotherapy was unnecessary has been the discovery that when post-treatment surgical staging is undertaken on all patients who have residual tumour either in the chest or abdomen after 3 months' treatment, more than two-thirds had no evidence of viable malignancy in the excised specimen and do not need any further chemotherapy (Oliver *et al.*, 1983; Rowland and Donohue, 1984). More than half of those with viable malignancy could be salvaged by giving additional second line chemotherapy (Rowland and Donohue, 1984). The therapeutic value of the surgery on its own is marginal, as only 20% of patients who had excision of viable malignancy without post-surgical chemotherapy survived. Post-

Table 20.5 Impact of experience on results of cytotoxic chemotherapy in metastatic malignant teratoma

		No.	*Long-term disease free* (%)
BV	1974 Samuels *et al.* (1976)	50	26
	1978 Samuels *et al.* (1979)	92	42
BVP	1977 Einhorn and Donohue (1977) 1980 Einhorn and Williams (1980)	50	58
Etoposide combination	1982 Oliver (unpublished observations)	15	67
	1984 Oliver (unpublished observations)	21	95
Charing Cross	1980 Newlands *et al.* (1980)	43	66
	1984 Newlands *et al.* (1984)	69	83
Memorial VAB IV	1981 Vugrin *et al.* (1981)	41	60
Memorial VAB VI	1983 Vugrin, Whitmore and Golbey (1983)	25	80

B: bleomycin
V: vinblastine
P: cisplatin

treatment surgical staging, however, has played an immense role in educating clinicians treating germ cell tumours to the fact that it is not necessary to go on using toxic chemotherapy until all signs of scar tissue at the site of metastases have disappeared. Ultimately, given the extensive nature of the surgery sometimes necessary, the aim must be to develop better non-invasive methods such as magnetic resonance imaging (n.m.i.) to determine when it will be safe to stop treatment.

The place for radiotherapy in the chemocurable malignancies

In childhood leukaemia, with better definition of patients with a low risk of CNS relapse, some centres have shown that it is safe to rely on prophylactic intrathecal chemotherapy alone (Freeman *et al.*, 1983), although, in terms of patient tolerance, cranial radiation is probably a less distressing treatment. Because of its possible interference with bone growth in vertebrae, as well as marrow depression the need for craniospinal irradiation, if no intrathecal treatment is given is a less viable option in young children.

In Hodgkin's disease, the principal reasons for not using chemotherapy in early stage disease are the damaging effect of chemotherapy on the gonads, the risk of a second malignancy and the overall toxicity, although this is somewhat less when chlorambucil is substituted for mustine, and vinblastine for vincristine (McElwain, 1978). When chemotherapy was compared with radiotherapy in randomized trials in patients with comparable disease, i.e. stage 3, the relapse rate was higher after radiotherapy, but as most of the failures could be salvaged by chemotherapy, the overall survival was identical (Lister *et al.*, 1983) (*see* Chapter 8). Recently, a similar trial comparing chemotherapy with radiotherapy in poor prognosis stage 1 and 2 cases has been undertaken (Young, 1984 personal communication). So far there have been no relapses among 30 patients randomized to receive six courses of MOPP chemotherapy, while nearly one-quarter of those receiving radiotherapy have relapsed. Although the protocol called for six courses, all patients receiving chemotherapy had no clinical evidence of disease after one course. The dilemma now is that, given the recent discovery that two courses of mustine chemotherapy produces substantially less interference with fertility (daCunha *et al.*, 1984) and in theory, although no data are available to confirm it, less serious risk of malignancy, is it safe to consider using two courses of combination chemotherapy with the less toxic chlorambucil, vinblastine, prednisolone and procarbazine (Chl VPP) (McElwain 1978) as a first line treatment for early-stage poor risk cases? Possibly the safest and quickest way to resolve the issue would be to set up a randomized trial comparing two courses of Ch VPP, versus radiotherapy alone using post-treatment surgical staging to confirm the completeness of response.

Another area where radiotherapy could be used in Hodgkin's disease is as an adjunct to sites of bulk tumour in patients with advanced disease. Although there have been several studies the data are not conclusive (Rosenberg *et al.*, 1978; Crowther *et al.*, 1984). These studies have suffered the same difficulties of interpretation as similar trials in metastatic teratoma (Duchesne and Peckham, 1984) and childhood solid tumours (Lemerle *et al.*, 1983) i.e. it is unclear whether there is any malignancy in the mass by the time radiotherapy is given. The other difficulty has been that this type of scheduling offers the least opportunity for drug–radiation interaction as the drugs and radiation are given at a different time, although as Peckham's group have demonstrated, this is the safest time to use irradation in order to keep normal tissue damage to a minimum (Yarnold *et al.*, 1983). As there is no real evidence of advantage, radiation is no longer used to treat sites of bulk disease in patients with metastatic maligant teratoma and is being less often advocated in Hodgkin's disease, childhood malignancy and even seminoma, where it has recently been demonstrated that using cisplatin as a single agent may be as effective in curing patients as combination chemotherapy or radiotherapy alone (Oliver, Hope-Stone and Blandy, 1983, 1984).

The results from the use of cisplatin in the treatment of metastatic seminoma have provided the first situation in oncology where it may be possible to compare the effect of a single chemotherapeutic agent with radiation. When cisplatin-containing cytotoxic drug combinations had been shown to cure patients with metastatic teratoma, they were tested in patients with metastatic seminoma before there was adequate information on the activity of cisplatin as a single agent. Another complicating factor was that given the high cure rate of metastatic seminoma with radiation, most cases treated with drugs had already failed with radiation. This, combined with the relative rarity of metastatic seminoma, at first masked the fact that this tumour is even more sensitive to chemotherapy than malignant teratoma and close to 90% of patients may be curable using cisplatin alone (Oliver, Hope-Stone and Blandy, 1984). Although the current studies have used 3 months' treatment, as in the early stage Hodgkin's disease trial discussed above, the most significant unknown is how little treatment is needed. A substantial proportion of patients with seminoma achieved remission with only one treatment, and this would be a realistic alternative to test against radiotherapy after orchidectomy as an adjuvant for early stage cases.

In malignant teratoma patients with stage 1 disease, increasingly sophisticated staging procedures have made it possible to consider not using retroperitoneal lymph node dissection or radiotherapy as prophylaxis (*see* Chapter 3). Although using either procedure prophylactically does reduce the relapse rate by 5–10%, 75% are cured by orchidectomy alone and close to 100% of relapses can be salvaged by chemotherapy, thus the need for prophylactic treatment is being increasingly questioned (Peckham *et al.*, 1983: Oliver, Hope-Stone and Blandy, 1983). Given the fact that the cure rate of stage 2 disease is close to 100% with chemotherapy alone, and only 50–60% with radiotherapy or surgery once prognostic factors for relapse can be defined, the next trials for stage 1 patients will be some form of adjuvant chemotherapy, possibly only using one or two courses.

Radiation fractionation through the eyes of a medical oncologist

Since the data of Schabel on the kinetics of tumour and normal tissue response to chemotherapy were first published (Skipper *et al.*, 1950), medical oncologists have accepted the concept of intermittent pulses of treatment with repair time in between to protect normal tissues, although most of the chemotherapy-induced normal tissue damage studied was an early rather than a late effect. Today more attention is paid to late effects, as increasing long-term follow-up is available. Subclinical damage to stem cell compartments in the bone marrow after CCNU and cisplatin is one example of this, as are the problems of chronic graft versus host disease after bone marrow transplantation and loss of fertility in patients treated for Hodgkin's disease.

In contrast, most of the data on radiotherapy schedules have long recognized the importance of waiting for the data on late effects before accepting that a new schedule is safe. There is little doubt that the 5 days a week fractionation with daily doses up to 200 cGy, have proven safest in terms of maintaining the highest cure rate with the minimum of normal tissue damage, notably skin and central nervous system, when radiotherapy has been used with curative or prophylactic intent (Fowler, 1983). In the last few years increasing interest has focused on exploiting the observation that 90% of subclinical radiation-induced DNA damage is repaired within 2 hours (Elkind *et al.*, 1965; Douglas and Fowler, 1976; Masuda, Hunter and Withers, 1980). This has made possible new radiation schedules, either hyperfractionation with treatment three times a day using lower fraction size for a conventional 6-week period (Littbrand and Edsmyr, 1984), or accelerated fractionation two or three times a day in pulses of 2–3 days' treatment repeated every 2–3 weeks (Van dem Bogaert *et al.*, 1982). The long-term follow-up of these studies in terms of both tumour cure and late damage is not yet available, although it is likely that there will be some increase in late damage compared to conventional schedules (Masuda, Hunter and Withers, 1980). So far these regimens have been demonstrated to have equivalent early reaction and tumour control rates (Van dem Bogaert *et al.*, 1982) but logistic difficulties within radiotherapy departments have been the principal reason restricting widescale investigations of these methods, particularly the continuous hyperfractionation approach. However, as can be seen from *Table 20.6*, the accelerated fractionation schedules involve almost the same number of actual 'treatment set-ups' of the patient as conventional daily treatment regimens. Although the radiation treatment time is also the same, the time the patient spends in travelling to hospital is much reduced. This might produce important revenue consequences with saving on admission charges or transport costs for those having outpatient treatment. All of these advantages are relatively minor compared to the critical one of the accelerated fractionation schedule giving the maximum chance for interaction with cytotoxic drugs. This approach has already shown some promise in animal studies (Looney and Hopkins, 1983; Joiner, Bremner and Denekamp, 1984) and will be considered in the next section.

History of drug–radiation interaction

Conventional cytotoxic chemotherapy

Despite nearly 30 years of attempts to investigate drug–radiation interaction in clinical and laboratory research, there has been very little evidence for an increase in response compared to the best results obtainable with the most active of the two modalities used alone. In the experimental animal models for most drugs, the best evidence of potentiation rather than addition of antitumour effect of the two modalities is seen when the drug is given either 2–5 days before or after radiation, although there is some suggestion that for CCNU the best potentiation is seen when the drug is given at the same time as the radiation (Kann *et al.*, 1980).

In the clinical context it has been much more difficult to translate this synergistic effect into a real increase in cure rate because, in most situations, there has also been enhancement of normal tissue damage (Steel and Peckham, 1979). Thus there is evidence of increased lung damage when bleomycin and radiation are combined, increased bladder toxicity with cyclophosphamide and radiation, and increased cardiac toxicity with hydroxydaunorubicin and radiation. Similar interactions can be demonstrated in experimental studies, although for two drugs, cyclophosphamide and cytosine arabinoside, pretreatment with these drugs has been

Table 20.6 Experimental accelerated radiation fractionation schedules (modified from Van den Bogaert *et al.*, 1985)

Schedule number	*Fraction size (cGy)*	*Irradiations per day*	*Irradiations per course*	*Total days for each treatment*	*Interval between courses (days)*	*No. of courses*	*Total dose (cGy)*	*Total time (days)*	*Total no. of treatments*
1	200	1	30	30		1	6000	42	30
2	160	3	30	10	21–28	2	7200	49	45
3	200	3	15	5	21–28	2	6000	42	30
4	160	3	15	5	14	3	7200	49	45
5	200	4	8	2	14	4	6400	44	32

shown to protect normal bone marrow from radiation damage (Millar, Blackett and Hudspith, 1978).

Most evidence suggests that radiation acts by a mechanism similar to alkylating agents and many of the clinical studies of drug–radiation interaction have been with alkylating agents. For the future, there is a need for more detailed studies of the interaction of radiation with non-alkylating agent chemotherapeutic drugs used singly, particularly with the radiation given in intermittent pulses using the new schedules of multiple fractions per day.

Other drugs

With evidence of increased damage to malignant cells from interaction between hypoxic radiation sensitizers and cytotoxic drugs this approach is currently the most interesting area where drug–radiation interaction is being explored. One interesting pilot series has suggested increased activity for this approach in non-small cell carcinoma (Abratt, 1984), although the problem will be to show that the synergy has been achieved without any increase in normal tissue damage.

Immunotherapy

As was mentioned above on the treatment of acute myelogenous leukaemia, although there was some benefit from the various trials of BCG, most of this was from the non-specific effect of improving residual normal bone marrow tolerance to chemotherapy (Oliver, 1977). This was also the conclusion from the use of thymic hormone preparation in a combined radiotherapy/chemotherapy trial in oat cell carcinoma (Cohen *et al.*, 1979).

There have been few trials of immunotherapeutic agents in combination with radiotherapy despite several studies showing that radiotherapy does produce more marked immunosuppression after conventional 5-day a week treatment than after single large fractions (MacLennan and Kay, 1978). There is no firm evidence that this minor degree of immunosuppression has any effect on the clinical behaviour of human tumours. However, in breast cancer there has been some suggestion (Sternswald *et al.*, 1972) that although controlling local recurrence, post-radiotherapy immunosuppresson might accelerate the growth of tumour in those patients with metastases already present. This might explain why despite the benefit in terms of local control there is no survival advantage from using prophylactic radiotherapy. The only trial where immunotherapy has been given in a randomized fashion to patients receiving conventional radiotherapy was conducted by Pines (1976) who treated 40 patients with squamous cell carcinoma of the lung with radiation with or without BCG, and showed superior survival for those receiving BCG. Further trials of this type might be worth consideration possibly using interferon, given that there is evidence that it can potentiate radiation reaction (Dritschilo *et al.*, 1982).

Reappraisal of the role of medical as opposed to radiotherapeutic oncologists

Today surgeons are responsible more frequently than any other hospital specialist for discovering malignant disease. Most of this is found at the level of the district general hospital. If the criterion of cure as opposed to palliation is used to justify provision of cancer services in this day and age of cost effectiveness, the majority of cancer patients in terms of absolute numbers, i.e. those with breast, squamous cell, lung and gastrointestinal tumours, could be managed without referral to specialist oncological centres. Using the same criterion there would be little place for drug treatment compared to radiotherapy, although the fact that drugs do cure some patients means that it would be necessary to make provision for it on a small scale. This scenario of course accurately reflects the current organization of cancer treatment in the UK, though less so in the USA. In the latter country the travelling distances involved and the large capital costs of radiotherapy equipment have mitigated against the large centres and in favour of the community oncologist.

There are two questions which need to be clarified to resolve the issue of what should be the appropriate relationship between medical and radiotherapeutic oncology. The first is whether malignancies as a collective group of illnesses would benefit from having a generalist in the district general hospital familiar with the natural history of tumours in every organ; and more importantly whether such a person would have to be efficient in the use of all the diagnostic instrumental techniques such as laryngoscopy, fibreoptic gastroscopy, cystoscopy, colonoscopy and bronchoscopy which are neccessary to diagnose and monitor the patient's progress.

The second question for clarification is whether training and experience is necessary in order to treat cancer patients with cytotoxic drugs, or can they be used by any clinician under guidance of someone giving advice, as for example a bacteriologist does for antibiotics? The fact that these drugs can be lethal if used inappropriately, and the evidence from at least three of the chemocurable tumours, (Hodgkin's disease, children's tumours and testicular teratoma) that the results are favourably effected by the greater experience of the centre giving the treatment (Oliver *et al.*, 1983; Kramer *et al.*, 1984; MRC Testicular Tumour Working Party, 1985), both argue in favour of treatment being given by specialists trained in their use.

For the future, the challenge for the non-surgical oncologist will be to develop new treatments which are relevant to the problems posed by the cancer epidemic. Although there are increases in the incidence of malignancies in young people, the major factor in the overall increase in malignant disease is that cancer is a disease of old age and the population is living longer. The challenge, in the face of increasing acceptance of the concept that infinite resources cannot be available for health care, will be to develop treatments which improve throughput and may, in addition, improve quality as well as quantity of life. It is in this context that the progress in developing new fractionation procedures and radiation sensitizers will make a major impact and could produce a 20–30% increase in the numbers of patients who can be treated with the present facilities (*see* Chapter 2).

In terms of the science of cancer, the new work on oncogenes and their gene products is opening up a whole new area of understanding of growth control of different organs and the neoplasms which arise from them. The observation that malignant oncogene products are often closely related to normal growth factors and may only have a single amino acid difference from the normal product (Premkumar Reddy *et al.*, 1982) suggests that it may eventually be possible to produce anti- or superactive-growth factor analogues to interfere with the proliferation of the cancer cell.

Against this background the concept of distinguishing between a radiotherapeutic oncologist and a medical oncologist is rather sterile. The need for the specialist non-surgical oncologist to have a training which enables him to have a broad understanding of the biology and natural history of malignancy as well as the pharmacology of anticancer drugs, and in addition to know how to use a megavoltage machine with the assistance of a radiographer and physicist, is obvious. Equally, with the escalating cost of providing megavoltage equipment and the need to treat more patients, the specialist cancer treatment centre will need an academic component with clinical facilities for trials to monitor new innovations in treatment and provide a nursery for new drug development. From the point of view of the service at district level, it is unrealistic to conceive of a general oncologist in every one. There is, however, a need to use the academic component within the cancer centre to contribute to the training of the specialists who work in the district in the treatment of the types of malignancy within their speciality, so that due weight is given to the fact that malignancy is responsible for more than one-quarter of all deaths.

Conclusions

For the most part, the history of chemotherapy drug interaction has been a frustrating catalogue of failure, mainly due to an increase in local normal tissue effects without any increase in local cure. Although this is disappointing in terms of improving cancer cure rates, what has not been focused on (with one notable exception in a trial of bleomycin and radiation in head and neck cancer (Shanta and Krishnamurthi, 1977)), is whether the combination allows less total doses of radiation to be given with maintenance of the cure rate, thus reducing treatment attendances with benefit to both the patient in terms of travelling time and reduction of actual treatment costs.

This chapter has reviewed the evidence on which scheduling of drugs and radiation has been developed. The possibilities of exploiting the new intermittent hyperfractionated radiation schedules and the development of new treatments using antagonists of the products of oncogenes have been highlighted as areas for exploration in the future.

References

ABRATT, R. P. (1984) Radical radiation of lung cancer with

concurrent chemotherapy and misonidazole. *Abstracts of the European Society for Therapeutic Radiology and Oncology*. 3rd Annual Meeting, Jerusalem, p.58

BEGENT, R. J. H. and BAGSHAWE, K. D. (1982) The management of high-risk choriocarcinoma. *Seminars in Oncology*, **9**, 198–203

BELL, R., ROHATINER, A. Z. S., SLEVIN, M. L., *et al.* (1982) Short term treatment for acute myelogenous leukaemia. *British Medical Journal*, **284**, 1221–1229

BERKOWITZ, R. S., GOLDSTEIN, D. P., JONES, M. A., MAREAN, A. R. and BERNSTEIN, M. R. (1980) Methotrexate with citrovorum factor rescue. Reduced chemotherapy toxicity in the management of gestational trophoblastic neoplasms. *Cancer*, **45**,423–426

BONADONNA, G., ROSSI, A., VALAGUSSA, P. *et al.* (1977) The CMF program for operable breast cancer with positive axillary nodes. *Cancer*, **39**, 2904–2915

BONADONNA, G., VIVANI, S., BONFANTE, V., VALAGUSSA, P. and SANTORO, A. (1984) Alternating chemotherapy with MOPP/ABVD in Hodgkin's disease: updated results. *Proceedings of the American Society of Clinical Oncology*, p.254

BRITISH NATIONAL LYMPHOMA INVESTIGATION (1975) Initial treatment of stage IIIA Hodgkin's disease. Comparison of radiotherapy with combined chemotherapy. *Lancet*, **2**, 991–995

BROWMAN, G. P., ARCHIBALD, S. D., YOUNG, J. E. M. *et al.* (1983) Prospective randomized trial of one-hour sequential versus simultaneous methotrexate and 5 fluorouracil in advanced and recurrent head and neck cancer. *Journal of Clinical Oncology*, **1**, 787–792

BRUCE, W. R., MEEKER, B. E. and VALERIOTE, F. A. (National Cancer Institute) (1966) Comparison of the sensitivity of normal hematopoietic and transplanted lymphoma colony-forming cells to chemotherapeutic agents administered *in vivo*. *Journal of National Cancer Institute*, **37**, 233–245

CHABNER, B. A. and MYERS, C. E. (1982) Clinical pharmacology of cancer chemotherapy. In *Cancer: Principles and Practice of Oncology*, edited by V. T. DeVita, S. Hellman and S. A. Rosenberg, pp. 156–197. Philadelphia, Toronto: J. B Lippincott and Co

CLARKSON, B. D. (1972) Acute myelocytic leukemia in adults. *Cancer*, **30**, 1572–1582

COATES, A. S., TATTERSALL, M. H. N., SWANSON, C. *et al.* (1984) Combining therapy with methotrexate and 5 fluorouracil: a prospective randomized clinical trial of order of administration. *Journal of Clinical Oncology*, **2** , 756–761

COHEN, M. H., CHRETIEN, P. B., IHDE, D. C. *et al.* (1979) Thymosin fraction V and intensive combination chemotherapy. Prolonging the survival of patients with small cell lung cancer. *Journal of the American Medical Association*, **241**, 1813–1815

CROWTHER, D., POWLES, R. L., BATEMAN, C. J. T. *et al.* (1973) Management of adult acute myelogenous leukaemia. *British Medical Journal*, **1**, 131–137

CROWTHER, D., WAGSTAFF, J. *et al.* (1984) A randomized study comparing chemotherapy alone with chemotherapy followed by radiotherapy in patients with pathologically staged IIIA Hodgkin's disease. *Journal of Clinical Oncology*, **2**, 892–897

daCUNHA, M. F., MEISTRICH, M. L. FULLER, L. M. *et al.* (1984) Recovery of spermatogenesis after treatment for Hodgkin's disease: limiting dose of MOPP chemotherapy. *Journal of Clinical Oncology*, **2**, 571

De VITA, V. T. and SERPICK, A. (1970) Combination chemotherapy in the treatment of advanced Hodgkin's disease. *Annals of Internal Medicine*, **73**, 891–895

DOUGLAS, B. F. and FOWLER, J. R. (1976) The effect of multiple small doses of X-rays on skin reactions in the mouse and a basic interpretation. *Radiation Research*, **66**, 401–426

DRITSCHILO, A., MOSSMAN, K., GRAY, M. and SREEVALSAN, T. (1982) Potentiation of radiation injury by interferon. *American Journal of Clinical Oncology*, **5**, 79–82

DUCHESNE, G. and PECKHAM, M. J. (1984) Chemotherapy and radiotherapy in advanced testicular nonseminoma. 2. Results of treatment. *Radiotherapy and Oncology*, **1**, 207–215

EINHORN, L. H. and DONOHUE, J. P. (1977) Cis-diaminedichloroplatinum, vinblastine and bleomycin combination chemotherapy in disseminated testicular cancer. *Annals of Internal Medicine*, **87**, 293

EINHORN, L. H. and WILLIAMS, S. D. (1980) Chemotherapy of disseminated testicular cancer: a random prospective study. *Cancer*, **46**, 1339

ELKIND, H. M., SUTTON-GILBERT, H., MOSES, W. B. *et al.* (1965) Radiation response of mammalian cells in culture. *Radiation Research*, **25**, 359–376

FOWLER, J. F. (1983) Fractionation and therapeutic gain. In *The Biological Basis of Radiotherapy*, edited by G. G. Steel, G. E. Adams and M. J. Peckham, pp. 181–194. Amsterdam, New York, Oxford: Elsevier

FOWLER, J. F., HILL, S. A. and SHELDON, P. W. (1980) Comparison of tumour cure (local control) with regrowth delay in mice. *British Journal of Cancer*, **41**, (Suppl. IV), 102–103

FREEMAN, A. I., WEINBERG, V., BRECHER, M. L. *et al.* (for CALGB) (1983) Comparison of intermediate-dose methotrexate with cranial irradiation for the post-induction treatment of acute lymphocytic leukemia in children. *New England Journal of Medicine*, **308**, 477–484

GLASHAN, R. W., HOUGHTON, A. L. and ROBINSON, M. R. G. (1977) A toxicity study of the treatment of T3 bladder tumours with a combination of radiotherapy and chemotherapy. *British Journal of Urology*, **49**, 669–672

HAIJE, W. G., MEERWALDT, J. H., TALERMAN, A. *et al.* (1979) The value of sensitive assay of carcinoplacental alkaline phosphatase in sera of patients with hepatocellular carcinoma. *Clinica et Chimica* Acta, **40**, 67

HIGBY, D. J., WALLACE, H. J., ALVERT, D. J. and HOLLAND, J. F. (1974) Diaminedichloroplatinum: a phase I study. *Cancer*, **33**, 1219

HOWELLS, A., BUSH, H., GEORGE, W. D. *et al.* (1984) Controlled trial of adjuvant chemotherapy with cyclophosphamide, methotraxate, fluorouracil for breast cancer. *Lancet*, **2**, 307–311

JOINER, M. C., BREMNER, J. C. M. and DENEKAMP, J. (1984) The therapeutic advantage of combined X-rays and melphalan. *International Journal of Radiation Oncology, Biology and Physics*, **10**, 385–392

KANN, H. E., BLUMENSTEIN, B. A., PETKAS, A. *et al.* (1980) Radiation synergism by repair-inhibiting nitrosoureas in L1210 cells. *Cancer Research*, **40**, 771

KRAMER, S., MEADOWS, A. T., PASTORE, G. *et al.* (1984) Influence of place of treatment on diagnosis, treatment, and survival in three pediatric solid tumours. *Journal of*

Clinical Oncology, **2**, 917–923

LEMERLE, J., VOUTE, P. A., TOURNADE, M. F. *et al.* (1983) Effectiveness of preoperative chemotherapy in Wilms' tumour: results of an international societity of paediatric oncology (SIOP) clinical trial. *Journal of Clinical Oncology*, **1**, 604–609

LISTER, T. A., DORREEN, M. S., (1983) The treatment of stage IIIA Hodgkin's disease. *Journal of Clinical Oncology*, **1**, 745–749

LISTER, T. A., WHITEHOUSE, J. M. A., OLIVER, R. T., D. *et al.* (1980) Chemotherapy and immunotherapy for acute myelogenous leukaemia. *Cancer*, **46**, 2142–2148

LITTBRAND, B. and EDSMYR, F. (1984) Hyperfractionated radiotherapy of carcinoma of the bladder. In *Abstracts of European Society for Therapeutic Radiology and Oncology*. 3rd Annual Meeting, Jerusalem: p.139

LOONEY, W. B. and HOPKINS, H. A. (1983) A new approach for the more effective utilization of combined chemotherapy and radiotherapy. *International Journal of Radiation Oncology, Biology and Physics*, **9**, 137

MASUDA, K., HUNTER, N. and WITHERS, H. R. (1980) Late effect in mouse skin following single and multifractionated irradiation. *International Journal of Radiation Oncology, Biology and Physics*, **6**, 1539–1544

McELWAIN, T. J. (1978) Chlorambucil, vinblastine, prednisolone, procarbazine, a combination of low toxicity for treatment of Hodgkin's disease. *Cancer Treatment Reviews*, **6**, 133–138

McELWAIN, T. J. and SELBY, P. J. (1984) Etoposide in combination treatment of Hodgkin's disease. In *Etoposide (VP-16)*, edited by B. F. Issell and F. Muggia, pp. 293–299. New York: Academic Press

MacLENNAN, I. C. M. and KAY, H. E. M. (1978) Analysis of treatment in childhood leukemia. The critical association between dose fractionation and immunosuppresion induced by cranial irradiation. *Cancer*, **41**, 108–111

MILLAR, J. L., BLACKETT, N. M. and HUDSPITH, B. N. (1978) Enhanced postirradiation recovery of the haemopoietic system in animals pretreated with a variety of cytotoxic agents. *Cell and Tissue Kinetics*, **11**, 543–553

MORSTYN, G., IHDE, D. C., LICHTER, A. S. *et al.* (1984) Small cell lung cancer 1973–1983: early progress and recent obstacles. *International Journal of Radiation Oncology, Biology and Physics*, **10**, 515–539

MRC TESTICULAR TUMOUR WORKING PARTY (1985) Report on prognostic factors in advanced non-seminomatous testicular germ-cell tumours. *Lancet*, **1** 8–11

NEWLANDS, E. S., BEGENT, R. H. J., KAYE, S. B., RUSTIN, G. J. S. and BAGSHAWE, K. D. (1980) Chemotherapy of advanced malignant teratoma. *British Journal of Cancer*, **42**, 378

NEWLANDS, E. S. BEGENT, R. H. J., RUSTIN, G. J. S., PARKER, D. and BAGSHAWE, K. D. (1983) Further advances in the management of malignant teratomas of the testis and other sites. *Lancet*, **1**, 948

NICHOLSON, W. M., BEARD, M. E. J., CROWTHER, D. **et al.** (1970) Combination chemotherapy in generalized Hodgkin's disease. *British Medical Journal*, **3**, 7–10

OLIVER, R. T. D. (1977) Active specific and non-specific immunotherapy for patients with acute myelogenous leukaemia. *Proceedings of 3rd International Congress Immunology. Progress in Immunology III*. pp. 572–578. Canberra: Australian Academy of Science

OLIVER, R. T. D. (1980) The place of chemotherapy in the treatment of patients with invasive carcinoma of the bladder. In *Bladder Tumours and Other Topics in Urological Oncology*, edited by Paveone-Macaluso *et al.* p. 381. New York: Pleumn Publishing Co

OLIVER, R. T. D. (1985) Testicular germ cell tumours — a model for a new approach to treatment of adult solid tumours. *Postgraduate Medical Journal*, **61**, 123–131

OLIVER, R. T. D., BLANDY, J. P., HENDRY, W. F., PRYOR, J. P., WILLIAM, J. P. and HOPE-STONE, H. F. (1983) Evaluation of radiotherapy and/or surgico-pathological staging after chemotherapy in the management of metastatic germ cell tumours. *British Journal of Urology*, **55**, 764

OLIVER, R. T. D., HOPE-STONE, H. F. and BLANDY, J. P. (1983) Justification of the use of surveillance in the management of stage 1 germ cell tumours of the testis. *British Journal of Urology*, **55**, 760–763

OLIVER, R. T. D., HOPE-STONE, H. F. and BLANDY, J. P. (1984) Possible new approaches to the management of seminoma of the testis. *British Journal of Urology*, **56**, 729–733

PECKHAM, M. J., BARRET, A., HORWICH, A. and HENDRY, W. F. (1983) Orchiectomy alone for stage 1 testicular non-seminoma. A progress report. *British Journal of Urology*, **55**, 754–759

PINES, A. (1976) A 5-year controlled study of BCG and radiotherapy for inoperable lung cancer. *Lancet*, **1**, 380–381

PINKEL, D., HERNANDEZ, K., BORELLA, L. *et al.* (1971) Drug dosage and remission duration in childhood lymphocytic leukemia. *Cancer*, **27**, 247–256

POWLES, R. L., RUSSELL, J., LISTER, T. A. *et al.* (1977) Immunotherapy for acute myelogenous leukaemia. A controlled clinical study 2.5 years after entry of last patient. *British Journal of Cancer*, **35**, 265–275

PREMKUMAR REDDY, E., REYNOLDS, R. K., SANTOS, E. and BARBACID, M. (1982) A point mutation is responsible for the acquisition of transforming properties by the T24 human bladder carcinoma oncogene. *Nature*, **300**, 149–152

PRICE, L. A. and HILL, B. T. (1981) Safer cancer chemotherapy using a kinetically based approach: clinical implications. In *Safer Cancer Chemotherapy*, edited by L. A. Price, B. T. Hill and M. W. Ghilchik, pp. 9–18. London: Baillière Tindall

REIMER, R. R., HOOVER, R., FRAUMENI, J. F. Jr. *et al.* (1977) Acute leukaemia after alkylating-agent therapy of ovarian cancer. *New England Journal of Medicine*, **297**, 177–181

ROSENBERG, S. A., KAPLAN, H. S., GLATSTEIN, E. J. and PORTLOCK, C. S. (1978) Combined modality therapy of Hodgkin's disease: a report on the Stanford trials. *Cancer*, **42**, 991–1000

ROWLAND, G. R. and DONOHUE, J. P. (1984) Cytoreductive surgery in testicular cancer. *World Journal of Urology*, **2**, 48

SAMUELS, M. I., LANZOTTI, V. J., HOLOYE, P. Y. *et al.* (1976) Combination chemotherapy in germinal cell tumours. *Cancer Treatment Review*, **3**, 185

SAMUELS, M. L., SELIG, D. E., OGDEN, S., GRANT, C. and BROWN, B. (1981) IV hyperalimentation and chemotherapy for stage III testicular cancer: a randomized study. *Cancer Treatment Reports*, **65**, 615-627

SANTORO, A. and BONADONNA, G. (1979) Prolonged disease-free survival in MOPP-resistant Hodgkin's disease after treatment with adriamycin, bleomycin, vinblastine and dacarbazine (ABVD). *Cancer Chemotherapy and Pharmacology*, **2**, 101–105

SANTORO, A., BONFANTE, V., VIVIANI, S., VALAGUSSA, P. and BONADONNA, G. (1984) Salvage chemotherapy (CT) in relapsing Hodgkin's disease. *Proceedings of the American Society of Clinical Oncology*, p.254

SHANTA, V. and KRISHNAMURTHI, S. (1977) Combined therapy of oral cancer bleomycin and radiation: a clinical trial. *Clinical Radiology Bombay*, **28**, 427–429

SIMON, R. M. (1982) Design and conduct of clinical trials. In *Cancer, Principles and Practice of Oncology*, edited by V. T. De Vita, S. Hellman and S. A. Rosenberg, pp. 198–225. Philadelphia, Toronto: J B Lippincott Co

SIMONE, J. V. (1979) Childhood leukemia as a model for cancer research. The Richard and Hinda Rosenthal foundation award lecture. *Cancer Research*, **39**, 4301–4307

SIMONE, J. V. (1984) The treatment of neuroblastoma (editorial). *Journal of Clinical Oncology*, **2** , 717–718

SKIPPER, H. E., SCHABEL, F. M. Jr, MELLET, L. B. *et al.* (1950) Implications of biochemical, cytokinetic, pharmacologic, and toxicologic relationships in the design of optimal therapeutic schedules. *Cancer Chemotherapy Reports*, **54**, 431–450

STEEL, G. G. and PECKHAM, M. J. (1979) Exploitable mechanisms in combined radiotherapy chemotherapy: the concept of additivity. *International Journal of Radiation Oncology, Biology and Physics*, **5**, 85–91

STERNSWALD, J., JONDAL, M., VANKY, F., WIGZELL, H. and SEALY, R. (1972) Lymphopenia and change in distribution of human B and T lymphocytes in peripheral blood induced by irradiation for mammary carcinoma *Lancet*, **1**, 1352–1356

SUTCLIFFE, S. B., WRIGLEY, R. F., PETO, J. *et al.* (1978) MVPP chemotherapy regimen for advanced Hodgkin's disease. *British Medical Journal*, **1**, 679–683

TUCKER, D. F., OLIVER, R. T. D., TRAVERS, P. and BODMER, W. F. (1985) Serum marker potential of placental alkaline phosphatase-like activity in testicular germ cell tumours evaluated by H17E2 monoclonal antibody assay. *British Journal of Cancer*, (in press)

VALAGUSSA, P., SANTORO, A., FOSSATI BELLANI, F. *et al.* (1982) Absence of treatment-induced second neoplasms after ABVD in Hodgkin's disease. *Blood*, **59**, 488–494

VAN en BOGAERT, W., VAN der SCHEUREN, E., VAN TONGELEN, C. *et al.*, (1985) Late results of multiple fractions per day (MFD) with misonidazol in advanced cancer of the head and neck. *Radiotherapy and Oncology*, **3**, 139–144

VUGRIN, D., CVITKOVIC, E., WITTES, R. E.and GOLBEY, R. B. (1981) VAB-4 combination chemotherapy in the treatment of metastatic testis tumours. *Cancer*, **47**, 833

VUGRIN, D., WHITMORE, W. E. Jr. and GOLBEY, R. B. (1983) VAB-6 combination of chemotherapy without maintenance in treatment of disseminated cancer of the testis. *Cancer*, **51**, 211

YAGODA, A., WATSON, R. C., NATALE, R. B. *et al.* (1979) A critical analysis of response criteria in patients with prostatic cancer treated with cisplatinum. *Cancer*, **44**, 1553–1557

YARNOLD, J. R., HORWICH, A., DUCHESNE, G. *et al.* (1983) Chemotherapy and radiotherapy for advanced testicular non-seminoma. 1. The influence of sequence and timing of drugs and radiation on the appearance of normal damage. *Radiotherapy and Oncology*, **1**, 91–99

YOUNG, R. C., KNAPP, R. C. and PEREZ, C. A. (1982) Cancer of the ovary. In *Cancer, Principles and Practice of Oncology*, edited by V. T. De Vita, S. Hellman, and S. A. Rosenberg, pp. 884–913. Philadelphia, Toronto: J. P. Lippincott Co

Index

Accelerated fractionation, 8
  effects, 10
Acromegaly, 357
Actinic keratosis,
  treatment of, 284
Actinomycin,
  in children's tumours, 436
  in osteogenic sarcoma, 251
  in rhabdomyosarcoma, 249
Acquired immunodeficiency syndrome, (AIDS), 298
Adenoid cystic carcinoma, 119
Adenomatosis, 313
  multiple endocrine, 314
Adrenalectomy, medical, in breast cancer, 87
Adrenal tumours, 311–313
  cortex, 311
  histology, 312
  medulla, 311, 312
  metastases, 312
Aesthesioneuroepithelioma, 109
Afterloading systems,
  Cathetron, 211, 212, 216
  in cervical cancer, 209
  component distribution, 215
  component loading, 215
  component size, 214
  curietron, 212
  protection and, 417, 419
  radium and Selectron compared, 214
  remote systems, 210–211
  Selectron, 211, 212, 213
  for uterine cancer, 227
Age,
  effect on survival in bladder cancer, 37
  uterine cancer and, 225
Aldosterone, 312
Aminoglutethimide, in breast cancer, 88
Amputation, for sarcoma, 138, 139
Anal carcinoma, 330–332, 379
Ankylosing spondylitis,
  radiotherapy for, 386
    risks of, 384
Apudomas, 313–314
Asbestosis, 164
Astrocytoma,
  differentiated, treatment of, 342
  malignant, treatment, 342
  of spinal cord, 361
  retreatment, 340
Auditory canal, malignant disease of, 289
Axillary node metastases,
  from breast cancer, 70
    radiotherapy, 77
    treatment of, 72, 83
Azathioprine, for polymyositis, 392

Basophil adenoma, 361
Bence-Jones protein, 271
Benign conditions, 384–399
  radiotherapy in,
    discussion with patient, 385
    rationale of, 385
    scope of, 386
Bile duct carcinoma, 325
Biliary system, extrahepatic, carcinoma of, 325
Bladder,
  lesions complicating cervical cancer therapy, 220, 221, 222
  radiation effects on, 36
  radiation-induced malignancy, 223
  radiation tolerance, 231
  telangiectasia of, 222
Bladder cancer, 2, 27–38, 402
  adenocarcinoma, 28
  chemotherapy in, 38
  classification, 27
  cystectomy for, 33
  cystodiathermy for, 28
Bladder cancer (*cont.*)
  grading, 27
  indications for treatment, 28
  influence of smoking, 27
  involving prostate, 33
  lung metastases, 28
  lymph node invasion, 28
  lymphoma, 28, 34
  metastases from, 28, 30, 433
    treatment and, 30
  palliative treatment, 34
  preoperative irradiation, 33, 36
  radiosensitivity of, 28, 33
  salvage cystectomy, 29, 37, 38
    indications for, 36
  schistosomiasis and, 27, 28
  spread to penis, 65
  staging, 27
    treatment and, 28
  treatment techniques, 29
    causes of failure, 38
    downstaging effect, 28
    effect of age on, 37
    external beam irradiation, 29
    follow-up, 36
    hyperfractionation, 33
    importance of correct dose levels, 37
    interstitial irradiation, 29, 381
    isodose curves, 30, 32, 34
    London Hospital technique, 29
    metastases and, 30
    morbidity of, 36
    multiple fields, 33
    neutrons, 33
    oxygenation in, 33
    results of, 36
    rotation, 33
    use of radiosensitizers, 20
Bleomycin,
  in cancer of maxillary antrum, 108
  in germ cell tumours, 253, 436
  in head and neck cancer, 95

Bleomycin (*cont.*)
in Hodgkin's disease, 190
in malignant teratoma, 437
in ovarian cancer, 236
Blood, malignant disease of, 258–279
Blood flow,
effect of radiation on, 5
role in radiosensitivity, 21
Blood vessels, radiation injury, 5, 6
Body image, changes in, 409
Bone,
chondrosarcoma, 137, 141–142
giant cell tumour, 137, 142
involvement in Hodgkin's disease, 178
irradiation induced cancer, 385
lymphoma, 142, 196
metastases in,
adrenal tumours, 312
breast cancer, 84
chordoma, 363
lung, 161
prostatic cancer, 43
rhabdomyosarcoma, 250
soft tissue sarcoma, 134
osteosarcoma, 137–141
aetiology, 138
Cade treatment, 138
chemotherapy, 139
clinical picture, 138
incidence, 137
limb-sparing treatment, 139
management of, 138
metastases from, 140
radiotherapy, 141
site of, 138
spread of, 138
plasmacytoma of, 275
radiation damage, 134
sarcomas, 137–144
tumours, in children, 250–253
Bone marrow, aplasia, 53
Bone marrow metastases, from rhabdomyosarcoma, 250
Bone marrow transplantation, 10
dosage of radiation, 261
in leukaemia, 259, 260, 264
London Hospital technique, 261
side-effects of radiation, 262
technique, 260
total body irradiation in, 260
Bowel,
lesions complicating cervical cancer therapy, 222
radiation effects, 220
in bladder cancer, 36
in cervical cancer, 216
in prostatic cancer, 45
reactions, during treatment, 408
Bowen's disease, 64, 281, 282
treatment of, 284
Brachial plexus, involved in bronchial carcinoma, 159
Brachyteletherapy, 12
Brachytherapy, 415–417
Brachytherapy (*cont.*)
CT scanning in, 417
dosimetry, 416
radiation protection, 429
role of physicist, 411
Brain,
haemangioma of, 397
metastases in,
adrenal tumours, 312
breast cancer, 86, 363
lung, 161, 164, 363
melanoma, 293, 363
soft tissue sarcoma, 135
microgliomatosis, 354
necrosis, 338
radiation effects on, 338
safe levels, 339
radiation tolerance, 338, 340
suprasellar germinomas, 346
tumours,
adjuvant chemotherapy, 345, 353
astrocytomas, 342
chemotherapy, 365
combined treatment, 365
fast neutron irradiation, 365
general policy, 340
gliomas, 342
lymphoma, 354
management problems, 340
medulloblastoma, 347
meningioma, 353
metastatic, 353, 363
new methods of treatment, 365
oligodendroglioma, 344
pineal, 345
radiation techniques, 342
radioactive implants for, 365
radiotherapy, 342
results of radiotherapy, 353
safe dose levels, 339
sensitizers in treatment, 365
reticulum cell sarcoma, 354
third ventricle tumours, 345
treatment, 340
vascular, 355
Brain stem tumours, 346
Breast,
radiation tolerance of, 71
Breast cancer, 69–92
adjuvant chemotherapy, 75, 84, 88
axillary node metastases, 70
chemotherapy, 88
combination chemotherapy for, 89
endocrine therapy, 84, 86
adjuvant, 90
side-effects, 88
hormone receptors in, 70
incidence of, 69
inflammatory, 69, 70
interstitial therapy, 81, 380
locally advanced, radiotherapy for, 84
in males, 90
mastectomy, cosmetic result, 82, 83
medullary, 69
Breast cancer (*cont.*)
megavoltage radiotherapy, 73
metastases from,
bone, 84
brain, 86, 363
causing spinal cord compression, 85
eye, 86
liver, 86
pelvis, 85
radiotherapy for, 84
in spinal cord, 364
treatment of, 72
oestrogen receptors in, 70
oophorectomy for, 87
ovarian irradiation in, 87
pathology of, 69
polygonal, 69
post-irradiation 'salvage' mastectomy, 79
quadrantectomy, 83
radiosensitivity, tumour size and, 79
radiotherapy, 77
after surgery, 82
cosmetic result, 82, 83
following mastectomy, 71
history of, 72
role of, 71
side-effects, 81
survival rates, 74, 79, 80
technique, 75
radium treatment, 78
recurrence,
after mastectomy, 73, 74
after radiation, 81
scirrhous, 69
screening for, 69
staging, 70
surgical operations for, 70, 71
history of, 72
results of, 78
radiotherapy after, 82
radiotherapy following, 71
'salvage', 79
survival rates, 70, 71, 73, 78, 80
Bronchial carcinoma, *see Lung cancer*
Brown-Sequard syndrome, 85
Buccal mucosa, cancer of, use of radiosensitizers, 21
BUdR, as radiosensitizer, 24
Burkitt's lymphoma, 241
dosage for, 10
Busulfan,
in leukaemia, 263, 264
in myelofibrosis, 270
in polycythaemia, 268, 269

Caesium-137,
in afterloading systems, 209, 210, 418
in brachytherapy, 416
for implants, 370
half life, 211
Californium-252, 219, 371

Cancer,
  discussion with patient, 403
  spread of, patient's fears, 404
Carcinogenesis, radiation causing, 53
Carcinoid syndrome, 313–314
Carcinomatous meningitis, 365
Cataract, radiation, 119
Cataract formation in bone marrow transplantation, 263
Cathetron, 211, 212, 216, 418
Cells,
  hypoxic, 15, 16
    radiosensitization of, 20
  kinetics, 20
  malignant,
    oxygenation in, 12, 14
    radiovulnerability of, 4
  metabolic process of, 4
  mitosis, radiation effects, 12
  proliferation kinetics, 19
  radiovulnerability of, 4
Cell death, 4, 5, 19
  in central nervous system, 337
Central nervous system,
  Hodgkin's disease of, 189
  malignant disease of, 337–368
    see also specific regions and organs
    classification, 338
  metastases in, 162
  radiation effects, 337
  radiotherapy of,
    in children, 239, 256
    growth hormone deficiency following, 256
  treatment of, 415
Cerebral cortex,
  radiation tolerance, 340
  tumours in, 343
Cerebral oedema, in treatment of brain tumour, 340, 341
Cervical cancer, 203–224
  as model in radiobiological research, 219
  clinical assessment, 204
  exophytic tumours, 204
  extension of, 207
  external pelvic irradiation in, 217
  histology, 204
  incidence of, 203
  infiltrative tumours, 204
  intracavitary therapy, 207
    complications of, 220
  in situ, 203
  morphology, 204
  presentation, 204
  radiation-induced second malignancy, 223
  radioactive afterloading, 209, 210
  Cathetron, 211, 212, 216
    comparisons, 214
    component distribution, 215
    component loading, 215
    component size, 214
    Curietron, 212
    Selectron, 211, 212, 213
Cervical cancer (*cont.*)
  screening for, 203
  treatment,
    advanced disease, 217
    dosimetry, 206
    Manchester system, 205
    Paris method, 206
    radiosensitizers in, 16, 20, 23
    stage 0, 1 and 2, 205
    Stockholm method, 205
  ulcerative tumours, 204
  uniform pelvis irradiation, 219
Charged particles, in treatment of uveal melanoma, 120
Cheek,
  cancer of, 100
    interstitial therapy, 378
    survival rates, 101
  iridium-192 implants, 373
Chemicals, skin cancer from, 280
Chemotherapy, *see also specific compounds, etc.*
  cancer cure with, 432
  combination, 433
  criteria of response to drugs, 432
  hair loss from, 402
  interaction with radiotherapy, 432–444
  reappraisal of, 440
  response to single agent, 433
  subclassification of drugs, 433
  toxicity of drugs, 435
Chest wall, invasion of bronchial carcinoma, 160
Children,
  acute lymphoblastic leukaemia in, 239
  bone tumours in, 250–253
  care of during treatment, 408
  changes in body image, 409
  communication with, 401
  Ewing's sarcoma, 251-253
  germ cell tumours, 253
  hair loss in, 409
  histiocytosis X, 253
  Hodgkin's disease in, 242
  immobilization of, 409
  keloids in, 395
  leukaemia in, chemotherapy, 435
  medulloblastoma, 347
  neuroblastoma in, 245–257
  non-Hodgkin's lymphoma in, 241
  osteogenic sarcoma in, 250
  radiotherapy in, 238
    late effects of, 255
    to central nervous system, 239
  retinoblastoma, 254
  rhabdomyosarcoma, 247–250
  terminal care of, 238
  treatment of, 408
  tumours in, 238–257
    chemotherapy, 435
    incidence of, 238
Chlorambucil,
  in Hodgkin's disease, 190
  in leukaemia, 265
Chlorambucil (*cont.*)
  in non-Hodgkin's lymphoma, 198, 199
  in polycythaemia, 269
Chloroma, 266
Chordoma, 362
Choroidal metastases, from breast cancer, 86
Choroid plexus papilloma, treatment, 344
Chromium-51, in brachytherapy, 416
Chromophobe adenoma, 360
Cisplatin,
  as radiosensitizer, 24
  in germ cell tumours, 253, 436
  in head and neck cancer, 95
  in malignant teratoma, 437
  in osteogenic sarcoma, 251
  in ovarian cancer, 236
  in seminoma, 438
  in soft tissue sarcoma, 136
Cobalt-60, 14
  in afterloading systems, 210
  in brachytherapy, 416
  in Cathetron, 216
  half life, 211
Colon,
  carcinoma of, metastases, 363
  lesions complicating cervical cancer therapy, 220, 222
  radiation effects, 317
Computers, use of, 416, 420, 422
Computer-controlled tracking technique, 415
Conformation therapy, 415
Conn's syndrome, 312
Cornea,
  benign conditions of, 395
  radiation damage, 119
Corticosteroids, in leukaemia, 265, 266
Craniopharyngioma, 355
Cryotherapy, in retinoblastoma, 254
CT scanning, 411
  in brachytherapy, 417
  in oesophageal carcinoma, 169
  in radiotherapy, 424
  in treatment planning, 420
Cunningham's model for photons, 423
Curietron, 211, 212, 214, 418
Cushing's syndrome, 312, 358, 361
Cyclophosphamide,
  bladder toxicity, 439
  chemotherapy, 260
  in childhood tumours, 436
  in Ewing's tumour, 252
  in gastric cancer, 319
  in germ cell tumours, 253
  in lung cancer, 163
  in multiple myeloma, 273
  in neuroblastoma, 246
  in non-Hodgkin's lymphoma, 241
  in osteosarcoma, 139
  in polycythaemia, 268
  in rhabdomyosarcoma, 249
  in soft tissue sarcoma, 136, 137

Cyclophosphamide (*cont.*)
in thyroid lymphoma, 306
in Wilms' tumour, 244
Cytostatic drugs, 432
Cystectomy,
for bladder cancer, 33
salvage,
in bladder neoplasms, 29, 36, 37, 38
Cystitis,
irradiation, 36, 221
Cystodiathermy, in bladder cancer, 28
Cytosine arabinoside, in leukaemia, 258, 260
Cytotoxic drugs,
as radiosensitizers, 23
classification, 434
criteria of response, 432
interaction with radiation, 432, 439
site of action, 434
toxicity, 435
versus cytostatic drugs, 432

Dacarbazine, in melanoma, 293
Demyelination syndrome, 338
3,4-Dihydroxyphenylalanine, 313
Diarrhoea, following treatment of cervical cancer, 222
DNA synthesis, cytotoxic drugs and, 434
Dosage and dosimetry, 421
accelerated fraction, 8, 10
alpha/beta ratios, 8
in brachyteletherapy, 12
chemical adjuvants modifying, 14
dose-rate effects, 10
fractionation schemes, 6
hyperfractionation, 8, 9, 10
intercavitary therapy, 12
interstitial treatment, 12
ionization chambers, 421
multiple fractions per day, 8
nominal standard dose, 7
reduction factors, 16, 17
sensitivity of instrument, 422
split-dose experiments, 7
thermoluminescent, 421
tissue response to, 3
two dose levels, 1
Dose-effect,
differences in, 3
single doses, 2
Dose effect curves, 8
Dose rates, clinical importance of, 10
Dose-rate effects, 10
Dose reduction factors, 16, 17
Duodenum, radiation effects of, 316
Dysphagia,
following radiotherapy, 105
in post-cricoid carcinoma, 114
in radiation oesophagitis, 155
Dysuria, from treatment of bladder cancer, 36

Ear,
carcinoma of, 106, 290
Ear (*cont.*)
malignant disease of, 289, 290
Ectopic ossification, radiotherapy for, 392
Electron-avid compounds, 14
Endocrine system, tumours of, 300–315
see also specific organs
Endocrine therapy, for breast cancer, 87
Endometrial carcinoma, 381
Endometrial cancer, 224
adjuvant hormone therapy, 231
differentiation, 224
intracavitary postoperative radiotherapy, 230
postoperative radiotherapy, 230
preoperative radiotherapy, 225
remote afterloading treatment, 227
spread of, 224
Eosinophilic adenoma of pituitary, 357
Ependymoma,
of spinal cord, 362
treatment, 344
Epidermolysis bullosa, 281
Epilation, 402, 405
in children, 409
radiotherapy for, 397
Erythropheresis, in polycythaemia, 269
Ewing's sarcoma, 137, 196
in children, 251–253
secondary tumours following, 255
External beam therapy, 412–415
acceptance of machine, 413
beam quality, 413
computer-controlled tracking, 415
conformation therapy, 415
dosimetry, 412
development, 414
post-acceptance, 414
involvement of physicist, 412
quality assurance tests, 413
radiation protection, 429
Eye, *see also Orbit*
malignant disease of, 287
metastases in, from breast cancer, 86
protection during radiotherapy, 287
radiation damage, 119
retinoblastoma, 254
uveal melanoma, 120
Eyelid, malignant disease of, 287, 289

Femur, metastases from prostatic cancer, 43
α-Fetoprotein, 253
Fibroids, 393
5-Fluorouracil,
in anal carcinoma, 331, 332
in bladder cancer, 38
in carcinoid syndrome, 314
in carcinoma of stomach, 319
in head and neck cancer, 95
in pancreatic cancer, 322, 324
in rectal cancer, 327
5-Fluorouracil (*cont.*)
response to, 435
5-Fluorouracil ointment, 284
Fractionation,
chemotherapy and, 439
increased, effect on dose effect curves, 10
radiosensitizers and, 23
schemes, 6
trials, 6

Gall bladder, carcinoma of, 325
Ganglioneuroblastoma, 247
Gastrinoma, 313
Gastrointestinal carcinomas, 316–336
see also specific organs
Gastrointestinal syndrome, 10, 53
Germ cell tumours, 253
chemotherapy, 436
Gestational choriocarcinoma, 432
Gliomas,
treatment, 342
radiosensitizers in, 15, 16, 23
Glomus jugulare tumour, 106
Glottis, carcinoma of, 109, 110, 111
Glucagonoma, 313
Glutathione, 16
Gold-198,
for implants, 370, 381
in brachytherapy, 416
in pituitary tumours, 358
in rheumatoid arthritis, 387
Golfer's elbow, 388
Gorlin's syndrome, 281
Graft versus host disease, 263
Granulocytic sarcoma, 266
Granulomatous thymomas, 178
Growth hormone deficiency, postradiotherapy, 256
Gynaecological radiotherapy, 203–237
care of patient during, 408
interstitial therapy, 381
Gynaecomastia, 397

Haemangioblastoma, 355
Haemangioma, radiotherapy for, 396
Haematological syndrome, 11
Hair loss, 397, 402, 405
in children, 409
Halogenated pyrimidines, as radiosensitizers, 24
Hashimoto's thyroiditis, 301, 302
Head and neck, *see also under specific organs and regions*
cancer, 93–123
chemotherapy, 95
choice of management, 93
fractionation, 94
lymph nodes, 96, 97
metastases from, 93
neutron therapy, 94
postoperative radiotherapy, 94
preoperative radiotherapy, 93
radiosensitizers in, 20, 22, 23
radiotherapy, 94, 95
soft tissue sarcoma, 132

Head and neck (*cont.*)
cancer (*cont.*)
surgery in, 94
Hodgkin's disease of, 189
non-Hodgkin's lymphoma of, 195
plasmacytoma of, 275, 276
salvage interstitial therapy, 382
Hepatic ducts, carcinoma of, 325
Herpes, in cervical cancer, 203
Herpes zoster, radiotherapy for, 397
Histiocytosis X, 253
Hodgkin's disease, 177–191
A and B symptoms, 182, 183
biopsy, 179, 181
bone involvement, 178
central nervous system, 189
chemotherapy, 186, 190, 191, 436
in children, 242
chemotherapy and radiotherapy in, 438
classification, 179
combined chemotherapy, 190, 196
CT scanning, 181
diagnostic laparotomy, 181
external beam therapy, 415
extranodal involvement, 178
factors influencing prognosis,
age and sex, 183
blood picture, 183, 185
staging, 182
general features, 177
haematological investigation, 180
histology, 179
prognosis and, 183
in children, 242
second malignancy after treatment, 256
intermittent syndrome, 178
investigation, 179
isotope scanning, 180
liver involvement, 178
lymphocyte depletion, 179
lymphocyte predominance, 179
lymphography, 180
metastases from, 364
mixed cellularity, 179
nodular sclerosis, 179
pulmonary involvement, 178
radiotherapy, 185, 191
at special sites, 189
causing thyroid cancer, 300
dosage, 185
extent of, 185
head and neck, 189
inverted Y, 188
mantle, 188
prophylactic, 188
techniques, 187
total nodal, 188
skin lesions, 298
staging, 182, 242
stomach, 189
surgery for, 191
survival rates, 186
treatment, 185–191
ultrasound scanning, 180
Hormone therapy, for breast cancer, 86, 90
Horner's syndrome, 159
Hurthle cells, 302
Hydroxydaunorubicin,
in acute lymphoblastic leukaemia, 239
in bladder cancer, 38
in carcinoid syndrome, 314
in Ewing's sarcoma, 252
in gastric cancer, 320
in Hodgkin's disease, 190, 436
in leukaemia, 258, 260
in lung cancer, 163
in non-Hodgkin's lymphoma, 198, 241
in osteogenic sarcoma, 251
in osteosarcoma, 139
in ovarian cancer, 236
in soft tissue sarcoma, 136, 137
in Wilms' tumour, 244
Hydronephrosis, 223
5-Hydroxytryptophan, 313
Hydroxyurea, as radiosensitizer, 24
Hyperbaric oxygen, 20
Hyperfractionation, 8, 9
effects of, 10
Hyperparathyroidism, 313
Hypopharynx, carcinoma of, 114
Hypothyroidism, 301

Ileitis, radiation, 221
Ileum, lesions complicating cervical cancer therapy, 221
Imaging techniques, localizing, 405
^{131}I-meta iodobenzylguanidine, 313
Immunoglobulins, in multiple myeloma, 271, 272
Immunotherapy, 440
Impotence, following treatment of prostatic cancer, 45
Infertility, following irradiation, 53
Inguinal lymph nodes, in anal carcinoma, 332
Inhomogeneities, in radiotherapy treatment planning, 425, 427
Inner canthus, malignant disease of, 287
Insulinoma, 313
Intercavitary therapy, 12
Intermittent syndrome in Hodgkin's disease, 178
Interstitial therapy, 12, 369–383
after previous external radiation, 369
contraindications, 369, 370
for salvage therapy, 382
general indications, 369
indications for, 377
isotopes for,
characteristics, 371
for implants, 370
patient's view of, 403
perioperative implants, 370
primary treatment with, 369
results of, 377
Intestine,
non-Hodgkin's lymphoma of, 195
radiation effects on, 316, 317
Intrathoracic tumours, 145–176
see also under specific regions and organs
Iodine-125, 370
in brachytherapy, 416
in brain tumours, 366
in pancreatic cancer, 324
in prostatic cancer, 381
Iodine-131, 403
Ionization chambers, 421
Iridium-192
implants, 371
distribution rules, 374
dosimetry, 374, 375, 377
duration of, 377
hairpin technique, 372
moulds, 374
plastic tube loop technique, 372
plastic tube miniature technique, 373
plastic tube technique, 371
radiation protection requirements, 377
template technique, 373
treatment with,
anal carcinoma, 330
bladder cancer, 381
in brachytherapy, 416
breast cancer, 381
carcinoma of penis, 380

Juvenile angiofibroma, of nasopharynx, 105

Kaposi's sarcoma, 298
Keloids,
radiotherapy for, 393
dosage, 395
Keratitis, solar, 282
Keratocanthoma, 281
Kidney, *see also heading Renal*
neoplasms of, 55
metastases from, 364
radiation damage to, 53, 235
Wilms' tumour, 242–245
Klatskin tumours, 325
Klinefelter's syndrome, 90

Lacrimal gland tumours, 119
Laryngeal palsy, in bronchial carcinoma, 146, 158
Laryngectomy, salvage, 111
Laryngopharyngectomy, 114, 115
Larynx,
carcinoma of, 109–113
adverse effects of treatment, 113
diagnosis and staging, 109
lymph node involvement, 110
patient care during treatment, 113
radiotherapy dosage, 110
recurrence, 111
results of treatment, 112

Larynx (*cont.*)
 carcinoma of, (*cont.*)
  salvage surgery, 110, 111
  surgery for, 112
  treatment, 110
 oedema, post treatment, 113
Lentigo maligna, 293
Leukaemia, 258–266
 acute, 238
 acute lymphoblastic, 238, 239, 259
 acute non-lymphocytic, 258
 bone marrow transplantation, 259, 260
 chemotherapy, 258, 259, 263, 265
  in children, 435
 chronic granulocytic, 263
 chronic lymphocytic, 264
 extramedullary deposits, 266
 incidence, following radiotherapy, 384, 386
 myeloid, chemotherapy, 436
 radiotherapy and chemotherapy in, 438
 treatment, 415
L'Hermitte's syndrome, 53
Limbs,
 irradiation of, 128
 soft tissue sarcoma, 128
Linear accelerators, 413
 acceptance tests, 414
Lip,
 carcinoma of, 98, 289
  interstitial therapy, 378
Liver,
 in Hodgkin's disease, 178
 metastases in,
  adrenal tumours, 312
  breast cancer, 86
  lung, 161, 162
  soft tissue sarcoma, 135
 radiation damage, 263
 radiosensitivity, 316
Lomustine, in melanoma, 293
Lung,
 carcinoid syndrome, 314
 involved in Hodgkin's disease, 178
 involvement in neuroblastoma, 247
 metastases in,
  adrenal tumours, 312
  bladder neoplasms, 28
  Ewing's sarcoma, 251
  osteosarcoma, 140, 250
  renal cell tumour, 55
  rhabdomyosarcoma, 250
  soft tissue sarcoma, 134
  testicular tumours, 52
  thyroid cancer, 305
  Wilms' tumour, 244, 245
 oatcell carcinoma, 146, 150
 radiation effects, 53
 radiation-induced malignancy, 223
 radiotherapy, in Wilms' tumour, 244, 245
 squamous cell carcinoma, 146
  see also under Lung cancer
Lung cancer, 145–164
Lung cancer (*cont.*)
 adenocarcinoma, 146
 chemotherapy, 163
 classification of, 145
 curative treatment, 146
 dysphagia in, 157
 incidence of, 145
 invading chest wall, 160
 invading oesophagus, 157
 investigations, 145
 laryngeal palsy in, 146, 158
 metastases from, 145, 155
  bone, 161
  brain, 363
  central nervous system, 162
  liver, 162
  skin, 162
  spinal cord, 364
  treatment of, 161
 oat cell, 146, 150, 433
 palliative radiotherapy, 150, 151
  care of patient, 155
  technique, 152
 Pancoast syndrome, 158
 pleural effusion in, 160
 radical radiotherapy, 146
  as adjuvant to surgery, 149
  care of patient, 149
  radiosensitizers in, 20, 21
  technique, 147
 respiratory obstruction, 156
 selection of patients, 145
 small-cell, 163
 superior vena caval obstruction in, 155
 surgery for, 146
  adjuvant radiotherapy, 149
 systemic treatment, 163
Lymph node invasion,
 from bladder neoplasms, 28
 from breast cancer, 86
Lymphoedema, following irradiation, 45
Lymphoepithelioma, 103, 171
Lymphoma (non-Hodgkin's), 177, 192–202
 biopsy, 194
 BNLI classification, 192
 in brain, 354
 Burkitt type, 241
 chemotherapy of, 196, 198, 199
 in children, 241
 diffuse, 192
 diffuse lymphocytic intermediate, 193
 diffuse lymphocytic mixed, 194
 follicular, 192
 histiocytic cell, 194
 histology, 192
 investigations, 194
 management, 192
 palliation, 199
 primary extranodal, 195
 primary nodal, 196
 radiotherapy, 177, 196
  total body, 197
Lymphoma (non-Hodgkin's) (*cont.*)
 total nodal, 197
 of skin, 298
 surgery of, 199
 of thyroid, 302, 306, 307
Lymphoma cutis, 299

Malabsorption, following intracavitary treatment, 222
Magnetic resonance images, 420
Manchester system for treatment of cervical cancer, 205
Mandible,
 cancer of, 99
 osteoradionecrosis of, 103
 resection, 100
Mastectomy,
 for breast cancer, 70, 71, 78, 79
Maxillary antrum,
 carcinoma of, 106–109
Mediastinal germ-cell tumours, 173–174
Mediastinal irradiation, for testicular tumours, 50
Mediastinal metastases, from breast cancer, 86
Mediastinitis, radiation, 173
Mediastinum, germ cell tumours, 253
Medical adrenalectomy, in breast cancer, 87
Medulloblastoma, 347–353
 adjuvant chemotherapy, 353
 radiotherapy, 347
  London Hospital technique, 347
  long-term side-effects, 352
  results, 353
 recurrence after treatment, 353
 treatment, 340, 346, 415
Melanomas, 281, 292–293
 brain metastases, 363
 chemotherapy, 293
 diagnosis, 292
 prognosis, 292
 radiotherapy, 293
 spreading, 292
Melphalan,
 in multiple myeloma, 273, 274
 in osteosarcoma, 139
Menadiol (Synkavit), 21
Meninges, haemangioma, 397
Meningioma, 353–354
Meningitis, carcinomatous, 365
Menopause, induction of, 393, 405
Menorrhagia, radiotherapy for, 393
6-Mercaptopurine, in leukaemia, 239
Methotrexate,
 as radiosensitizer, 24
 response to, 435
 treatment with,
  bladder cancer, 38
  brain tumours, 365
  cancer of maxillary antrum, 108
  gastric cancer, 319
  head and neck cancer, 95
  leukaemia, 239
  lung cancer, 163

Methotrexate (*cont.*)
  treatment with (*cont.*)
    osteosarcoma, 139, 251
    for polymyositis, 392
    soft tissue sarcoma, 136
Methyl CCNU, in gastric cancer, 320
Metronidazole, 14
Micturition, frequency of, 402
Misonidazole, 22
  as radiosensitizer, 15, 16
  at beginning and end of treatment, 23
  results of treatment with, 23
  with every fraction, 22
  with multiple small fractions, 23
Mitomycin C,
  in anal carcinoma, 331, 332
  in gastric cancer, 319
Mitosis, radiation effects, 12
Motor neurone disorder, 338
Mould room, patient in, 406
Mouth,
  cancer of, 98–101
    anterior faucial pillar, 100
    buccal mucosa, 100
    diagnosis and staging, 98
    floor, 99, 101
    interstitial therapy, 378, 383
    lower alveolus, 100, 101
    radiotherapy, 99
    retromolar trigone, 100
    soft palate, 103
    treatment, 99
  care of, during treatment, 407
  iridium-192 implants, 373
Multiple myeloma, 270–275
  clinical features, 270
  cytotoxic therapy, 273
  diagnosis, 271
  maintenance chemotherapy, 273
  palliative therapy, 274
  prognostic factors, 272
  relation to plasmacytoma, 275
  staging, 272
  treatment, 273
    regimens, 274
    results of, 275
Mustine, in Hodgkin's disease, 186, 242, 436
Mutation, 384
Mycosis fungoides, 293–298
  electron beam therapy, 295
  treatment, 294
Myelitis, radiation, 52, 85, 337, 338
Myelofibrosis, 269–270
Myelosclerosis, 269

Nasal cavity,
  entrance to, malignant disease of, 289
Nasal fossa,
  tumours of, 109
Nasopharynx,
  anaplastic carcinoma of, lymph node metastases, 97
  cancer of,
    diagnosis and staging, 104
Nasopharynx (*cont.*)
  cancer of (*cont.*)
    interstitial therapy, 379
    results of treatment, 105
    treatment, 104
  juvenile angiofibroma of, 105
Nelson syndrome, 358, 361
Nephritis, radiation, 53
Nephrotic syndrome, in Hodgkin's disease, 178
Neuroblastoma, 245–247
  chemotherapy, 246, 436
  diagnosis, 246
  incidence, 245
  radiotherapy, 246, 247
  symptoms and diagnosis, 246
Neurofibromatosis, 312
Neurofibrosarcoma, 125
Neurotoxicity, from radiosensitizers, 22, 23
Nitrogen mustard,
  in Hodgkin's disease, 190
  in lung cancer, 152, 163
4-Nitroimidazoles, 16, 21
Nominal standard dose, 7
Nose, malignant disease of, 289

Oesophagitis, radiation, 155, 170
Oesophagus,
  carcinoma of, 166–170
    care of patient in radiotherapy, 170
    CT scanning in, 169
    involving lower part, 170
    preparation of patient for treatment, 166
    radiotherapy, 166
    surgery for, 166
  compression of, in bronchial carcinoma, 157
  tumour invasion of, from bronchial carcinoma, 157
Oestrogen receptors, 70
Olfactory neuroblastoma, 109
Oligodendroglioma, treatment, 344
Omentectomy, 234
Oophorectomy, in breast cancer, 87
Optic nerve glioma, 353
Oral cavity, carcinoma of, 98
Orbit,
  carcinoma of, from maxillary antrum, 108
  effects of radiotherapy, 119
  lacrimal gland tumour, 119
  lymphoma of, 117
  pseudotumour, 119
  rhabdomyosarcoma, 118
  tumours of, 117–119
Oropharynx,
  cancer of, 101–103
Osteogenic sarcoma,
  in children, 250
  secondary following treatment, 256
Osteonecrosis, 134
Osteosarcoma, 137
  aetiology, 138
  age and sex incidence, 137
Osteosarcoma (*cont.*)
  clinical picture, 138
  management of, 138
    Cade treatment, 138
    chemotherapy, 139
    limb sparing techniques, 139
    metastases, 140, 141
    radiotherapy, 141
  metastases from, 140
  radiation induced, 385
  site of, 138
  spread of, 138
Ovarian antigens, 234
Ovarian cancer, 234–237
  chemotherapy, 234, 236, 433
  palliative treatment, 236
  radiotherapy, 235
Ovary,
  germ cell tumour, 253
  irradiation, in treatment of breast cancer, 87
  lesions complicating cervical cancer therapy, 223
Oxygen, hyperbaric, 1, 2, 14
Oxygenation,
  effects, 20
  in tumour cells, 12
Oxygen effect, 14
  importance of, 20
Oxygen mimics, 22

Paget's disease, 138
  extramammary, 283
Painful heel syndrome, 388
Palate, cancer of, 379
Pancoast syndrome, 158
Pancreas,
  carcinoma of, 321–324
    chemotherapy and radiotherapy, 322, 324
    metastases, 363
  radiation pathology, 318
Parametrium, radiation, 221
Para-nitroacetophenone (PNAP), 22 22
Paraplegia, radiation induced, 337
Paratesticular tumours, in rhabdomyosarcoma, 250
Paris system, 374
Paroidectomy, 115, 116
Parotid gland, pleomorphic adenomas, 115
Paterson-Kelly syndrome, 114
Patient,
  bowel reactions during treatment, 408
  cancer and, 403
  communication with, 401
  during gynaecological treatment, 408
  during pelvic treatment, 408
  during treatment, 409
  follow-up clinics, 410
  guidelines for, 407
  hostel accommodation, 402
  instructions to,
    care of skin, 406

Patient (*cont.*)
 instructions to (*cont.*)
  cleansing, 407
 management of, 400–410
 in mould room, 406
 mouth care, 407
 position of, 405
 questions asked, 401, 402, 403
 talking and listening to, 400
Pelvic bath technique, 85
Pelvic metastases,
 from breast cancer, 85
 from lung cancer, 161
Pelvis, treatments on, care of patient, 408
Penis,
 carcinoma of, 57–65
  external radiation for, 62
  interstitial therapy, 379
  mould technique of treatment, 59
  palliative treatment, 64
  radiation problems, 61
  results of treatment, 63
  secondary, 64
  spread of, 63
  stage 1, 59, 63
  stage 2, 62, 64
  stage 3, 63, 64
  stage 4, 63
  staging, 58
Pericarditis, radiation, 173
Phaeochromocytoma, 312
Pharyngeal cancer, 115
 treatment, 23
^{32}Phosphorus, in polycythaemia, 267, 268
Photons, calculation for, 423
Physicist, role of, 411–431
Pigmented villonodular synovitis, radiotherapy for, 392
Pineal tumours, 345, 346
Pinna, malignant disease of, 290
Pituitary tumours, 357–361
 basophil adenoma, 361
 chromophobe adenoma, 360
 eosinophilic adenoma, 357
 implant therapy, 359
 malignant, 361
 prolactinoma, 360
 proton beam irradiation, 358
 radiation techniques, 357, 360, 361
Plantar fasciitis, 388
Plantar warts, 395
Plasma cell tumours, 194
Plasmacytomas, 275, 276
 in multiple myeloma, 273, 274
 solitary, 275
Platinum, as radiosensitizer, 24
Pleomorphic adenoma, 115, 119
Pleural effusion, in bronchial carcinoma, 160
Pleural mesothelioma, 164–166
Pneumonitis,
 interstitial, 263
 radiation, 53, 305
Poikiloderma, 294
Polychondritis, relapsing, 387
Polycythaemia rubra vera, 267, 268
Polymyositis, 392
Pontine glioma, 340
Post-cricoid carcinoma, 114
Proctitis, in treatment of cervical cancer, 220
Prolactinoma, 313, 360
Prostatic cancer, 39–46
 from bladder, 33
 hormone therapy, 43, 46
 interstitial therapy, 381
 metastases from, 39, 43, 433
  general bone, 43
  skeletal, 43
  skin infiltration, 45
  in spinal cord, 364
 palliative treatment, 43
 radiosensitivity, 39
 spread to penis, 65
 staging, 39
 surgery of, 46
 treatment techniques, 40
  bowel affected by, 45
  for skeletal metastases, 43
  future management, 46
  impotence following, 45
  interstitial irradiation, 41
  isodose curves, 41, 42
  London Hospital technique, 40
  radical irradiation, 40
  results, 45
  side-effects, 45
Pterygium, 395
Pulmonary embolism, from pelvic disease, 236
Pyriform fossa, carcinoma of, 114
Pyrimidines, halogenated, as radiosensitizers, 24

Quadrantectomy, 83
Queyrat's erythroplasia, 64, 282

Radiation,
 effect on gastrointestinal tissue, 316
 interaction with cytotoxic drugs, 432
 skin effects, 280
Radiation distribution charts, computation of, 422
Radiation effects,
 hepatitis, 316
 ileitis, 221
 mediastinitis, 173
 myelitis, 52, 85, 337
 nephritis, 53, 235
 oesophagitis, 155, 170
 pericarditis, 173
 perichondritis, 113
 pneumonitis, 53, 263, 305
 thyroiditis, 303
Radiation protection, 428–430
 during afterloading, 209, 212, 417
 in brachytherapy, 415
Radioactive implants, 370
Radioactive sources, for brachytherapy, 416
Radiobiology, 1–18
Radioiodine,
 in follicular carcinoma of thyroid, 304, 305
 protection aspects, 310
 thyroid failure following treatment with, 5
 in thyrotoxicosis, 311
 unsealed source, 306
Radiosensitizers, 2, 19–26
 cytotoxic drugs as, 23
 criteria for, 22
 definition of, 19
 development of, 16
 electron-avid compounds, 14
 hyperbaric oxygen, 14, 20
 hypoxic, 15, 16
 hypoxic cells and, 20
 neurotoxicity of, 22, 23
 oxygen, 20
 role of blood flow, 21
 therapeutic index, 19
Radiotherapy,
 automation and, 421
 in benign conditions, 384–399
 chemocurable malignancies and, 438
 computers in, 416, 420, 422
 correcting for density, 427
 CT scanning in, 424
 interaction with chemotherapy, 432–444
 magnetic resonance images in, 420
 patient and, *see under Patients*
 planning, *see under Treatment planning*
 research and development, 429
 risks of, 384
Radium, 209, 415
Radium-226, for implants, 370
Radium implants, 369
Razoxane, as radiosensitizer, 24
Rectovaginal fistula, 222
Rectum,
 carcinoma of, 326–330
  classification, 326, 327
  fast neutron therapy, 330
  hyperbaric oxygen in therapy, 330
  interstitial therapy, 379
  metastases from, 326
  palliative therapy, 327
  radiotherapy, 327, 328, 329
  recurrence, 327, 329
  spread of, 65, 326
 lesions complicating cervical cancer therapy, 222
 radiation effects, 317
 radiation-induced malignancy, 223
Reed-Sternberg cells, 179
Renal cell carcinoma, 55
Renal pelvis, transitional cell carcinoma, 56
Research and development, 429
Respiratory obstruction, in bronchial carcinoma, 156
Retinoblastoma, 125

Retinoblastoma (*cont.*)
  in children, 254
Retinopathy, radiation, 120
Retroperitoneal sarcomas, 132, 134
Rhabdomyosarcoma,
  in children, 247–250
    prognosis, 250
    radiotherapy, 249
    staging and diagnosis, 248
    treatment, 249
  paratesticular tumours, 250
Rheumatoid arthritis, 386, 387
Ribs,
  involvement in bronchial carcinoma, 160
  metastases, from prostatic cancer, 43
  radiation fractures, 134
Ruthenium plaques, in retinoblastoma, 254

SR2508, as radiosensitizer, 23
Sacrococcygeal germ cell tumours, 253
Salivary fistula, 397
Salivary gland tumours, 115–117
Scars, cancer developing on, 280
Schistosomiasis, effect on bladder cancer, 27, 28
Sebaceous glands, carcinoma of, 282
Selectron, 211, 418
  Christie Hospital experience, 213
  dosimetry, 213, 214
  features of, 211
Semiconductors, in dosimetry, 421
Sexual function,
  following carcinoma of penis, 61
  following treatment of testicular tumours, 53
Shoulder, capsulitis, 388, 389
Sickness, after treatment, 402
Single-dose response curves, 2, 3
Sipple's syndrome, 313
Sjögren's syndrome, 302
Skeleton,
  metastases, 43, 52
Skin,
  acute reaction, 10
  anatomy of, 281
  avoidance of friction after treatment, 407
  basal carcinoma, 284
  care of, 406
  lesions complicating cervical cancer therapy, 223
  lymphoma, 298
  malignant disease of, 280–299
    aetiology of, 280
    genetic causes, 281
    infiltration, 285
    interstitial therapy, 379
    of special sites, 287
    pathology of, 281
    staging of, 283
    treatment of, 285
  metastases, 86, 162
  premalignant conditions, 282, 284
Skin (*cont.*)
  radiation effect, 5, 7
    depth dose curves, 296
    late effects, 291
  squamous carcinoma, 284
  temperature and, 407
Skin appendage tumours, 282
Smoking, bladder cancer and, 27
Soft palate, cancer of, 103
Soft tissue sarcoma, 124–137
  aetiology, 125
  age and sex incidence, 125
  biopsy, 126
  bone metastases, 134
  chemotherapy, 136
  clinical assessment, 125
  CT scanning, 126
  development of, 125
  histology, 126
    classification, 124
  incidence of, 124, 125
  investigation of, 126
  lung metastases, 134
  management of, 125
  metastases, 125
  peripheral tumours, 128
  radiography of, 126
  radiotherapy, 128
    acute reaction, 132
    adjuvant chemotherapy, 137
    fast neutrons, 136
    late reactions, 133
    palliative, 134
    patient assessment, 128
    planning and dosage, 129
    policy, 128
    postoperative, 128
    preoperative, 136
    radiosensitizers in, 24
    results of, 137
    techniques, 128
    under hypoxic conditions, 135
  recurrence, 128
  site of, 125
  spread of, 125
  staging, 127
  surgical treatment, 127
    postoperative radiotherapy, 128
    preoperative radiotherapy, 136
  treatment,
    choice of, 127
    policy, 127, 128
Solar keratitis, 282
Somnolence syndrome, 338
Spinal artery compression, in Hodgkin's disease, 189
Spinal cord,
  astrocytoma, 361
  chordoma, 362
  compression, 85, 163, 274, 305, 397
  ependymoma, 362
  glioma, 362
  haemangioma, 397
  medulloblastoma, 348
  metastases in, 364
Spinal cord (*cont.*)
  radiation damage, 337
  safe levels of radiation, 339
  tumours of, 361–363
Spinal metastases, from lung, 161
Spleen,
  irradiation,
    in leukaemia, 264
    in myelofibrosis, 270
Splenectomy in leukaemia, 265
Split dose experiments, 7
Stewart's granuloma, 109
Stilboestrol-associated adenocarcinoma of vagina, 231
Stomach,
  adenocarcinoma, 170
  carcinoma of, 318
    chemotherapy, 319, 320
    classification, 318
    spread of, 318
  Hodgkin's disease of, 189
  non-Hodgkin's lymphoma of, 195
  radiation effects on, 5, 317
Strontium-90,
  for ophthalmic use, 395
  in mycosis fundoides, 296
Subglottis, carcinoma of, 109, 110, 112
Submandibular tumours, 116
Sunlight,
  keratotic changes from, 282
  malignant effects, 280
Supraglottis, carcinoma of, 109, 110, 112
Suprasellar germinomas, 346
Surgery, radiation effects and, 6
Sweat glands, tumours of, 282
Synovitis, pigmented villonodular, 392

Tamoxifen, in breast cancer, 88
Tantalum-182, in brachytherapy, 416
Taste, loss of after radiotherapy, 100, 105
Tennis elbow, 388
Teratomas, 253
  chemotherapy, 436, 438
Testis,
  disease of, in acute lymphoblastic leukaemia, 240
  germ cell tumours, 253, 432
  lymphoma of, 49, 196
  post radiotherapy effects on, 256
  seminoma, 438
  tumours, 46–55
    chemotherapy, 49, 54
    classification, 46, 47
    CT scanning in, 47
    future management, 54
    investigation, 46
    mediastinal irradiation, 50
    metastases from, 52, 364
    palliative irradiation, 52
    results of, 53
    seminoma, 48, 50, 53, 54, 438
    side-effects of treatment, 52
    sexual function following treatment, 53

Testis (*cont.*)
  tumours (*cont.*)
    staging, 46
    surgery of, 46, 49
    teratoma, 49, 50, 53, 55
    treatment policy, 47
    treatment techniques, 49, 52
    ultrasound in diagnosis, 47
Thalamus, tumours of, 346
6-Thioguanine, in leukaemia, 260
Thiosulphates, as radiosensitizers, 17
Thymic tumours, 170–173
  classification and diagnosis, 171
  granulomatous, 178
  radiotherapy, 171
Thyroid gland,
  anaplastic carcinoma, 302
    management of, 305
  anatomy, 300
  cancer of, 300–311
    clinical and diagnostic aspects, 301
    following brain tumour irradiation, 352
    incidence, 300
    management, 302, 305
    metastases from, 302
  failure, after radioiodine treatment, 5
  follicular carcinoma, 302
    chemotherapy, 305
    external beam radiotherapy, 308
    metastases from, 304
    prognosis, 306
    management of, 303
  irradiation of, risks of, 385
  lymphoma, 302
    external beam radiotherapy, 307
    management of, 306
    prognosis, 306
  medullary carcinoma, 302, 313
    external beam radiotherapy, 308
    management of, 305
    prognosis, 306
  papillary carcinoma, 301
    prognosis, 306
  radiotherapy,
    external beam, 307
    radioiodine, 306, 310
    technical aspects, 306
Thyroid stimulating hormone, 301
Thyroiditis, radiation, 303
Thyrotoxicosis, treatment with radioiodine, 311
Thyroxine, 301
Tissue,
  acute reaction, 4, 19
  late reacting, 5, 19
  normal response of, 3
  radiation effects, 7, 19
Tomato tumours, 294
Tongue,
  cancer of, 99
    interstitial therapy, 377

Tongue (*cont.*)
  cancer of, (*cont.*)
    results of treatment, 101, 103
  iridium-192 implants, 373
Tonsil, cancer of, 102, 103
Tonsillar fossa, cancer of, 279
Transitional cell carcinoma of renal pelvis, 56
Treatment,
  automated technique, 421
  computers in, 420
  CT scanning in, 424
  magnetic resonance images in, 420
  planning, 404
    computer methods, 424
    guidelines for, 404
    in homogeneities in, 425, 427
    involvement of physicist, 418
    simulation procedures, 420
    steps in, 420
Trichofolliculoma, 282
Tricoepithelioma, 282
Tuberculous lymph nodes, radiotherapy for, 397
Tumeur d'emblée, 294

Ultraviolet radiation, effects of, 280
Ureter,
  lesions complicating cervical cancer therapy, 223
  transitional cell carcinoma of, 56
Urethra,
  carcinoma, 57, 381
  hairy, 398
  rhabdomyosarcoma, 248
Urinary tract, radiation effects, from treatment of prostatic cancer, 45
Urological malignancies, 27–67
  See also under specific regions and organs
Uterus,
  cancer, 224–231
    adjuvant hormone therapy, 230
    differentiation, 224
    intracavitary treatment, 225, 230
    Manchester system, 226
    postoperative radiotherapy, 228–229
    preoperative radiotherapy, 225
    primary radiotherapy, 226
    remote afterloading systems for, 227
    spread of, 224
    staging, 224
    survival, 229
  involvement in cervical cancer, 207, 220
  perforation of, 220
Uveal melanoma, 120

Vagina,
  carcinoma of, 231–232
    interstitial therapy, 381
  involvement in cervical cancer, 207

Vagina (*cont.*)
  involvement in rhabdomyosarcoma, 248
  lesions complicating cervical cancer therapy, 221, 222
Vaginal vault, in uterine cancer, 229, 230
Vascular permeability, changes in, 6
Vascular tissues, radiation injury to, 5
Vena caval obstruction, in bronchial carcinoma, 155
Vesico-vaginal fistula, 222
Vinblastine,
  in germ cell tumours, 436
  in Hodgkin's disease, 436, 438
  in malignant teratoma, 437
Vincristine,
  treatment with,
    acute lymphoblastic leukaemia, 239
    brain tumours, 345, 353
    cancer of head and neck, 95
    childhood tumours, 436
    Ewing's sarcoma, 252
    gastric cancer, 319
    Hodgkin's disease, 186, 190, 242, 436, 438
    leukaemia, 435
    lung cancer, 163
    neuroblastoma, 246
    non-Hodgkin's lymphoma, 241
    osteosarcoma, 139
    rhabdomyosarcoma, 249
    soft tissue sarcoma, 136
    thyroid cancer, 306
    Wilms' tumour, 244, 245
VIPoma, 313
Viral warts, 395
von Recklinghausen's disease, 312
Vulva, carcinoma of, 232–233

Waldeyer's ring,
  Hodgkin's disease of, 189
  non-Hodgkin's lymphoma of, 195
Wegener's granulomatosis, 109, 119
White reflex, in retinoblastoma, 254
Wilms' tumour, 242–245
  chemotherapy, 243, 244, 436
  clinical features, 243
  diagnosis, 243
  histology, 243
  incidence of, 242
  radiotherapy, 243, 244
  staging, 243
Wound healing, 6

Xeroderma pigmentosa, 281

Yttrium-90,
  for pituitary tumours, 359, 361
  for rheumatoid arthritis, 387

Zollinger-Ellison syndrome, 313